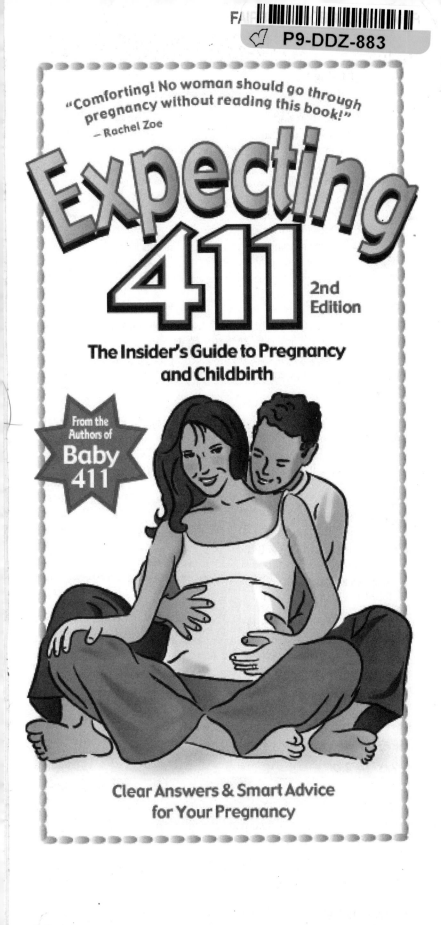

Copyright Page

Cover/interior design and keyboard solo by Epicenter Creative
Index by New West Indexing
Author photography by Dana Patrick and Tracy Trahar.
Catering by Mark Brown
Illustration assist by Julia Brown
Special thanks to Tanya Remer Altmann, M.D.

Dr. Hakakha would like to thank:
Neil: thank you for reading and reading and re-reading!
Mike: thank you for being by my side no matter what. I love you.
Leila & Ava: thank you for teaching me how to be a mommy. I love you both so much.

To buy this book, order online at Expecting411.com or call 1-800-888-0385. Questions or comments? Email us at authors@Expecting411.com.

The latest info on this book is online at Expecting411.com

Brown, Ari, M.D.
Hakakha, Michele, M.D.
   Expecting 411: Clear Answers & Smart Advice for Your Pregnancy/
Michele Hakakha, M.D., Ari Brown, M.D.
   608 pages.
   Includes index.
   ISBN 1-889392-42-1

Cataloging-in-Publication data for this book is available from the Library of Congress.

Windsor Peak Press
436 Pine Street
Boulder, CO 80302
www.windsorpeak.com

Version 2.0

Do you have an old copy of this book? Check our web site at Expecting411.com to make sure you have the most current version (click on "book" and then "which version?").

OVERVIEW

From the moment you discover that positive result on the home pregnancy test, your mind is filled with questions. This section explores what to do first, including meeting your practitioner, prenatal care and all of the decisions you have to make (Birthing classes? Where to have the birth? Hiring a doula?). We'll take a week by week look as you go through your first, second and third trimesters. And we'll prepare you for what lies ahead. Finally, let's look at what's normal (and what's not) for your changing body, plus all of those tests you'll take over the next nine months.

You've adjusted to the shock and awe of pregnancy and now reality sets in. What do you need to eat for a healthy pregnancy? What environmental hazards should you avoid? What about exercise during pregnancy? Sex? Travel? Work? This section covers it all, plus answers to whether it is safe to color your hair, whiten your teeth, get your nails done and more.

Prepping for parenthood is more than picking out a crib. You also have to stare down a myriad of decisions: Bank your baby's cord blood? Circumcision? Expanded newborn screen? And how do you pick a pediatrician? This section covers it all, plus looks at going back to work (childcare options), breastfeeding versus formula and a key hot topic: vaccinations for your child. Finally, this section looks at the home stretch: getting ready for delivery, childbirth classes, how to tell if you are in labor and more.

Show time! We cover your labor day with a detailed look at both vaginal deliveries and C-sections. What to expect at the hospital, home birth or birthing center. Then it's everything you wanted to know about epidurals, but were afraid to ask. After the baby is born, we look at your baby's first few minutes, days and weeks. We also discuss other key postpartum issues, such as care for mom after delivery, weight loss, baby blues and more.

Let's hope you don't have to read this section. But if you need it, you can find info on the top 12 emergencies during pregnancy plus the 51 most common pregnancy complications. Sickness happens—so we cover the most common infections, colds/flu and girl problems. Are you over age 35? We look at the special issues with "advanced maternal age" pregnancies, plus provide a detailed view of preterm labor and babies. Multiples have their own special challenges . . . we cover this in-depth with info on twins, additional testing and more. Finally, When It Doesn't Work covers miscarriage and stillbirth. Plus we have a detailed glossary, index and info on our other books.

TABLE OF CONTENTS

Chapter 4

Is This Normal?

Chapter 5

Tests

SECTION TWO: LIFE GOES ON

Chapter 6

NUTRITION

Chapter 7

THE ENVIRONMENT AND YOUR BABY

Chapter 8

LIFESTYLES

Chapter 9

SPA TREATMENT

SECTION THREE: GETTING READY FOR THE BIG EVENT

Chapter 10

PARENTHOOD PREP

Chapter 11

BREASTFEEDING

Chapter 12

HOME STRETCH

SECTION FOUR: THE BIG EVENT

Chapter 13

LABOR DAY

Chapter 14

POSTPARTUM: WHAT'S NEXT?

SECTION FIVE: SPECIAL CONCERNS & PROBLEMS

Chapter 15

PREGNANCY 911

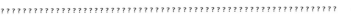

Chapter 16

THE COMPLICATED PREGNANCY

Chapter 17

INFECTIONS

Chapter 18

ADVANCED MATERNAL AGE

Chapter 19

PRETERM LABOR & BABIES

Chapter 20

MULTIPLES

Chapter 21

WHEN IT DOESN'T WORK

Appendices

MEDICATIONS, GLOSSARY, FOOTNOTES, INDEX

WHY READ THIS BOOK?

Foreword

Congratulations! You have a precious little being growing within you for whom you are now responsible. And he hasn't even peed on you yet . . . or asked for the car keys.

Everyone tells you that becoming a parent will change your life—and they're right. But what you may not realize is that the change happens *now*. We're not talking about nine months down the road—we're talking about this very moment. Your health during pregnancy affects your baby. So your first job as a parent is to take good care of yourself.

For the person carrying the bundle of joy, welcome to *Invasion of the Body Snatchers*. You will look in the mirror sometimes and wonder who is staring back at you.

For the person supporting that pregnant gal, you too may wonder who is staring back at you (and occasionally yelling and crying . . . while simultaneously demanding a foot massage).

After 40 weeks of aches, pains, and emotional outbursts, you will be rewarded with the most amazing experience of your life. And if that wasn't enough, you'll next embark on life's most challenging, frustrating, uplifting, delightful journey—parenthood!

As the mothers of four young children, we know what you are going through. And if you are anything like us, you quickly realize pregnancy is both equal parts exciting . . . and terrifying.

Most of all, we realize you have questions. Lots of questions. And that's why we are here.

You need solid advice on what's best for you and your baby. And you want the *latest* information and research about pregnancy, not outdated advice from ten years ago or, worse . . . from your mom's generation!

Of course, there's no shortage of advice for pregnant women—you hear it from your friends, office co-workers, or strangers at the grocery store. Then there's the web...and the zillions of other pregnancy books out there.

So, why write another book on pregnancy? What can we possibly say here that hasn't already been said in those other thick pregnancy tomes? And can't you just get advice online for free?

Funny you should ask! Let's discuss.

Does the world need another pregnancy book?

Yes, it does.

Sure, there are dozens of other pregnancy books out there. You could flip through the pregnancy section on Amazon and go into labor before you're done.

But take a closer look at the other pregnancy books. As experts on pregnancy and babies, we found many pregnancy books to be . . . well, *lacking*.

Some are out-of-date, leaving you to base important decisions on ancient medical history (that is, anything we knew before 2012).

Other books are written by well-meaning authors who don't deliver babies for a living. It is one thing to *research* pregnancy, labor and delivery . . . and another to actually dedicate your career to caring for pregnant women and their babies! Trust us, there's a big difference.

And then there is the original sin of too many pregnancy books: *the freak-out factor*. Their aim to catalog every possible terrible thing that can go wrong with pregnancy ends up scaring the bejesers out of every reader. But what's often missing is *perspective*—how common are these complications? Is a risk real . . . or merely hypothetical?

So that's why we decided to write *Expecting 411*. Our goal: give you the most up-to-date advice on pregnancy and childbirth—while taming the freak-out factor. Best of all, this advice is from two women who spend their days and nights caring for pregnant women and their babies.

Meet the authors

Healthy pregnancies produce healthy babies. So, it's key to get the facts straight. You need a reliable source you can trust.

Who better to write a book about giving birth than an obstetrician . . . and a pediatrician? While that sounds obvious, *Expecting 411* is the first pregnancy book to be authored by BOTH a baby doc and a doc who delivers babies. The combined expertise gives you a 360 degree view of this crazy process we call having a baby.

Let's take a second to introduce you to Dr. Michele Hakakha, OB/GYN and Dr. Ari Brown, pediatrician.

MEET DR. H
OB/GYN, MOM

I'm an obstetrician/gynecologist who has been practicing in Beverly Hills, CA for ten years. I received my training at UCLA/Cedars Sinai Medical Center in Los Angeles. In addition to authoring several articles on pregnancy, I also appeared in *Little Man*, an award-winning documentary on preterm labor and premature birth.

I decided to become an obstetrician because I love the bond that develops between a woman and her OB/GYN—the ups and downs of puberty, pregnancy and childbirth, even menopause (but who wants to think about that right now!). And it's an absolute honor to be present to help women through labor and delivery.

After having two kids of my own, I bring a real-world perspective to pregnancy and delivery that they don't teach you in medical school. Morning sickness, heartburn, varicose veins, labor pains—yes, I've been there, done that!

And I am passionate about educating pregnant couples. It has been a labor of love to share my knowledge and expertise with you!

MEET DR. B
PEDIATRICIAN, MOM

I am a pediatrician in practice for 16 years after training at Harvard Medical School/Boston Children's Hospital. I practice in Austin, TX and started writing books in 2003.

Besides authoring the best-sellers, *Baby 411* and *Toddler 411*, I am also a spokesperson for the American Academy of Pediatrics and a medical advisor to *Parents Magazine*. And I have two children. (Fortunately, I never need to sleep). My kids are a little older than Dr H's, but believe me, I remember my pregnancies just like yesterday!

I love my job because I get to participate in a family's birth experience and help babies grow up healthy and thrive.

Why do we have *both* an OB and pediatrician authoring this book? We share the same patient—your baby. Dr. H (the OB) handles moms-to-be and the baby-in-the-womb and Dr. B (the pediatrician) handles care once the baby is born. Both of us combine our expertise on the best things you can do during pregnancy to ensure a healthy baby. And we can prepare you for newborn issues and decisions that arise before or shortly after delivery. Having two expert perspectives makes this book unique.

We've also recruited additional experts for special must-read sections. For breastfeeding, we turned to a certified lactation consultant. For home births, a certified midwife will walk you through this experience.

FOREWORD

Seven reasons to buy this book!

Now that you've met the authors, let's talk about what makes this book different.

1 **EASY-TO-FIND ANSWERS.** You've got questions—and you want to find the answers quickly. We've organized the basics of your pregnancy into three chapters (First Trimester, Second Trimester, Third Trimester). But many questions don't fit so easily into a week by week or month by month format.

That's why the rest of the book is organized by *topics* so you can actually find the information you need. If you are wondering if a symptom is normal, check out the "Is it Normal?" chapter. Curious about a test your doctor has ordered? Yep, that's in a chapter cleverly titled "Tests." And you'll easily be able to find info on exercise in "Lifestyles."

2 **BETTER THAN GOOGLE.** Yes, there's a lot of free pregnancy advice online. But that free advice is often worth the price you've paid.

Why? Most web sites have short, pithy answers to questions about pregnancy—that's nice, but sometimes you want a more detailed answer (the pros and cons of a certain test, for example). This book gives you the depth you need to make wise decisions.

Of course, many pregnancy web sites are supported by advertising—as a result, their advice is carefully calibrated to avoid offending any sponsor. We don't accept corporate sponsorship, so we tell you like it is.

3 **FREQUENT UPDATES.** Medicine moves at light speed these days— upending what was common practice just a few years ago.

We update *Expecting 411* every two years. When you buy the most recent edition of the book, you can be assured you are not reading advice that is dated.

We also have a detailed web page (Expecting411.com) with updates *between* editions. Read the latest breaking news on our blog, subscribe to our Twitter feed and check the wall on our Facebook fan page. Our free e-newsletter also provides detailed updates for readers. Plus, check out our online bonus materials and our popular reader message boards.

4 **PARANOIA, TAMED.** Nothing is more terrifying than reading about the myriad of things that can go wrong with pregnancy. Even if these complications are rare, you can lose endless hours of sleep worrying about your baby (as if you didn't have enough issues with getting some shut-eye!).

To solve this problem, we put all the scary stuff into one section at the end of this book. That way, you don't have to read about these problems unless it is absolutely necessary.

And to help lower the fear level, we also mark other potentially unsettling content with a special warning icon. Feel free to skip these sections, which are included for readers who want the whole story.

Another key point: when it comes to risks to your pregnancy, we separate the hypothetical from reality. We'll tell you if science backs up a warning . . . or not.

? ?

FOREWORD

5 **QUESTIONS YOU ARE TOO EMBARRASSED TO ASK.** Let's be honest—when you are face-to-face with your OB, it can be embarrassing to discuss what's really on your mind.

As two mamas who've been there, we know you wonder about items that seem silly to discuss with your doc. Like . . . can you wax down there? How about oral sex? No, it won't kill you (contrary to what other books might say!) We've got answers to more embarrassing questions than anyone else!

6 **YOUR PARTNER WANTS TO READ TOO!** There's a reason there are two people on the cover of this book. We know that partners are much more involved in pregnancy and childbirth than past generations. And you want "insider tips" that go beyond "be supportive" and "hold mom's hand during labor."

That's why we've scattered partner tips throughout this book—we assume both of you are reading it. And we promise to treat you with the intelligence and respect you deserve. (Now go make that midnight run for Twinkies, you numbskull!)

7 **PARENTHOOD PREP.** Yep, your job as parents starts when you conceive. While you may spend eight months picking out that perfect paint hue for your baby's nursery, what happens when you actually hold that newborn in your arms for the first time?

Many of us are clueless when it comes to preparing to be a parent. (We sure were when we were first parents). Newborn screening. Cord blood banking. Childcare. Breastfeeding. Circumcision. Vaccinations. These are just a few decisions that lie ahead. Don't worry—we will walk you through all of these topics since you often have to make these decisions while you're still pregnant. As always, the secret sauce of the 411 series is reader feedback. Many of the questions you see in this book are real-life queries from Dr. H and Dr. B's patients. You'll also note that we put our email address in the back of this book. How many other pregnancy books let you email the authors?

How to Use this Book

Before we get rolling, let's go over a few details on how to get the most out of *Expecting 411*.

First, this book contains some BIG UGLY LATIN WORDS. You can't discuss medical issues and pregnancy without whipping out a few complex medical terms, which conveniently are often in Latin. What? You didn't study Latin in college?

Okay, to keep the jargon from overwhelming you, we have a handy glossary at the end of this book. When you see a **BIG UGLY LATIN WORD** in bold small caps, turn to the back to get a quick definition.

Second, if you flip through the chapters, you'll note boxes with opinions from Dr. H or Dr. B. As it sounds, these are the authors' opinions on several hot button issues. Feel free to disagree with these thoughts, but they are based on years of seeing real-world patients and delivering hundreds of babies. Unlike some other pregnancy books, we think readers deserve to know where the line is drawn between fact and opinion. You can then decide what works for you and your partner.

Finally, let's talk footnotes—we've footnoted the sources used throughout this book. These references are at expecting411.com/extra in case you want to read more about a particular study or source.

No Ads? No Plugs?

Yes, that's true—as with all our books, this guide contains ZERO ads, spam or commercial plugs. No pharmaceutical or formula company has paid the authors to plug their products in this book. Dr. H and Dr. B do NOT go on all-expense paid junkets to Aruba to learn about the latest drug or medical research. When you go to our web site at Expecting411.com, you won't see ads for cord blood banks or pregnancy tests.

We do this to remain objective—this ensures that the info you get here is based on the best scientific research, not who pays us a commission, ad fee or royalty.

Full disclosure: Windsor Peak Press, the publisher of this book, does offer a "custom publishing" program that allows companies, non-profit organizations and government agencies to purchase bulk copies of our books to give away to their customers, patients or employees. These books are often specially printed with a company or organization logo and (sometimes) a customized title page. Such arrangements do NOT imply an endorsement or recommendation of the company or its products by Windsor Peak Press, this book or its authors.

Major Legal Disclaimer

No medical book is complete without that ubiquitous legal disclaimer . . . so here's ours:

The information we provide in this book is intended to help you understand the medical issues around pregnancy and childbirth. It is NOT intended to replace the advice of your doctor. Before you start any medical treatment, always check in with your doctor who can counsel you on the specific needs for your pregnancy and baby.

We have made a tremendous effort to give you the most up-to-date medical info available. However, medical research is constantly providing new insight into maternity healthcare. That's why we have an accompanying website (Expecting 411.com) to give you the latest breaking updates.

Okay, enough of the introductions. First up: It's Blue—Now What Do You Do?

ICONS

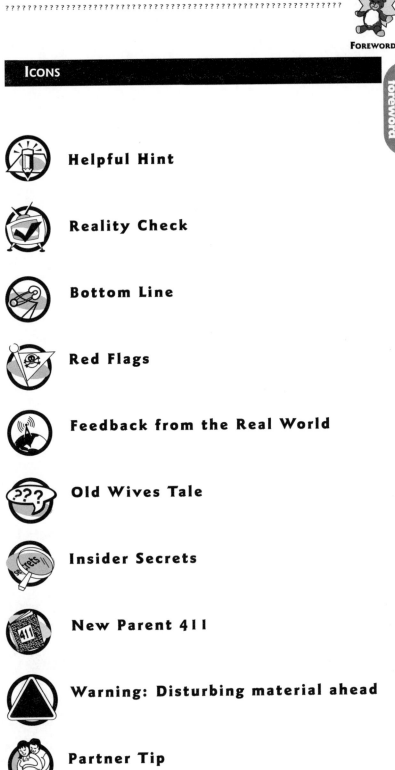

Helpful Hint

Reality Check

Bottom Line

Red Flags

Feedback from the Real World

Old Wives Tale

Insider Secrets

New Parent 411

Warning: Disturbing material ahead

Partner Tip

It's Blue ...
Now what do I do?
Introduction

*"It sometimes happens, even in the best of fami-
lies, that a baby is born. This is not necessarily
cause for alarm. The important thing is to keep
your wits about you and borrow some money."*
~ Elinor Goulding Smith

What's in this Chapter

- ◆ **Are you really pregnant?**
- ◆ **Calculating Your Due Date**
- ◆ **The Birds and the Bees**

There's probably one big question running through your mind
right now: "I think I'm pregnant.
Now what?"

For many of you (and trust us, we felt
this way too) seeing those two lines on the
pregnancy test is quite a shock. So let's
take a deep breath and then read on.

Some pregnancies are strategically
planned, others just . . . happen.

In an ideal world, a woman and her
partner have a pre-conception visit (a visit
that occurs prior to pregnancy) with the
woman's practitioner. The practitioner
reviews the woman's medical conditions,
previous pregnancy or gynecological
issues, immunization history, list of medications she is taking, lifestyle issues that may
be risky for an unborn baby and mom-to-
be (drug use, alcohol use, smoking, envi-
ronmental/work exposures), nutrition,
exercise habits, and both partners' family
medical histories to assess for potential
genetic disease risks.

Then the practitioner recommends that
the woman interested in becoming pregnant start taking prenatal vitamins and
change any poor lifestyle habits.

Wouldn't it be nice if we all did this?
Let's get real. For many of us, pregnancy
just happened . . . without starting those
prenatal vitamins or changing bad habits.
Don't panic. That's why we are here—we
will bring you up to speed.

? ?

IT'S BLUE!

This introductory chapter is a crash course in pregnancy before we discuss your life for the next 40 weeks. Yes, some of this is pretty boring stuff (especially if you never liked science or health class). But it is helpful for you to understand what is going on with your body and your baby right from the start. So let's get rolling.

Am I really pregnant?

This question will hit you when you either a) miss your period, b) feel like you ate some bad sushi, or c) yell at your loved ones for no apparent reason. Then, like all of us, you will run out and buy one (or three) home pregnancy tests to confirm your suspicions.

If your test is clearly positive, congratulations! You can pass go and skip to the next section. But sometimes it's not that clear cut. Let's talk about how those home pregnancy tests work.

Q. What does the pregnancy test actually test for?

The test looks for **HUMAN CHORIONIC GONADOTROPIN (BETA-HCG)** in the urine. Beta-hCG is a hormone the body makes during pregnancy. It circulates through the body and then gets eliminated in the urine. In most normal pregnancies, the levels of beta-hCG more than double every 48 hours until about ten weeks of pregnancy. So, by the time a woman misses her period, there is plenty of beta-hCG in her urine to make a test turn positive.

Your practitioner can also order a blood test that measures beta-hCG (obviously not something one does in your own bathroom).

Q. When is the most accurate time to do a home pregnancy test?

Any time after a missed period. I know it's hard to wait, especially if you have been trying and are anxious to see if those two lines are there. Truthfully, many home pregnancy tests can detect beta-hCG a few days *before* a missed period. But doing the test too early may give you inaccurate results. In English: you're pregnant but the test doesn't detect it yet. Besides being unnecessarily disappointed and wasting a few bucks, testing too early may lead you to resume habits that could be dangerous for a new pregnancy (like drinking alcohol).

Bottom Line
Be patient. Wait until you miss your period to do the test.

Q. What if the first home pregnancy test is negative but I really feel pregnant?

Early in pregnancy, some women feel the way they do just before they get their period. You may have tender breasts, cramps, moodiness, and cravings.

If you have these symptoms, miss your period, and your first pregnancy test is negative, you've got two options.

IT'S BLUE!

◆ Option 1: Wait a few days and take another urine pregnancy test at home.
◆ Option 2: See your practitioner and get a blood pregnancy test. Because the blood test looks at actual blood levels of beta-hCG, it detects this pregnancy hormone a few days sooner and confirms pregnancy earlier than a urine pregnancy test.

Q. What if there is only a faint line?

A faint line means that there is some beta-hCG in your urine.

You may get one of those "faintly positive" tests (where you have to squint your eyes and put the stick up to the sunlight to see the line) if you do a home pregnancy test a few days before a missed period or very close to the date of the missed period. Or you may have ovulated later than you thought, so you are not as far along as you anticipated. This is common in women who have menstrual cycles that are longer than 28 days.

It's common for the first few home pregnancy tests to be light (where the test result line is lighter than the control line) because the hormone levels are lower in the early stages of pregnancy. I say "the first few tests" because if you are like most women, you will not take just one test. You will take TEN before you even get to your first doctor's visit! Some women test multiple brands to make sure that they all are positive. I've even had a patient make her husband pee on one to act as the "control!"

Regardless of which test kit(s) you use, it is important to follow the instructions correctly. A key point: you are supposed to read the test results within five to ten minutes.

Reality Check

If you let the pregnancy test sit for an hour and then go back to read it (or pull it out of the trash can to check just one more time—it's ok, I did that too), you may see a faint line that is actually a false positive. The faint line does not mean anything if the test has been sitting for an hour.

Q. What if the first one is faintly positive and the next one is negative?

The most likely reason is that you *were* pregnant but you had an abnormal pregnancy. Many women have what doctors informally call **"CHEMICAL PREGNANCIES."** A chemical pregnancy means your body made enough beta-hCG to produce a positive test but not a viable baby. You actually were pregnant, but there was a very early miscarriage that occurred before anything could even be detected by ultrasound. This is common. The good news: it doesn't usually happen repeatedly. You don't have to see your practitioner if this happens, but you should call the office and let her know.

IT'S BLUE!

What's My Due Date?

Q. How do I figure out my due date?

A full term pregnancy is about 40 weeks or 280 days long. Docs start counting from the first day of your last menstrual period. Back in the good old days before ultrasounds and pregnancy tests, a birth date or due date was calculated by this equation:

Take the first day of your **LAST MENSTRUAL PERIOD** (LMP).
Subtract 3 months.
Add 7 days.

That date is your estimated due date or **ESTIMATED DATE OF DELIVERY** (EDD). This is also sometimes referred to as the **ESTIMATED DATE OF CONFINEMENT (EDC)**, which is an old Victorian term used when women really were confined for birth.

While this is an easy way to do it, it's not perfect. It assumes that a woman has a 28-day menstrual cycle (which many of us don't) and doesn't consider leap years or months with less than 31 days.

If you and math haven't gotten along since 8th grade algebra, you can use a due date calculator such as one found at womenshealth.gov (click on health tools, then due date calculator).

Your practitioner has something called a "pregnancy wheel" that is kind of a cheat sheet for us. We routinely whip one of these plastic wheels out of our white coats many times during the course of your pregnancy and intensely spin it around to calculate how far along you are. In fact, we are pretty incapacitated without one!

Nowadays, we calculate a patient's due date by using a combination of the first day of the last known menstrual period (LMP), a pelvic exam, and an ultrasound.

Don't be alarmed if you can't remember when your last period was or if you have irregular periods. Your practitioner can make a pretty good approximation after doing an exam and ultrasound. It may sound odd, but your practitioner will have a better idea on dates the *earlier* an ultrasound is performed.

Women who have conceived with assisted reproductive technology (like in vitro fertilization) have their due date calculated by their fertility specialist. That date is based on the date of the procedure, the stage of the embryo being implanted (for IVF), and early ultrasounds.

Bottom line: *it's crucial to have accurate dates for a pregnancy because most tests need to be done during a specified window of time during pregnancy.*

To figure out when you need to make your first prenatal appointment, call your practitioner's office and give them your LMP (the first day of your last menstrual period) and the date of your first positive pregnancy test. They will then know when to schedule the appointment.

Reality check

If you are in Vegas, do not bet on your due date being your baby's birthday. You have a 5% chance of actually delivering on that day. You read that right; that wasn't a typo. In fact, I

IT'S BLUE!

PREGNANCY LINGO 411

it's blue

Yes, there is a whole glossary of Big Ugly Latin Words in the back of this book for you to reference at your leisure, or to use as a sleeping aid. But here are a few terms that are routinely tossed around so you can follow along in this chapter.

Conception: The big event. This is when the sperm and egg meet. It's also sometimes called fertilization.

C-section (Cesarean section): This is a surgical procedure used to deliver a baby. The obstetrician makes a small cut or incision in a woman's lower abdomen and uterus to remove the baby.

Ectopic pregnancy: An embryo implants in the wrong place. Instead of the embryo setting up shop and growing in the uterus (womb), it settles elsewhere—most commonly in the Fallopian tube. Ectopic pregnancies cannot go to completion and are medical emergencies.

Embryo: This is what your unborn baby is called from the time of conception through the first eight weeks of development.

Fetus: This is what your unborn baby is called from nine weeks of development until he is born.

Gestation: The period of time that the embryo/fetus develops in the womb. Gestational age refers to the number of weeks or days the embryo/fetus has been in the womb.

Placenta: Organ that forms after fertilization occurs. It is your baby's life support system. It brings in nourishment and removes waste from the unborn baby (fetus). The umbilical cord, which contains blood vessels, is the conduit between the placenta and the fetus.

Postpartum: The six-week window after a woman gives birth.

Practitioner: To simplify things, we will refer to your healthcare provider as "your practitioner." This refers to your obstetrician ("OB"), family practitioner, nurse practitioner, nurse midwife, or lay midwife who serves as your main healthcare provider during the course of your pregnancy.

Preconception: Before you are pregnant.

Prenatal: The time from conception until birth.

Trimesters: Your pregnancy lasts about 40 weeks. That time is divided into three stages or trimesters, and each is about 13 weeks. The first trimester is 0-13 weeks; second is 14-27 weeks; third is 28-40 weeks.

Uterus: The female organ commonly known as the womb. It is where the developing baby grows until she is born.

Vaginal delivery: A baby is delivered after traveling through the birth canal (the vagina). The vagina is basically a muscular tube that goes from the uterus and cervix to the outside.

IT'S BLUE!

? ?

know a local obstetrician who won't even give his patients a due date. Instead, he gives them a two-week window when the probability is highest that they will deliver. But this nebulous date should at least give you a ballpark idea of when to have your nursery ready.

Factoid: The time between when a woman ovulates (releases a mature egg for fertilization) and when she menstruates (gets her period) is remarkably consistent for all of us. It is usually 14 days. It's the time between when you get your period and when you ovulate that varies a bit—which explains why one woman may have a 28-day cycle and another might have a 34 day cycle. We mention this, just in case you want (or don't want) to get pregnant again! Subtract 14 days from the first day of your last period and you will know how many days into your cycle you are ovulating.

Old Wives Tale

You'll have better odds of conceiving if the guy is on top (missionary position).

The truth: You'll have better odds of conceiving if you make love while you are ovulating, no matter which position you are in.

Q. How long am I actually going to be pregnant?

280 days. That is divided up by three "trimesters", ten lunar months, or 40 weeks. Any way you slice or dice it, it's a long time. By the end, you will be wishing you were a seahorse, one of the few species where the males carry the babies!

Q. Why do you refer to everything in weeks instead of months?

This can be very confusing. Pregnancy is not exactly nine months, and the number of days in each month varies. So, it's more accurate to follow your pregnancy by the week and not the month. A pregnancy that goes to term (also called **FULL TERM**) is 37 to 40 weeks.

Bottom line: Just tell your girlfriends how many weeks along you are and let them figure out when to plan your baby shower.

The Birds and the Bees

Fair warning: this may sound suspiciously like the "talk" you had in fifth grade. You remember the day they separated the girls from the boys and made you watch embarrassing videos.

Q. How does a baby become, well, a baby?

A typical woman releases an egg from one of her two **OVARIES**. Her female hormones elegantly control this monthly event. Once the egg is released, it leaves the **OVARY** and travels through the **FALLOPIAN TUBE**. That's called **OVULATION**.

Once that egg starts its journey, it's got about 24 hours to find a nice sperm to pair up with while it is in the fallopian tube. If the sperm do not reach and penetrate the egg, the egg dies and a woman menstruates (i.e., gets her **MENSTRUAL PERIOD**) about 14 days later.

If a man's sperm finds the egg, which seems easy enough because there are usually anywhere from 20 million to 200 million per batch, voila! Fertilization can occur.

This is, however, a difficult feat for sperm...they have to navigate through the top of the **VAGINA** into the **CERVIX** (a few good men are lost there). Then, they swim up into the body of the **UTERUS** and some choose the wrong fallopian tube, while others choose the right one.

This is as tough as it sounds. There are no road signs or GPS systems to rely on. And sperm, being of the male gender, won't ask for directions! (Just kidding on that last one).

Of the remaining sperm that make it into the correct fallopian tube, only one (and in rare cases two) actually break down the hard outer shell of the egg (the zona pellucida) and fertilize it. That's called **CONCEPTION**.

The fertilized egg (**EMBRYO**), then enters the woman's **UTERUS** and attaches (called **IMPLANTATION**) to the uterine lining about seven days later. That little fertilized egg is now your baby.

Of course, that's the old-fashioned way. Today, there are more options to accomplish this goal! There is a whole chapter devoted to multiples (twins or more) in Chapter 20, Multiples. We'll explain how Mother Nature makes that happen (and how your friendly fertility specialist can do the same thing).

Fertilization and Implantation

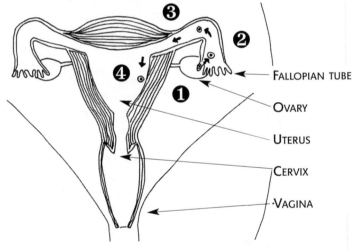

KEY

1. Egg travels from ovary to fallopian tube (ovulation).

2. Egg meets sperm in fallopian tube (fertilization).

3. Fertilized egg moves through fallopian tube.

4. Fertilized egg attaches to uterine lining.

Factoid: Sperm can live in a woman's body for as long as five days. Eggs are on a tighter time schedule, however. Once an egg heads out of the ovary, it has to be fertilized by a sperm within 24 hours. *(ACOG)*

???

Factoid: Of the millions of sperm that are released during sexual inter-course, less than 200 get anywhere near that little egg. And only one (or, rarely two) is the lucky winner that gets to fertilize it. *(Hacker NF)*

Reader Alert: Confusing Math Ahead!

There are two ways to follow your growing baby's development.

HOW IT ALL WORKS: NITTY GRITTY DETAILS

So how does a human become a human? Let's do a brief review in case you were sleeping through your high school biology class.

◆ Chromosomes are our body's blueprints. They carry genetic material (our genes) made from DNA (deoxyribonucleic acid).

◆ Human cells have 23 pairs (or 46 total) of chromosomes.

◆ The two chromosomes that make up each pair of Pairs 1 to 22 are identical.

◆ The two chromosomes that make up the 23rd pair are the sex chromosomes. Girls have two identical X sex chromosomes. Boys have one X and one Y sex chromosome.

◆ The egg (ovum) and the sperm are special human cells because they are the only cells in the body that have half the number of chromosomes that all other cells do. So, eggs have 23 chromosomes (22 plus an X sex chromosome). Sperm have 23 chromosomes (22 plus either an X or a Y sex chromosome).

◆ When an egg and a sperm meet, their single chromosomes pair up with each other. Pairs 1 to 22 find each other as does Pair 23. If the 23rd pair is XX, she will be a girl. If the 23rd pair is XY, he will be a boy. Each baby gets half of their genetic blueprints from mom and half from dad. However, the X or Y carrying sperm is what ultimately determines the sex of the baby.

◆ Once the egg and sperm unite, the fertilized egg starts divid-ing and growing about 24 hours later to become a ball of cells.

◆ This little ball follows its highly complex blueprint to become a human and enters the world about 37 weeks later.

Egg & Sperm	Genetic material meets	Chromosomes pair up	New cell	Cell divides

4 Easy Steps

1. Egg and sperm genetic material meet.
2. The chromosomes pair up.
3. A new cell is made.
4. The cell divides.

There will be a quiz on this next Monday.

IT'S BLUE!

it's blue

◆ *FERTILIZATION AGE*: Day 1 starts when the egg and sperm meet (that is, fertilization or conception). It takes 266 days or 38 weeks for a fetus to complete its development.

◆ *GESTATIONAL AGE:* Day 1 starts on the first day of your last menstrual period (LMP). For the sake of simplicity, this is used because we don't usually know the exact day that fertilization/conception hap-

---

Tales from the womb: Your growing baby (Sadler TW)

GESTATIONAL AGE (weeks)	SIZE (inches)	WEIGHT (oz/lbs)	MILESTONE (FOR BABY)
Embryo			
Day 1			First day of last menstrual period
1 week			Egg not yet released from ovary
2 weeks			Egg and sperm meet (fertilization)
3 weeks			Implantation
4 weeks	0.06*		Brain/spine/nerves develop
5 weeks	0.1*		Heart/eyes/ears/budding arms
6 weeks	0.2*		Face/arms/organs form, heart beats
7 weeks	0.3*		Lower legs, intestines, bladder
8 weeks	0.6*	0.04 oz	4 chamber heart, throat, teeth buds
9 weeks	0.8*	0.07 oz	Inner ear, nose, fingers
10 weeks	1.3*	0.14 oz	Doppler detects heartbeat
Fetus			
11 wks	1.9*	0.3 oz	Eyelids fused together
12 wks	2.4*	0.5 oz	Some organs working, mouth forms
14 wks	3.4*	1.5 oz	External genitals visible
16 wks	4.7 *	3.8 oz	Suck thumb, swallow, breathe, pee
18 wks	5.5*	7 oz	Bones harden, ovaries make eggs
22 wks	10.9 in	1 lb	Head/body hair, body fur, fetal kicking
24 wks	11.8 in	1.4 lbs	Hearing, rapid eye movements
26 wks	14.2 in	1.8 lbs	Lungs begin maturing, fingernails
28 wks	14.8 in	2.2 lbs	Eyes open and close
30 wks	15.7 in	2.9 lbs	Bone marrow works
32 wks	16.7 in	3.7 lbs	Pupils respond to light
34 wks	17.7 in	4.6 lbs	Eyes close with sleep
36 wks	18.6 in	5 lbs	Lungs mature, testes descend
38 wks	19.6 in	6.4 lbs	Fat accumulates, breasts protrude
40 wks	20.2 in	7.5 lbs	Ready to go!

Key:
*CRL=Crown Rump Length. Your practitioner measures your baby's length from his head to his hiney (Crown Rump Length, or CRL) on ultrasounds until about 14 weeks. Starting at 20 weeks, it's possible to estimate your baby's length from head to toe.

(All measurements are averages. Don't obsess about them.)

---

pened. It takes 280 days or 40 weeks to complete development if you look at it this way. This is how your practitioner follows your baby's progress, so that's what we will do in this book. Confusing, we know. It's true, you are not carrying a fertilized egg for the first two weeks of this time period—but any time you get two free weeks without nausea or the urge to pee, consider it a blessing!

Putting it All Together—and What About Me?

We have a handy table (see previous page) of your growing baby. Below is a table of *your* growing body for the next 40 weeks, just to give you the big picture of it all. And here is a rough timeline of the changes to come:

WEEK (GESTATIONAL AGE)	HOW YOUR BODY CHANGES

First trimester (0-13 weeks)

4 weeks	Home pregnancy test positive
6 weeks	Sore breasts, frequent urination
8 weeks	Nauseated, grumpy (okay—bitchy), severe fatigue, constipated
10 weeks	Enlarging breasts, enlarging waistline (pants that buttoned in the morning will NOT close by late afternoon)
12 weeks	Uterus can be felt above the pelvis, increased vaginal discharge
13 weeks	Risk of miscarriage diminishes, baby bump may appear

Second trimester (14-27 weeks)

14 weeks	Nausea usually ends, bitchiness may not, more energy
16 weeks	Growing and feeling good, increased appetite, onset of heartburn, aches and pains
20 weeks	Center of gravity changes, clumsiness, start to feel fetal movement
24 weeks	Skin changes, swollen feet at the end of a long day

Third trimester (28-40 weeks)

28 weeks	Back pain, leg cramps
30 weeks	Heartburn worsens, constipation returns, swollen veins around the anus (**HEMORRHOIDS**) bless us with their presence
32 weeks	Leaking early breast milk is possible, practice contractions may begin
34 weeks	Fatigue returns, shoes don't fit, stretch marks may appear
36 weeks	Vaginal discharge increases AGAIN, may start to leak urine
37 weeks	Practice contractions begin or continue, mucous blocking cervix may come out, hard to find a comfortable position
38 weeks	Peeing every 1 to 2 hours, hemorrhoids enlarge, can't sleep
39 weeks	Everything we've already said taken to another level!
40 weeks	You'll be praying to every holy being in every religion to please make you go into labor!

Now that you've overcome the shock and awe, let's talk about the weeks ahead. Up next: the first trimester.

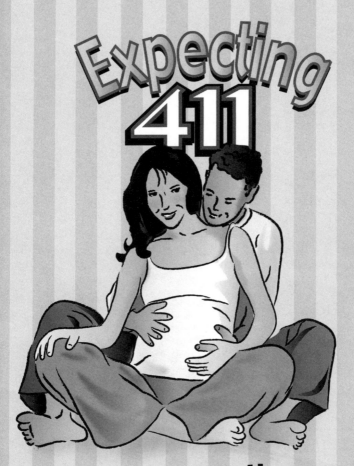

Expecting 411

section one

I'm pregnant!
Now what?

THE FIRST TRIMESTER

Chapter 1

"Always end the name of your child with a vowel, so that when you yell, the name will carry."
~ Bill Cosby

Welcome to your first trimester of pregnancy!

Here's our goal for this chapter (and the two that follow). By trimester, we'll look at body changes, common questions, your healthcare needs (called prenatal care), decisions you will need to make, and what is going on with your growing baby. And we will guide you to where you will find info on specific topics covered in later chapters.

You: The First Trimester

Let's start with an overview of what's to come over the next several weeks.

0-2 weeks

Technically, you haven't even conceived yet. But the 40-week countdown begins on the first day of your menstrual period. You get two free weeks right at the start!

3 weeks

This is the week the fertilized egg implants into your womb (uterus). Some women experience light spotting (a few drops of blood that stain a panty liner or undies) when this happens. This is called **IMPLANTATION BLEEDING**. You probably don't even realize that you are pregnant at this point because you have not missed your period yet. If you have been trying to become pregnant, you should already be avoiding unhealthy habits and taking prenatal vitamins.

1ST TRIMESTER

? ?

4-5 weeks

Congratulations! You miss your period and discover you have a positive pregnancy test. Enjoy the elation.

Signs of pregnancy are heading your way soon. If you aren't already taking daily prenatal vitamins, put this book down right now and go buy some (later in this chapter we offer tips on which ones to buy). Stop any habits that are bad for you and even worse for your unborn baby. See Chapter 7, Environment for details.

Call your practitioner to set up your first prenatal visit. For most of you, your first appointment will be when you are between seven to ten weeks pregnant. If you have a chronic medical condition, your first appointment will be sooner than that.

If you have any vaginal bleeding or severe abdominal pain, don't wait for your first prenatal appointment. Call your practitioner now. (See Chapter 21, When It Doesn't Work and Chapter 15, Pregnancy 911 for symptoms of **MISCARRIAGE**).

If you have conceived with the help of a fertility specialist, that doctor will probably care for you until eight to 12 weeks. At that point, you see your practitioner for the first visit.

Contemplating sushi or continuing with your lattes during pregnancy? Check out Chapter 7, Environment. Wondering if you need to cancel your hair highlights or manicure/pedicure appointments? See Chapter 9, The Spa Treatment.

Curious to know if you can still take that Caribbean cruise when you are pregnant? See Chapter 8, Lifestyles. Want to know how to eat a healthy diet and gain the right amount of weight during pregnancy? It's all there in Chapter 6, Nutrition.

6-7 weeks

One of the first clues you are pregnant is that your breasts will be sore and tender. See Chapter 4, Is This Normal? for ways to relieve your discomfort. You will also need to pee more than usual. You may need to get up a few times a night to urinate. Again, see Chapter 4 for what is normal and what warrants a visit to your practitioner. You may also start having quite a bit of vaginal discharge. Sorry, but this will continue throughout your pregnancy.

8-9 weeks

Pregnancy should be in full swing now. Many women experience severe fatigue, all-day nausea (who are we kidding by calling it morning sickness?), and general grumpiness. Some women also experience mild pelvic cramps. See Chapter 4, Is This Normal? to sort out what to do about these typical symptoms. You'll have to live with some of these unpleasant issues for the next four weeks or so.

If you have excessive vomiting, you need to call your practitioner now. See Chapter 15, Pregnancy 911 and Chapter 16, Complications for details on morning sickness gone south (**HYPEREMESIS GRAVIDARUM**).

You'll have your first prenatal visit this week or soon after. Be sure to bring your partner with you to this visit, and block out your morning or afternoon (it's usually a long appointment). Check out details in this chapter for a list of questions to ask your practitioner.

Yes, lab tests are a fact of life for all pregnant moms. See Chapter 5, Tests, for details on all the routine tests as well as optional ones you may want to request.

Plan on routine appointments with your practitioner about once a month until you are 28 weeks.

10-11 weeks

This is the week of the enlarging breasts and waistline. Your partner will enjoy looking at your new chest but your breasts will likely be so tender that they'll be off limits. See Chapter 4, Is This Normal? for some reassurance and tips to relieve discomfort.

You will notice that you can button your pants in the morning, but not in the afternoon. If you haven't spilled the beans to family, friends, or your boss, you won't be able to hide your body changes much longer. Read later in this chapter for concerns about telling family and friends. See Chapter 8, Lifestyles, about telling your boss and to learn more about employee medical leave rights.

If you are 35 years of age or older (a.k.a. "Advanced Maternal Age", ugh!), you may want to learn about optional tests that screen for chromosomal abnormalities like the **FIRST TRIMESTER SCREENING TEST, CHORIONIC VILLUS SAMPLING (CVS),** or **AMNIOCENTESIS.** See Chapter 5, Tests for all you need to know about these specialized tests. Even if you are under 35, you may want to read this section.

The first trimester screening test is done between ten and 13 weeks and a CVS is done at about the same time, so get reading.

12-13 weeks

You are almost done with your first trimester! Hooray! If you have made it this far, it's much less likely you will miscarry. Your little baby bump may start to appear . . . yes, you are really going to have a baby.

Your practitioner will begin listening to your baby's heartbeat with a Doppler device at each visit. This is really fun (and very reassuring) to hear. You'll start showing between 13-20 weeks, depending on your body stature, whether this is your first baby or not, and how many babies you are carrying. Normal complaints in the first trimester include headaches, lightheadedness, forgetfulness, all-day nausea, constipation, excessive gas and burping, lots of vaginal discharge, lots of peeing, acne, and of course, moodiness and fatigue. You'll be happy to head into your second trimester. Pregnant life does get better!

Aches, pains and changes the **FIRST TRIMESTER (0-13 WEEKS)**
Common symptoms:
- ◆ Moody, emotional ◆ Tired
- ◆ Headaches ◆ Gas, burping, constipation
- ◆ Difficulty sleeping ◆ Tender, growing breasts
- ◆ Frequent urination, urinating at night
- ◆ Nausea, vomiting (morning sickness)
- ◆ Vaginal discharge starts and continues for the duration
- ◆ Acne, splotchy marks on the face

1ST TRIMESTER

? ?

Common Questions About the First Trimester

We know you've got a million questions right now! And you won't be seeing your healthcare provider for a little while. So this section should ease your mind until that first appointment.

Q. My home pregnancy test was positive. When should I schedule an appointment with my practitioner?

Most practitioners see newly pregnant patients anywhere between seven to ten weeks of pregnancy. You can calculate this from the first day of your last menstrual period (see "How do I figure out my due date?" in the Introduction, It's Blue).

If you conceived by assisted-reproductive technologies, like in-vitro fertilization (IVF), your fertility specialist will see you at frequent intervals during the early part of your pregnancy. You will then be "released" into the care of your practitioner anywhere between eight and 12 weeks of gestation.

If you have a **HIGH-RISK PREGNANCY** (see box below), you may need to see your practitioner sooner rather than later. Not sure if you fit into that category? Check out our handy box below or call your practitioner. She can tell you when to come in for that first appointment.

Q. Are there any foods or beverages I need to avoid now that I am pregnant?

Short answer: Yes.

The long answer to what you should and shouldn't eat gets an entire chapter later in this book (Chapter 7, The Environment). But here's a list to review before you see your practitioner for the first time so you don't have any early anxiety attacks.

Prime example: I received an emergency page from a patient's husband on a Friday night. Why? His wife ate some soybeans that had been sitting in the same take-out box as his sushi. Did this put the pregnancy at risk?

DO I HAVE A HIGH-RISK PREGNANCY?

The answer is YES if you:

◆ Are having twins, triplets, or even more multiples.
◆ Have a history of repeated miscarriages.
◆ Conceived by assisted reproductive technology/with the help of a fertility specialist.
◆ Are having vaginal bleeding.
◆ Have chronic medical issues like lupus, pre-existing diabetes or high blood pressure.
◆ Have a complication arise during your pregnancy (like placenta previa).
◆ Are 35 years old or older (I know, that seems extreme) although some docs consider only women over age 40 to be high-risk.
◆ Have a history of an ectopic pregnancy.

(Answer: no!)

So, given the high anxiety level about this topic, here's the brief 30-second version of what to avoid eating when pregnant:

- *Avoid eating fish with high mercury levels—and limit the amount of fish with moderate and low mercury levels.* That list is featured in Chapter 7, The Environment.

- *Avoid raw or undercooked meat.* Sorry, that means sushi is a no-no. Seared fish and rare meat are also off limits. And avoid anything made with raw eggs. That includes freshly made Caesar salad dressing, hollandaise sauce, and homemade egg nog.

- *Avoid unpasteurized dairy products.* Some fancy cheeses fit into this category. These can include brie, Camembert, feta, gorgonzola, queso blanco and Roquefort.

- *Wash all fruits and vegetables thoroughly before eating.*

- *Thoroughly cook pre-sliced deli meat and hot dogs before eating (microwave until steaming).*

- *Avoid alcoholic beverages.*

- *Avoid caffeine if possible.* If that sounds daunting (we're doctors, we understand caffeine), aim for limiting your consumption to one or at most two caffeinated beverages a day, especially in the first trimester.

- *Stop smoking.* If that has been tough, talk with your practitioner about other options to help quit. (This one we won't budge on.)

Your practitioner will discuss and/or give you a list of all the banned food and beverages during pregnancy at your first visit. But you can get started with your new pregnancy diet having this information in hand. We will explain WHY you have to avoid all these foods in detail when you get to Chapter 7, The Environment.

Reality check

If you smoke, drink alcohol or use drugs, now is the time to stop.

Q. Are there any medications I need to stop using now that I am pregnant?

The short answer is yes.

There is an expansive list at Expecting411.com/extra that covers both over-the-counter and prescription medications with safety ratings for pregnancy and breastfeeding.

Certain medications are absolute no-no's, especially in the first trimester (13 weeks) because they can cause medical problems for an unborn baby.

For other medications, the risk to the unborn baby must be weighed against the benefit of the mother-to-be's health. The practitioner handling your pregnancy can discuss possible alternative medications with your other healthcare providers if there is a significant risk with what you are currently taking.

If you have health or mental health issues that require you to take daily medication, call the physician who is prescribing that medication and notify him or her of your pregnancy right now—just in case you need to stop that medicine. And you or your physician can always call your obstetrician to double check on medications that are safe to take during pregnancy.

Q. How about herbal medication? Can I continue or start taking those meds?

Check with your practitioner if you are currently taking or want to start taking any herbal, homeopathic or alternative medicine. Seemingly innocuous supplements such as ginseng and St. John's wort have the potential to cause bleeding and should not be used in pregnancy. Check out the list of alternative remedies and their safety/risks during pregnancy at Expecting411.com /extra.

Until you have your first prenatal appointment, I suggest holding off on these products.

Q. Are there any vitamins or nutritional supplements I need now?

Yes! Until you visit your practitioner and get her advice, I recommend taking a daily dose of any over-the-counter prenatal vitamin containing 300 mg of DHA (fish oil or "omega-3 fatty acid"), at least 400 mcg of folic acid, and *less than* 5,000 IU a day of Vitamin A. I also recommend picking up a calcium/Vitamin D supplement. A calcium supplement of 500 mg to 600 mg is a good addition to the calcium that's already in your prenatal vitamin and diet.

If you planned this pregnancy, you should already be taking prenatal vitamins. The latest research shows that taking prenatal vitamins containing at least 400 mcg of folic acid for three months before conception lowers the risk of certain birth defects (**NEURAL TUBE DEFECTS**) and some pregnancy-associated health issues, such as preterm births. If your pregnancy was a pleasant surprise, put down this book and go buy some prenatal vitamins.

Don't get overwhelmed when you go to the pharmacy. There are several choices when it comes to prenatal vitamins and most pills are similar. Some contain a stool softener (which is usually a welcome treat in the first trimester as constipation is a frequent side effect of pregnancy). Some contain DHA, which has health benefits for both mom and baby. What's most important is to check for the amount of folic acid and Vitamin A.

We cover prenatal vitamins and other supplements in greater depth in Chapter 6, Nutrition. So, pop over there for some very helpful tips!

After you go to your first prenatal visit, you may also need to take an iron supplement if you are anemic. Your practitioner will let you know based on a blood test taken at your first visit.

Insider Secret

Take your prenatal vitamin and calcium supplement at different times during the day so the calcium is more effectively absorbed.

Insider Secret

Do prenatal vitamins make you feel queasy? The label on your prenatal vitamin probably tells you to take the pill on an empty stomach so the vitamins will be better absorbed. This will, ten times out of ten make you vomit. Believe us, we've tried it! We suggest taking your prenatal vitamin on a full stomach, with your biggest meal of the day. Or at least have some pudding or crackers to coat your stomach first.

Q. When am I going to start gaining weight and how much should I gain?

Read about this topic in depth in Chapter 6, Nutrition. Here is the quick answer: the amount you should gain depends on your pre-pregnancy weight. And yes, you will start to gain weight in your first trimester.

If you were a healthy weight (normal Body Mass Index or BMI), you should gain about three to five pounds in this trimester. See our web site Expecting411.com (click on Bonus) to check your BMI.

Q. Will I start feeling bad before I get in to see my doctor?

Probably. Most women see their practitioners between seven and ten weeks of pregnancy. And some women begin having pregnancy symptoms right away. Here are some things you might suffer from . . . uh, we mean experience, before you get to see your practitioner:

1 FATIGUE. And we mean severe fatigue…like the life has been sucked out of you. Don't be surprised if you are ready to go to bed at 6:30pm. Try to catch a nap if you can. Your body needs it.

2 CRAMPING IN YOUR LOWER BELLY. You may feel like you're having menstrual cramps. Most of the time, you feel this because your uterine muscles are stretching and growing. Occasionally it can be a sign of a problem—especially if you are having vaginal bleeding with those cramps or pain only on one side. See the Red Flags section below for details and to see whether you need to call your practitioner.

3 LOTS OF PEE. Pregnant women pee a lot. And yes, that happens even in the early stages of your pregnancy. You may need to get up two or three times a night to use the bathroom. If it hurts or burns when you urinate, call your practitioner. You need to be tested for a bladder infection.

4 BIG, TENDER BREASTS. You may be used to getting some breast tenderness before your period. But you ain't seen nothing like this. Some women's breasts and nipples are so tender that water running over them in the shower or a sheet sitting on them in bed is excruciating. Needless to say, your partner can gaze, drool, and even take pictures (if you are so inclined), but touching will be off limits! You may also notice that the veins on the skin of your breasts and surrounding chest area become very prominent and often resemble a road map. No need to worry—that's to accommodate the increased blood flow to your "naturally enhanced" breasts.

5 **SENSITIVITY TO ODORS.** You and your dog can now compete for who smells food first. Pregnant women have bionic powers of smell and can pick up a scent a mile away. That sounds cool, except that most of those smells (that never bothered you before) may send you running for the nearest place to vomit. When I was pregnant, I was bothered by the metal smell of my keys. I had to hold my nose until I placed the keys in the ignition or into the front door of my house. I'm sure my neighbors thought I was odd, but that was better than throwing up in my car or on my lawn everyday.

6 **"MORNING" SICKNESS.** If only it happened just in the morning, hah! Many pregnant women feel nauseated or have queasy stomachs all day long. In fact, it is often worse at the end of the day. Some women just *think* they are going to puke, and others are unlucky enough to actually do it. This feeling starts around the sixth or seventh week of pregnancy and usually lasts until the first trimester ends. I'll see some women in my office for their first prenatal visit who claim to feel great—but it's a different story when I see them for their next visit a few weeks later. Look for tips on combating morning sickness in Chapter 4, Is This Normal?

7 **EMOTIONAL ROLLERCOASTER.** Pregnant women should have a sign posted on them that says, "Pregnant woman—stay back 200 feet." Take those PMS symptoms you are used to and multiply them by 1000. You may go through periods of feeling weepy, bitchy, elated and detached all in a span of thirty minutes. And yes, your partner is often the recipient of this hormonal behavior—so you might want to issue a warning! We hurt the ones we love the most. All of these feelings are normal. Since all those hormones start surging right at the beginning of pregnancy, so will these emotional up's and down's. You (and your partner) should know that things start to smooth out by week 14.

Bottom Line

Yes, you may "feel" pregnant before you see your practitioner for the first visit. However, here is a key fact: 30% of women don't have any symptoms of pregnancy other than a missed period. Don't panic: lacking symptoms isn't a sign that something is wrong.

Feedback from the Real World
Dr. B and Mrs. Hyde

My husband and I rarely fight, but one night we had a real shouting fest. I don't even remember what we were fighting about, but I assure you it was something utterly ridiculous. It was so ridiculous, my husband decided that I either had some alter ego he was previously unaware of or that I had to be pregnant. He shouted, "Either something's wrong with you or you must be pregnant!" I resisted the temptation to hurl a frying pan at him and did a home pregnancy test. It was blue. I hate it when he's right, but he usually is!

Q. People say I am eating for two. But with this morning

sickness, I can't even eat for one right now!

We won't lie: you can feel pretty queasy during the first trimester. Around ten weeks, you will feel like you want to crawl into a hole and wake up next spring.

Many women are extremely nauseated and eat only what makes them feel better. Whether that is Taco Bell (Dr H's first pregnancy) or Coke and Cheetos (Dr H's second pregnancy), you do what you've gotta do to get through it. We don't recommend the Coke and Cheetos diet, however, once you have gotten over morning sickness!

Focus on diet and nutrition in the *second* trimester when your gut feels better and life returns to something closer to normal. We'll cover all of your nutrition questions and concerns in Chapter 6, Nutrition.

For your first trimester, remember that when people say you are "eating for two," you are actually eating for one and a few millimeters. . . so you do need to eat more, but within reason.

Q. I am having food aversions. Anything that has a strong smell makes me sick to my stomach. Is this normal? Why does this happen?

It is very common, particularly in the first trimester, to have very strong aversions to smells.

Your stomach might turn with the fainted whiff of cigarette smoke, meat and fish, or anything overwhelming in the kitchen pantry. Think of it as nature's way of preventing pregnant women from ingesting potentially dangerous things.

Here's the theory: hundreds of years ago (before refrigeration and the FDA), our ancestors relied on their sniffers to determine if something was rotten or poisonous. In other words—something you shouldn't eat. Since a pregnant woman has a greater risk of harm (to herself and the unborn baby) from ingesting something bad, your sense of smell is now in overdrive.

Of course, our food supply today is quite a bit safer and we can read labels to avoid potentially dangerous foods. Yet our instincts often take over despite modern society.

DR H'S TRUE STORY

One of my patients (who is also a great friend) couldn't come within a mile of chicken with her pregnancy. Seeing, touching, smelling or eating chicken was impossible. To this day, she steers clear of chicken, which is comical since her family is in the meatpacking business!

Red Flags: Danger signs in first few weeks

Here are the big red flags for the first few weeks of pregnancy (contact your practitioner immediately):

◆ *Vaginal Bleeding.* Most of the time, a little spotting does not mean

? ?

1ST TRIMESTER

something serious is going on. But call your practitioner if you have ANY bleeding from your vagina and let your practitioner decide what to do. Heavy bleeding, like the volumes you see when you get your period, can be a sign of loss of pregnancy (**MISCARRIAGE**), the embryo implanted in the wrong place (**ECTOPIC PREGNANCY**), or a separation of the placenta (from the wall of the uterus). Your practitioner will need to see you, do an exam, check your blood type, and most of the time, perform an ultrasound. Miscarriage and ectopic pregnancies are discussed in detail in Chapter 21, When It Doesn't Work.

If all is well upon exam and testing, the heavy bleeding is presumed to be from a placental separation, and you might be placed on bed rest or asked to limit your activity (modified bed rest).

◆ *Severe Cramps.* Most pregnant women have occasional cramps in their pelvic area, most noticeably in the first trimester. These feel like menstrual cramps, and are usually normal.

Severe pain isn't normal. Pain located on one side more than the other also isn't normal. Call your practitioner. This can be a sign of miscarriage or ectopic pregnancy—especially if severe, painful cramps go along with heavy vaginal bleeding.

◆ *Persistent Vomiting.* Pregnant women are nauseated. And some pregnant women vomit. But a few can't stop vomiting (**HYPEREMESIS GRAVIDARUM,** see Chapter 16, Complications, complication #1). Those women are dehydrated and malnourished because nothing will stay down. Sometimes hospitalization is required to break the vomiting cycle and help rehydrate a woman with nutrition and fluid given through a vein (**INTRAVENOUS FLUID**). Call your practitioner if you can't keep anything down.

Red Flags for ectopic pregnancy

An ectopic pregnancy occurs when a fertilized egg implants in the wrong place, outside of the uterus. This is a dangerous medical complication. Symptoms include: severe abdominal pain, particularly on just one side, or even painless vaginal bleeding with a missed period and positive pregnancy test. See Chapter 15, Pregnancy 911 and Chapter 21, When It Doesn't Work for details.

Prenatal Care

As we discussed earlier, the first visit is about seven to ten weeks from the first day of your last menstrual period. Once your home pregnancy test(s) is positive, go ahead and schedule your first "prenatal" appointment. (Prenatal care is the official term for all those healthcare appointments prior to labor and childbirth.) Yes, those few weeks before you see your practitioner feel like forever!

Wondering which practitioner you should see for your prenatal care? We cover that in the Decisions section later in this chapter.

? ?

1ST TRIMESTER

Q. Are there any reasons why I might need to see my practitioner before the standard first visit?

Yes. See if you fit into any of these categories below. If so, call your practitioner as soon as you know you are pregnant.

1. You have a chronic medical condition, such as lupus, diabetes, heart disease or high blood pressure.
2. You are having vaginal bleeding.
3. You have severe abdominal (belly or lower belly) pain.
4. You cannot stop vomiting.
5. You conceived by assisted reproductive technologies—IUI (Intrauterine Insemination) or IVF (In Vitro Fertilization).
6. You know you are carrying multiples (twins, triplets, etc).
7. You are taking prescription medication.

Those of you in categories #5 and #6 have a fertility specialist who will probably continue to care for you until you are eight to 12 weeks gestation at which time you will be released into the care of your obstetrician for your prenatal care.

Insider Secret

If you have pre-existing medical problems, call your practitioner as soon as you know you are pregnant. Pregnancy can make some medical conditions worse, and it can make some conditions better. Your practitioner can advise you right at the start once she knows you are pregnant. She may want to see you earlier than seven to ten weeks. This is especially important if you are having a flare-up of your disease, or need to take medication on a daily basis.

Q. What happens at the first visit?

I'll walk you through what I do for a typical first visit. While this may vary a little from practitioner to practitioner, this should give you the basic idea of what an obstetrician will do. Let's pretend you are my patient:

I start by visiting with you (and hopefully your partner) in my office before going into an exam room. I find it easier to have a conversation with you when you aren't naked, sitting under a wispy paper gown in a freezing exam room!

I thoroughly review your personal medical history, dad-to-be's medical history, both of your family medical histories and discuss any potential issues such as never having had chickenpox or having cats at home. This helps me determine if this is a high-risk pregnancy and allows me to advise you of any special concerns.

Then we move into an exam room to do a breast exam, pelvic (internal) exam, and then an ultrasound.

During the pelvic exam, I take a few swabs from the cervix (opening of the womb/uterus) to test for infections like gonorrhea and Chlamydia. I'll also do a Pap smear if one has not been done recently. I then do a bimanual exam

? ?

1ST TRIMESTER

(placing one or two fingers in the vagina and the other hand on top of the lower abdomen) to assess the size of the uterus, ovaries and fallopian tubes.

Next, a **TRANSVAGINAL ULTRASOUND** is done (see Chapter 5, Tests for a more complete explanation) if this is your first visit early in your pregnancy. The ultrasound probe is inserted into your vagina (as opposed to placing the probe on top of your belly) because at this point the fetus is too small to see any other way.

This ultrasound tells me several things: I can see that the growing fetus is in the uterus where it should be and is not implanted in the wrong place (see **ECTOPIC PREGNANCY**). I can figure out if the size of the fetus is appropriate based on the date of your **LAST MENSTRUAL PERIOD** (**LMP**). I can document if the fetus has a detectable heartbeat. (This depends on how many weeks along you are when you have your first visit). And I can see that the other internal female organs (fallopian tubes and ovaries) are normal.

Occasionally, twins or other multiples can be seen during this ultrasound too. The excitement over seeing your baby for the first time will probably make you forget that you have a probe in your vagina!

Next, you get your blood drawn for several screening tests (details in Chapter 5, Tests). Some of my patients dread this more than the transvaginal ultrasound! When the lab results are completed several days later, you'll get a phone call.

Assuming all is well, we go back into my office (with paper gown in the trash and clothes back on!) and I give out my standard pregnancy do's and don'ts advice sheets (good news: they are included in this book!), information on the hospital where I perform deliveries, the reason for and dates of upcoming screening tests and resources for childbirth/breastfeeding/first aid classes. You'll schedule your next appointment in two to four weeks.

FYI: That breast exam at the first visit is pretty uncomfortable because most women have extremely tender breasts in the first trimester.

Reality Check

Be sure to take off a morning or afternoon from work for your first appointment—you will be there for a while! I also suggest that you eat a good breakfast, drink a lot of water, and turn your head the other way when you get your blood drawn!

Helpful hints for your first visit

◆ Bring a list of medications you are taking.
◆ Compile a family health history for both you and your partner to give your practitioner.
◆ Compile your own health history (we have a fill in the blank form at Expecting411.com, click Bonus) to share with your practitioner.
◆ Bring your partner!

Q. What are the standard tests done in the first trimester?

The American Congress of Obstetricians and Gynecologists (ACOG) recommends several screening tests during pregnancy. These tests will be explained in full detail in Chapter 5, Tests. But here is the basic rundown:

TEST	WHEN IT'S DONE
Blood pressure, weight and urinalysis	every visit
Prenatal blood panel*	first or second prenatal visit
Pap smear	first prenatal visit
Cervical cultures	first prenatal visit

Complete blood count, blood type, infectious disease panel (HIV, syphilis, Hepatitis B, rubella)

Q. Are there any optional tests that can be done?

Yes. There are other tests that may be useful, depending on your personal medical history, age, or ethnicity. These may raise (or lower) the risk of certain disorders. Chapter 5, Tests, provides a full explanation of your choices. But these are the tests to consider:

1. **First Trimester Screening Test.** A blood test and an ultrasound calculates the odds of having a baby with Down Syndrome (Trisomy 21) or Trisomy 18. Test occurs between ten to 13 weeks.
2. **Chorionic Villus Sampling (CVS).** A physician performs a minor procedure to obtain tissue from the placenta. The test diagnoses 99% of all chromosome abnormalities, and some other disorders. Test occurs at ten to 13 weeks.
3. **Additional Infection Panel.** These specific tests identify exposure and/or immunity for other infections. Example: cat owners may get tested for toxoplasmosis. Tests occur at first visit or whenever necessary.
4. **Other screening tests.** Tests for sickle cell anemia carriers, cystic fibrosis carriers, and other screens may be recommended, depending on your health history and ancestry. Tests are done either prior to pregnancy or at the first prenatal visit.

Q. Will I have a pelvic (internal exam) every time?

No. That's the good news!

It's standard protocol to have a pelvic exam during the first appointment. Then, as long as there are no particular concerns, there won't be another pelvic exam until the home stretch of your pregnancy.

Q. Will I get an ultrasound each time?

No.

Although you might want to sneak a peek at your baby every time you visit your practitioner, this isn't necessary for routine pregnancies.

Most docs do an ultrasound at the first visit, and sometimes one at the next visit.

There are a couple of screening tests that also utilize ultrasounds—one is called the first trimester screening test (done at ten to 13 weeks) and the other evaluates all the fetus' body parts at 20 to 22 weeks. Those studies are discussed in Chapter 5, Tests.

However, there are special situations that call for an ultrasound as part of each visit. Example: women with twins or triplets.

Q. How often will I see my practitioner after the first visit?

Although all practitioners do things a little differently, here is the American Congress of Obstetricians and Gynecologists (ACOG) recommended schedule of routine visits for a typical pregnancy:

Office visit every four weeks from seven to ten weeks up to 28 weeks
Office visit every two weeks from 28 weeks to 36 weeks
Office visit once a week from 36 weeks until delivery

If you have a high-risk pregnancy, such as carrying twins or having high blood pressure, you get to visit your practitioner more often. And if any problems arise (fever, pain with urination, etc.) between those routine visits, you may have a few more appointments.

Q. After the first visit, what usually happens at prenatal appointments?

You will get used to the routine when you walk into your practitioner's office. Yes, this varies depending on your practitioner, but this is what will happen in most cases if you are seeing a physician or nurse practitioner.

First, you will get handed a plastic cup for a urine sample. Believe it or not, we can learn a lot from your pee. We can make sure you don't have a bladder infection (UTI), which can be relatively symptom-free in pregnancy. And we can tell if you are dehydrated or in need of some extra calories.

Next, you get to weigh in. I'm not going to lie—this isn't fun. You will start to see weights on the scale you have never seen before. At one point during my second pregnancy, I weighed more than my brother-in-law and made the mistake of telling him that. To this day, I have never lived it down! The important thing here is to know that you are supposed to gain weight in pregnancy and your practitioner will make sure you are gaining the right amount.

You'll also get your blood pressure measured at every visit.

Next, your practitioner will visit with you, feel your belly, and listen for the baby's heartbeat. Finally, there is an opportunity to ask any burning questions that are keeping you up at night. So write down your list and remember to bring it in to your appointment (or jot it in your iPhone, Blackberry, etc).

Q. When can I hear the baby's heartbeat?

It depends. Hearing your baby's heartbeat is different than seeing it. If your first appointment is at seven weeks of pregnancy and you have an ultrasound, you should be able to see the baby's heartbeat. Some ultrasound machines have an audio component that allows you to hear the heartbeat at this point, but most do not.

Most practitioners use a hand-held Doppler ultrasound after eight to ten weeks that is placed on Mom-to-be's belly. Your baby's heartbeat is much faster than yours. It's ticking at about 120-160 beats per minute and sounds like a galloping horse. The Doppler may also pick up your own, much slower, heart rate of 60-90 beats per minute. After having several of these, you will learn the difference in the rates and noises.

? ?

1ST TRIMESTER

Q. Can I buy my own Doppler?

Yes, but we don't recommend it.

First of all, they are very expensive (around $500 to purchase; $25 to $50 a month to rent). Secondly, using the Doppler requires the experienced hands of someone who has used one about a thousand times. And even in those experienced hands, it can be hard to find the baby's heartbeat, especially early in pregnancy.

What ends up happening is that the pregnant couple can't detect the baby's heartbeat at home and they frantically rush into their practitioner's office. Other times, couples listen cheerfully to mom's pulse instead of baby's heartbeat!

So, skip the panic (you'll have your share of that as new parents) and save your money—you'll need it for the college fund.

Q. Should I bring my spouse/partner with me to every visit? Are there some that are more important than others?

It's nice to have both members of the pregnant couple present at every visit, but let's face it, that isn't always possible. It's often hard enough just to fit all those prenatal visits into one person's crazy schedule—coordinating two schedules may be impossible sometimes. (By the way, this will prepare you for juggling your child's future baseball games, dance lessons, and band practice into your own busy lives and getting everyone where they need to be on time and fed . . . but we digress.)

You may have to pick and choose which visits are the most important ones for both partners to attend. Here are the visits I think are the critical ones for the first trimester:

1 **FIRST PRENATAL APPOINTMENT.** This is key, especially if this is your first child. The information dispensed is both important, and sometimes overwhelming. Four ears hear more than two. This way, everyone's questions get answered (yes, spouses and partners have questions too) and both of you can together see your baby for the first time. Yes, he/she may look like a "blob", "speck of dust", "blueberry", or "peanut"—but it's your peanut!

2 **FIRST TRIMESTER SCREENING TEST.** FYI: This is not a routine test, so it doesn't apply to everyone. And there are several different strategies to approaching these tests—here's a brief overview.

This is typically a visit with a genetic counselor and perinatologist (high-risk obstetric doctor) that occurs between ten and 13 weeks of pregnancy. The genetic counselor thoroughly reviews both of your families' medical histories, genetic problems, and potential exposures to chemicals, medications or drugs (**TERATOGENS**) that could be harmful to your unborn baby/fetus.

The perinatologist then performs an ultrasound. She checks the overall size of the fetus, the thickness of the back of the fetus' neck (**NUCHAL LUCENCY**) and whether or not the nasal bone is present. These assessments help the perinatologist determine if a fetus is at risk for certain genetic syndromes, birth defects, or miscarriage. More on this in Chapter 5, Tests.

Then, be prepared for more blood to be drawn.

It's really important for the couple to be present so that a thorough medical history can be obtained from both of you. If you have an egg donor or a sperm donor, bring all the medical information about the donor. And together, you can be advised of any high-risk pregnancy issues. Occasionally, an abnormality is found and additional testing is recommended on the spot. It's nice to have your partner there (or your mom, sister, best friend) to help make decisions if need be.

INSIDER TIP: It's also helpful for your partner to be present at the 20 to 22 week ultrasound and the 32 to 34 week prenatal visit. We'll explain why in the chapters covering the second and third trimesters.

Partner Tip

Find out what the person carrying the baby REALLY wants you to do. She might say she doesn't mind if you can't make it to an appointment (but she really does...you know how that goes!) Then try your best to be there!

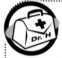

DR H'S OPINION:
PARTNERS AND PRENATAL VISITS

Most of the other prenatal visits are pretty routine. If your partner is able to be there for all the visits, that's great! You may or may not want your partner there for your weigh ins, blood draws, and urine tests—which, by the end of your pregnancy should be considered an Olympic sport. Crouching over the toilet trying to aim your pee into a teeny, tiny cup gets harder and harder as you get bigger and bigger!

Decisions

As parents-to-be, you will have MANY decisions to make. Being major planners ourselves, we think it's a good idea to be prepared so you and your partner don't have any surprises. We will put these items on your radar screen for each trimester (and head over to Chapter 10, Parenthood Prep for even more decisions to make)! Our advice: make decisions as a couple. Believe us, unilateral decision-making is not great for maintaining good relations with your beloved. Here are some good conversation starters:

Q. Should we tell all our family and friends we are pregnant or is it better to wait until I am further along in the pregnancy?

This is a question that comes up often—pretty much with every newly pregnant couple. And it's not an easy answer. We'll give you the facts, and then you can decide for yourself.

Most **MISCARRIAGES** (loss of pregnancy) occur before the 8th week of pregnancy. Here are the stats: there is a 15 to 33% chance of having a miscarriage when someone knows they are pregnant.

There are even more miscarriages that happen before someone knows they are pregnant or has taken a pregnancy test. When you add those undiscovered pregnancies into the mix, some experts estimate that up to 50% of all pregnancies don't make it.

Obviously, the risk of miscarriage is higher in women who have had previous miscarriages, medical problems, or ongoing drug or alcohol use. The risk of miscarriage is also higher for women in their 30's and 40's, especially those turning to assisted-reproductive technologies (IUI or IVF) to conceive.

Women who are pregnant with multiples (twins, triplets, or more) also have a higher rate of miscarriage.

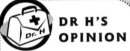

DR H'S OPINION

"I suggest waiting at least until your first prenatal visit when a heartbeat is detected on a pelvic ultrasound before you announce the pregnancy."

Now, you may be so excited to discover you are pregnant that you've already told your parents, siblings, the mailman, and everyone in line at your local grocery store. But if you haven't blabbed yet, here is what those stats mean for you. Your practitioner will likely do an ultrasound at your first prenatal visit (seven to ten weeks of pregnancy). The ultrasound determines if the baby's size matches the date of your last menstrual period (LMP). If a heartbeat is detected and the baby's size is equivalent to how many weeks you are supposed to be, the risk of miscarriage is much lower. That may be all you need to hear before you tell the world the good news.

For other women who fit into the "advanced maternal age" (that is the over-age-35 club, don't take it personally) or fertility specialist-assisted pregnancy categories, you may want to wait a few more weeks until more tests are done (**FIRST TRIMESTER SCREENING TEST** and **EXPANDED-AFP TEST**, explained in Chapter 5, Tests) before everyone finds out your little secret.

Once you've made it to 13 weeks, the odds are very low that you will miscarry and very high that you won't be able to hide that growing bulge for much longer. So, if you really want to wait until the last minute to

DR B'S OPINION: SHARING THE NEWS WITH A YOUNG CHILD

If you already have a young child/children at home, I suggest waiting to share the news with her/him until you are actually showing. Pregnancy itself is a fairly abstract concept to a young child. Having a visual aid to follow is helpful! Waiting until after 13 weeks also increases your odds that the pregnancy is successful. (It's very sad and confusing for the older sibling-to-be if you have to tell her/him that the baby is "no longer in mommy's tummy.")

I always remind parents that young children have no concept of time—hence the famous, "Are we there yet?" line you will hear incessantly from the back seat of your car. Once you tell your older child that a new baby is coming, the sibling-to-be will be rather impatient for that day to come. The later in pregnancy this is announced, the less you will have to deal with the daily explanation!

divulge, you'll have to endure some lengthy stares while people wonder if are you pregnant or just getting thick around the middle.

Obviously, this is your call—just remember that if you decided to announce your pregnancy and then have a miscarriage, you will have to deal with the inevitable questions. While some couples feel it is therapeutic to share their grief with family and close friends, others find talking about a miscarriage to be a painful reminder of their loss. Consider how both of you might handle this situation.

Reality Check

Here are the stats on spilling the beans to co-workers and employers from a BabyCenter.com survey:

◆ 23% tell immediately.
◆ 23% wait a few weeks until reality sets in.
◆ 36% wait until after the first trimester (13 weeks).
◆ 14% wait until they are starting to show.

Q. Which practitioner should I use for my pregnancy and delivery?

There are many different types of healthcare providers who care for pregnant women. Some provide prenatal care and deliver babies, while others provide prenatal care or support, but don't actually do deliveries. Let's review the different types of providers, and explain their training and background.

◆ **Obstetricians** ("OB" or "OB/GYN" for short) are medical doctors (M.D.) or doctors of osteopathic medicine (D.O.) who have at least eight years of medical training after completing a bachelor's degree in college. They complete four years of medical school, four years in a specialty residency in obstetrics and gynecology, and then complete licensing and board certification. Obstetricians provide prenatal care, perform deliveries (both vaginal and Cesarean) and postpartum care. Most OB's take care of both low-risk and high-risk pregnancies, but this varies in different parts of the country. OB's deliver babies in hospitals and carry malpractice insurance.

◆ **Family practitioners** are also medical doctors (M.D.) or doctors of osteopathy (D.O.). After graduating from college, they complete four years of medical school, three years of family practice residency, then licensing and board certification. Some, but not all, programs offer training in obstetrics. Simply put, not all family practice docs take care of pregnant women and deliver babies. Family practitioners who practice obstetric medicine typically only care for routine pregnancies (not high-risk ones). Family practice docs also deliver their babies in hospitals and carry malpractice insurance.

◆ **Nurse practitioners** (NP) are registered nurses who have completed additional advanced nursing education (generally a master's degree). In the United States, NP's have state licensing and board certifications. They see patients on their own, under the supervision of a physician. Most nurse practitioners do not deliver babies, although they do provide prenatal and postnatal care. If you use an obstetrician for your prenatal care, your doc may have an NP who sees you for one or more of your visits (especially if the doc has to run out to deliver someone else's baby during office hours!).

◆ *Midwives*. There are actually many different types of midwives: Certified Nurse Midwives (CNM), Certified Professional Midwives (CPM), Registered Midwives (RM), Licensed Midwives (LM), Certified Midwives (CM), Traditional midwives.

◆ *Certified nurse midwives* (CNM) graduate from college, then complete nursing and midwifery training. Some CNM's have a master's or doctoral degree in nurse-midwifery. They attend births in hospitals (although not all hospitals allow midwives to deliver), birthing centers and at home. CNM's either practice under the supervision of a physician or independently. They offer prenatal and postnatal care. CNM's do not perform Cesarean sections. Almost all CNM-assisted deliveries occur in a hospital setting. All 50 states require CNM's to be licensed. Some accept health insurance and all of them must carry malpractice insurance.

◆ *Certified professional midwives* (CPM) either train at an accredited midwifery school or through an apprenticeship, meeting standards of the North American Registry of Midwives (NARM) and the Midwives Alliance of North America (MANA). Individual states regulate credentialing, so there is some variability in the way CPM's practice in each state. CPM's practice independently. They offer prenatal care, home deliveries and postpartum care. CPM's typically do not take insurance, nor carry malpractice insurance.

◆ *Certified midwives* (CM) have no requirement for previous nursing training or experience. They do have formal midwifery train-

BEHIND THE SCENES: WHO IS ACOG ANYWAY?

ACOG stands for the American Congress of Obstetricians and Gynecologists, a non-profit organization that represents over 50,000 obstetricians (doctors who treat pregnant women) and gynecologists (doctors who treat women's health issues). ACOG makes recommendations for the highest standards of medical care for women, including during pregnancy.

To become a member or "fellow" of ACOG, doctors must graduate from an accredited medical school, complete a residency in obstetrics and gynecology, have an active license to practice medicine, and successfully pass the national board examination in obstetrics and gynecology. Basically, doctors who are fellows of ACOG should know their stuff. Look for the letters FACOG after a doctor's name as proof of his or her credentials.

Being a Fellow of ACOG myself, I will refer to ACOG guidelines for pregnancy throughout the book. If you are in the market to find an ACOG doctor, you can go to acog.org/member-lookup/ and find a list of doctors in your hometown.

1ST TRIMESTER

? ?

ing. Not all states certify or license CM's. *Licensed midwives* and *registered midwives* are titles used in some states for the same thing.

♦ *Traditional midwives (lay midwives)* learn their trade from other midwives or on their own. They rely mainly on the wisdom of thousands of years of midwives before them. Traditional midwives may not have a college degree or any certification. They may perform deliveries in the home or at a birthing center. Let's be clear: there's no requirement to have any formal medical training to call yourself a midwife. Over time, the number of lay midwives in this country has declined.

♦ Lastly, there are *doulas*. Doulas do not provide prenatal care or deliver babies. They are women who offer prenatal and post-partum support, education, breastfeeding counseling and "labor support." Simply put, a doula will help coach you through your labor. Doulas are great additions to the labor team, especially if a woman wants to attempt labor and delivery without pain medication.

DR H'S OPINION:
WHO SHOULD DELIVER YOUR BABY?

So, what type of practitioner should deliver your baby? This is strictly my opinion and I admit that I am biased based on the method in which I was trained. Here's my take: most deliveries should occur in a hospital with an obstetrician. My sister is a midwife and she will disagree (apologies in advance, Heather).

Why do I feel this way? I trained at Cedars-Sinai Medical Center where approximately 7,000 deliveries take place each year. After four years of work, I saw it all—the good, the bad and the ugly.

Most of the time, deliveries go great. Mom feels fine . . . baby is perfect . . . bonding occurs… everyone goes home elated.

But when something does go wrong in obstetrics, there isn't much time to act. Often times a seemingly normal, low-risk delivery has a completely unforeseen complication at the last minute that takes everyone by surprise. When this happens, it is my opinion that the safest place to be is at a hospital.

Yes, the list of possible complications is long (and we'll discuss these in more detail later in this book). But just consider one possibility: bleeding so severe after delivery (**POSTPARTUM HEMORRHAGE**) that the mother needs a blood transfusion and requires a surgical procedure in an operating room. You can't do that at home.

Again, the point is not to scare you. The truth is 95% of the time, none of the scary stuff happens. However, you should make an educated decision about who assists you during birth and where your baby is born.

DR B'S OPINION: DITTO THAT

As a pediatrician, I agree with Dr H, and also admit to being biased as a doctor who has seen it all!

While most deliveries are fairly textbook, the occasional emergency is a real emergency. Bad things can happen within the first five minutes of a baby's life that have potential life-long consequences (brain damage from lack of oxygen) . . . or can even be fatal. From a pediatrician's perspective: do you really want to deliver anywhere that is more than five minutes away from a neonatologist (a medical doctor who cares for premature and high-risk newborns) or a neonatal intensive care unit (NICU)?

I delivered both my kids at a hospital that had a NICU right down the hall from the newborn nursery. I never needed their services, but I was glad they were there. This is particularly important if you have a high-risk pregnancy (like having twins). You are more likely to need a NICU and you won't want to be at one hospital and have your baby/babies transferred to another.

Top 10 questions to ask yourself when deciding on a practitioner

1 **WHERE DO YOU WANT TO DELIVER?** Do you have a preference of delivering in a hospital, birthing center, or at home? That may influence your provider choice. For instance, if you want to deliver in a hospital, having a midwife may not be an option (it depends on the hospital's policies). If you want to have your baby at home, know that most if not all OB's carry malpractice insurance that will NOT cover home deliveries. And if you have your heart set on one particular hospital, make sure your practitioner does deliveries there. One more thing to consider: some community hospitals do not have in-house anesthesiologists, neonatologists and neonatal intensive care units (NICUs). Larger city hospitals and academic institutions routinely have these features available 24/7. Find out what your prospective delivery site offers.

2 **WHO DID YOUR FRIENDS USE?** If all roads point to the same practitioner in your circle of friends, you will probably like this person too. However, if you are the first among your friends to have a baby, call the hospital where you plan to deliver and ask to speak to a friendly labor and delivery nurse. L & D nurses know better than almost anyone which practitioners are competent and nice (even at 3am).

3 **ARE YOU A HIGH-RISK PREGNANCY?** Take a look at the high-risk pregnancy box earlier in this chapter. If the answer is yes, you need an obstetrician and you should deliver at a hospital.

Of course, it's possible to start out as a routine, low-risk pregnancy and become high-risk if you develop a condition along the way (see Chapter 16, Complications). If you want to deliver with a midwife or your family practitioner, you'll need to have a backup plan for an obstetrician and a delivery hospital if this happens.

4 **WHAT TYPE OF OBSTETRIC PRACTICE ARE YOU LOOKING FOR?** Obstetric practices come in several flavors. There are solo practitioners, small group practices, and large group practices.

Some doctors do their own patients' deliveries on weekdays, and let the on-call OB handle deliveries on weekends. Others have a delivery-doc-of-the-day, everyday. And a few doctors, like me, deliver (almost) all their own babies.

Spoiler Alert for the movie *Knocked Up*: even if your doctor does all her own deliveries, she may still take an occasional vacation or attend a Bar Mitzvah in San Francisco when you go into labor.

In any obstetric practice, it's possible to have one doctor do all your prenatal care visits and end up with the Doc-du-jour doing your delivery. Yes, you may be meeting that person for the first time when you are in labor. When you are in the midst of pushing, you probably won't care who the heck is there, as long as that person gets you and your baby through it!

Some practices utilize nurse practitioners to keep your appointment from being cancelled when your doc gets called to a delivery ten minutes before your appointment time. These same nurse practitioners sometimes handle postpartum care (hospital visits after birth). This might be fine . . . or you may prefer a practice where only your doc sees you for all your appointments, knowing that there is a good chance you will have at least one or two appointments rescheduled because someone else's baby is coming.

BOTTOM LINE: Find out with whom your doctor shares on-call responsibilities so you know who may be there for your delivery. Ask to be introduced to the other doc(s).

5 **HOW AM I GOING TO PAY FOR THIS?** Some practitioners accept health insurance; others don't. Even if you have health insurance, you may have to pay a deductible or a portion of the costs for your prenatal visits and delivery. So be sure to check your insurance benefits carefully. When people say having a baby is expensive, they aren't just talking about the cost of diapers!

All-cash practices (that is, those docs who don't accept insurance) may offer longer office visits and other added services (such as a pledge by your doc to be there at delivery, barring a natural disaster).

6 **DO YOU PREFER A MALE OR FEMALE PRACTITIONER?** If you have a major preference here, remember to find out with whom your prospective practitioner shares on-call responsibilities. You may or may not be able to control the gender of the practitioner who does your delivery.

7 **IF YOU CHOOSE A PHYSICIAN, IS HE/SHE BOARD-CERTIFIED? IF YOU CHOOSE A MIDWIFE, IS SHE CERTIFIED?** While there are no absolute guarantees in life, having a practitioner who is certified should mean she has a certain level of competency and knows her stuff.

8 **HOW MUCH EXPERIENCE DOES THE PRACTITIONER HAVE?** Has this practitioner done ten deliveries or 1000? Being the delivery attendant during medical training counts in these numbers. So even if your obstetrician has entered private practice recently, she's probably logged in at least a couple hundred deliveries during her training. Obstetricians definitely have more hands-on experience (particularly in high risk pregnancies and deliveries) than family practitioners just by the nature of the medical training they receive.

9 **DOES THE PRACTITIONER HAVE CHILDREN?** This is certainly not a requirement, but it helps! One doesn't need to have undergone quadruple-bypass surgery to be a great cardiac surgeon. But I can tell you that I learned an enormous amount from going through two pregnancies myself.

This doesn't just pertain to female practitioners. My husband is also an OB/GYN (you can only imagine our dinner table conversations—on second thought, don't) and he has told me that he absolutely approaches his pregnant patients differently, with more empathy and with more helpful advice since we've had children.

Being pregnant or living with a pregnant person is on-the-job training. There is so much that isn't taught in school or in textbooks. Bottom line: going through a pregnancy changes your perspective!

10 **DO YOU FEEL COMFORTABLE WITH THE PRACTITIONER?** By far, this is the most important question. After your first appointment, ask yourself—is this practitioner a good fit?

Having a child is one of the most amazing experiences you will ever have. You want someone you trust and who will take good care of you.

Q. When I interview prospective practitioners, what questions should I ask?

You and your selected practitioner need to have the same vision for your birth experience. This is an opportunity to see if this is a good fit.

We'll put it all together in 40 questions to consider asking:

For doctors

1. Will I see you for all my prenatal visits?
2. Do you have nurse midwives, or nurse practitioners on staff?
3. Are there other doctors in your practice?
4. Are there other doctors outside your practice with whom you share on-call responsibilities?
5. What gender are the doctors in your on-call group? (If this is important to you.)
6. If you may not be delivering me, will I have a chance to meet all of the doctors in your practice or on-call group?
7. Where will I deliver?
8. If you perform deliveries in a hospital, is it a teaching hospital or academic center?
9. Will there be residents and medical students present and participating in my labor or delivery?
10. How long have you been in practice?
11. How many deliveries have you done?

12. How do I reach you in case of an emergency?
13. What are your recommendations on pregnancy nutrition, vitamins, and how much weight I should gain?
14. When do you recommend I stop traveling?
15. I work as a _____ (fill in the blank). Are there any risks for my pregnancy due to my occupation?
16. I smoke, drink alcohol, or _____. (Be honest here!) What risks do I face? Do you have any suggestions to help me stop?
17. I take _____ medications regularly. Are these safe to take during pregnancy?
18. I have _____ disease/disorder. Are my symptoms going to worsen during my pregnancy? Will it affect my pregnancy?
19. I had _____ with a previous pregnancy. Is this something I need to worry about with this pregnancy?
20. I have a family medical history of _____. Do I need to have any special tests done during my pregnancy?
21. My spouse/spouse's family has _____ medical problem. Do I need to have any special tests done during my pregnancy?
22. How do you feel about inducing my labor?
23. How do you feel about doing an "elective" or scheduled **CESAREAN SECTION** (surgical procedure to remove baby) without a medical reason for it (if this interests you)?
24. How do you feel about using an **EPIDURAL** (pain medication that numbs the lower part of the body)?
25. Do you work with doulas? Do you have any you recommend?
26. Do you work with acupuncturists? Chiropractors?
27. Do you accept my health insurance plan?
28. If you don't accept my health insurance plan, how much is your fee? Will you help me get reimbursed by my insurance plan?
29. What are the general costs for a vaginal delivery and for a Cesarean section?
30. Are there any other costs for prenatal care, labor, and delivery I should anticipate? (These include blood tests, cultures, imaging studies like ultrasounds, hospital charges, anesthesiologist, etc).

For midwives and home births

1. How much experience do you have?
2. What was your training like?
3. Are you licensed or certified?
4. Do you work with other midwives?
5. Do you cover for one another?
6. Will you have someone with you at the time of my delivery or will you be alone?
7. Which prenatal tests do you perform or recommend for your patients?
8. What happens if there is an unexpected complication/emergency during delivery?
9. Do you have an obstetrician you work with in case a problem arises with my pregnancy or delivery?
10. Where is the nearest hospital and what type of emergency transportation do you have lined up should my baby or I need immediate medical attention?

What's Going on Down There?! The First Trimester

For each trimester, we'll give you the 411 on your growing baby. There are some pretty amazing things going on inside your body right now—let's take a look.

1 week. *The egg.*
The 40 week countdown for **GESTATIONAL AGE** has already started, even though the egg and sperm haven't met yet.

2 weeks. *The egg and sperm meet (fertilization).*
Fertilization occurs in the fallopian tube. The fertilized egg begins rapidly dividing, making new cells while it travels toward the uterus.

3 weeks. *Implantation.*
The ball of rapidly dividing cells (your future baby) is called a morula at this stage. Later, it's called the embryo...then the fetus...then Bob or Suzy. The cellular ball attaches to the lining of the uterus and gets cozy. Three membranes start to form to protect and feed the embryo (technical terms: yolk sac, amnion, chorion). Specialized cells invade the wall of your uterus to begin forming the placenta.

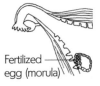

Fertilized egg (morula)

4 weeks. *The embryo.*
You can call the ball of cells an embryo now. The embryo already has the crude beginnings of a brain, spinal cord, and nerves (called the **NEURAL TUBE**).

Neural tube

5 weeks. *The embryo.*
The embryo has a top end (cranial neuropore) and a bottom end (caudal neuropore). The heart, eyes, ears, and budding arms begin to develop.

Neuropore

6 weeks. *The embryo.*
The face, arms (including elbows and fingers), and legs start to develop. The crudely formed heart beats (it doesn't have four chambers yet nor a circulatory system to transport blood).

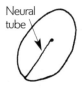

Head

Tail

7 weeks. *The embryo.*
Your embryo (baby) now has the beginnings of a nose, mouth, throat, intestines, pancreas, liver, bladder, fingers, and toes. Your embryo also has a little tail (don't worry, that will go away). And his intestines bulge into the umbilical cord.

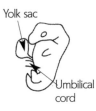

Yolk sac

Umbilical cord

8 weeks. *The embryo.*
The girl or boy parts finally start to grow, even though the sex of the embryo was determined way back at fertilization. The heart has four chambers now. The throat forms. The teeth begin forming, although you won't see them for several months after birth.

9 weeks. *The embryo.*
All body organs and systems are present. At this point, they develop more and begin functioning. The inner ear develops. Your baby has a nose with nostrils, and an anus that is open. He has fingers, but his toes are still webbed.

10 weeks. *The fetus.*
Your baby is now a fetus. You can hear his heart beating by Doppler. His tail is gone, and his taste buds are forming.

Critical periods in your baby's development

Weeks of pregnancy		Embryo			
3	4	5	6	7	8
	Nervous System:	Neural tube defects, intellectual disability			
	Heart:		Structural heart defects		
	Upper Limb:		Whole or partially missing limb		Less sensitive pe
	Lower Limb:		Whole or partially missing limb		Less sensitive pe
	Upper Lip:			Cleft lip	
	Ears:			Low set ears, malformed, deafness	
	Eyes:			undeveloped, cataracts, glaucoma	
	Teeth:				
	Roof of Mouth:				
	External Genitals:				
All or nothing*		Major birth defects			

Either the damage is so great that the embryo dies or it has little effect and baby develops without defects.

12 weeks.
Your baby's mouth is forming. He has vocal cords (although you won't hear what he has to say for a while). Some body organs, like the liver, gallbladder, and pancreas are working. Arms and legs bend at the elbows and the knees.

1st trimester

Q. What's the difference between an embryo and a fetus?

An **EMBRYO** is your baby for the first eight weeks after fertilization. Lots of cells divide and organize into future body organs and systems . . . and believe it or not, most of this organization is complete after just eight short weeks.

After ten weeks gestation, your baby is now called a **FETUS** (pronounced FEE-tus). In many ways, the die has already been cast. The brain and nervous system, however, are still sensitive to injury throughout pregnancy.

The main job of the fetus is to grow and mature. The fetus will have the most growth in length from three to five months. And he will gain the most

	9	10	Fetus 11	18	34	40
					Less sensitive period	
	Less sensitive period					
	...riod					
	...riod					
	Less sensitive period					
			Less sensitive period			
		Less sensitive period				
	Underdeveloped enamel, staining		Less sensitive period			
	Cleft palate		Less sensitive period			
	Female parts become masculinized		Less sensitive period			
			Minor defects or function defects			

weight at eight to nine months. His head will be half of his body size at eight weeks. At birth, it will be about 1/4 of his entire body size.

Reality check

Unfortunately, you may not even realize that you are pregnant while your baby is in this critical window. So, naturally, you might start to freak out here.

Here's our message: relax. Odds are your baby will still be born with ten fingers and ten toes . . . even if you had a martini last week or an x-ray at the dentist.

There's something called the "all or nothing effect" when it comes to potential **TERATOGENS** (something that has a negative effect during embryo/fetal development) early in the first trimester. That is, pregnancies where embryos have a significant amount of damage often end up miscarrying rather than going to term and resulting in a newborn with a major abnormality.

Of course, if you actually find out you're pregnant around four to five weeks, it's time to make some healthy lifestyle changes.

Your baby is most susceptible to exposures that can lead to improper development or malformations (birth defects) during weeks five to ten of gestation—that's the critical period of development. By exposures, we are talking about infections, medications, drug use, vitamin/nutritional deficiencies, environmental toxins, x-rays/radiation, etc.

Q. How does the baby get nutrition while he/she is growing in the womb?

The **PLACENTA** is the middleman between mom and baby. It grows from cells that are originally part of the embryo. The placenta becomes a full-fledged body organ (as you will see at delivery, if you dare!). A blood vessel network is formed between the placenta and the uterus.

The **UMBILICAL CORD** is the tissue that connects the placenta to the baby with three blood vessels. One blood vessel (the umbilical vein) sends in the food, oxygen, and your antibodies (cells that help fight infection) to the baby. Two blood vessels (the umbilical

Umbilical Cord

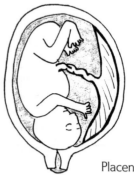

Placenta

arteries) send the baby's waste products (including carbon dioxide) back to the placenta. The placenta processes the waste and dumps it back into mom's blood stream for removal.

This elaborate system allows mom's body to feed and supply oxygen to the baby and allows baby to eliminate waste, usually without a direct mingling of mother and baby's blood. There are certain situations where direct mingling occurs, and that's covered in Chapter 16, Complications. The placenta also makes hormones that nurture pregnancy and initiate labor and delivery.

When your baby is born, he stays attached to the placenta by the umbilical cord. Someone (your healthcare provider or maybe your support person) will cut the cord after placing two clamps on it so the baby will not lose any blood from the blood vessels that remain temporarily intact. And FYI, after you deliver your baby, you will then have to "deliver" the placenta about three to 15 minutes later. While it's not nearly as large as the baby (it's about a pound or so), it does have to come out too.

Reality check

The good news is that your antibodies travel through the placenta and protect your baby. The bad news is that the placenta is not perfect and some infections, as well as certain drugs and medications, use that same transit system. Most infections (like the common cold) have no significant health effect on your baby. The ones that can cause problems for your baby are discussed in Chapter 17, Infections. There are also certain medications that can cross the placenta—these should be avoided. See Medications at Expecting411.com/extra for details.

Factoid: The umbilical cord is about 50 centimeters long (just under two feet).

Q. Does the fetus actually breathe?

This is a trick question. Yes, your fetus practices breathing while in the womb. But, no, she won't breathe in air and get oxygen the way you do.

Your fetus gets her oxygen from your blood when she is hanging out in your uterus. You breathe oxygen into your lungs and that oxygen enters your bloodstream. Your red blood cells carry it through the arteries of your body to all of your organs.

If you are pregnant, the oxygen-rich red blood cells also travel to your placenta. It's here (through an amazing system) that oxygen leaves your red blood cells, attaches to fetal red blood cells, then travels through the umbilical vein to your fetus.

AMNIOTIC FLUID 411:
YOUR BABY'S PRIVATE SWIMMING POOL

Your unborn baby is swimming around in a watery substance called amniotic fluid. After about ten weeks, it is composed of a liquid containing proteins and other vital minerals and nutrients.

Early on, the placenta makes amniotic fluid—although some of it comes from fetal urine (more on that later). By the end of pregnancy, most of the amniotic fluid is composed of fetal urine.

The amniotic fluid levels are maintained by mom's fluid intake and by the fetus' intact digestive tract (esophagus/stomach/intestines/anus) and urinary system (kidneys/ureter/bladder/urethra). The fetus drinks the amniotic fluid and it then goes through its digestive tract, helping the fetus to form **MECONIUM** (the baby's first poop).

The fetus makes urine in his kidneys the same way that we do and after it's eliminated via the bladder and urethra, it adds to the pool of amniotic fluid. The fetus also "breathes" amniotic fluid in and out of his lungs. In fact, this is essential for normal lung development.

You may catch your fetus breathing on an ultrasound—where her chest wall moves in and out. She's actually taking amniotic fluid into her lungs, not air. This is very reassuring to see on ultrasound. In fact, it is one of the things we look for if we are concerned about the well-being of a baby. "Practice breathing" is one part of fetal life that tells us your baby is healthy.

When your baby takes her first breath at birth, she'll begin to get rid of all of that fluid from her lungs. She will also cough and sneeze to help get it out too, and that's kind of cute to watch! That first breath also triggers a major change in blood flow (circulation) to the lungs to let your baby breathe in air and exchange oxygen for carbon dioxide.

Q. Does the fetus eat, sleep, pee or poop?

Yes, yes, yes, and hopefully, no.

Yes, your fetus eats, but not through his mouth. There's an all-you-can-eat buffet available 24/7 (like a cruise, minus the food poisoning) through mom's bloodstream. Everything that you take into your body is processed, absorbed into your bloodstream, filtered by the placenta and taken via the umbilical vein straight to baby. This continues up until birth when the umbilical cord is cut. That's the first time your baby will actually have to exert some energy and work to eat—breast milk or formula.

Yes, your fetus sleeps. In fact, some researchers think fetuses may start dreaming as early as 24 weeks gestation, because they begin to have rapid eye movements around this time *(Birnholz JC)*. Fetuses have sleep cycles that can last up to 90 minutes, but unfortunately, they don't always correspond to your sleep patterns. So, you might have a sleeping fetus at 2pm and an active one at 2am!

Yes, your fetus urinates. That urine dumps right into the amniotic sac and helps make up some of the **AMNIOTIC FLUID**. The fetus also drinks almost 1/2 quart a day of amniotic fluid. It's kind of gross to think about drinking recycled urine, but it's clean stuff. What we mean by "clean" is that there are no waste products (remember, you and your placenta filter out all the waste) and no bacteria. That same sterile fluid goes in and out of the lungs.

While your fetus does have the ability to poop while inside the womb, he usually doesn't—and no one wants him to! See information in Chapter 16, Complications.

Whew! That was a lot of information to digest. But hopefully you got a nice overview of the the first trimester. And you can feel better having some knowledge before your first prenatal visit.

Next up: The second trimester.

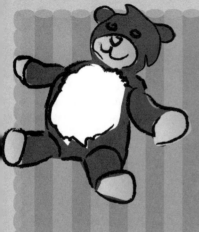

THE SECOND TRIMESTER

Chapter 2

"Women who miscalculate are called mothers."
—*Abigail Van Buren*

Welcome to your second trimester (14 to 27 weeks)! You're probably feeling a bit more confident and used to being pregnant at this point. But we know you still have a ton of questions. What's going on with your body? When will you start to show (if you haven't already)? How much weight will you gain? So, here we go.

You: The 2nd trimester

14-15 weeks

Ahh. This is the beginning of the trimester where you will feel your best. Morning sickness should end and you will feel more energetic than you have for the past several weeks. If you had a healthy body mass index (BMI) before pregnancy, you should gain about one pound a week from here on out—sometimes a little more, sometimes less. See Chapter 6, Nutrition for the scoop on that and our web site Expecting 411.com for a Body Mass Index (BMI) chart.

Enjoy being intimate with your partner while it is still fun. See Chapter 8, Lifestyles, for some take home tips. Many women develop vaginal infections during pregnancy, so if you have itching or burning down there, check out Chapter 17, Infections, for some troubleshooting on yeast infections and other causes of

? ?

unpleasant vaginal discharge.

You will be offered the option of specialized testing (Second Trimester Screen, Amniocentesis) to screen for and/or diagnose chromosome abnormalities. These tests are done between 15 and 20 weeks. For details, see Chapter 5, Tests.

16-17 weeks

"Are you going to finish that?" You never thought liver and onions would look appealing and now you want seconds. Your appetite will really pick up and strange cravings may begin. Visit Chapter 6, Nutrition to get a handle on what it means to have a healthy pregnancy diet now that you feel like eating again.

While we are on the subject of mealtime, you also may get some heartburn (and that's not just if you overindulge on Taco Bell). See Chapter 4, Is This Normal? for details.

18-20 weeks

Let the aches and pains begin. Some women start to have back pain, side pain, groin pain, and leg cramps. Not to mention shooting pain around the belly button. Fun, no? See Chapter 4, Is This Normal? to figure out if you are just pregnant, or if your symptoms need to be checked out further.

With your expanding belly, your center of gravity starts to change. You will suddenly feel clumsy. Be careful to support yourself and wear comfortable shoes (no more heels, ladies) to avoid falls.

Between 18 and 22 weeks, you will start to feel your baby kicking. Women who have been pregnant before often feel it by 15 to 16 weeks. At first, it might feel like gas. But it will become clear as time goes on that you've got an active baby on your hands.

Your practitioner will begin measuring your baby bump at each visit with a tape measure (**FUNDAL HEIGHT**). Somewhere between now and 22 weeks, you'll likely have a detailed ultrasound to thoroughly assess all of the baby's body parts.

21-23 weeks

Some women experience mild pelvic cramping (like period cramps) in the second trimester. Sometimes it's just the uterine muscle cramping due to the baby's growth. Or, it's early practice contractions (**BRAXTON HICKS CONTRACTIONS**). Rarely, it is a sign of preterm labor. The cramps usually go away with some rest and drinking lots of fluids. But you should always let your practitioner decide—pick up the phone. See Chapter 4, Is This Normal? and Chapter 15, Pregnancy 911 for details.

The same rule goes for any time you have spotting or vaginal bleeding during your pregnancy.

Talk to your practitioner about sleeping on your back and the proper use of seat belts.

24-25 weeks

If you deliver today, your baby has good odds of surviving. But we do want you to keep that bun in the oven a little while longer.

??

Between now and 28 weeks, you'll take a test to screen for gestational diabetes (see Chapter 5, Tests).

If this is not your first pregnancy, you might start feeling practice contractions (**BRAXTON HICKS CONTRACTIONS**) now. See Chapter 4, Is This Normal? and Chapter 15, Pregnancy 911. If there is any concern that you might be having signs of preterm labor, call your practitioner.

Between 24 to 26 weeks, you should feel your baby moving around regularly. That's when it's a good idea to check **FETAL KICK COUNTS** every day. The official recommendation says you should relax for an hour and feel TEN movements. A more realistic goal: you should feel movement within every 12-hour period. If you don't sense any movement, lie down on your left side, hydrate, have a sugary snack and see what happens over the next hour. If there is little or no movement, call your practitioner right away. Check out Chapter 5, Tests, for a complete discussion.

26-27 weeks

You might start having some odd complaints. Here are a few of them: feelings of pins and needles (or numbness) in the legs/feet/hands, a constantly stuffy nose, or frequent nosebleeds and bleeding gums. Yep, we warned you these are weird. Check out Chapter 4, Is This Normal? to see if you are, indeed, normal.

You have very good odds of having a viable baby if he is born right now. If you go into preterm labor (or deliver a premature baby), you will want to read Chapter 19, Preterm Labor for your special concerns.

A few women start to develop high blood pressure as they enter their 3rd trimester. Just as she has been doing the whole time, your practitioner will check your blood pressure at every visit for this reason. If you do encounter this problem, check out Chapter 16, Complications (see complications #20 and 21).

Remember to do daily fetal kick counts, or at least be aware of your baby's movements every 12 hours.

Aches, pains and changes the **SECOND TRIMESTER (14-27 WEEKS)**
Common symptoms:

◆ Stuffy nose	◆ Nosebleeds
◆ Hemorrhoids	◆ Heartburn
◆ Swollen/bleeding gums	◆ Itching in outer genital area
◆ Darker nipples	

◆ Feet swelling, if you are on your feet all day
◆ Belly pain, hip pain, groin pain, back pain, wrist pain, leg cramps
◆ Itching, chafing, skin tags, red palms and soles, stretch marks

 ### Old Wives Tale
Rubbing a pregnant woman's belly gives you good luck.
False. It may work for Buddha, but we can't promise the same fortune after rubbing a pregnant woman's belly. This won't stop people, though. Folks from all walks of life will stroll up to you and—often without permission—reach a hand out to stroke your tummy.

Be prepared with a courteous way to say, "Hands off."

Common Questions About the Second Trimester

Q. When am I going to start showing? Right now I just look and feel fat!

This depends on if this is your first pregnancy, if you are carrying one baby or multiples, and your pre-pregnancy body stature. A tall woman carrying one baby with her first pregnancy may not have a baby bump until 20 weeks. A short woman, carrying twins with a second pregnancy, may show as early as ten weeks and will be cursing her less vertically challenged friends. *On average, women start showing between 13 and 20 weeks.*

Unfortunately, for women of all shapes and sizes, you will look chunky—not pregnant—before that cute little baby bump appears. You will have to endure that chunky look (and feeling) through the first trimester and part of the second trimester. Buy a t-shirt that says, "Yes. I am pregnant!" if it makes you feel better.

If this is your first pregnancy, you may not fit into maternity clothes until your second trimester. That's when it will be obvious you have a baby on board. If it's not your first rodeo, pull out those maternity clothes earlier!

Q. How much weight am I supposed to gain this trimester?

Read Chapter 6, Nutrition for all the details. It depends on what you weighed (your body mass index or BMI) before you were pregnant. But do not get obsessed about it as these are general guidelines.

Women at a healthy BMI before pregnancy should gain about one pound per week.

Women who are underweight to begin with should probably gain a little more than the standard goal (about one to two pounds per week). Women who are carrying twins or multiples will also gain more.

Women who were overweight or obese before pregnancy should gain less than one pound per week.

Partner Tip

Both members of the expectant couple often gain weight during pregnancy. If you want to avoid the equivalent of the proverbial "Freshman 10" for pregnancy, watch what you eat. You are NOT eating for two!

Q. I am definitely having food cravings! Is this normal? Why does this happen?

Yes, this is very normal. And the basis for all those pickles and ice cream pregnancy jokes.

But why do you crave the strangest foods? Your pregnant body needs more calories and you will feel much more hungry than before.

And sometimes, you will find yourself needing to eat the strangest things. . .and we mean NEEDING. Some women go for weeks at a time just wanting to eat citrus fruits (it was tangerines in Dr. H's case). Others only want pasta. Some can't get enough burgers or fast food (Taco Bell is

? ?

2ND TRIMESTER

a particular favorite among pregnant women for some reason).

Occasionally, your body will need certain vitamins or nutrients. As an example, it is not uncommon for vegetarians to start craving meat because the body says it needs more iron. Although docs don't know exactly what causes some of the stranger cravings, you can probably blame elevated hormone levels circulating in your body.

The take-home message: aim for a well-balanced diet, plus a craving indulgence here or there.

Reality Check

If you begin craving and chewing ice, it may be a sign of iron-deficiency anemia. Let your practitioner know so she can decide whether or not you need a blood test. FYI, as strange as it sounds, sometimes an anemic patient will even begin eating detergent, clay, soil, chalk, paper, salt or soap.

Q. I've heard it's unhealthy for me to sleep on my back. Is this true?

After 20 weeks, avoid lying on your back all night. This prevents your big ol' pregnant uterus from putting pressure on your major blood vessels (the aorta and vena cava). It's best to lie on your left side for optimal blood circulation but the right side is okay as well.

If you wake up and realize you have ended up sleeping on your back, don't panic! Just roll over, get comfy, and go back to sleep.

Q. When will I feel my baby kicking?

If this is your first pregnancy, you should feel the baby moving (called **QUICKENING**), between 18 and 22 weeks. If you've done this pregnancy thing a time or two already, you may feel quickening as early as 15 to 16 weeks.

The first time you feel this sensation, you may think it's gas. It may feel like little bubbles, little thumps, or perhaps a flick against your belly. But you won't be able to see action happening on the outside of your belly—yet. That type of movement, which will begin to look like something out of the movie *Aliens*, won't happen until you are about 28 weeks.

If you were overweight pre-pregnancy or if your placenta lies closer to your belly and in front of the baby (anterior placenta), rather than under the baby (posterior placenta), it may take a few more weeks before you feel this sensation.

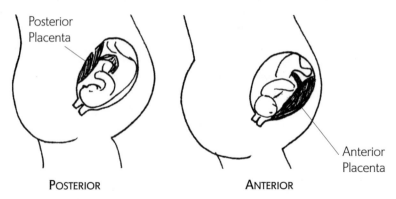

Posterior
Placenta

Anterior
Placenta

POSTERIOR   **ANTERIOR**

Q. When is it possible to determine the sex of the baby?

It depends on what testing you have done. If you want to know your baby's gender (and you are lucky), your doc can sometimes identify the girl or boy parts as early as 12 weeks on an ultrasound. A later ultrasound done between 16 to 17 weeks has better odds of showing the family jewels.

Don't get your hopes up, though. The fetus has to be willing to show off. If you have a more modest fetus, who sits with his/her legs crossed, you may not be able to see anything. (That was the case with both of Dr H's kids. Dr B wanted to be surprised.)

If you have **CHORIONIC VILLUS SAMPLING** (see Chapter 5, Tests) between ten to 13 weeks, you can find out without question whether your baby has XX (girl) or XY (boy) chromosomes. **AMNIOCENTESIS** (see Chapter 5, Tests) at 15 to 20 weeks, can determine gender by the chromosomes as well.

Today, many parents-to-be want to find out the baby's gender in advance. Dr H rarely gets to say "It's a boy" or "It's a girl" at the delivery anymore, as did OBs of yesteryear. That said, there are no rules here on whether you should know or not. It's helpful if you want to know which color to paint the nursery or if you need to make a circumcision decision. However, this is a personal decision that you need to make as a couple. We don't recommend having one partner know, while the other partner's in the dark. The secret is bound to slip out!

Speaking of which, if you *don't* want to know the sex of your baby, tell your practitioner to write in BIG BOLD LETTERS across the top of the chart, "Patient does not want to know sex of baby!" And, feel free to remind anyone remotely involved with ultrasounds, looking in your chart or providing you with lab results.

Old Wives Tale
You can tell whether you are having a boy or girl depending on how fast their hearts beat.

False. The heart rate of a fetus is usually between 120 to 160 beats per minute. Just like us, that rate increases with activity. So, a faster heart rate might mean you have an active baby on your hands—but it doesn't tell you the *gender* of your baby.

Old Wives Tale
You can tell if you are having a boy or girl based on how you are carrying.

False. The way you "carry" (the shape and distribution of your baby bump) during your pregnancy is based on a few things, but the baby's gender isn't one of them.

A woman with a deep pelvis can hide a pregnancy longer and look like she is carrying lower. A woman who is heavier than her ideal body weight pre-pregnancy may have more fatty tissue over her belly and this can change the shape. And carrying multiples definitely alters how a woman carries.

Bottom line: People can guess about gender, but your shape won't predict whether you are having a boy or girl.

? ?

2ND TRIMESTER

Six really helpful pregnancy purchases

1 GRANNY PANTIES. When you already feel bad about how you look, it can be really demoralizing to outgrow your sexy little thong undies. You may end up biting the bullet if you find it more comfortable to wear maternity underwear. However, we've come a long way in the underwear department, baby! There are a few styles of thong underwear that are actually comfortable to wear during pregnancy. For example, Hanky Panky and Cosabella brand thongs are low enough that they sit below a blossoming belly. Some pregnancy stores even sell maternity thongs.

2 MATERNITY BELT. Meet your new best friend. As your belly grows, it can start to ache—both in the front and back.

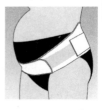

The curvature of your spine changes, and so does your center of gravity. The bigger your belly gets, the more you will feel the aching. This usually happens earlier and earlier with each subsequent pregnancy.

I am a big believer in maternity belts. You can buy them at most maternity stores. They really help lift the belly up and relieve some of the pressure and discomfort. But you have to wear them correctly to get relief. You need to try on many different styles and decide what fits best before you purchase. Don't buy one online!

Note: an extra pair of hands are invaluable when trying to put on the belt. You will need to lift your belly up and the extra pair of hands you are borrowing for the day (your partner, friend, neighbor or completely uninterested 3rd grader) can adjust the Velcro on the belt.

It can be a real quality-of-life-saver for pregnant women who have belly, back, and leg pains.

3 NURSING PADS. Although you won't be breastfeeding until after delivery, your breasts may start to make and leak fluid (**COLOSTRUM**) as early as the end of your second trimester. If you'd like to keep your breast incontinence (i.e. wet spots on your blouse) a secret from co-workers and friends, nursing pads are a wise investment. And even if you don't use them much now, you'll definitely need them after delivery.

4 SUPPORT HOSE. This is another unattractive fashion accessory for the well-dressed pregnant gal. TED (Thrombo Embolic Deterrent) hose is just one of several brands of support stockings that help reduce swelling in your feet, and improve blood flow in your legs. They come in white, beige or black knee-highs and white only thigh-highs (there's no need for a garter belt—they have tight elastic at the top). You can buy them at most pharmacies. Some women wear them only at night, others wear them all day long. You'll thank us for recommending them around the beginning of your third trimester or anytime you take a plane trip.

5 BRA EXTENDERS. Here's a cheap way to extend the life span of your existing bras. Buy a bra extender (for about $1.50; sold in stores or online at Amazon) to increase the band size (34, 36, 38 etc) until you outgrow your cup size (A, B, C, etc). Your breasts will probably enlarge at least one cup size during your pregnancy (and potentially beyond with breastfeeding). You'll still end up having to buy new bras, but this might tide you over until your size stabilizes.

6 **BELLY BAND.** When your belly is too big to button your waistband but you are not ready for maternity jeans, a belly band is a lifesaver— it covers the unbuttoned waist band of your jeans and that gap between your top and bottom. The Belly Band is a seemless knit band of fabric that runs about $17.

Prenatal Care

You will visit your practitioner every four weeks in the second trimester. If you have an uncomplicated pregnancy, typically you'll have a total of four visits. Although it varies a bit, plan on appointments around 14 to 15 weeks, 18 to 19 weeks, 22 to 23 weeks, and 26 to 27 weeks of pregnancy.

Q. What happens at my prenatal appointments during this trimester?

These visits are pretty routine if all is going well. You will get weighed (you don't have to look) and you will need to pee in a little cup (you do have to look) at every visit. You'll also get your blood pressure measured at every visit. Some women have high blood pressure before pregnancy. Others may develop it during pregnancy. So doing this simple test makes sure any elevation is detected.

Next, your practitioner will visit with you, feel your belly, listen for the baby's heartbeat, and, if you are beyond 20 weeks, measure the baby's size by measuring the **FUNDAL HEIGHT** (see box below). Then you can ask questions and discuss aches, pains, and other fun body changes you are experiencing.

Q. Are there any routine tests done in the second trimester?

Yes. There are two important tests:

♦ *The One hour Glucola test.* This involves drinking a sugary liq-uid and then getting your blood drawn to assess for pregnancy-related diabetes (GESTATIONAL DIABETES). This test occurs between 24 to 28 weeks.

♦ *Fetal Kick Counts.* Your practitioner will instruct you to tune in to your baby's movements on a daily basis, starting at 24 to 26 weeks. This is a critical indicator that your baby is thriving, and it's kind of fun.

We will discuss both of these tests in detail in Chapter 5, Tests.

Q. Are there any additional tests that I need to ask my practitioner about?

Yes, and you should learn more about these tests in Chapter 5, Tests.

FUNDAL HEIGHT 411

Fundal height is the measurement from the pubic bone to the top of the uterus (called the uterine fundus).

Your practitioner will get out a little tape measure and push on the top of your belly to determine the fundal height. It is a very old, but useful technique to estimate the size of both the baby (fetus) and the other contents of the uterus (placenta, amniotic fluid). Fundal height is measured in centimeters (cm), starting at about 20 weeks, which is when the top of the uterus is at the level of your belly button. At each visit, the number measured in centimeters should be roughly equal to your pregnancy in weeks. For example, if you are 32 weeks along, your fundal height should be roughly 30 to 34 cm.

There are always exceptions to the rule, but in general, it is a quick and easy way to assess the growth of a fetus and uterus. For instance, if you have been on target with all of your measurements and suddenly measure three weeks smaller in cm than would be appropriate for your dates, an ultrasound would be warranted to make sure your baby is growing well and that there is an appropriate amount of amniotic fluid.

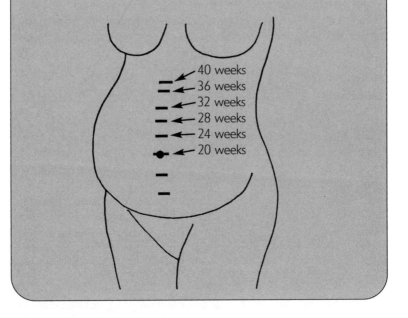

◆ **Second Trimester Screen** (also known as AFP, Expanded AFP, QUAD screen, Full Integrated screen). This blood test assesses the chances of a fetus having Down syndrome, Trisomy 18, and a few serious abnormalities. Testing occurs between 15 and 20 weeks.

◆ **Ultrasound.** While it isn't routine, it is very common to perform a comprehensive ultrasound between 20 to 22 weeks to examine all the body parts of the fetus.

◆ **Amniocentesis.** By a minor procedure, a doctor obtains amniotic fluid that can diagnose chromosome defects and some medical conditions in the fetus. Testing occurs between 15 and 20 weeks.

Q. Are there any more ultrasounds?

Many (but not all) practitioners will perform an ultrasound at 20 and 22 weeks.

There are also special situations that require ultrasounds at every visit. For example, women who have had preterm labor with a previous pregnancy may need regular ultrasounds to assess the length of their cervix. This may also apply to women who have had procedures on their cervix (LEEP, conization) or who have a history of **CERVICAL INSUFFICIENCY** (incompetence). We'll pontificate about issues of the cervix later in this book (see Complication #34 in Chapter 16, Complications).

Q. Which visits are the most important for my partner to attend?

We personally vote for the 20 to 22 week ultrasound. If you did not have a first trimester ultrasound, this is a great time to catch your baby looking like a baby for the first time on screen. But beware, from some angles, your baby will look. . . well, extraterrestrial (you'll know what we mean when you see the ultrasound pics).

But seriously, this ultrasound evaluates every little part and organ of your baby from the brain to the toes. It's amazing to see your baby moving around on the screen. In fact, it's priceless.

Decisions

This section covers the classes we recommend taking before going into labor. The only decision you need to make is when you and your partner can both attend!

◆ *Childbirth classes.* If this is your first baby, take these classes. Note: there are different ways to approach labor and the childbirth process. Do your homework by reading Chapter 12, Home Stretch to see which type of class is right for you. It's best to take these classes between 28 to 34 weeks of pregnancy. Sign up now so you can graduate from childbirth class before you go into labor! You have a couple of options here.

1. Community hospitals usually offer small group sessions that meet several times over a period of weeks or one mega-weekend/couples retreat. If you and your partner have busy schedules, it can be a challenge to coordinate. That leads to Option #2.

2. Hire a childbirth educator to come to your home for a private class.

◆ *Breastfeeding class.* This class helps to prepare for breastfeeding before baby arrives. Now you have time to take a class, scope out breast pumps and identify a lactation consultant. Your OB and/or pediatrician can provide recommendations, if need be.

While your body may be naturally prepared for breastfeeding, your brain is not. Think of a breastfeeding class like driver's ed. You won't get to use your skills until you get behind the wheel for the first time!

The best time to take a breastfeeding class is 32 to 38 weeks. And yes, the class is for BOTH partners. The non-breastfeeding partner will learn how to aid the breastfeeding partner and baby.

◆ ***Infant CPR class.*** All new parents should take an infant CPR class. Of course, it's easiest to carve out time to take it before your baby is born. You'll thank us for telling you to do this when your baby crawls over to the dog food bowl, digs in, and chokes on a morsel. Yes, this happened to Dr B with her first baby!

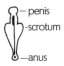

Partner tip

We suggest you read this next section so you can impress your baby-carrying mate when you accompany her to the ultrasound appointments. Trust us, you will prove how much you are into this pregnancy thing if you throw out some technical jargon here and there!

What's Going on Down There?! The Second Trimester

Girl parts

Boy parts

14 weeks.

Big news! Your baby's genitals have declared themselves. If you have a boy, you might catch a glimpse of his penis and scrotum on ultrasound. Don't be disappointed if your practitioner can't tell you what you are having yet, though, as it's often tough to see until about 16 weeks. The testes sit inside the abdomen for several more weeks, and then migrate down to the scrotum as your fetus nears the end of his development. For girls, the clitoris and labia form on the outside and the ovaries mature inside the abdomen.

16 weeks.

The fetus can suck his thumb, swallow, "breathe,"and pee. His lungs practice inhaling and exhaling, even though amniotic fluid (not air) is going in and out. The circulatory system (that transports blood throughout the body) functions now. And your baby's kidneys start making urine.

20 weeks.

A cheesy covering (**VERNIX**) appears, protecting the skin from the watery environment of the amniotic fluid. Your baby has head and body hair, including eyebrows. He is making brown fat, which he will use for heat production as a newborn. His bones are hardening.

24 weeks.

Viability. It's possible that your baby could survive life outside the womb if he delivers prematurely. The fetus can use his ears to hear, and his legs to kick (you'll feel that "quickening" occasionally!). He now has rapid eye movements, and blinks/startles in response to noise.

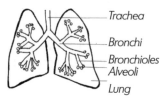

Trachea

Bronchi

Bronchioles
Alveoli

Lung

The Lungs

26 weeks.

SURFACTANT is the big news this week. Special cells in the lungs make a soapy substance called surfactant, which keeps the tiny airways open. Surfactant is critical to helping lungs do their job outside the womb. (Remember this when we discuss prematurity later on in the book.)

Q. When can a fetus survive outside the womb?

The official term is **VIABILITY**. It's based on both the **GESTATIONAL AGE** (number of weeks in pregnancy) and fetal weight. Here are the guidelines:

◆ Babies at 23 weeks gestation have a 30% survival rate.
◆ Babies at 25 weeks have a 75% survival rate.
◆ Babies whose birth weights are about one pound have an 11% survival rate.
◆ Babies who weigh between 1.5-1.75 lbs at birth have a 75% survival rate. For details, see Chapter 19, Preterm Labor.

Q. Is it true that my baby will recognize my voice when she is born?

Yes.

The ear is completely formed by 24 weeks gestation, but studies show that hearing may begin as early as 16 weeks. And a mother's voice reaches her fetus with much more strength and intensity than music, the dog barking, or even the jackhammer down the street. Your voice will even resonate above the sound of rushing blood in your blood vessels, your heart beating, and your gurgling digestive tract. It's a wonder that a fetus can sleep with this cacophony!

So, whether you are singing your unborn baby a lullaby or yelling at the car in front of you as they abruptly cut you off, your baby will hear you and recognize your voice at birth.

You've survived the second trimester! Onward to the third and last trimester.

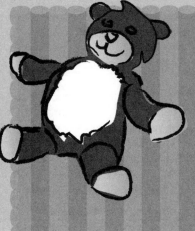

THE THIRD TRIMESTER

Chapter 3

"Children are a great comfort in your old age—and they help you reach it faster, too."
—Lionel Kauffman

This is it! Let's count down the final weeks of pregnancy.

You: The 3rd trimester

28 weeks

If you have a routine pregnancy, you will start visiting your practitioner every two weeks now until about 35 to 36 weeks, when visits become weekly.

Here is a little insight into your last trimester:

Your baby may start having hiccups, which you will feel. They can last for a few minutes or even a few hours. They might feel like little flicks or spasms against your belly. No worries.

You may start to feel short of breath as your enlarging uterus and baby push against the muscle that sits below your lungs. Swelling of the legs, feet, or fingers is common now. Your genital area may swell as well.

It's normal to retain some fluid, but check out Chapter 4, Is This Normal? to learn when a little swelling has become too much. You may also start to have low back pain, as the curvature of your spine changes. If you haven't discovered a maternity belt yet, get one now.

Some women become anemic around this time, so if you are feeling more fatigued (than usual) or begin craving or

? ?

3RD TRIMESTER

chewing ice, be sure to tell your doctor. See Chapter 16, Complications (Complication #13).

Your blood type was tested at your first prenatal visit. If your blood type is Rh negative, you will need an injection of the medication Rhogam at 28 weeks to prevent your body from mounting a potential immune response against any future babies. See Chapter 16, Complications, (Complication #14). You'll get another shot after delivery if your baby is Rh positive.

Start interviewing potential pediatricians. Take childbirth classes within the next six weeks. Consider taking a breastfeeding class and infant CPR class as well. While you probably have another ten to 12 weeks before you deliver, it's better to be prepared. Read Chapter 10, Parenthood Prep for details.

If you want to hire a doula (delivery assistant), now is the time to start doing interviews.

Be aware of fetal movements—continue checking fetal kick counts.

29 to 30 weeks

You might start to become constipated again (especially if you are taking iron supplements). And constipation only makes hemorrhoids worse—yes, hemorrhoids show up around this time. Work on increasing fiber and water intake. You may even need a stool softener.

This is the time in your pregnancy when your skin might change. Your nipples may get darker, or you might get a dark line from your belly button to your pubic hair. You may also see some strange hair growth on your face, arms, belly, or around your nipples. Great, huh? At least the hair on your head and your fingernails get some benefits while you are pregnant—they grow like weeds. See Chapter 4, Is This Normal? for details.

Check fetal kick counts every day.

31 to 33 weeks

You might start leaking fluid from your breasts (**COLOSTRUM**). That's just your body's way of preparing you for the weeks ahead. If you plan on breastfeeding, be sure to read up on things you can do now to make it a success. See Chapter 11, Breastfeeding.

Your uterus may harden up intermittently—and you'll feel it. These are called **BRAXTON HICKS CONTRACTIONS**. While these are technically contractions, they will feel different from the real deal when you are in labor. This chapter will help you figure out the difference. And check out Chapter 4, Is This Normal? for more info. If you have ANY concern that you might be in preterm labor, pick up the phone and call your practitioner.

Your baby is still swimming around in amniotic fluid. He will start moving to his planned position for birth in the next few weeks.

Now is the time to think about circumcision—will you want to have it done? Who will perform the procedure? You will want to discuss this with your practitioner.

Decide if you want your newborn to receive optional screening tests after birth—if so, you will need to order a collection kit. The same goes for cord blood banking. See Chapter 10, Parenthood Prep for details.

Check fetal kick counts every day.

? ?

3RD TRIMESTER

34 weeks

Any energy you had during your second trimester is a distant memory now. Fatigue returns to your body (which is a bit larger than your body of yesteryear) and it's difficult to get comfy for a good night's rest.

Stretch marks start to make their appearance. Your skin, especially your belly skin, might get itchy. Some women even get chafing around rolls of skin they never had previously. Check out Chapter 4, Is This Normal to see if it is okay and Chapter 9, The Spa Treatment, to see what you can do about it. You also may need to buy some new shoes because your pre-pregnancy ones might not fit anymore! While you are at it, pick up some support stockings to reduce wicked leg cramps and swelling.

If you deliver today (up until 37 weeks), you would have a **LATE PRETERM INFANT**. See Chapter 19, Preterm Labor for what that means for you and your baby.

Read Chapter 12, Home Stretch and Chapter 13, Labor Day to prepare for the big day. If you are a real planner, read Chapter 14, Postpartum Care. Your practitioner will probably sit down with you and discuss your labor and childbirth goals and desires around your 32-34 week office visit.

We know you know, but keep checking fetal kick counts daily.

35 weeks

If this is your first pregnancy, your baby may start to head downwards into your pelvis this week (**LIGHTENING**). Don't believe your friends when they tell you that once the baby drops, labor is right around the corner. Some babies drop five weeks in advance, others (especially when it's not your first baby) won't drop until labor begins. Once this happens, you may start to feel better. Why? Shortness of breath and heartburn may go away. But now your baby is pushing against your bladder so you will be urinating even more often (seems absolutely impossible, doesn't it?).

Between now and 37 weeks, your practitioner will do a culture to see if you carry a bacteria called Group B Strep. If you are a carrier, you'll need to take antibiotics, but only when you go into labor (see Chapter 5, Tests).

Keep checking daily fetal kick counts. Time to pack your hospital bag and get that car seat installed!

36 weeks

Feeling wet down there? It might be because your body is making even more vaginal discharge (if that's imaginable) or because you are leaking urine. Concerned your water may have broken? Look for "Wet Undies 411" in the common questions section in this chapter.

You are entering the home stretch! You will see your practitioner once a week until you deliver. You'll have an internal exam at most of these visits, so you can mentally prepare for that.

It's important to assess your body's readiness for delivery. Your practitioner will be able to tell if your cervix is ripening (getting softer and opening up). The exam also helps determine if your baby is starting to move down towards the exit and what position he plans to be in (hopefully, head first—called **VERTEX**). Spotting after an exam like this is frightening, but it's normal. See Chapter 16, Complications.

Keep up those fetal kick counts.

3RD TRIMESTER

? ?

37 weeks

Your baby is officially "Full-Term." Even so, every week counts. You may still be pregnant until your due date (or beyond). You'll be hot and sweaty from here until delivery day, even if you are fortunate enough to deliver in the winter.

You might discover a clear glob in the toilet after you've peed for the umpteenth time this week. That's your **MUCOUS PLUG,** which plugs your cervix and protects your uterus throughout pregnancy. As your cervix ripens (softens and opens), the plug might fall out. Sorry, but it doesn't mean you are in labor. It can fall out as your body makes its final preparations for childbirth. That could be tomorrow or in three weeks. Some women never see their mucous plug come out, and sometimes it comes out at delivery.

Make sure you read Chapter 12, Home Stretch, Chapter 13, Labor Day, and Chapter 14, Postpartum Care if you have not gotten around to it yet.

Have we mentioned to check fetal kick counts everyday?

38 weeks

You are probably peeing every couple of hours now. And thus, you are not sleeping more than a couple of hours at a time.

Even though you are more than ready to give birth, your baby may not be ready. Don't beg, plead, or try to bribe your practitioner into an early induction or scheduled C-section. Sometimes, dates are off and you might have a baby who is younger than billed. Those babies can potentially end up with longer hospital stays or problems not normally encountered with a full-term baby. Be patient. You are almost there.

Fetal kick counts!!

39 weeks

Don't plan any major events. You could go into labor any day! On the flip side, you could also be sitting around twiddling your fingers for another week or two.

If you start having regular contractions and pass blood-tinged discharge (**BLOODY SHOW**), you are going into labor. Congratulations! See Chapter 13, Labor Day for what happens next.

It's especially important now to continue checking daily fetal kick counts.

40 weeks

This may be the week you meet your baby for the first time (we hope!)…or maybe not. Your baby cannot stay in your womb until kindergarten, so it's just a matter of time. Hang in there!

You and your practitioner may start having a conversation about inducing labor if there's no activity going on down there. You may also be hooked up to a few monitors to have a non-stress test (NST) to make sure your baby can safely continue in the uterus. Read Chapter 12, Home Stretch to learn about the **BISHOP SCORE** that can predict if you will have a successful induction.

Check fetal kick counts until you deliver.

? ?

3RD TRIMESTER

41 weeks

Still pregnant? Check out information on post-term babies in Chapter 16, Complications (see Complication #49), and being induced in Chapter 12, Home Stretch.

Aches, pains and changes the **THIRD TRIMESTER (28-40 WEEKS)**

Common symptoms:

◆ Moody, tired, emotional again	◆ Trouble sleeping
◆ Stuffy nose	◆ Nosebleeds
◆ Swollen/bleeding gums	◆ Early breast milk leaking
◆ Heart palpitations	◆ Swollen hands, fingers, feet
◆ Spider veins, varicose veins	◆ Pelvic cramps

◆ Mild shortness of breath without chest pain

◆ Practice contractions (Braxton Hicks)

◆ Frequent urination, urinating at night, leaking

◆ Itching, chafing, stretch marks, sweaty

◆ Belly pain, hip pain, groin pain, back pain, wrist pain, leg cramps

◆ Enlarging breasts, with darker nipples, prominent veins, stretch marks

◆ Constipation, gas, burping, heartburn, hemorrhoids, shooting pain in the vagina and rectum

Common Questions About the Third Trimester

Q. How much weight am I going to gain?

In the final leg of this journey, you will probably gain about one lb. a week if you were at a healthy weight before pregnancy. Don't be surprised, though, if your weight plateaus near the very end. And occasionally, women may even lose a pound or two right before a due date is reached.

Q. I am having trouble sleeping. Any advice?

At some point during your pregnancy, you will dread going to bed at night. Trying to fall asleep (and stay asleep) will be priceless. Here are some tried and true tricks to help you sleep through the night:

Create a nest of pillows—one under your head, one between your knees, one to hug, and one under your feet. Buying a body pillow (sold at Target, Bed Bath & Beyond as well as online) may be a good investment—most cost $50 to $100. One reader favorite is the Leachco Snoogle Total Body Pillow ($50 on Amazon).

As you build a fortress of pillows around yourself to get cozy, your bed partner will get shoved further and further away—perhaps onto the couch or into another bedroom if you don't have a king-sized bed! Note to partners: remember, it's not about you.

Avoid caffeine altogether. Even having an iced tea at lunch can sometimes be enough to keep you up at night.

Empty your bladder right before hopping into bed (okay, we know, it's more of a rolling motion). Yes, you will still have to get up at some point to go to the bathroom, but at least you can get a few good hours in a row at the beginning of the night.

Avoid lying on your back all night. If you awaken and you are on your back, do not freak out—just roll over.

Reality check: no matter which side you wake up on, you will ache every morning as your pregnancy progresses. Chalk it up to the sacrifices of parenthood. Yes, it will all be worth it very soon.

Q. I feel my uterus tighten up occasionally. My OB says they are just practice contractions. How will I be able to tell the difference between these and the real thing?

Because your uterus has a large muscle layer, it contracts or tightens from time to time, whether you are pregnant or not. When you weren't pregnant, you probably only felt those contractions during your menstrual period or occasionally with an orgasm. **BRAXTON HICKS CONTRACTIONS** are the special name for uterine contractions NOT associated with labor.

It is very normal to experience Braxton Hicks contractions during your pregnancy. The more children you have had, the earlier in the pregnancy you may feel them. They tend to occur when you or your baby are moving around. They can also happen if you are dehydrated, have a bladder infection or after an orgasm.

If you've noticed several Braxton Hicks contractions in a row, kick your feet up and relax with a nice big glass of water. They eventually go away.

Real uterine contractions prepare your cervix for the birth process. Your cervix will start to thin out and open with these contractions.

Will you be able to tell the difference between these contractions and the real deal contractions? That can be tricky sometimes, but here are some key differences:

Braxton Hicks contractions
◆ These usually don't hurt.
◆ Your belly gets hard (like your chin), then relaxes and softens again.
◆ You can sit, breathe, and talk through them.
◆ They happen sporadically.
◆ They do not get more intense over time.
◆ They occur more often as your pregnancy progresses.

Real labor pains
◆ These hurt—like really bad menstrual cramps or terrible low back pain.
◆ You won't want to sit, breathe, talk (or do much of anything) during one.
◆ They happen at more regular intervals.
◆ Their intensity and frequency increase with time.
◆ They most often occur in the third trimester, although they are possible at any point in the pregnancy.

If you aren't sure which contractions you are having, it is always a good idea to check in with your practitioner.

Q. I am leaking fluid from my breasts. Is it breast milk?

While you won't make mature breast milk until two to five days after delivery, you might produce and leak some early milk (called **COLOSTRUM**) at the end of your second or early in your third trimester.

We'll talk more about colostrum and preparation for breastfeeding in Chapter 11, Breastfeeding. But for now, don't be alarmed if you see a thin, clear-yellow substance leaking from your nipples. You also shouldn't be alarmed if you don't see it! Some pregnant women leak while other women start after delivery when their baby begins to nurse. Leaking during pregnancy does not determine whether or not you will breastfeed successfully.

Reality Check: Nursing pads

If you are leaking, it's time to buy some nursing pads. There are two options: disposable pads or reusable (washable) 100% cotton pads. There are pros and cons to each option.

Disposable pads are cheap and you can just throw them away once they are used. But they can make you look a little lumpy in a tight fitting shirt. You can pick up a pack of 60 disposable pads for about $10 at Target.

Reusable pads are softer and a bit more form fitting. But they are more expensive and you have to wash them every day—you'll have to buy several unless you like doing laundry all the time. You also have to watch out that they don't migrate out of your bra, since they have no adhesive backing. It's not so attractive to have a nursing pad make its way to daylight during a business meeting or while grocery shopping!

We have an entire discussion of the best nursing pads in our other book, *Baby Bargains* (see back of this book for details). In brief, readers like the Lansinoh and Johnson & Johnson disposable pads best. For reusable pads, top honors went to Medela and Avent.

Q. Um, my undies are a little wet. Did I just pee or did my water break?

Wet undies are due to one of three things: 1) urine, 2) vaginal discharge, or 3) amniotic fluid (water bag breaking). Early in pregnancy, it's usually #1 or #2. To help you figure it out, we present to you:

Wet Undies 411

1 **URINE.** It's never fun to be incontinent, but this is something that can happen throughout pregnancy. As your baby gets bigger, he/she puts more pressure on your bladder. That pressure can be more than the muscle that prevents leakage can handle. Your baby's movements can also trigger leakage. Either way, the urine just comes right on out and you'll be darting for the nearest place to change your underwear. For the first time in your life, you'll actually be jealous that you can't wear a "Stadium Pal" (yes, it is true—a contraption billed as "a portable urinal" so guys don't have to miss an important 4th down play during a football game).

2 **VAGINAL DISCHARGE**: Both the cervix and the vagina make and secrete more discharge during pregnancy. This looks yellowish-white

and can be thick and mucousy on the underwear. Urine and amniotic fluid are more watery.

3 **AMNIOTIC FLUID.** If your "water breaks" (called **RUPTURE OF THE AMNIOTIC SAC**), you'll see clear, watery fluid. It doesn't look or smell like urine. It can happen at any point during pregnancy and needs to be immediately diagnosed and addressed by your practitioner. Always call your practitioner if you aren't sure. There is a simple test that can be done to figure it out.

It's really tough to know sometimes. As an OB/GYN, I have seen many patients in the office and sent a few to the hospital (in the middle of the night) because the complaint is "wet underwear" or leaking water from the vagina. If you are unsure, the best thing to do is to call your practitioner, describe your symptoms, and let him or her decide with a few tests.

Here's how practitioners figure it out:

First, we look inside the vagina with a speculum to see if there is any "pooling." We will ask you to cough and if your bag is broken, a lot of fluid often pools in the vagina.

Then we take a swab of fluid with a sterile Q-tip and look at it on a slide under the microscope. Once the fluid on the slide dries, actual amniotic fluid usually has something called a "ferning" pattern.

We also put some of that fluid on litmus-like paper, testing its pH. Amniotic fluid has a pH of 7-7.5 and our little yellow piece of paper turns dark blue. That's what we are looking for.

Your OB may also perform an ultrasound to see how much amniotic fluid still remains inside your uterus around your baby.

A newer test option called Amnisure can be done in the office or in the hospital. The fluid is tested for a protein that is only found in amniotic fluid. Because it is new, Amnisure isn't offered everywhere.

Taking all this information into account, your practitioner will be able to decide if you have in fact ruptured your amniotic sac or if the less important (but more embarrassing) condition has occurred: you peed in your pants.

Q. I used to have a cute "inny" belly button. Now I have an "outty." Is this permanent?

No, it's probably not permanent. Chances are, it will look (relatively) normal again as your body returns to its pre-pregnancy shape.

As your uterus starts to grow, it pushes your belly out. With that expansion, your belly button (officially, the **UMBILICUS**) may disappear and become flush with the rest of your skin, or may pop out. This is one of the reasons we recommend taking out your belly button piercing, if you have one. See Chapter 9, Spa Treatment for details.

Your belly button will return to something similar to its original shape after delivery, but it might be a little bit bigger. So as much as we would love to, we can't guarantee you will look exactly the same in a string bikini before and after childbirth.

? ?

3RD TRIMESTER

Q. Are there any products I can use to prevent stretch marks?

We are all desperate when it comes to preventing stretch marks and will do just about anything to avoid getting them. I used a crazy combination of creams and oils, one on top of another, that made me smell like a slightly minted rosemary-eucalyptus tree when I went to bed at night. . . just one of the sacrifices my husband made during both of my pregnancies! But remember this: there is no one "wonder cream" that will prevent stretch marks (despite all the hype out there).

Prenatal visits

You will visit your practitioner every two weeks from 28 to 36 weeks, and then once a week until you deliver. You will be an old pro at this point. Get weighed. Pee in a cup. Roll up your sleeve and check blood pressure. Listen to baby's heartbeat. Measure fundal height.

But your practitioner will add a pelvic (internal) exam to this routine, starting at the 36-week visit . . . and at most weekly visits until you deliver. Good times. You won't look forward to these exams because they are fairly uncomfortable. Your practitioner will probably say something like, "You're going to feel a little bit of pressure," to prepare you for it.

FYI: The word "pressure" in obstetrics is code for "this is going to be pretty darn uncomfortable."

But it's important to do these exams in the last stage of pregnancy so your practitioner can figure out if your body is getting ready for delivery. Your practitioner can determine if your **CERVIX** is starting to open up and soften (we call it ripening—yes, like a fruit).

The exam also helps your practitioner know what position your baby plans to be in (95% of the time, that is head first—called **VERTEX**).

At one of these visits, you (and your partner, hopefully) will sit down with your practitioner to discuss your upcoming labor and delivery. This is also your chance to discuss the childbirth experience: your desires, etc.

Q. Are there any more routine tests?

Yes. Between 35 and 37 weeks, your practitioner will do a swab of your vagina/rectum for a **GROUP B STREPTOCOCCUS OR "GBS" CULTURE.** The details of this test are in Chapter 5, Tests. In short, if you are a carrier of this bacteria, you will need antibiotics during labor to prevent spreading it to your baby in the birth process.

And you need to keep monitoring your baby's fetal kick counts, which are also covered in Chapter 5, Tests.

Q. Any more ultrasounds?

If you have a routine pregnancy, the answer might be no. Some OB's also do one more ultrasound at 28 to 32 weeks to assess the baby's size and to be sure there is an appropriate amount of fluid that surrounds the baby (**AMNIOTIC FLUID**).

Q. Which visits are the most important for my partner to attend?

If you can only pick one, go for the 32 to 34 week visit. This is the big "what will happen in delivery" talk. Check with your practitioner to see when they like to have this discussion.

In my practice, this is the visit when I discuss all the nitty-gritty details about labor and delivery. That includes: what going into labor feels like, when to call me, when to go to the hospital, what your pain control options are, how I monitor mother and baby during labor, what interventions are used for complicated deliveries, and why Cesarean sections happen. Then, I answer all the who/what/when/where/why questions you have about the big day.

You can see why both of you should be at this appointment!

Decisions

There are some pretty important health and parenting decisions that you and your partner need to tackle—ideally, before your baby arrives. For some decisions, your healthcare team needs to know what you want at or just after delivery (which is no time to make rational decisions)! For others, you need to plan ahead so you will have the most options available to you. Bottom line: You are about to become parents and you can no longer procrastinate.

You can find detailed information on these topics in Chapter 10, Parenthood Prep, but here are the highlights:

◆ **Circumcision.** Even if you don't want to find out your baby's gender before delivery, you and your partner should decide if you'd want a son to be circumcised (have the foreskin surgically removed).

Yes, it is weird to discuss the fate of your future son's penis—but you should. Have a discussion with your OB and your future pediatrician who can explain the medical benefits and risks.

Because circumcision is routinely done before a newborn leaves the hospital, you'll need to find out who will do the procedure. Sometimes the obstetrician or family practitioner does the circumcision, other times it is the pediatrician. If you are Jewish and plan to use a mohel, you'll need to get that person lined up in advance.

Bottom line: make this decision between 32 and 36 weeks of pregnancy.

◆ **Cord blood banking.** The pitch is emotional: should you bank your baby's umbilical cord blood to possibly save your child's life (or someone else's) in the future?

You'll have several options: skip the banking, bank with a private bank or donate the cord blood to a public donation program (depending on where you live and your medical history).

After you read our take on cord blood banking, surf the major cord blood bank sites and talk with your practitioner. Your baby's pediatrician can also weigh in if you have a consultation (prenatal visit) with him/her before delivery.

The key: make your decision BEFORE delivery day. If you pick a private bank, the company will send you a collection kit—yes, you have to remember to bring this with you to the hospital. Some hospitals may stock collection kits from major banks . . . but don't rely on this option!

◆ *Expanded newborn screening.* State health departments routinely test every newborn's blood for medical disorders that might otherwise go undetected until irreversible damage has been done (which is why it is so important to do the testing). Many of these tests look for problems that the baby has in metabolizing fats, sugars, and proteins.

All 50 states screen for the 29 most common treatable disorders. There are 25 *additional* tests that you may choose to do (or your state may mandate), but there is no treatment for these diseases once a diagnosis is made. Those 25 tests may or may not be done in your state—each state weighs the cost of the test and the potential benefit. To see what your state mandates, go to our website at Expecting411.com; click on Bonus Material.

If you live in a state that does limited testing, you can pay a private lab to perform an expanded newborn screening for the entire panel of 54 possible tests.

You should make a decision on whether you are doing expanded newborn screening between 32 to 36 weeks. Why? If you use a private lab for expanded screening, they'll send you a collection kit that needs to be taken to the hospital. You need to leave time for the kit to arrive before delivery.

◆ *Hiring a doula.* What's a doula? This is a person who is trained to provide emotional, physical and educational support during pregnancy and delivery (and shortly after delivery).

Some couples decide they want to have a doula in addition to their practitioner at one or all phases of their birth experience. Doulas are invaluable if you are planning to go through labor without pain medication. Of course, it would be wise to make sure both of you want have a doula.

Ask your practitioner for recommendations—you'll want to make sure that if the doula has worked with your practitioner before, they have a good relationship.

You can also talk to friends who have used doulas during their pregnancies. Start interviewing doulas at about 28 weeks of pregnancy and meet with as many as you need to until you both feel comfortable with one.

See Chapter 12, Home Stretch for a more detailed discussion on doulas.

◆ *Picking a pediatrician.* That little peanut growing inside of you will eventually need his or her own doctor. And you may not realize that your baby's first exam with the pediatrician happens shortly after delivery. So, it's important to select a practitioner for your baby BEFORE you deliver!

We have a full section on how to select a pediatrician in Chapter 10, Parenthood Prep. Start interviewing practitioners between 28 and 34 weeks of pregnancy.

Many pediatricians offer prenatal meetings or consultations for prospective parents. A prenatal visit not only helps you decide if you feel comfortable with that person, but also may provide insight on other decisions—like cord blood banking, circumcision, etc. It is well worth your time to do it.

◆ *Going back to work/childcare options.* Daycares and preschools with the best reputations often have waiting lists with parents signed up BEFORE baby is born. Crazy, we know. . . but don't say we didn't warn you at the very start!

What's Going on Down There?! The Third Trimester

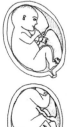

28 weeks.
The eyes open and close. She can show off her eyelashes.

32 weeks.
Your baby's pupils respond to light now. She's getting bigger and more cramped in her little home—so she curls into a ball called the fetal position.

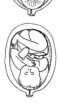

36 weeks.
Your baby's lungs are now mature and could function outside the womb. For boys, testes have migrated into the scrotum. Your baby starts fattening up.

40 weeks.
Good to go.

Now that you've seen the big picture of pregnancy, we'll cover all the nitty-gritty details. Next up: Is This Normal? We answer 50 of the most common questions on aches, pains, and strange hair growth—from head to toe.

IS THIS NORMAL?

Chapter 4

Sid: "My feet are sweaty."
Manny: "Do we have to get a newsflash every time your body does something?"
—Ice Age

WHAT'S IN THIS CHAPTER

- ◆ WHY ARE MY FEET SWELLING?
- ◆ WHEN TO WORRY, WHEN TO CALL YOUR DOC
- ◆ AND 50 MORE WEIRD THINGS YOU WORRY ABOUT FROM HEAD TO TOE

Your body is undergoing a major metamorphosis. Okay, that's not exactly a surprise. What you may not realize, however, is your *whole body* is changing—not just the female parts! And as long as you have a growing human being inside, you will not feel normal.

For instance, your heart and blood vessels have to accommodate the increased blood flow to your growing baby. Your gut has to deal with hormones that will increase heartburn and decrease bowel movements. You'll have aches and pains in places you've never felt before. Those are just a few examples of the *many* changes to come.

This chapter will tell you what is normal and what is not, so you'll know when you need to call your practitioner . . . and when you can relax.

And since some of these symptoms aren't the most pleasant to endure, we'll also cover what to do about them (other than just living with them—which, unfortunately, is sometimes the answer).

Below is a little synopsis of your body changes for the next 40 weeks, so you won't be alarmed when these weird symptoms arise.

Yes, this is a lengthy chapter. To make it easier to use, we have divided it by body system—from head to toe.

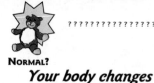

Your body changes

Table of common body changes/complaints*

Symptom	When it happens, by trimester
BRAIN	
Moody	1st and 3rd trimester
Headaches	1st trimester
Dizzy	1st and 3rd trimester
Fatigue	1st and 3rd (if 2nd, it may be due to anemia)
Trouble sleeping	1st and 3rd trimester
Forgetfulness	The whole damn time
EYES	
Blurry vision	Throughout pregnancy
EAR, NOSE, THROAT	
Stuffy nose	Late 2nd and 3rd trimester
Nosebleeds	2nd and 3rd trimester
Gums swollen/bleeding	2nd and 3rd trimester
BREASTS	
Tenderness	1st and early 2nd trimester
Enlargement	1st and 3rd trimester
Darker nipples	2nd and 3rd trimester
Blue veins	Throughout pregnancy
Leaking early milk (colostrum)	2nd and 3rd trimester
Stretch marks	3rd and after breastfeeding is completed
LUNGS	
Shortness of breath	Late 2nd and 3rd trimester
HEART AND BLOOD VESSELS	
Swollen body parts (**EDEMA**)	2nd (if you are on your feet all day), 3rd trimester
Heart palpitations	Anytime (always see your practitioner)
STOMACH AND INTESTINES	
Morning sickness (nausea/vomiting)	1st, early 2nd, rarely through 3rd trimester
Constipation	1st and 3rd trimester
Hemorrhoids	2nd and 3rd trimester**
Gas	1st and 3rd trimester
Burping	1st and 3rd trimester
Heartburn (acid reflux)	Rarely 1st, mainly 2nd and 3rd trimester
Umbilical pain	2nd trimester
Shooting pains in vagina/rectum	3rd trimester

NORMAL?

SYMPTOM	WHEN IT HAPPENS, BY TRIMESTER

GIRL PARTS

Pelvic cramps	Throughout pregnancy
Braxton Hicks contractions	Usually 3rd, but 2nd trimester if it's not your first baby
Vaginal discharge	Throughout pregnancy
Varicose veins in outer genitals	Late 2nd and 3rd trimester
Spotting	Anytime (always see practitioner)
Swelling/discomfort	Late 2nd and 3rd trimester
Shooting pains in vagina/rectum	3rd trimester
Itching in outer genital area	Often 2nd and 3rd trimester (always call practitioner)

KIDNEYS AND BLADDER

Frequent urination	1st and 3rd trimester
Leaking urine (**INCONTINENCE**)	Late 2nd and 3rd trimester
Urinating at night	1st and 3rd trimester

SKIN, HAIR, NAILS

Increased hair growth	Throughout pregnancy
Nail growth	Throughout pregnancy
Glowing skin	For some women throughout, and for others never.
Acne	1st trimester
Blotchy marks on face (**MELASMA**)	1st, 2nd and 3rd trimester
Dark line on belly (**LINEA NIGRA**)	Late 2nd and 3rd trimester
Stretch marks	2nd and 3rd trimester
Itching	2nd and 3rd trimester
Red palms and soles	2nd and 3rd trimester
Skin tags	2nd and 3rd trimester
Darker, more prominent moles	2nd and 3rd (always see practitioner)
Chafing/intertrigo	2nd and 3rd trimester
Spider veins	2nd and 3rd trimester
Varicose veins	2nd and 3rd trimester
Sweaty	2nd and 3rd trimester

MUSCLES, BONES, AND NERVES

Hip pain (round ligament pain)	Late 1st and early 2nd trimester
Groin pain	2nd trimester
Pubic/leg pain	3rd trimester
Low back pain/sacral pain	Late 2nd and 3rd trimester
Sciatic pain	Late 2nd and 3rd trimester
Leg cramps	Late 2nd and 3rd trimester
Wrist pain (carpal tunnel syndrome)	Late 2nd and 3rd trimester

IMMUNE SYSTEM

Illnesses last longer	The whole time

* With your second pregnancy, all these body changes happen earlier!
** If you escape them during pregnancy, they will appear while pushing at delivery!

Factoid: Your body changes with pregnancy, and it may not return to exactly your same ol' body when the pregnancy is over.

NORMAL?

A word about Red Flags

The detailed information to follow explains all the common and normal things that may happen to you, why they happen, and what to do about them. You'll also see Red Flags called out with each symptom. As you would guess, Red Flags are NOT normal and need to be addressed immediately. You can find details on these complications in Chapter 15, Pregnancy 911. Bottom line: if you have a Red Flag issue, you need to call your practitioner.

ACHES AND PAINS BY THE TRIMESTER

Here is a little snapshot of your pregnant body for each trimester. It's not exactly a sales pitch for becoming pregnant. But since you're here already, you might as well know the truth!

FIRST TRIMESTER (0-13 WEEKS)

Common symptoms:

- ◆ Moody
- ◆ Headaches
- ◆ Tender, growing breasts
- ◆ Gas, burping, constipation
- ◆ Frequent urination, urinating at night
- ◆ Nausea, vomiting (morning sickness)
- ◆ Vaginal discharge starts and continues for the duration
- ◆ Acne, splotchy marks on the face
- ◆ Tired
- ◆ Difficulty sleeping

SECOND TRIMESTER (14-27 WEEKS)

Common symptoms:

- ◆ Stuffy nose
- ◆ Hemorrhoids
- ◆ Swollen/bleeding gums
- ◆ Nosebleeds
- ◆ Heartburn
- ◆ Itching in outer genital area
- ◆ Darker nipples, leaking early milk
- ◆ Feet swelling, if you are on your feet all day
- ◆ Belly pain, hip pain, groin pain, back pain, wrist pain, leg cramps
- ◆ Itching, chafing, skin tags, red palms and soles, stretch marks

THIRD TRIMESTER (28-40 WEEKS)

Common symptoms:

- ◆ Moody, tired, emotional again
- ◆ Stuffy nose
- ◆ Swollen/bleeding gums
- ◆ Heart palpitations
- ◆ Spider veins, varicose veins
- ◆ Trouble sleeping
- ◆ Nosebleeds
- ◆ Early breast milk leaking
- ◆ Swollen hands, fingers, feet
- ◆ Pelvic cramps
- ◆ Mild shortness of breath without chest pain
- ◆ Practice contractions (Braxton Hicks)
- ◆ Frequent urination, urinating at night, leaking
- ◆ Itching, chafing, stretch marks, sweaty
- ◆ Belly pain, hip pain, groin pain, back pain, wrist pain, leg cramps
- ◆ Enlarging breasts, with darker nipples, prominent veins, stretch marks
- ◆ Constipation, gas, burping, heartburn, hemorrhoids, shooting pain in the vagina and rectum

Brain

- Moody
- Dizzy
- Trouble sleeping
- Baby blues

- Headaches
- Fatigue
- Forgetfulness

Q. I'm 8 weeks pregnant and my husband tells me I am acting like I'm getting my period—really moody and short-tempered. Is this normal?

Symptom: Moodiness. You yell at your partner for not getting dinner and rubbing your feet at the same time.

Usual time of onset: 1st trimester. It can last throughout pregnancy.

Cause: Changes in your hormone levels, particularly elevations of estrogen and progesterone trigger moodiness.

Treatment:

- Have an open conversation with your partner and be thankful this person loves you.
- Exercise.
- Get more sleep.
- Rarely, some women benefit from antidepressant medication.

Red Flags:

- Crying all the time.
- Cannot carry out activities of daily living (bathing, cooking, eating, dressing, working).
- Unable to get out of bed.
- Loss of appetite or weight loss.
- Withdrawal from friends or loved ones.
- Thoughts of harming yourself or others.

If you have any of the above "Red Flag" symptoms, talk to your practitioner immediately.

Partner Tip

Your partner is growing a human being inside of her and may not seem like herself anymore. The dramatic hormonal surges occurring in her body are changing her emotions faster than an Indy 500 racecar. Be patient. Be calm. Help her as much as you can. Don't take it personally. It's not about you. This will end (at some point)!

Q. I am getting really bad headaches. Is there anything I can take for them?

Symptom: Headaches.

Usual time of onset: 1st trimester.

Cause: Thank your elevated hormone levels again. Other causes include dehydration, increased stress, abruptly ending your caffeine intake, or a change in your sleep habits. Occasionally, pregnancy causes the shape of the lens in your eye to change, resulting in strained vision. This can give you a headache, too.

Treatment:

- Sleep more.
- Exercise.
- Stay well hydrated.
- Ask your partner for a massage (or pay for one).
- Medication options: acetaminophen (Tylenol) or a caffeinated beverage.
- Consider getting your vision checked.

Red Flags:

- The worst headache you have ever had.
- Headache that wakes you up from sleep.
- Headache that doesn't go away with hydration and pain meds.
- Headache that lasts more than a few hours or returns frequently.
- Abdominal pain with a headache.
- Vision changes with a headache.
- Fever with a headache.

Reality Check: Migraines and pregnancy

If you are a migraine sufferer, take note. Migraines, like many other chronic medical issues, follow the "Rule of Thirds" in pregnancy: 1/3 of pregnant migraine sufferers say that symptoms improve, 1/3 stay the same, and 1/3 worsen.

Unfortunately, ibuprofen (Motrin, Advil) is **not** recommended during pregnancy.

It's safe to take acetaminophen (Tylenol) but most migraine sufferers do not get relief from Tylenol alone.

If you are one of the unlucky ones, there are some prescription migraine medications that are acceptable to take if nothing else is working. See Medications at Expecting411.com/extra for details. Bottom line: always check with your practitioner *before* taking any prescribed migraine medication.

Since your medication options are limited, try putting a cold towel on your head and resting in a quiet, dark room once a migraine hits.

As for prevention, avoid things that you know may trigger your migraines such as cheese, chocolate, stress and lack of sleep. You may also want to try meditation, yoga, acupuncture or a regular exercise program.

Q. I have moments of feeling really lightheaded, like I am going to faint. What can I do to prevent this feeling?

Symptom: Dizziness or lightheadedness.
Usual time of onset: 1st and 3rd trimesters.
Cause: Hormones and/or dehydration. High levels of the hormone progesterone can cause your veins to dilate and blood pressure to drop. Especially if you are standing up, you may have less blood flow to your head and more to your feet. That can make you dizzy or lightheaded. If you are dehydrated, there is less volume circulating in your bloodstream, which can also make you feel lightheaded.
Treatment:

- Sit or lie down.
- Drink more water.
- Consider wearing support stockings if this happens regularly.

- If symptoms persist, put your head between your knees (so it is lower than your heart). This will bring blood back to your head, relieving your symptoms in most cases. (Memo: we realize this is easier in your first trimester than in your last one!)

Red Flags:
- Dizziness and shortness of breath.
- Dizziness and chest pain.
- Dizziness and calf or leg pain.
- Dizziness and heavy vaginal bleeding.
- Actual fainting.

Q. I am tired constantly. Is anything wrong with me?

Symptom: Fatigue... as if the life is being sucked out of you!

Usual time of onset: Worst in the 1st, returning in the 3rd trimester.

Cause: Most of your energy stores are being used to grow a human being inside of you. That doesn't leave much energy for you.

Treatment:
- Exercise. That will be the last thing you want to do, but it may help you recharge.
- Rest. Take a nap when you are tired (if your schedule permits) and go to bed early to get a good night sleep.
- No matter what you do, it gets better with time. The severe fatigue you have in the first trimester goes away as you enter into the second trimester. It does return in your third, but not to the degree you experienced in the first trimester.

Red Flags:
- Fatigue during the 2nd trimester.
- Severe fatigue upon awakening (especially 2nd or 3rd trimester).
- Fatigue and depressed mood.

Q. I just can't get a good night's sleep. What can I do about it?

Symptom: Sleep disruption. Constant waking and difficulty returning to sleep.

Usual time of onset: 1st and 3rd trimesters

Cause: There are several reasons.
- It's hard to get comfortable and then stay comfortable.
- You need to pee all the time.
- Relentless heartburn that is worse when you are lying down.
- Feeling slightly short of breath until the baby drops down into your pelvis (**LIGHTENING**) towards the end of pregnancy.
- Anxiety. Many women report not being able to fall back to sleep because they have racing thoughts about what lies ahead.

All of these issues conspire to turn your evening's rest into a real nightmare.

Treatment:
- Buy a body pillow.
- Sleep with your head slightly elevated (particularly if you are suffering from heartburn).
- Take a relaxing bath before bed.
- Get a massage just before bed.

◆ Exercise during the day—not right before bed.
◆ If all else fails, talk to your OB about using a medication like diphen-hydramine (Benadryl), doxylamine (Unisom) or in very severe cases, Ambien. See Medications at expecting411.com/extra.

Red Flags:
◆ Unable to fall asleep without medication.
◆ Getting less than four to five hours of sleep a night on a chronic basis.
◆ Disrupted sleep with weepy/sad mood, lack of interest in activities.

Insider Secret

Some pregnant women suffer from obstructive sleep apnea. If your partner complains about your snoring, tell your doctor (even if it's embarrassing). You may need help!

Q. Sometimes I feel like I am losing my mind, and I'm not a forgetful person. Does this get better after I deliver?

Symptom: Forgetfulness. You can't find your keys, remember your neighbor's last name, or recall the questions for your practitioner that you just thought of five minutes ago.

Usual time of onset: 1st, 2nd and 3rd trimesters (and even into the postpartum period).

Cause: During pregnancy, it may be due to those elevated hormone levels. The "Mommy Brain" or "placenta brain" as one of Dr H's patients likes to call it, persists after delivery thanks to having a newborn in the house. Anything that interferes with having a solid night's sleep for three to four months (or more) can make anyone a bit forgetful.

Treatment: Write everything down. If you have trouble remembering what your practitioner told you after you've left the office, ask for handouts or booklets to take home, or take notes while she talks.

Red Flags: None.

Q. I've heard about women having postpartum depression, but I'm still pregnant and already feeling the blues. Shouldn't I be excited about having this baby?

Symptom: Depressed mood.

Usual time of onset: 3rd trimester, although it's possible at any point in the pregnancy.

Cause: Let's see, you are about to deliver a baby (which can cause anxiety, even if you have done it before), you are about to be totally responsible for a helpless little being, you get disrupted sleep every night and your hormone levels are off the charts. If it is your 2nd child, sprinkle in some guilt about having to divide your love. Is that enough? Those emotions and hormones can override the excitement for what lies ahead. Also, if you have a personal history of depression, medication dosages and types may have changed or you may not be on any medication at all at this point. This can lead to an increase in the severity of your symptoms.

Treatment: Exercise (we know you're sick of us saying this by now). Talk about your feelings with your partner. Tell your practitioner how you feel. People can't help you if they don't know what is going on.

NORMAL?

Red Flags:
- ◆ Crying all the time.
- ◆ Cannot perform activities of daily living (bathing, dressing, working).
- ◆ Cannot get out of bed.
- ◆ Loss of appetite or weight loss.
- ◆ Withdrawing from friends.

Eyes

- ◆ Blurry vision

Q. I wear glasses/contacts. All of a sudden things seem blurry. Is that normal?

Symptom: Blurry vision, change in vision. It may be associated with a mild headache.

Usual time of onset: 1st, 2nd or 3rd trimester.

Cause: Elevated hormone levels can make the lenses in your eyes swell. This is temporary but can cause significant changes in your vision, particularly if you already wear glasses or contacts.

Treatment: Get a cheap new pair of eyeglasses from your eye doctor. Don't waste your money on a super expensive pair because your vision will probably go back to baseline after you deliver! Always tell your OB about any vision changes so he can check for potential medical issues.

Red Flags:
- ◆ Sudden onset of blurry vision.
- ◆ Seeing flashes of light or blind spots.
- ◆ Severe headache and blurry vision/vision changes.
- ◆ Abdominal pain and vision changes.

Ear, Nose, Throat

- ◆ Stuffy nose
- ◆ Swollen, bleeding gums
- ◆ Nosebleeds

Q. My nose is constantly stuffy. I don't feel sick or have any other allergy symptoms, it's just my nose. What do I do?

Symptom: Stuffy nose or nasal congestion.

Usual time of onset: 2nd and 3rd trimesters.

Cause: Elevated levels of estrogen and progesterone cause many body parts to swell, including your sinus and nasal passages.

Treatment:
- ◆ Use saline nose spray as often as needed to loosen nasal secretions.
- ◆ Put a humidifier in your bedroom to help loosen mucus.
- ◆ It is okay to use diphenhydramine (Benadryl) periodically, but it may not help. Check with your practitioner about using other antihistamines.

Red Flags:
- ◆ Fever and congestion.

NORMAL?

? ?

- ◆ Severe facial pain/headache and congestion.
- ◆ Persistent sore throat and congestion.

Q. I've started having nosebleeds. Is this unusual?

Symptom: Nosebleeds.

Usual time of onset: 2nd and 3rd trimesters.

Cause: Elevated estrogen and progesterone levels enlarge and soften your blood vessels. As a result, those blood vessels become more fragile. So, just blowing your nose or breathing in dry, cold air can irritate the lining of your nose and cause a nosebleed.

Treatment:

- ◆ Prevention: Keep the skin inside your nostrils nice and moist.
- ◆ Use saline nose drops or nasal spray liberally (several times daily).
- ◆ Use a Q-tip to apply petroleum jelly or Aquaphor (a personal favorite) to the lining of your nostrils twice daily—especially at night.
- ◆ Sleep with a warm-mist humidifier in your room.

Red Flags:

- ◆ Daily nose bleeds.
- ◆ A nosebleed that you cannot control or stop after 20 to 30 minutes. This kind of nosebleed likely requires medical attention.

How to handle a nosebleed: lean forward slightly and pinch your nose, squeezing your nostrils together for five minutes. If bleeding continues, repeat. Decongestant nose spray (like Afrin) can stop a nosebleed, but you should only use it after asking your practitioner. The decongestant shrinks the blood vessels in the nose, but if used frequently, it can have the same effect on the blood vessels in the placenta. Afrin can also become addictive.

Q. I brush and floss my teeth regularly, but my gums are swollen and bleeding. Am I doing something wrong?

Symptom: Swollen and bleeding gums.

Usual time of onset: 2nd and 3rd trimesters.

Cause: Elevated hormone levels increase blood flow and cause your gums to swell. Swollen gums bleed more easily.

Treatment:

- ◆ Brush regularly (at least twice a day) with a soft bristle toothbrush.
- ◆ Floss. Yes, every day.
- ◆ See your dentist for routine check-ups and cleanings.
- ◆ Rinse your mouth periodically with a warm water and salt rinse.

Red Flags:

- ◆ Severe pain with brushing.
- ◆ Pain or bleeding in only one area.
- ◆ Pain or bleeding and fever.

Insider Secret

Take care of your teeth and gums. Continue getting regular dental exams and cleanings. And FLOSS! According to my dad (who also happens to be a dentist), it's even more important than brushing! If a problem arises, see your dentist. Periodontal disease and abscesses may lead to preterm labor and delivery.

NORMAL?

Breasts

◆ Tenderness	◆ Enlargement (growth)
◆ Dark nipples	◆ Blue veins
◆ Leaking milk (colostrum)	◆ Stretch marks

Q. I'm outgrowing my bras. My breasts are also really tender. When will this growth spurt end?

Symptom: Breast enlargement and tenderness. Your nipples may be especially sensitive. You'll get those boobs you've always dreamed of (temporarily) when you are pregnant.

Usual time of onset: 1st and 3rd trimesters.

Cause: Elevated hormone levels (particularly estrogen) make milk ducts and breast tissue grow and enlarge.

Treatment:

◆ Wear a bra to bed for extra support. Bras without underwires are best, such as an exercise bra.

◆ Avoid hot water in the shower.

◆ Apply vitamin E directly to your nipples.

◆ Time. Most women get some relief after the first trimester is over.

Red Flags:

◆ Breast mass.

◆ Nipple discharge (although it's usually early milk, which is normal—see **COLOSTRUM**).

◆ Nipple or breast tissue dimpling.

◆ Significant skin discoloration, other than darkening of the areolae and nipples.

Insider Secret

It's difficult to do self-breast exams during pregnancy because there is so much growth of your breast tissue. But do let your practitioner know if something looks or feels odd.

Q. My nipples have suddenly become discolored. Any concerns?

Symptom: Dark nipples.

Usual time of onset: 2nd and 3rd trimesters.

Cause: Pregnancy increases **MELANIN** production (the pigment that makes skin color). This excess melanin causes certain areas on the body that are already pigmented to become darker, including your nipples.

Treatment: None. It usually goes away on its own about three to six months after delivery.

Red Flags:

◆ Skin changes on the breast other than the nipple and areola (that circular area around the nipple).

Reality check: Seeing black

You may find several body areas get darker—underarms, vagina, **VULVA** (outer genital area), belly button and even the line from your belly button to your pubic hair (see **LINEA NIGRA** in the skin section later in this chapter.) Occasionally, women get a dark line on the back of their legs mimicking the seam of a pair of panty hose! If you have olive toned or dark skin to begin with, you're more likely to see these changes.

Old Wives Tale
You can't get breast cancer while you are pregnant.

False. Breast cancer diagnosed during pregnancy is RARE but possible. It is estimated to occur only once in every 3500 pregnancies. But any change in color or dimpling of the breast tissue itself should be checked out, as should any new lumps. If you notice any of these symptoms, you should have your practitioner take a look.

Q. I am also starting to see some big veins popping up on my chest. Is this permanent?

Symptom: Blue veins. You may begin to look like a road atlas.
Usual time of onset: 1st trimester.
Cause: Elevated hormone levels cause both the breast tissue and the vessels within them to expand.
Treatment: None. After you deliver and stop breastfeeding, those veins shrink back to their old size again.
Red Flags: None.

Q. I've been told that leakage coming from my breasts is a sign of breast cancer. I have a clear fluid leaking from them now. Do I need to worry?

Symptom: Colostrum production. Nope, you don't need a mammogram. You need some bra pads. Your body is now making the early stages of breast milk.
Usual time of onset: Occasionally 2nd trimester, but usually 3rd.
Cause: Hormonal changes tell your breast tissue to make colostrum. Your body starts making it and it may start to leak out.
Treatment: None. Just wear nursing bra pads to soak everything up so that everyone on the street doesn't know you are leaking colostrum!
Red Flags:
- ◆ Bloody or blood tinged discharge from nipples.
- ◆ Green discharge from nipples.
- ◆ Nipple discharge and pain, skin changes or a breast mass.

Q. As my breasts grow, I am starting to develop stretch marks. Will these go away?

Symptom: Stretch marks usually start out looking like dark purple or red streaks on the skin. Over time, they often fade to a lighter pink, white or silver color.
Usual time of onset: 1st or 3rd trimesters, as well as right after delivery.
Cause: Hormones, again. They make your breasts grow rapidly. And that rapid growth causes the dermis (the layer of skin under the top layer, or

epidermis) to tear, leading to stretch marks.

Treatment: Moisture and support. Keep skin moistened with lotions, oils or creams. Wear a bra that supports your enlarging breasts. See the section on stretch marks later in this chapter (in the skin section). Although they may fade, unfortunately, they don't really ever go away completely.

Red Flags: None.

Lungs

◆   Shortness of breath

Q. I'm having difficulty catching my breath, even at rest. Should I call my doctor?

Symptom: Shortness of breath.

Usual time of onset: Late 2nd and 3rd trimesters.

Cause: As your uterus gets bigger, it starts to push on your diaphragm (no, not the birth control device, but the muscle that sits below your lungs that shares the same name). Pushing the diaphragm upwards reduces the volume of air you can breathe into your lungs. At the same time, your pregnant body needs more oxygen. To accommodate, your body forces you to take more frequent breaths.

Treatment:
◆   Rest as much as possible.
◆   Sit up straight with shoulders back and take a few deep breaths.
◆   Breathe in slowly and really expand your chest.
◆   Take yoga classes, which can help focus on breathing.
◆   Avoid situations that are physically exerting, like climbing stairs or vigorous exercising.

Red Flags:
◆   Rapid and labored breathing.
◆   Chest pain and shortness of breath.
◆   Heart racing (palpitations) or a rapid pulse (see Chapter 15, Pregnancy 911; How to Check Your Pulse) and shortness of breath.
◆   A bluish discoloration around your lips or fingers and shortness of breath.
◆   A cough and shortness of breath with or without fever/chills.
◆   Coughing up blood and shortness of breath.
◆   Pain or swelling in one or both legs and shortness of breath.
◆   Shortness of breath in people with asthma whose flare-ups have become more severe, more often, or more difficult to control.

If you have any of the above Red Flag symptoms, talk to your practitioner immediately.

Heart & Blood Vessels

◆   Swelling (**EDEMA**)   ◆   Heart racing (palpitations)

Q. I can't wear my regular shoes anymore because my feet are so swollen. Will I ever get back into my Manolo's?

Symptom: Swelling of body tissues (**EDEMA**). Layman's term: fluid retention. Usually, swelling occurs in the legs and feet. Sometimes your hands, fingers and face will swell too.

Usual time of onset: 2nd and 3rd trimesters.

Cause: The answer is complicated, but it boils down to two things: extra water and extra salt. A pregnant woman has a greater volume of blood in order to meet the needs of the growing fetus. We're talking between 1.5 and two liters of extra fluid. A pregnant woman also retains more sodium (salt) due to a process that controls blood pressure. While your body is doing what it is supposed to, you get the unwelcome side effect of fluid retention.

Treatment: See the Swollen Feet 411 below.

Red Flags:

- ◆ Severe swelling that develops overnight.
- ◆ Rapid swelling in one leg or foot more than the other, with or without pain.
- ◆ Severe swelling in the hands and face.
- ◆ Chest pain and severe swelling.
- ◆ Blurred vision or a severe headache and swelling.

Real World Tip

You may want to wear your wedding ring on a necklace if your fingers get swollen. I have seen the diamonds-go-a-flying in the ER when a pregnant woman waits too long to take off a beloved ring and ends up having an ER doc cut the ring off with a small saw. Don't wait.

Swollen Feet 411

Virtually all pregnant women find that their feet swell during pregnancy (**EDEMA**)—it is particularly noticeable at the end of a long day. Expect it to get worse if you spend all day on your feet or if you wear shoes that are too tight.

Here are a few tips that can help:

- ◆ *Get bigger shoes.* Wear comfortable, good fitting shoes. Yes, you may have to buy a pair that is a half or whole size bigger than normal and they probably shouldn't be Christian Louboutins. Think Birkenstocks (or a comfy pair of sneakers or clogs).
- ◆ *Cut the salt.* Cut back on excess salt in your diet. You may have to kiss chips and salsa good-bye temporarily.
- ◆ *Pick your feet up.* Elevating your legs on a pillow or two when you are sitting can help.
- ◆ *Buy some lovely TED hose.* Purchase support stockings (also

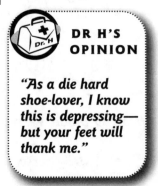

DR H'S OPINION

"As a die hard shoe-lover, I know this is depressing— but your feet will thank me."

called TED hose). Available in most pharmacies, TEDs help reduce swelling. Some women benefit from wearing them at night, while others wear them all day long. And no, they aren't the sexiest hose on the market—but they'll help you feel better!

The only thing that permanently solves your swelling problem is giving birth. But don't panic if your legs and feet are even more swollen a few days *after* delivery. It's normal to have edema for seven to ten days after you deliver. All that excess fluid from pregnancy needs time to be eliminated (a nice way to say you will pee it out).

When to contact your doctor: If there is rapid, painful swelling in one leg, it can signal a **DEEP VENOUS THROMBOSIS** (DVT) or blood clot. Also, sudden onset of swelling in your legs, feet, hands and face can be a symptom of **PREECLAMPSIA** (high blood pressure with accompanying protein in urine). This may be the only symptom you notice. These are both good reasons to call your practitioner in a jiffy. See Chapter 16, Complications (Complication #18 and #20).

Q. Every once in a while, I feel my heart racing. It's pretty unsettling. Should I worry about this?

Symptom: Heart palpitations. It feels like your heart is beating out of your chest—similar to how you would feel after drinking a double shot espresso.

Usual time of onset: Any time during the pregnancy, but particularly in the 1st and 3rd trimester.

Cause: Remember, you've got an extra 1.5 liters of blood that has to be moved around. Your heart works extra hard to pump that excess volume. It beats faster to accomplish this goal.

Treatment: Rest. Drink plenty of water. And yes, anything that contains caffeine can make the palpitations worse. Avoid coffee and other caffeinated beverages as well as excessive amounts of chocolate (sorry)!

Red Flags:
- Chest pain and heart palpitations.
- Shortness of breath and heart palpitations.
- An irregular heart beat and palpitations.
- Dizziness and heart palpitations.
- Underlying heart disorder and palpitations.

Stomach & Intestines

- Morning sickness
- Hemorrhoids
- Burping
- Umbilical pain
- Constipation
- Gas
- Acid reflux/heartburn

Q. I'm in my first trimester and I feel queasy on and off all day long. Is this "morning" sickness?

Symptom: Morning sickness (nausea and/or vomiting). Don't be fooled by the name—many women suffer from nausea ALL DAY LONG. It happens more often in women who are pregnant with multiples, women who get queasy easily (particularly when taking birth control pills) and, anecdotally, in women carrying girls.

Usual time of onset: Six to 14 weeks.

Cause: The triple shot of raging pregnancy hormones: beta-hCG, estrogen and progesterone. Progesterone in particular relaxes the smooth muscles that line your entire gastrointestinal tract. The result: belching, nausea, vomiting, heartburn, gas and constipation.

Treatment:

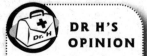

DR H'S OPINION

"I had a patient who was so nauseated in her first trimester that she carried a lemon with her at all times so she could scratch and sniff it to combat her urge to purge. You have to do whatever works!"

- Eat several small meals throughout the day.
- Eat the moment you awaken.
- Try ginger tea or candy.
- Keep saltine crackers at your nightstand.
- Add some lemon juice to water or suck on a lemon drop or sour candy.
- Exercise (yes, it works for just about every malady).
- Take over the counter Vitamin B6, 25 to 50 mg, three times a day.
- Try Sea-Bands (acupressure bands worn on the wrists).
- Consider acupuncture.
- Use an over-the-counter antihistamine like diphenhydramine (Benadryl) or doxylamine (Unisom). Note: both of these can make you pretty sleepy, so only use them at night.
- If you are in agony, ask your doctor for a prescription anti-nausea medication, such as Reglan or odansetron (Zofran). See Medications at expecting411.com/extra.

Red Flags:

- Vomiting repeatedly for more than six hours.
- Urinating less than once every eight hours.
- Weight loss of more than 5% of your pre-pregnancy weight.
- Vomiting daily and unable to keep down food or liquids.
- Vomiting blood.
- Fever and vomiting.
- Severe abdominal pain and vomiting.
- Diarrhea and vomiting.
- 2nd or 3rd trimester nausea/vomiting long after morning sickness is over.*

*Nausea and vomiting in the 2nd or 3rd trimester is probably something other than morning sickness.

 Feedback from the Real World

Smelling or tasting sour things often helps combat nausea.

Reality Checks

1 **YOU ARE MORE LIKELY TO HAVE MORNING SICKNESS IF YOUR MOM SUFFERED FROM IT.** If your mom or sister had morning sickness or excessive vomiting (**HYPEREMESIS GRAVIDARUM,** see red flag below), you are more likely to have it, too.

2 **IT IS MORE COMMON TO GET MORNING SICKNESS WITH MULTIPLES.** Research suggests that higher levels of a specific pregnancy hormone (beta-hCG) lead to morning sickness. The more babies you are carrying, the more beta-hCG you produce and the more nauseated you get.

3 **IF YOU HAVE MORNING SICKNESS, YOU ARE HAVING A GIRL.** Maybe! There is a study currently underway looking at this interesting phenomenon to see if it's actually true (and if so, why). Don't paint the nursery pink because you are puking, however—many women carrying boys have terrible nausea as well. But Dr H can tell you from professional and personal experience that in general, girls make their moms sicker than boys do!

4 **IF YOU SUFFER FROM MIGRAINES, YOU ARE MORE LIKELY TO HAVE MORNING SICKNESS.** Migraine-prone women have a greater chance of suffering from both morning sickness and excessive vomiting. Motion sickness-prone women also have more morning sickness.

5 **YOU ARE LESS LIKELY TO MISCARRY IF YOU FEEL SICK.** If there is any silver lining to all this vomit…you probably have a well-functioning placenta that produces higher levels of hormones. Numerous studies show that you're less likely to miscarry if you have morning sickness.

Red Flag: Excessive Vomiting

Up to 75% of pregnant women have morning sickness . . . but only about five in 1000 pregnant women are unlucky enough to go above and beyond typical morning sickness (**HYPEREMESIS GRAVIDARUM**).

These women vomit so much that they lose at least 5% of their pre-pregnancy weight and have nutritional and metabolic abnormalities. Practitioners need to rule out other medical causes and aggressively treat this condition. See Chapter 16, Complications (see Complication #1).

Q. I've never had a problem having regular bowel movements until now. Normal?

Symptom: Constipation.

Usual time of onset: Worst in 1st trimester. Also shows up in the 3rd trimester.

Cause: Elevated levels of progesterone relax the smooth muscle lining the gastrointestinal tract, making it move in slow motion. Added bonus: iron supplements (taken to treat anemia) can make things even worse.

Treatment:
- Eat more fiber. See Chapter 6, Nutrition for high-fiber food list. To get you started: try blueberries, stewed prunes, and high-fiber cereals.
- Drink more water.

- Try Metamucil or Benefiber natural fiber supplements.
- Take an over-the-counter stool softener like docusate (Colace).
- Ask your doctor for lactulose (Kristalose), a prescription laxative.
- If you need to take iron supplements, consider trying a less consti-pating type, such as Slow Fe or iron prepared in a liquid solution.

Red Flags:
- Pooping less than once every four to five days.
- Severe abdominal pain and constipation.
- Bloody poop and constipation.
- Really black (not dark brown) poop and constipation.*

*Iron supplements can make your poop (stool) color turn dark brown.

Q. I think I might have a hemorrhoid. There is a little bit of blood when I wipe after a bowel movement. What can I do about it?

Symptom: Hemorrhoids. Constipation and hemorrhoids go hand in hand. Hemorrhoids are just swollen veins (**VARICOSE VEINS**) around the anus.

Usual time of onset: They only get worse as pregnancy progresses and even if you aren't blessed with them during your pregnancy, they often appear when pushing during labor. They are nearly impossible to avoid!

Causes:
- When you're constipated, you push harder to get the poop out. Pushing makes the veins around the anus swell up.
- Increased body weight and an enlarged uterus put pressure on these veins and interfere with blood circulation in the lower part of your body. This makes all the veins dilate (that's why you can get varicose veins in the feet, legs, vulva, vagina, and rectum).
- That darn progesterone dilates all your blood vessels, including those around your butt.

Treatment:
- Avoid severe constipation (see tips above in constipation section).
- Use a stool softener like docusate (Colace) to limit pushing while pooping.
- Use soothing witch hazel pads (brand name: Tucks Medicated Pads).
- Apply numbing/anti-inflammatory cream (for example, Preparation H, Anamantle, Analpram, Rectogel—you gotta love these names!) See Medications at Expecting411.com/extra.

Red Flags:
- Sudden, severe pain in the hemorrhoid (yes, it's a pain in the ass).
- Hemorrhoid(s) that is extremely tender to the touch.

Q. I'm burping and passing gas quite a bit. Is it from all the fiber I'm taking to avoid constipation?

Symptom: Burping and excessive gas. You could easily win a sports bar belching contest.

Usual time of onset: Burping/belching, 1st trimester. Gas happens the whole way through!

Cause: Your GI tract is in slow motion, thanks to your progesterone surge.

Treatment: Avoid foods that will add to the problem: beans, other legumes, dried fruit, carbonated drinks, broccoli. (Yes, this is a contradiction—high-fiber foods like beans help avoid constipation . . . but then contribute to this issue!).

Red Flags: No real red flags here. But your other half may wave the white flag of surrender after being in the same room as you for a few minutes!

Q. I have an uncomfortable sensation in my chest and I can sometimes taste food I've eaten hours ago. What is this?

Symptom: Acid reflux/heartburn/**GERD**. Burning pain in upper abdomen or chest. Occasionally people complain of a chronic cough or a bitter, metallic taste in the back of the throat or mouth, instead of heartburn.

Usual time of onset: 1st, 2nd or 3rd trimester.

Cause: Three reasons.

◆ There's a muscle at the junction of the esophagus and stomach called the lower esophageal sphincter (see illustration at right) that usually keeps stomach acid where it belongs. Pregnancy hormones relax that muscle, allowing the acid to move up into the esophagus (reflux).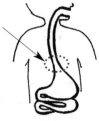

◆ The whole gastrointestinal tract slows down in pregnancy, giving both food and stomach acid more time to sit around and move up into the esophagus.

◆ The growing fetus and uterus push up on the stomach, which doesn't help matters.

Treatment:

◆ Avoid food and drinks that can worsen symptoms: caffeine, chocolate, citrus fruits, acidic foods, tomatoes and tomato sauce, greasy or fried food. We know, all the good stuff!

◆ Sleep with your head and chest slightly elevated, on pillows or a wedge.

◆ Try over-the-counter antacids like Tums, Maalox, or Mylanta.

◆ Consider over-the-counter "H2 blocker" acid reducers like ranitidine (Zantac), famotidine (Pepcid), or cimetidine (Tagamet).

◆ Probiotics may be helpful—these are pills, powders or liquids.

◆ If you are miserable, ask your doc about taking a prescription "proton pump inhibitor" acid reducer, such as Prevacid. Or a medication called metoclopramide (Reglan) that helps food move more quickly through the stomach. See Medications at Expecting411.com/extra.

Red Flags:

◆ Severe chest pain that isn't related to meals.

◆ Vomiting blood and heartburn or chest pain.

◆ Shortness of breath and chest pain.

 Old Wives Tale
If you have heartburn, you will have a hairy baby.
Maybe. Heartburn-afflicted pregnant women usually make more

progesterone than their friends. It is the high levels of progesterone that act to relax and open the lower esophageal sphincter, allowing acid to creep up out of the stomach and cause heartburn. That same progesterone also stimulates hair growth in the fetus. So, yes, if you have really bad heartburn, you just might deliver a baby with a full head of hair!

FYI: It is fairly common for pregnant women to experience sharp pain or an uncomfortable sensation around their belly buttons. Some pregnant belly buttons are very sensitive to touch, similar to your nipples. This usually happens somewhere smack dab in the middle of the second trimester. If you aren't having any other symptoms (nausea, vomiting, pain elsewhere in your abdomen or back, diarrhea, fever or pain with urination), don't worry. This will go away soon.

Note: If you are experiencing shooting pains in your rectum, you'll find the info you need in the gynecologic section to follow.

Girl Parts

- ◆ Pelvic cramps
- ◆ Braxton Hicks contractions (practice contractions)
- ◆ Vaginal discharge
- ◆ Varicose veins in outer genital area (vulva)
- ◆ Spotting
- ◆ Swelling/discomfort
- ◆ Shooting pains in vagina/rectum
- ◆ Itching of outer genital area (vulva)

Q. I'm seven weeks and having some mild cramps, like when I get my period. Is this okay?

Symptom: Pelvic cramps.
Usual time of onset: 1st trimester.
Cause: Your uterus is growing to accommodate the fetus. Since most of the uterus is made up of muscle, it often "cramps" during this process.
Treatment: None, its totally normal.
Red Flags:
- ◆ Vaginal bleeding and pelvic pain.
- ◆ Severe pelvic pain.
- ◆ Pelvic pain on one side (left or right) rather than in the middle.

Contact your practitioner if you have one of these red flag symptoms and read Chapter 15, Pregnancy 911 for details.

Q. I'm 22 weeks and having some mild cramps, like when I get my period. Is this normal?

Symptom: Pelvic cramps.
Usual time of onset: Late 2nd trimester.
Cause: Several possibilities.
- ◆ Often, it's the same reason as before: your baby is growing, causing your uterus to expand—again, feels like mild cramps.

NORMAL?

- Sometimes, the uterus is practicing for labor (**BRAXTON HICKS CONTRACTIONS**).
- Occasionally, a bladder infection can cause uterine cramping as the bladder sits right on top of the uterus. This may be your only symptom.
- Sometimes, the uterus can contract after intercourse, particularly if you had an orgasm.
- Rarely, it's premature labor.

Treatment: Rest, drink lots of fluids, and notify your practitioner. Most of the time, there is nothing to worry about and you may have just overdone it during the day . . . but let your practitioner decide.

Red Flags:
- You feel your uterus getting hard with or without vaginal bleeding and pelvic cramps.
- Increased vaginal discharge and pelvic cramps.
- Vaginal bleeding with pelvic cramps.
- Watery fluid leaking from the vagina and pelvic cramps.
- Severe, constant abdominal pain.
- Painful urination and pelvic cramps.
- Vomiting and pelvic cramps.
- Fever and pelvic cramps.
- Diarrhea and pelvic cramps.

Q. I'm 35 weeks and having some mild cramps, like when I get my period. Is this normal?

Symptom: Pelvic cramps.

Usual time of onset: 3rd trimester.

Cause: Braxton Hicks contractions or real labor contractions. This may just be your uterus doing calisthenics as a warm-up for the big day—or it may be real labor. Remember: Braxton Hicks contractions happen sporadically, they don't usually hurt, and you can sit, breathe, and talk through them.

Treatment: Rest. Drink lots of fluids. And notify your OB just so she can help decipher what is going on.

Red Flags:
- You feel your uterus getting hard and pelvic cramps.
- Vaginal bleeding and pelvic cramps.
- Watery fluid leaking from the vagina and pelvic cramps.
- Severe, constant abdominal pain or pelvic cramps.
- Painful urination and pelvic cramps.
- Vomiting and pelvic cramps.
- Fever and pelvic cramps.
- Diarrhea and pelvic cramps.

Q. I'm noticing quite a bit of discharge on my underwear. Is that normal?

Symptom: Vaginal discharge. You may have so much that you're forced to wear a panty liner every day.

Usual time of onset: Right from the beginning . . . all the way until the end.

Cause: There's more blood flow to the vaginal area, which leads to an increase in the normal vaginal discharge.

Treatment: Unfortunately, there is no treatment except childbirth. Bring a change (or two) of underwear with you each day so you can do a midday swap. Some women feel more comfortable wearing a panty liner every day. Caution: Daily panty liner use can lead to irritation of your outer genital area (vulva and vagina).

Red Flags:
- Itching and increased vaginal discharge.
- Burning and increased vaginal discharge.
- Painful urination and increased vaginal discharge.
- Abdominal pain and increased vaginal discharge.
- A change in the color or odor of your typical vaginal discharge.
- Bloody vaginal discharge.
- Watery vaginal discharge.

Q. I noticed a little bit of blood on the toilet paper when I was wiping myself. Is everything okay? I am panicking.

Symptom: Spotting or minimal vaginal bleeding.

Usual time of onset: Any point during the pregnancy.

Cause: Yes, this is scary to see when you are pregnant. Most of the time, it's not serious. It can be due to a broken blood vessel in the vagina or on the cervix, a yeast infection, recent intercourse or a tiny bit of bleeding from the area where the placenta meets the uterus. You may also see blood from other places in the vicinity of the vagina—like from the urethra with a bladder infection or from the anus in the case of a hemorrhoid. You can also have a bit of spotting if you just had a recent exam by your practitioner.

SPOTTING IN EARLY PREGNANCY. IS IT A PERIOD?

Yes, you can have some spotting. No, it's not a period.

The word "period" (or **MENSTRUAL PERIOD**) refers to the end of a monthly menstrual cycle when an egg is not fertilized, does not implant, and therefore, a pregnancy does not occur. When a woman's body realizes it is not going to nurture a pregnancy, part of the **ENDOMETRIUM** (inner lining of the uterus) sloughs off and some vaginal bleeding occurs for two to seven days.

If an egg is fertilized by a sperm and does implant, a period does not occur because the hormones change and the endometrium is needed to nourish and sustain the pregnancy.

That said, you can still have some spotting (a few drops of blood that stain a panty liner or undies) or light bleeding during a normal pregnancy. It's just not a "period." If this occurs between week three and four, it is often due to **IMPLANTATION BLEEDING**, when the embryo finds a good spot and nestles into your endometrium. There are other causes of bleeding during pregnancy, but these are not "periods" either.

Bottom line: Even though there may not be a problem, you should always discuss *any* vaginal bleeding during pregnancy with your practitioner.

? ?

NORMAL?

External genitalia

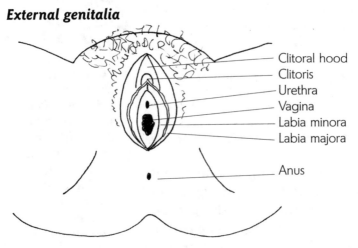

Clitoral hood
Clitoris
Urethra
Vagina
Labia minora
Labia majora

Anus

normal!?

Treatment: Always talk to your practitioner. A little bit of blood with no other symptoms can wait until normal office hours—unless you are a high-risk pregnancy, in which case you should notify your practitioner at the time of bleeding.

Red Flags:

◆ A lot of blood (the same amount or more than a light period).
◆ Severe abdominal pain/cramping and spotting.
◆ Watery vaginal discharge and spotting.
◆ Painful urination and spotting.
◆ Fever/chills and spotting.
◆ Dizziness and spotting.
◆ Diarrhea and spotting.
◆ Known high-risk pregnancy and spotting.*

* This refers to women with a **PLACENTA PREVIA,** preterm labor, **CHRONIC PLACENTAL ABRUPTION, SUBCHORIONIC HEMATOMA**, shortened cervix with or without a cerclage or those carrying multiples.

Q. My genital area feels swollen and tender. Did I do something wrong? Will there be any problems with delivery?

Symptom: Swollen **VULVA** (the collective term for your external girl parts—labia, clitoris, outer part of vagina—see illustration).

Usual time of onset: Late 2nd and 3rd trimesters.

Cause: During pregnancy, more blood flows to the entire female genital tract, including the vulva. This makes the area swell. Some women may also get varicose veins in the labia (lips), and that makes things even more swollen and tender. Rarely do these issues cause a problem during delivery.

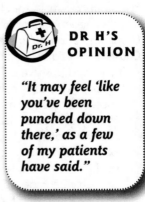

DR H'S OPINION

"It may feel 'like you've been punched down there,' as a few of my patients have said."

Treatment: Rest and wear a properly adjusted maternity belt. This lifts the uterus up and takes pressure off of every-

NORMAL?

? ?

thing below it. Look for one with "vulvar support" if you have severe swelling or significant varicose veins of the vulva.

Red Flags:

- ◆ Itching and swollen vulva.
- ◆ Burning and swollen vulva.
- ◆ A change in your typical vaginal discharge and swollen vulva.
- ◆ Vaginal bleeding and swollen vulva.

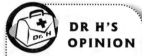

DR H'S OPINION

"One of my patients was horrified after looking at her genital area with a mirror. She said the outside of her vagina looked like a baboon's backside. Look at your own risk."

Q. I was sitting at dinner with my husband the other night and I started getting very sharp shooting pains in my vagina and rectum. They only lasted a few seconds but they were very painful. Is that normal?

Symptom: Knife or lightening-like shooting pain in the vaginal and rectal area. It lasts a few seconds, and is often repetitive.

Usual time of onset: Late 2nd and 3rd trimesters.

Cause: The baby puts pressure on the nerves that live in that area. A growing uterus and a moving baby conspire here as well.

Treatment: Get up and move around. That encourages the baby to move and (hopefully) alleviates the pain. Sitting or standing for long periods of time can trigger this pain. Try lying down on your side to see if that relieves the discomfort.

Red Flags:

- ◆ Pain that lasts more than a few minutes.
- ◆ Abdominal pain and shooting vaginal/rectal pain.
- ◆ Bleeding and shooting vaginal/rectal pain.
- ◆ Leaking watery vaginal discharge and shooting vaginal/rectal pain.

Q. I often feel itchy down there, like when I have a yeast infection. Is that normal?

Symptom: External vaginal itchiness, known as garden variety **VAGINITIS** (inflammation and irritation of the vagina, but no infection).

Usual time of onset: 2nd and 3rd trimesters.

Cause: Increased swelling of the vagina and increased vaginal discharge. If you used to shave or wax your pubic hair and now you've stopped, the hair is itchy as all heck as it grows back in. However, infection is still a possibility. Yeast loves pregnant women. There's more sugar in your vaginal discharge so that means your vagina is a great place for yeast to grow. *Treatment:* See your practitioner. She can take a look at your discharge under the microscope and tell you if there is an infection or not. If it's *not* an infection:

- ◆ Change underwear at least once throughout the day.
- ◆ Avoid wearing tight-fitting clothing, wearing underwear at night,

bubble baths and hot baths.

◆   Apply 1% hydrocortisone ointment to temporarily relieve the itching.
Red Flags: None.

Kidneys & Bladder

◆   Increased urination, night-time urination
◆   Lack of bladder control (incontinence)

Q. I need to pee all the time. Do I have a bladder infection or diabetes?

Symptom: Frequent urination. You may get up at night once, twice or even
   three times.
Usual time of onset: 1st and 3rd trimesters, but often throughout.
Cause: Elevated hormone levels and the pressure of the ever-enlarging
   uterus on the bladder. The bladder literally sits right on top of the uterus
   and as the uterus grows, the bladder is stretched. Once you enter your
   third trimester, you usually have extreme pressure on your bladder from
   your baby's head as well. Most pregnant women are very thirsty and
   pee all the time. This does not mean that you have diabetes.
Treatment: Because you need to be well-hydrated during pregnancy,
   there isn't much you can do. Avoid drinking right before bed (we know,
   its almost impossible because you are so darn thirsty all the time). Avoid
   caffeine. Empty your bladder just before getting into bed at night even
   if you don't have the urge to go.
Red Flags:
   ◆   Painful urination and frequent urination.
   ◆   Blood in your urine, frequent urination, fever, back pain.

Q. Every time I laugh or cough, I leak a little urine. Will this end after pregnancy?

Symptom: Lack of bladder control. You may leak urine so often that you

Your Body Organs

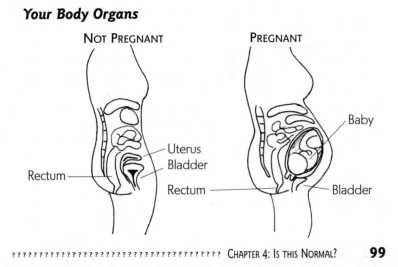

NORMAL?

? ?

need to wear a panty liner for that and your vaginal discharge too.

Usual time of onset: Late 2nd and 3rd trimesters. If this is not your first pregnancy, it may happen earlier. Sorry!

Cause: The pressure of the growing uterus on your bladder interferes with its ability to hold urine. Anything that increases your abdominal pressure (coughing, laughing, sneezing) will be the tipping point for your ure-thral sphincter (the muscle that prevents urine leakage until you decide it's time to release it). Your baby's kicking or moving can do it as well.

Treatment: Empty your bladder every two to three hours even if you feel like you don't have to go. Wear a panty liner or bring a change of under-wear in your purse. This is temporary. (After you deliver, you'll exchange the undies for a baby diaper in your purse for the next three years!)

Red Flags:

- ◆ Leaking urine when you haven't been laughing, coughing, or sneezing.
- ◆ Leaking urine while at rest.
- ◆ Painful urination and leaking urine. If there is pain, make sure your doc confirms you don't have a bladder infection.
- ◆ You'll want to be sure that the leaking liquid is urine and not amniotic fluid (your water bag). This is especially true if it happens spontaneously.

Skin, Hair & Nails

- ◆ Strange hair growth
- ◆ Glow
- ◆ Black line (linea nigra)
- ◆ Itching
- ◆ Skin tags and moles
- ◆ Spider veins
- ◆ Sweaty
- ◆ Dark splotches (melasma/chloasma)
- ◆ Hair and nail growth
- ◆ Acne
- ◆ Stretch marks
- ◆ Red palms and soles
- ◆ Chafing (intertrigo)
- ◆ Varicose veins

Q. I have hair growing in some strange places. Do I need to buy a mangroomer?

Symptom: Hair growth, often involving your face, arm, belly, and around the colored part of your nipples (**AREOLAE**).

Usual time of onset: 2nd and 3rd trimesters.

Cause: Yes, once again the elevated hormone levels that are responsible for so many other fun things that happen to your body work their magic here too.

Treatment: Shaving, plucking, waxing are all okay. Steer clear of hair removal creams (for example, Nair) and laser removal since we don't know if they are safe to use during pregnancy. Warning for waxers: Your skin may be much more sensitive to waxing right now. Ask your practitioner about applying a numbing cream (such as EMLA) before the wax job.

Red Flags: None, for the most part.

? ?

NORMAL?

Q. My hair and nails are growing much faster than normal. Is this okay?

Symptom: Accelerated hair and nail growth. It's good news—your hair and nails may get thicker (temporarily).

Usual time of onset: 2nd and 3rd trimesters.

Cause: Elevated hormone levels trigger most hair follicles to grow. Hormones also thicken nails and make them grow faster. Additionally, this may be the first time in your life that you are taking a multivitamin, extra calcium and a DHA supplement. These can all aid in hair and nail growth.

Treatment: No treatment needed. Enjoy the new you! You can still get regular manicures/pedicures and see your hairstylist (see Chapter 9, Spa Treatment for do's and don't during pregnancy).

Red Flags: None. However, hair LOSS during pregnancy can be a red flag. See box below.

Reality Check

You get a beautiful mane during pregnancy because most of your hair grows all at once. However, that same hair is also lost all at once (instead of losing hair in phases, which happens when you aren't pregnant). About three months after you deliver (the range is one to five months), be prepared for A LOT of hair to drop out in clumps both in the shower and your hairbrush. Dr H: Yes, it is alarming—even I was alarmed when I saw what was falling out in my shower and I do this for a living!

HAIR LOSS DURING PREGNANCY

As if pregnancy isn't enough to deal with, other health issues can crop up, too. If your hair is thinner, more brittle, or falling out during pregnancy, tell your practitioner. Thyroid disease, vitamin and mineral deficiency, certain collagen vascular diseases (example: lupus) and other rare disorders like **ALOPECIA AREATA** can all cause hair changes. It's most concerning if you have bald patches, balding in the front (male-pattern baldness), or massive hair loss.

Treatment obviously depends on what's causing the hair loss. But here are some general tips for everyone:

♦ Avoid chronic styling (and heating) of your hair with a blow dryer or curling/straightening iron.

♦ Avoid braids, weaves, or anything that pulls hair tightly and puts stress on the hair follicles.

♦ Use biotin-containing shampoos.

♦ Use a conditioner each time you wash your hair.

♦ Do not brush your hair while it's wet (if possible).

♦ Drink plenty of water, and eat fruits and vegetables (never a bad idea).

NORMAL?

? ?

Q. I've always heard about having a pregnancy "glow." I haven't seen mine yet. Does it happen to everyone?

Symptom: A healthy appearing shiny face and skin. Not everyone gets it, so no worries.

Usual time of onset: 2nd and 3rd trimesters.

Cause: Elevated hormone levels get your oil glands revved up to make more oil. Plus, you also have 50% more blood volume compared to your non-pregnant friends—that blood circulation makes your cheeks and face look rosier and healthier.

Treatment: Enjoy it! If your face gets too oily you can switch to an oil-free daily cleanser and moisturizer. Try using an astringent occasionally (it can be drying if you use it too often).

Red Flags: Too much "glow" (oil) leads to acne. And although this is not a "red flag" from a medical standpoint, it can be a red flag from a personal and social standpoint! See details on acne next and in Chapter 9, Spa Treatment.

Q. Help I have acne!

Symptom: Acne. Unfortunately ladies, not everyone is blessed with the pregnancy "glow"! If you suffered with acne before pregnancy, it may get even worse now. But even women who have perfect complexions may see their skin change for the worse. You may be forced to face the world looking like a teenager again.

Usual time of onset: 1st through 3rd trimesters.

Cause: Elevated hormones make the oil glands in your body secrete more oil. Oil clogs pores and causes acne.

Treatment:

- ◆ Keep your skin clean with twice-daily washes.
- ◆ Avoid sleeping in makeup.
- ◆ Avoid certain foods like nuts and chocolate (okay, it may be a myth, but it's worth a try!)
- ◆ Use topical acne medication sparingly, only on affected areas. Products containing salicylic acid, benzoyl peroxide and finacea (azelaic acid) are safe to use in SMALL amounts. Lathering them on can potentially lead to absorption into your blood stream—don't do it!
- ◆ Proactiv is okay to use in severe cases (but always check with your healthcare provider first).
- ◆ Use a moisturizer that's made for oily skin.
- ◆ If you are having persistent, worsening acne, consult a dermatologist and together with your practitioner they can come up with a plan to help. Check out Chapter 9, Spa Treatment for details.

Red Flags: None.

Q. I have developed an odd, dark discoloration on my face. What is this?

Symptom: Melasma/chloasma/mask of pregnancy. They are splotchy dark areas on your face, most often on your cheeks and forehead. Up to 40% of pregnant women get it in varying degrees.

Usual time of onset: 1st, 2nd and 3rd trimesters.

Cause: Increased melanin production that occurs during pregnancy. Exposure to the sun and UVA/UVB light makes it worse.

Treatment: Wear sunscreen (at least SPF 20) everyday and avoid sun exposure on your face. Wear a hat and sunglasses, and stay in the shade. If your melasma does not fade after your pregnancy ends, see your dermatologist. Skin docs have a few tricks to help remove or minimize the dark areas on your face.

Red Flags: None. Melasma is completely harmless and may fade after your pregnancy ends.

Q. There is a dark line extending from my pubic bone up to beyond my belly button. None of my pregnant friends have this. What is it?

Symptom: **LINEA NIGRA** (English translation "black line"): a dark line extending from the pubic bone to the belly button and in some cases, above the belly button.

Usual time of onset: Late 2nd and 3rd trimesters.

Cause: There is something called the **LINEA ALBA** (which literally means "white line" in Latin) that is present in everyone, but it's invisible when you're not pregnant. It extends from the pubic bone to well above the belly button. When you are pregnant, the increased pigment (melanin) production can temporarily "stain" this line, making it darker. The darker your skin color to begin with, the darker this line becomes. Occasionally in some women who are very fair, there is no visible line at all.

Treatment: No treatment necessary. It almost always fades in the months following your pregnancy.

Red Flags: None.

Partner Tip

If you point out that new black line and call it the "Happy Trail," you might end up sleeping on the couch. Never call attention to new skin marks on a hormonal pregnant woman.

Q. I am so worried about getting stretch marks. How common is it to get them?

Symptom: Stretch marks. If you have them, you're in good company. Approximately 90% of pregnant women get them somewhere. They are pinkish, reddish or purplish lines or streaks that occur most commonly on the breasts, abdomen, sides, buttocks or thighs.

Usual time of onset: Late 2nd and 3rd trimesters.

Cause: Stretching of the skin, particularly if the stretching is due to rapid or dramatic weight gain. Genetic predisposition is also a cause (if your mom has stretch marks, you may be more likely to develop stretch marks).

Treatment:
♦ Keep your weight gain gradual.
♦ Exercise regularly.
♦ Moisturize, moisturize, moisturize. Use daily lotions/creams/oils/butters to keep your skin soft and moist.

◆ Most stretch marks fade after delivery to look like whitish-silver lines. If they bug you, laser therapy is an option. Talk to a dermatologist when you are done making babies. See Chapter 9, Spa Treatment, for more details.

Red Flags: None.

Partner Tip
Pretend you don't see these marks, either.

Q. I'm itchy—all the time. What can I do?

Symptom: Itchy.

Usual time of onset: Late 2nd and 3rd trimesters.

Cause: Your belly is growing. As it grows, the skin stretches and tightens. This can lead to dryness, stretch marks, and yes, itching.

Treatment:

◆ Use a moisturizer twice a day and immediately after a shower or bath.

◆ Use anti-itch creams like calamine lotion, 1% hydrocortisone cream or diphenhydramine (Benadryl) cream.

◆ Avoid taking really hot showers which can dry out your skin.

◆ Drink plenty of water to stay well-hydrated.

◆ Try an oatmeal bath.

◆ Avoid long periods of time in hot weather or in the sun (which can make itching worse).

Red Flags:

◆ Nausea, vomiting, and itching.

◆ Severe fatigue and itching.

◆ Yellowing of your skin (particularly palms, soles, eyes) and itching.

◆ Any rash and itching.

Reality Check: PUPPS
Nope, it's not a new show on Animal Planet. PUPPS stands for Pruritic Urticarial Papules and Plaques. They are intensely itchy, large, raised red patches on your belly that can spread to your upper thighs, lower legs, and arms. PUPPS tortures one in 150 pregnant women. See Chapter 16, Complications for details.

Q. My palms and soles are red. Any problem?

Symptom: Red palms and soles. This is totally normal.

Usual time of onset: 2nd and 3rd trimesters.

Cause: Increased blood flow and circulation. Elevated estrogen levels.

Treatment: None.

Red Flags:

◆ Yellowing of palms and soles.

◆ Itching of only the palms and soles.

◆ Rash on palm and soles.

Q. I am noticing small growths of skin on my body, particularly under my arms. What are these and how do I get rid of them?

Symptom: Skin tags. These are small protruding growths of skin that usually show up on your neck, under your arms, on your breasts or in your groin area. They are usually flesh colored, although they can be a shade or two darker than your skin color.

Usual time of onset: 2nd and 3rd trimesters.

Cause: Yep, you guessed it, elevated hormone levels.

Treatment: Skin tags may disappear after your pregnancy ends. If they don't, your OB (or a friendly dermatologist) can freeze or snip them off. There is nothing to do about them now, unless they are large or get in the way of your clothing (such as right where your bra strap sits) and bother you.

Red Flags: Tell your doc about any large growth on any part of your body, flesh-colored or not.

Insider Secret

Your moles may get darker or more prominent. While this is a common pregnancy phenomenon, your practitioner should always check out changing moles and refer you to a dermatologist if there is a concern.

Q. I've got rolls of skin I never had before. And some of those skin areas are now red and sore. What do I do?

Symptom: Chafing (**INTERTRIGO**). These are red patches of skin usually in your armpits, under your breasts and in other skin folds.

Usual time of onset: 2nd and 3rd trimesters.

Cause: Elevated pregnancy hormone levels. Weight gain causing more skin folds than the Michelin Tire Man. We know—it's depressing, but it's temporary.

Treatment: Keep the skin in these areas extra clean and dry. Because skin folds are usually moist, they're a set up for yeast and other skin infections. If it's not infected, your doc can give you the green light to apply 1% hydrocortisone cream.

Red Flags:
- Chafing that is getting worse.
- Foul odor and chafing.
- Burning and chafing.
- Excessive itching and chafing.

Q. I have noticed a few patches of small bluish-purplish veins on my legs and feet. Do I need to worry about this?

Symptom: Spider veins on your lower extremities. They appear as broken blood vessels with a branching pattern on the skin's surface and are usually blue, purple or red.

Usual time of onset: 2nd and 3rd trimesters.

Cause: Elevated estrogen levels. You may be genetically predisposed (it runs in families).

NORMAL?

? ?

Treatment: Avoid crossing your legs when sitting down. Eating or drinking more Vitamin C may help (some studies show benefit). After delivery, most spider veins fade in a few weeks to months. If yours remain (and they bother you), dermatologists and/or vascular surgeons can treat them with local injections or laser therapy. Ask your practitioner for a referral.

Red Flags: Pain or swelling and a large area of discoloration.

Q. My mother got varicose veins when she was pregnant with me. Will I be prone to them as well?

Symptom: Varicose veins. They appear as bluish-purplish tortuous veins usually seen on the legs, but sometimes on the tops of the feet, vulva, rectum (hemorrhoids) and buttocks. Sometimes they ache a bit.

Usual time of onset: 2nd and 3rd trimesters.

Cause: Thank your genes. If someone in your family has them, you are more likely to get them during your pregnancy. Varicose veins also follow the laws of physics. When you are pregnant, the veins in the lower part of your body must work extra hard to return the blood back to your heart. Pretend your vein is a garden hose. Place a large boulder (the baby and uterus) in the middle of the hose. The part of the hose behind the boulder will bulge and possibly break as it tries to push the water against the boulder. This is what can happen to your veins during your pregnancy.

Treatment: The best treatment is prevention!

◆ Avoid sitting with your legs crossed.
◆ Avoid standing for long periods of time.
◆ When sitting, place your feet up on a few pillows so they are above the level of your body.
◆ Wear support stockings (they are far from sexy, especially in the summer time, but really help).
◆ Exercise.
◆ Take a vitamin C supplement.
◆ Avoid excessive weight gain during pregnancy.
◆ The good news: many veins drastically decrease in size over the first few weeks to months after delivery. If you want permanent removal when you're done with childbearing, get a referral to a vascular surgeon.

Red Flags:

◆ Entire leg is really painful.
◆ Swelling in one leg and varicose vein.

DR H'S OPINION: VARICOSE VEINS

I recently delivered a patient who had one of the worst cases of varicose veins I had ever seen. Yet, at her two-week postpartum check-up, I told her that I wouldn't have recognized her if I hadn't seen her face. There was such a dramatic change, with 80% improvement in her varicose veins! The take home message: delivering the baby fixes many of these pregnancy maladies!

? ?

NORMAL?

Q. I am hot and sweaty all the time despite sleeping without covers and having the air-conditioning on full blast. Will this last the whole pregnancy?

Symptom: Literally hot and sweaty 24/7.

Usual time of onset: Late 2nd and 3rd trimesters.

Cause: Elevated hormone levels make you and your menopausal mother feel the same way. View it as mother-daughter bonding. Carrying more weight around is also no friend to your thermostat.

Treatment: Buy a battery-operated fan, and take it with you everywhere. Dress in layers so you can easily adjust as the temperature changes throughout the day. Make sure you are drinking enough water. Freeze a water bottle every night so you have ice cold water the next day.

Red Flags: None.

Partner Tip
Pregnancy may be the only time that you and your partner's body thermostat are aligned. You may be able to sleep in the same bed together without a down comforter and an extra blanket. That is if her fortress of pillows doesn't come between you.

Muscle, Bone, and Nerves

◆ Round ligament pain
◆ Groin pain
◆ Pubic bone joint (symphysis) pain
◆ Low back pain
◆ Sciatic pain
◆ Leg cramps
◆ Wrist pain (carpal tunnel syndrome)

Q. I am having pain in my belly. There is a pulling or tugging pain on one side more than the other. Should I be concerned?

Symptom: Round ligament pain. Sharp pain in your abdomen or hip area, on one or both sides. The pain may occasionally extend into the groin area. Pain is brief and typically only lasts a few minutes. There are no other symptoms.

Usual time of onset: Late 1st and early 2nd trimester. It rarely occurs beyond that.

Cause: The rapidly growing uterus stretches the ligaments that attach the uterus to the sides of the abdominal wall. Any change in movement (like standing up or turning quickly) may also stretch this ligament(s) and cause pain.

Treatment: Unfortunately, there is no great treatment.

◆ Try to rest when it happens. Your body may be telling you that you're doing too much.
◆ Move and change positions more slowly.
◆ Try yoga or stretching exercises if round ligament pain happens reg-

ularly. Try this stretch: Place your hands and knees on the floor, while you lower your head to the ground and keep your tushie in the air.

◆ Try using a maternity belt.

Red Flags:

- ◆ Constant, unrelenting abdominal pain.
- ◆ Vaginal bleeding and abdominal pain.
- ◆ Watery vaginal discharge and abdominal pain.
- ◆ Vomiting and abdominal pain.
- ◆ Diarrhea and abdominal pain.
- ◆ Fever or chills and abdominal pain.

> **DR H'S OPINION**
>
> *"I used to tell my patients very casually, 'Oh, it's just round liga-ment pain,' until I experienced it with my first pregnancy. Wowser! It's not serious, but it can be very painful."*

Q. I am having pain in my groin. Do I have a hernia?

Symptom: Pain in the groin, particularly when walking or changing positions.
Usual time of onset: 2nd trimester.
Cause: Your pelvic and groin ligaments stretch and this often causes pain. Your pubic bones can also hurt. Another source for groin pain: round ligament stretching (see previous question). It is rare for this pain to be caused by a hernia (when a body organ—usually your intestines—pro-trudes through a weakness in your connective tissue).
Treatment: A maternity belt can help.
Red Flags:

- ◆ Mass or bulge and groin pain.
- ◆ Severe, persistent groin pain.
- ◆ Severe abdominal pain and groin pain.
- ◆ Vaginal bleeding and groin pain.

Q. My pelvis and hip bones hurt! They seem to be out of sync. Should this be happening?

Symptom: Symphysis pubic dysfunction/pain. Your pubic bone hurts or it hurts to stand or walk. At times, you may find it difficult to stand on one foot to wash the other one in the shower or even put on a pair of pants.
Usual time of onset: Late 2nd and 3rd trimesters.
Cause: In preparation for delivery, elevated hormone levels loosen the lig-aments that hold your pelvic bones together. This loosens your "joints" and can cause the above symptoms. Some unlucky women have the same problem with their hips or their sacroiliac joint in the back (where the hipbone and backbone meet).
Treatment:

- ◆ Wear a pelvic girdle (you can be fitted for one at certain mater-nity stores).
- ◆ Wear tighter, more supportive garments like exercise pants or Spanx undergarments.
- ◆ Ask for a referral to a licensed massage therapist or chiropractor.
- ◆ Try yoga.

Red Flags:
- ◆ Painful urination and severe pubic pain.
- ◆ Blood in your urine and severe pubic pain.
- ◆ Vaginal bleeding and severe pubic pain.
- ◆ Abdominal pain and severe pubic pain.
- ◆ Any skin changes (such as redness) in the area of the pain.

Q. My lower back is really starting to hurt. Any way I can avoid having this discomfort?

Symptom: Low back pain.

Usual time of onset: 2nd and 3rd trimesters.

Cause: As your pregnancy advances, the curvature of your spine changes. The added weight your body is carrying causes your center of gravity to shift. And loosening of ligaments (see above) contributes to back pain as well. Many pregnant gals also suffer from sciatic pain, because the sciatic nerve in their back is compressed. This feels like a sharp, shooting pain that goes from the lower back down to the legs. Not fun.

How to avoid it:
- ◆ Exercise.
- ◆ Avoid wearing high heels or completely flat shoes that do not offer any support.
- ◆ Squat to pick things up rather than bending over at the waist.
- ◆ Make a nest of pillows to get comfortable at night.
- ◆ Get enough rest.
- ◆ Work on your posture.

Treatment, once you've got it:
- ◆ Consider buying a maternity belt (around 20 to 28 weeks). Get fitted at a maternity store.
- ◆ Wear shoes with good support.
- ◆ Sleep on your side.
- ◆ Place a pillow between your knees while sleeping.
- ◆ Get a massage from a licensed massage therapist or chiropractor.
- ◆ Do stretching exercises upon waking and just before bed at night.
- ◆ Use a lumbar support pillow while sitting for long periods or driving.
- ◆ Use a heating pad.
- ◆ Take some acetaminophen (Tylenol).

Red flags:
- ◆ Painful urination and low back pain.
- ◆ Fever or chills and low back pain.
- ◆ Nausea or vomiting and low back pain.
- ◆ Abdominal pain and low back pain.
- ◆ Severe, constant low back pain that doesn't improve with any of the above treatments.
- ◆ Repetitive, rhythmic cramping pain in the back (concern: sometimes a sign of preterm or term labor contractions).

Old Wives Tale
Lifting heavy objects will cause a miscarriage.

NORMAL?

? ?

False. However, lifting heavy objects *will* cause back pain.

This is an international old wives tale, not just an American one. The story goes that lifting heavy objects can cause: a miscarriage, the baby to get tangled up in its umbilical cord, or the baby to turn into a breech (bottom or foot/feet first) position.

All of these are false.

But you are more likely to suffer a back injury during pregnancy if you lift heavy things. We don't recommend that you carry around your 35-pound toddler or rearrange furniture, even though we know it seems unavoidable. A word to the wise: no heavy lifting.

DR H'S TRUE STORY: MOVING FURNITURE AT 28 WEEKS

You should have seen the look on my husband's face when he saw his wife in her 28th week of pregnancy sitting in a completely "redecorated" home office, complete with a new location for the desk and bookcase. It seemed like a good idea at the time....

Q. I've started having shooting pain on my left (or right) side going from my buttocks down the back of my leg. Is this something to be worried about?

Symptom: Sharp, shooting pain or burning on the backside of either leg. It may feel like "pins and needles" in the lower back or leg, and/or numbness in the leg or foot. It begins near the buttocks and travels down the back of the leg, sometimes all the way to the foot.

Usual time of onset: Late 2nd and 3rd trimester.

Cause: Sciatic nerve pain. Swelling in the tissues where the sciatic nerve exits the pelvis or pressure on the nerve by the enlarging uterus are the causes. It's also possible to reactivate an old injury, if you've had one before.

Treatment:
- ◆ Avoid walking up or down hills.
- ◆ Skip the high heels and ballet flats. Wear comfortable shoes with some degree of support. Although they aren't glamorous, a good pair of tennis shoes or clogs are perfect.
- ◆ Rest more and lie on the side that doesn't hurt.
- ◆ Limit how much you stand up.
- ◆ Avoid heavy lifting.
- ◆ Take a warm bath, or place a heating pad on the area.
- ◆ Use acetaminophen (Tylenol) if necessary.
- ◆ Get a massage (by your partner or a professional).
- ◆ Buy a maternity belt.
- ◆ Get a physical therapy/chiropractor referral from your practitioner.

Red Flags:
- ◆ Severe, constant pain.
- ◆ A foot that drags or drops.
- ◆ Cannot walk.
- ◆ Swelling in one leg.

NORMAL?

Old Wives Tale
Your shoe size changes after pregnancy.

False, for most of us.

During pregnancy, your feet swell so much you may only be able to wear flip-flops, UGG boots or like one of my patients, her husband's orange crocs. But for most of us, foot swelling goes away a couple of weeks after delivery. You'll be back in your old shoes in no time.

A few women increase their foot size permanently. Elevated estrogen levels may lengthen the plantar ligaments in the feet.

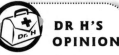

DR H'S OPINION

"Luckily, this wasn't the case for me because as my husband will tell you, I have invested way too much money in shoes!"

Q. I wake up in the middle of the night screaming because of cramps in my calf muscles. Do I need to take some vitamins or something?

Symptom: Severe leg cramps, most often in the calves, most often at night, leading you to scream out profanities and scare your significant other half to death. Don't be surprised if your calf muscle is still sore a day or two after a middle-of-the-night attack.

Usual time of onset: Late 2nd and 3rd trimesters.

Cause: No one really knows why pregnant women have more leg cramps or why they happen more often at night. It's possible that your leg muscles are tired from carrying around all of your extra weight. And remember that your expanding uterus changes your blood circulation. Your leg muscles may not like this change.

How to avoid it:
- Don't sit with your legs crossed for long periods of time.
- Stretch your calf muscles before bedtime.
- Walk or exercise daily.
- Keep well hydrated.
- Wear support stockings.
- Take a warm bath.
- Get a bedtime leg massage from your partner.

Treatment:
- Keep a leather strap by your bedside, insert into your mouth and bite down. (Just kidding—sorry, that's a bit of twisted OB/GYN humor).
- Try this stretch: straighten your leg by pushing out your heel first, then flexing your toes back towards your shin. This might not feel so great at first, but the spasm in your calf muscle will slowly ease.
- Apply local heat with a heating pad or warm washcloth.
- Try a magnesium supplement (if your practitioner thinks it's safe for you—check first). This won't treat the current cramp but may help prevent future episodes.

Red Flags:
- Muscle pain persisting for more than a day or two.

NORMAL?

? ?

◆ Swelling or tenderness in the leg and severe leg cramps—this would require immediate medical attention. Pregnancy puts you at higher risk for a blood clot. They are rare, but they are serious. Call your practitioner immediately for any of the "Red Flag" symptoms.

Q. My wrists and fingers have started to tingle and get numb. Why is that?

Symptom: Hand or fingers hurt or feel numb and tingle. But pain can also shoot up the forearm. It typically only involves the thumb, pointer and middle fingers. This is called Carpal Tunnel Syndrome (CTS). Symptoms are usually most intense at night and upon waking in the morning.

Usual time of onset: Late 2nd and 3rd trimester.

Cause: Swelling around your wrist puts pressure on the nerves and blood vessels that travel to your hand.

Treatment:

◆ Wear a wrist brace at night to relieve the discomfort.
◆ Limit your salt intake to decrease overall swelling.
◆ Avoid repetitive movements (like typing on a computer keyboard) that make it worse.
◆ Get physical therapy referral.

Red Flags:

◆ Pain in your neck and shoulders with hand pain/numbness.
◆ Loss of sensation in your hands and/or fingers.
◆ Unable to hold objects in your hand.

Immune System

See Chapter 17, Infections, for details on your body's immune system changes and all your questions about preventing and treating infections during pregnancy.

But here is a brief summary of what you need to know: Your immune system is seriously suppressed during pregnancy because it has to be. Yes, this is the only time that you can have foreign DNA (husband's, boyfriend's, partner's, the sperm donor's, etc.) in your body and not reject it.

If you got a kidney transplant, you would need serious immunosuppressive medication in order to not reject the donated kidney. Your body does this on its own during pregnancy. But a lowered immune system means that you are more susceptible to EVERYTHING . . . the common cold, cold sores, herpes outbreaks (if you have a history of these)—and everything your toddler brings home from preschool.

Now that you feel a bit more in touch with your body (for better or worse!), let's move on to all the poking and prodding you'll experience to ensure you and your baby are having a healthy pregnancy.

TESTS
Chapter 5

"First the doctor told me the good news: I was going to have a disease named after me."
—Steve Martin

Yes, you will have to endure many tests while you are pregnant. Good news: you don't have to study for any of them. But you may be curious as to *why* your practitioner needs a pint of your blood (okay, really a few tablespoons), makes you pee in a cup all the time, or in certain cases, recommends testing that's a bit more intrusive (like putting a needle into your uterus).

That's why this chapter is here. It covers the tests you'll be taking, from A to Z.

As you'll discover, some tests are routine (usually blood and urine tests) and recommended for all pregnant women to help ensure a healthy pregnancy. If a test comes back abnormal, your practitioner can investigate further and potentially offer treatment to protect you and your baby.

Other tests are optional and are more useful for certain women at risk for particular problems or complications.

Our goal: this chapter aims to make you an empowered parent-to-be, armed with the information you need to make decisions about having some or all of these tests.

Before we get going, a word about tests and their limitations—science and technology have come a long way since our moms were pregnant with us. Yet despite the dizzying array of tests, none of them can guarantee your baby will be 100% perfect when born. Nothing in life is guaranteed and that rule applies here too. That's why your baby's pediatrician examines your newborn shortly after birth to make sure everything is ok.

Lots o' tests, and when they're done

FIRST TRIMESTER TESTS	WHEN?	ROUTINE	OPTIONAL	ADDITIONAL
Blood tests				
Complete blood count (CBC)	First visit	✔		
Blood type; Rh/antibody screen	First visit	✔		
Hepatitis B testing	First visit	✔		
HIV testing	First visit	✔		
Syphilis	First visit	✔		
Rubella immunity testing	Before conception or first trimester		✔	
Varicella immunity testing (unless you've had chicken pox)	Before conception or first trimester		✔	
Cystic fibrosis screen	Before conception or first trimester		✔	
Fragile X carrier screening	First/second visit		✔	
Sickle Cell Anemia Screen	First visit		✔	
Hemoglobin electrophoresis	First trimester		✔	
Ashkenazi Jewish Panel	Before conception or first trimester		✔	
First trimester screen	10–13 weeks		✔	
Urine tests				
Urinalysis (U/A)	Every visit	✔		
Urine culture	First visit and when indicated	✔		✔
Other tests				
Ultrasound, vaginal	First visit and later if indicated		✔	✔
Blood pressure	Every visit	✔		
Pap smear (if you haven't had a recent one)	First visit	✔		
Cervical cultures (Chlamydia/Gonorrhea)	First visit	✔		
GBS vaginal culture (if having a CVS)	Within 2 weeks of CVS			✔
Chorionic Villus Sampling (CVS)	10–13 weeks		✔	✔

SECOND TRIMESTER TESTS	WHEN?	ROUTINE	OPTIONAL	ADDITIONAL
Second trimester screen (AFP/QUAD)	15–20 weeks		✔	
Ultrasound, abdominal	18–22 weeks		✔	✔
Ultrasound, vaginal	When indicated			✔
Amniocentesis	15–20 weeks		✔	✔
One hour Glucola	24–28 weeks	✔		
Three hour Glucose Tolerance (recommended if one hour Glucola is positive)	24–28 weeks			✔
Fetal Fibronectin	22–34 weeks			✔
Fetal kick counts	26–42 weeks	✔		

? ?

TESTS

THIRD TRIMESTER TESTS	WHEN?	ROUTINE	OPTIONAL	ADDITIONAL
Fetal kick counts	26–42 weeks	✔		
Ultrasound, abdominal	32–36 weeks			✔
Repeat CBC	32–36 weeks			✔
Repeat cervical cultures	32 weeks			✔
Repeat syphilis, HIV	32 weeks			✔
Non-stress test	28–42 weeks			✔
Contraction Stress Test	28–42 weeks			✔
Biophysical Profile	28–42 weeks			✔
Group B Strep vaginal/rectal culture	35–37 weeks	✔		

ADDITIONAL SPECIALIZED TESTS ADDITIONAL	WHEN?	ROUTINE	OPTIONAL	ADDITIONAL
Parvovirus titers	When indicated			✔
Toxoplasmosis titers	First visit or later			✔
CMV titers	First visit or later			✔
Herpes culture	First visit or later			✔

Key:

Routine Tests. These are screening tests recommended and routinely done on all pregnant women. Example: complete blood count (CBC).

Optional Tests. These are tests that may be useful for pregnant women whose individual medical history, age, or ethnic background puts them at risk for the disorders being tested. Example: Ashkenazi Jewish Screening Panel.

Additional Tests. These are tests done at your practitioner's discretion based on individual circumstances that arise during pregnancy. Example: A hemoglobin electrophoresis is an *additional test* that may be ordered by your practitioner based on your CBC results and ethnic background.

Chocolate Tests. These are tests involving the sampling of 67 varieties of chocolate. (Just kidding!)

FYI: A *screening test* identifies a person to be *at risk* for a certain disorder or complication. A positive screening test only means that more tests need to be done to make a diagnosis. A *diagnostic test* confirms that a person has a disorder or disease. Example: a woman who fails her "one hour glucola" screening test does not necessarily have pregnancy-related diabetes. She will end up doing a diagnostic test—in this case, a fun-filled three-hour glucose tolerance test—which determines if she has the disorder.

Heads up: This chapter is jam-packed with information, some of which is highly technical. We are going to do our best to explain it to you in English, in an organized fashion. We'll cover the tests in the order you will have them done or offered to you. And for each test, we'll note if it is routine, optional, or additional. If you are lost, just refer to the index to find the location of a specific test.

TESTS

? ?

TRUE POSITIVES VERSUS FALSE POSITIVES

Here's how to wrap your head around this concept.

Imagine a screening test is a fisherman's shrimp net. You want a net that catches all the shrimp ("true positive") and doesn't let them slip through the holes (that is, missing a true problem). But the net also picks up seaweed along with the shrimp. The seaweed is a "false positive" on a screening test.

Q. There are so many optional tests and many of them are expensive. How can I decide which tests I should do and which ones to skip?

Life was so much simpler when our parents were pregnant. As our moms like to remind us, they were never tested for diabetes nor did they have a single ultrasound during their pregnancies. They also casually mention that they didn't even put us in car seats when we were babies. We've come a long way, haven't we?

Today, there are so many tests it can make your head spin! While your gut says have every possible test done to check every possible thing, your pocketbook (or insurance company) may think otherwise.

The American Congress of Obstetricians and Gynecologists (ACOG) recommends certain tests in order to make sure all pregnant woman get high-quality obstetric care. It's likely your insurance will cover the costs of all of those tests.

If you are delivering with a doctor, he or she will tell you which tests ACOG recommends. Other tests are your call.

Some optional tests are a good idea for all pregnant women. Other tests are most useful for certain at-risk ethnic groups or certain ages. You should discuss these tests with your practitioner to find out which are most important for you. This chapter will help you consider your options.

Partner Tip

As you glance through this chapter, you'll notice a boatload of tests your pregnant other half will be enduring. Your job: be there and be supportive. It's the little things that count: holding a hand, making a joke to distract from the needle, etc. And when test results are returned, be the rock. Your pregnant partner will need calm reassurance that everything will be fine.

There are also occasional tests that can be done on either partner (cystic fibrosis testing for example). Offering to do one or more of these tests will win you some mighty big brownie points.

1st Trimester Tests

1st trimester, routine tests
BLOOD WORK, BLOOD PRESSURE, URINALYSIS, PAP SMEAR, CULTURES

TESTS

Q. I had tubes and tubes of blood taken at my first pre-natal appointment. Why?

There are certain tests that are recommended for every pregnant woman in order to identify potential health problems for mom and baby. The results of these tests are important to both your practitioner and your future baby's practitioner.

The standard tests include:

1 **COMPLETE BLOOD COUNT (CBC).** This test identifies women who have **ANEMIA** (see Chapter 16, Complications, complication #13).

People who are anemic carry less oxygen via their red blood cells to body tissues. There are many different causes of anemia, but it's most commonly due to iron-deficiency.

Your pregnant body requires more oxygen than your pre-pregnancy body. Plus, you will lose a good bit of blood during childbirth. So, it's particularly important to detect anemia and treat it as soon as possible. For iron-deficiency anemia, treatment is pretty simple. Eat iron-rich foods and take an iron supplement. (See Chapter 16, Complications for more info.)

Other abnormalities on a CBC alert us to check for inherited blood disorders (such as **SICKLE CELL DISEASE** and the **THALASSEMIAS**) that can potentially be passed on to the baby.

The CBC also tells us your platelet count. Platelets are the cells that help clot your blood when you are cut. Certain conditions reduce platelet levels, so practitioners need to be aware of these as well (see Chapter 16, Complications, complication #17).

2 **YOUR BLOOD TYPE AND RH.** Both your practitioner and your baby's pediatrician will want to know your blood type.

You've probably heard of blood types but how are these determined? Well, your blood cells have a protein that sits on the cell's surface. There are two proteins: "A" and "B." You can have one protein ("A" or "B"), both ("AB"), or no protein at all ("O").

Then, there is another group of proteins called the Rh factor (Rh stands for Rhesus). If you have Rh proteins, you are Rh-positive. If you don't, you are Rh-negative. FYI: 85% of all people are Rh positive.

So, for example, if you have both an A protein and a Rh protein on your blood cells, your blood type is "A positive." If you have no major blood type proteins or Rh proteins, your blood type is "O negative."

If mom's blood type is "Rh negative," her body could mount an immune response to her baby if he is "Rh positive" (this is not a good thing). Long before delivery, the baby can develop severe anemia. You'll need to receive an injection called **RHOGAM** during your pregnancy to prevent this response. (More info on Rhogam in Chapter 16, Complications, complication #14).

Your baby's doctor wants to know your blood type because if a baby is born with "A" or "B" blood type and you are "O," your newborn may be at greater risk for jaundice in the first few days of life (**ABO INCOMPATIBILITY**).

3 **INFECTIOUS DISEASE PANEL (HIV, HEPATITIS B, SYPHILIS (RPR), RUBELLA).** These diseases cause health problems for both the mother and the unborn baby. For example, a mother who had a previous Hepatitis B infection is now a carrier and can pass it on to her baby. Those babies need two shots shortly after birth to prevent Hepatitis B infection.

Bottom line: knowing whether or not you have/had one of these infections is critical for both you and your baby. Check out Chapter 17, Infections, for more details.

Insider Secret

ACOG does not recommend routinely testing for thyroid function. However, some doctors test their patients for this because altered thyroid function can lead to complications during pregnancy.

Real World Tip

It's extremely important for medical providers to know the results of the routine prenatal lab work when your baby is delivered. The lab results should be on your chart when you are admitted to the hospital.

But just in case things don't go as well as planned, ask for a copy of these test results so you can carry them to the hospital!

Q. Why is my blood pressure tested at every visit?

Your blood pressure is one of the most basic ways to assess your body's health—that's why docs always check it whether you are pregnant or not. It's even more important to check your blood pressure during pregnancy because (as you know from reading the last chapter) you aren't living in the same body you were before this baby came along.

Some women experience pregnancy-induced high blood pressure that needs to be monitored and occasionally treated (see Chapter 15, Complications, complications #20, 21). And some women have high blood pressure *before* becoming pregnant. That needs monitoring and treatment, too.

Practitioners check your blood pressure at the first office visit to make sure everything is normal. It is checked again at future visits to make sure it isn't getting too high.

By definition, 140/90 is high blood pressure (or **HYPERTENSION**). But when you are pregnant, trends are also important.

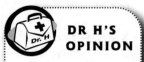

DR H'S OPINION

"My doc radar goes on red alert if I have a patient whose blood pressure was 90/60 in her first trimester and is now 130/80 in the third trimester. This is a patient that must be followed very closely!"

FYI: Your blood pressure. The first number (or the number on top) is the systolic (S) pressure, the force on the arteries when the heart is pumping. The lower number (the number on the bottom) is the diastolic (D) pressure, the force on the arteries when the heart is resting. Blood pressure is quoted as S/D.

There's a wide range of normal. For example, "normal" for you may be 90/60 or it could be 120/78. What's not normal: 140 or higher for the systolic pressure—or 90 or higher for the diastolic pressure.

TESTS

Q. Why is my urine tested at every visit?

It is amazing what a few drops of pee can tell us about you!

First, bladder infections. For non-pregnant gals, detecting a bladder infection is easy—it hurts like the dickens to pee, and you have the urge to go every ten minutes. But many pregnant women with bladder infections do not have any symptoms at all. If this isn't treated, it can become a kidney infection, which in pregnancy can lead to a bunch of other not-so-fun things like pneumonia, an infection in your bloodstream, and preterm labor.

Next, we look for sugar (glucose), fat (ketones), protein, and blood in the urine. It gives clues as to whether you are taking in enough calories, are dehydrated, or possibly diabetic.

Now that you know why it's so important, just smile and nod every time the nurse hands you that plastic cup and says, "You know the drill. Use the towelette to wipe from the front to the back and then catch your mid-stream urine in the cup."

Reality Check

A word of prenatal etiquette—it's nice to wipe the outside of the cup with a paper towel before you hand it back to the nurse!

Q. Why do I need a Pap smear on my first pregnancy visit?

If you haven't visited your practitioner for "well woman" care (a routine physical or check up) in the past year, you need a Pap smear. Your practitioner will be performing cervical cultures anyway, so it makes sense to screen for cervical cancer at the same time. Although it is relatively rare, about 3% of invasive cervical cancer is detected during pregnancy. Better to be safe and check it out!

If you have an abnormal Pap smear, your OB determines the next step based on the results, previous Pap smear results, your age, and if you have any other risk factors for cervical cancer. If there is a concern, you may need a simple procedure to look at the cells on the cervix.

If everything looks okay, your doc will either repeat the Pap test in six months or may even wait until six weeks after delivery. In some cases, a vaginal delivery actually removes abnormal cells from the surface of the cervix and you might have a normal Pap afterwards!

Q. Why do I need to be tested for sexually transmitted diseases if my partner and I are faithful to each other?

You are correct that you are not at risk if neither you nor your monogamous partner currently has an infection. The problem is that women can have either Chlamydia or gonorrhea without having any symptoms. So, it's technically possible for you to have a sexually transmitted infection and not know it. ACOG recommends that all pregnant women get this test done.

These infections can spell real problems for pregnancy and for a newborn whose mom is infected. Chlamydia and gonorrhea can cause pelvic infections and other complications, including miscarriage. Babies born to women with active infections involving either Chlamydia or gonorrhea are at risk for eye infections, blindness, and pneumonia. See Chapter 17, Infections, for details.

BOTTOM LINE: Even though you don't think you need to be tested for sexually transmitted diseases, it's worth doing it.

1st trimester, additional test
TRANSVAGINAL ULTRASOUND

Q. Will I have an ultrasound at my first visit?

Maybe.

Your practitioner may want to perform an ultrasound to confirm that your pregnancy is in the uterus and the due date is accurate.

But not every practitioner orders an early ultrasound. So don't be disappointed if you don't get to see your peanut at the first visit. And if your practitioner does order an ultrasound, don't be surprised if it is a *transvaginal* ultrasound.

Some women show up to their first OB visit with an excited grin, ready to see their bundle of joy on an ultrasound. That grin quickly turns to shock, when they are told to take off their undies for the test.

In the early stages of pregnancy, everything is *really tiny*. A fetus is usually three to five *millimeters* in length. Hence, a transvaginal ultrasound is the only way to see it and therefore, is the norm before about 12 weeks of pregnancy.

To perform the exam, a thin ultrasound probe (we know it looks really scary but it's not that bad) with a protective sheath is inserted into the vagina and voila! The beauty of the female reproductive system is displayed on the screen.

After 12 weeks, the ultrasound images come from moving a different type of probe over a woman's belly (like you see on TV and in movies). Docs only use transvaginal ultrasounds later in pregnancy for certain women who have high-risk conditions.

You'll find more info on ultrasounds in the 2nd trimester section of this chapter.

1st trimester, additional test
BETA-HCG

Q. I just had a positive home pregnancy test and now have some bleeding. My doctor has asked me to come in for a blood test. Why?

Yes, some women have spotting during a normal pregnancy. But it can also be a sign of an **ECTOPIC PREGNANCY** or a pregnancy that isn't developing normally.

In early pregnancy (before anything is visible on an ultrasound), your doctor can do a blood test to check rising beta-hCG levels to make sure your pregnancy is going in the right direction.

Your placenta makes beta-hCG, the "pregnancy hormone." In most normal pregnancies, the amount of beta-hCG more than doubles (66% increase) every 48 hours until reaching its highest level at ten weeks gestation.

Beta-hCG levels decrease, stay the same, or rise at a slower rate with most (but not all) ectopic pregnancies and pregnancies that are developing abnormally.

FYI: Doctors can't see much on an ultrasound before five weeks gestation. That's why the blood test is more effective when there is spotting or bleeding early in pregnancy.

1st trimester, optional tests
GENETIC SCREENING

Q. My doctor offered "genetic screening" to me. What are these tests?

While there are many tests for this, we'll focus on five optional tests used to screen for genetic disorders (diseases caused by a defective gene). We will spare you the genetics lecture, but here is the general idea: healthy people can be "carriers" for certain diseases. Carriers have one normal gene and one abnormal gene. (People with the disease have two abnormal genes.) If both parents are carriers, each of their children has a one in four chance of having the disorder.

Your practitioner or genetic counselor can advise you on which, if any, tests are worth doing with your ethnic background and family history…and on additional tests if you are carriers.

1 CYSTIC FIBROSIS (CF) CARRIER TESTING.

What is it? A disease affecting sweat and mucous production. It leads to problems with the lungs, pancreas, and digestive system. People with CF have a shortened life expectancy.

Who is at risk? Caucasians and Ashkenazi Jews are most likely to be carriers: the risk is about one in 25. Other ethnic groups are less likely to be carriers: Hispanic Americans have a one in 46 risk, African Americans have a one in 65 risk, and Asian Americans have a one in 94 risk. *(Gabbe SG)*

What is the test? A blood test. If both parents are CF carriers, doctors can test the fetus for cystic fibrosis via an amniocentesis or chorionic villus sampling (CVS). As of this writing, a CF carrier test costs between $150 and $300.

How accurate is the test? CF can result from over 1000 known gene mutations and the currently available tests can detect about 97 of them. So it is possible to have a negative screening test and have a baby with CF. Note: People of Asian and African descent have the least common CF mutations, so carrier testing is the least accurate in these ethnic groups.

Factoid: In the United States, 1 in every 4,000 Caucasian babies is born with cystic fibrosis. The rate is 1 in 15,000 African American babies and 1 in 32,000 Asian American babies.

2 ASHKENAZI JEWISH GENETIC PANEL (AJGP).

What is it? Test panels vary, but the panel Dr. H uses tests for carriers of up to 22 different disorders (including Tay Sachs, Gaucher's, Neiman-

Pick, Maple Syrup Urine Disease, and Canavan's disease). Tay-Sachs disease causes progressive neurologic deterioration and death in early childhood. Note: most AJGP tests include a Cystic Fibrosis carrier test because the risk of being a CF carrier is higher in this group. So be sure to ask what's included in the panel you are having done.

Who is at risk? These diseases are more common in Jewish families (Ashkenazi) who migrated from Eastern Europe—about 90% of Jewish Americans. One in every 30 Ashkenazi Jews is a carrier for Tay-Sachs. For Jewish couples, I suggest doing this test. That's also true even when only one partner is Jewish (although the risk is significantly lower of having a child with one of these diseases).

3 THALASSEMIA SCREEN.

What is it? Inherited blood disorders that cause anemia (when not enough normal red blood cells are produced). FYI: There are two types of thalassemia—"alpha" and "beta", depending on which protein abnormality is involved. Thalassemia disease can be mild (thalassemia minor) to severe (thalassemia major). Most people with thalassemia minor lead normal lives and are usually symptom free. The severe forms are treatable with frequent blood transfusions, but can cause fetal death.

Who is at risk? Mediterraneans (Italians, Greeks) and people of Middle Eastern ancestry (Iranians, Iraqis, Israelis) are more likely to be carriers of beta-thalassemia. Southeast Asian (Filipinos, Chinese, Vietnamese, Laotians, Cambodians) and African ancestries (African, Carribean) are more likely to be carriers of alpha-thalassemia, although people of European ancestry can also carry the trait. For more detailed info see Chapter 16, Complications, complication #16.

What is the test? A routine complete blood count (CBC) identifies people who may be carriers. Another blood test (**HEMOGLOBIN ELECTROPHORESIS**) confirms beta-thalassemia carriers. Amniocentesis and chorionic villus sampling (CVS) can diagnose a fetus with beta-thalassemia disease. For alpha thalassemia, you'll need more specialized genetic testing.

4 SICKLE CELL SCREEN.

What is it? Inherited blood disorder where red blood cells are "sickle" shaped (crescent shaped) instead of round. This causes severe anemia, pain, and lack of blood flow to some organs and body tissues.

Who is at risk? People of African, Central or South American (specifically Panama) descent as well as, those of Caribbean, Mediterranean (Turkey, Greece and Italy), Indian and Saudi Arabian ancestry. One in 12 African Americans is a carrier—one in every 500 African Americans has sickle cell *disease*.

What is the test? A routine complete blood count detects possible carriers. Further blood testing (**HEMOGLOBIN ELECTROPHORESIS**) confirms if someone is a carrier. Amniocentesis and CVS can diagnose the disease in the fetus.

5 FRAGILE X CARRIER SCREEN.

What is it? Fragile X syndrome is the most common inherited intellectual disability. It is named Fragile X because the gene defect is located on the X chromosome. (The gene abnormality is different than the previous disorders discussed.) There is a broad range of symptoms. Some children have mild learning disabilities, others have autism spectrum disorders. Males with Fragile X are more significantly affected because they only have one "X" chromosome, and it is abnormal. Females who have a Fragile X defect are either unaffected or mildly affected, because they have two "X" chromosomes (one gene is normal and one is abnormal).

Who is at risk? A woman with a family history of autism spectrum disorders or undiagnosed intellectual disability is more likely to be a Fragile X carrier. Testing is also helpful if either parent has an intellectual disability, developmental delay, or an autism spectrum disorder. (*Wilkins-Haug L.*)

What is the test? A blood test. If you are a carrier (one of your X chromosomes has the mutation) . . . there is a 50% chance that you will pass that X on to your offspring. CVS or amniocentesis can determine if your baby is affected.

1st/2nd Trimester optional tests
CHROMOSOME TESTING

Q. Should I do any extra tests during pregnancy because of my age?

It's probably a good idea. ACOG recommends that women who will be 35 or older at the time of delivery be offered prenatal testing to diagnose (or far more likely, to rule out) Down syndrome and other chromosome problems in the fetus.

And with modern medicine, every pregnant gal who is 35 or greater does not automatically need to have an amniocentesis. There are less invasive, safer tests that still give accurate results. Take a moment to read up on chromosomes and the different test options in this category. Then we will pull it all together for you at the end of this section.

Note: some tests are done in the first trimester and others are done in the second trimester. But for simplicity sake, all of them are covered here so you have a better feel for what your options are.

Q. Why would I want to test for chromosomal abnormalities if I am planning on having the baby no matter what?

Great question—and a very common one, we might add. Here are some things to consider:

◆ *It's nice to be prepared.* You can plan now for a baby that will need medical attention and extra help. The doctor can also prepare to have all the necessary people ready at birth (the pediatrician, and in some cases a neonatologist or pediatric surgeon). It also helps you and your family prepare mentally, emotionally, and financially.

???

CHROMOSOMES 411

Chromosomes are very thin strands of DNA (deoxyribonucleic acid—genetic building blocks) that are found in most cells in our body. A person normally has 23 pairs of chromosomes for a total number of 46. We get half of our chromosomes from our mother (23) and half from our father (23). They are numbered one through 22. The last pair (23rd pair) are the sex chromosomes and they determine if we are male or female. Females are 46 XX and males are 46 XY.

About one in every 200 babies will have abnormal chromosomes. These occur when there is either an abnormal number of chromosomes or an abnormal amount of information on the chromosomes (such as when there is an extra or missing piece of a chromosome).

"Trisomy" means there are three chromosomes instead of two, in a pair. The most common abnormality is Down syndrome (also called Trisomy 21 because the 21st pair has three chromosomes). Trisomy 13 and Trisomy 18 are also major chromosomal defects. These fetuses either miscarry early in pregnancy, become stillbirths later in pregnancy or die shortly after birth. Other defects are so severe that an embryo cannot survive—and become first trimester miscarriages.

Each abnormality has unique effects on a growing embryo/fetus/newborn, with varying degrees of intellectual impairment and birth defects.

How do these chromosome problems happen? There is usually an issue with the genetic material in either the egg or the sperm before conception even occurs. For women, our eggs developed when we were fetuses ourselves. Those eggs are continually exposed to environmental dangers for all of the years we've lived prior to pregnancy.

As women age, our chromosomes get "sticky." It is harder for them to separate and therefore, some eggs get an extra copy and some get too few. The older we are when we conceive, the higher the chances are that our eggs have abnormal chromosomes. We hate to tell you this, but our egg quality declines with time. We are born with all the eggs we will ever have and the older we get, the more likely our eggs will have issues.

Guys are not off the hook, however, even though their sperm is "fresh" (meaning that new sperm are made every day.) The older the guy, the more likely his sperm contains abnormal chromosomes (you can remind your guy of that if he chides you for having "advanced maternal age"). In fact, men over the age of 40 have a five times greater risk of having a child with an autism spectrum disorder, which is thought to be caused in part by genetic abnormalities.

Head to Expecting411.com/extra for a table on the risk of Down syndrome and other chromosome abnormalities based on a mother's age.

???

◆ *You might change your mind.* Some chromosomal abnormalities cause stillbirth—it may be psychologically difficult to continue the pregnancy when you know the outcome.

First Trimester Screening Test

Q. My doc offered me a "First Trimester Screening Test" to test for Down Syndrome. Should I do it?

Yes. The first trimester screening test is easy and safe to do, it's done early enough in pregnancy to make further decisions, and it calculates your personal odds of having a baby with Trisomy 21 (Down syndrome) or Trisomy 18 (and Trisomy 13 in some labs). The screening test identifies over 85% of fetuses that have one of these abnormalities.

This is a blood test that looks at certain hormone levels plus an ultrasound to assess the thickness of the back of the baby's neck (**NUCHAL LUCENCY**) and nasal bone. Although the timing of the test varies across the country, it is usually done between ten and 13 weeks.

Example: If you are 36, your general risk of having a baby with Down syndrome is 1 in 270. But based on the First Trimester Screening Test, your specific "risk ratio" may turn out to be a bit worse at 1 in 80 or in most cases, a bit better at 1 in 6,000. Based on these numbers, your doctor or genetic counselor will discuss whether or not he/she suggests further diagnostic testing such as chorionic villus sampling (CVS) or amniocentesis. If you have a low risk based on this test, you may decide against doing the more invasive tests (CVS and amniocentesis).

Remember, a positive screening test does not mean that your baby has a problem. It just means that there is a potential risk and you should consider additional testing. A negative first trimester screening test, on the other hand, means your baby has less than a 1% chance of having Trisomy 18 or 21. Although this test does not detect *all* chromosomal abnormalities and birth defects, you can probably rest easier with a negative test.

This is an optional test so your insurance company may not pay for it. And not all practitioners across the country offer it. An obstetrician, perinatologist (high-risk obstetric specialist), or obstetrically-trained ultrasonographer can do the test.

Insider Tip

If your pregnancy started out as twins and one miscarried, you may not be able to do the entire first trimester screening test.

If you miscarried one of the twins very early on and there is no fetus visible in the second sac, you can have the full first trimester screen (blood work and an ultrasound).

If, however, you miscarried one recently and there is still a visible fetus in the second sac, you will only be able to have the ultrasound portion of the test performed. The blood portion of the test cannot be done as the hormones made by the second fetus and placenta can impact your results and increase the chance of a false-positive screening result.

Chorionic Villus Sampling (CVS)

Q. **I'm over 35 and having my first baby. My doctor suggested that I have either a CVS (chorionic villus sampling) or amniocentesis. What are these tests?**

Both a CVS and an amniocentesis are diagnostic tests—meaning that the results will accurately diagnose a chromosome defect in the fetus 99% of the time. Both tests can also diagnose some genetic disorders like cystic fibrosis and thalassemia. Remember, if you did a **FIRST TRIMESTER SCREENING TEST,** which showed that you had a low risk of having a baby with Trisomy 21 or 18, you may decide to skip these tests.

Let's start with CVS, or chorionic villus sampling—now you see why we call it "CVS" for short! A high-risk obstetrics specialist (usually a perinatologist) performs the test in the first trimester, between ten and 13 weeks. She guides a very thin catheter into the uterus (while watching its movement via an ultrasound) and takes a tiny bit of tissue from the placenta. The catheter either enters the uterus through the cervix (trans-cervical) or through the abdominal wall via a needle (trans-abdominal).

The main advantage of CVS over amniocentesis is that it can be done earlier in pregnancy, so there is more time for a couple to make decisions if the results are abnormal. The disadvantage is that the procedure carries a slightly higher risk of miscarriage (0.5%) than with amniocentesis (0.2%).

Amniocentesis

An amniocentesis gives us the same information as a CVS, but it is done at a later point in pregnancy (around 15 to 20 weeks). Practitioners rarely do amniocentesis any earlier than 15 weeks because the chance of complications caused by the test is higher.

Either your obstetrician or a perinatologist performs the amniocentesis. The doctor guides a very thin needle through the skin into the uterus (while watching its movement on an ultrasound) and withdraws a little bit of amniotic fluid for testing.

Patients often worry that the needle will poke the baby during the procedure. Yes, it happens but it is exceedingly rare. The doctor will be looking on the ultrasound to make sure the needle is in the right spot, away from the placenta and the baby. Rarely, a fetus moves and bumps into the needle—that is really, really rare. And even if this happens, it's even more rare for something bad to happen as a result of this encounter.

The advantages of amniocentesis are that the procedure is a little safer and the test provides more information than CVS. Amniocentesis also checks the amniotic fluid for AFP levels, which screens for brain/spinal cord and stomach/intestine malformations. The disadvantage is that the procedure must be done later in pregnancy.

FYI: If you do an amniocentesis, you don't need a **SECOND TRIMESTER SCREENING TEST,** because both tests screen for the same problems. (Read about second trimester screening below.)

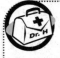

DR H'S OPINION: DOES AMNIOCENTESIS HURT?

Having had one of these myself, I'll tell you honestly. It's a combination of slight pain (like a pinch), a tickle, and the sensation of needing to pee all at once. The most common word my patient's have used to describe it is "weird." But it's over very quickly and you don't need anything more than a little band-aid to cover the area.

Reality Check

Does insurance cover these tests? Unfortunately, the answer for this varies by your state and insurance provider (most insurance policies cover needed tests during pregnancy). Example: California has a state program that pays for a CVS or amniocentesis if your first or second trimester blood screening tests show that you are at increased risk of having a chromosomally abnormal fetus. The state also covers the cost of the ultrasound and any genetic counseling that occurs as well.

Second Trimester Screening Test

Q. Are there any other non-invasive test options for chromosome problems?

Yes. The **SECOND TRIMESTER SCREENING TEST** is an optional (but recommended) blood test done between 15 and 20 weeks—although it is most accurate if done between 16 and 18 weeks. (To make things really confusing, this test is also called a multiple marker screening, an expanded AFP test, serum integrated screening, full integrated screening, a triple screen, or a quad screen! The names keep changing as more tests become available.)

The invasive tests (CVS and amniocentesis) are the only (nearly) foolproof ways to know if your baby has normal chromosomes. But the second trimester screen looks for Trisomy 21 and 18—and these two disorders account for half of all fetal chromosomal abnormalities.

This test helps to determine the likelihood that a fetus will have:

◆ Down syndrome (Trisomy 21) with 80% accuracy
◆ Trisomy 18 with 67% accuracy
◆ Brain/spinal cord defects—major spinal cord defects (**SPINA BIFIDA**) with 80% accuracy, major brain defects (**ANENCEPHALY**) with 97% accuracy
◆ Stomach/intestine malformations with 85% accuracy
◆ A very rare genetic defect called **SMITH-LEMLI-OPITZ** syndrome with 60% accuracy

Even if your **FIRST TRIMESTER SCREENING TEST** was normal, it's a good idea to do this test as it screens for additional problems. And there is enough time to do an amniocentesis if the screen is abnormal.

Although this test comes in different flavors (hence all those names), they basically test for levels of certain substances in mom's blood (alpha fetopro-

TESTS

? ?

tein, hCG, estriol, and inhibin A) and compare the amounts. Without getting too technical, the "Quad" screen is slightly better than the "Triple" screen because it tests more substances and provides more accurate information. And if you do both the **FIRST TRIMESTER SCREENING TEST** and **SECOND TRIMESTER SCREENING TEST**, the results can be combined to give you a better risk assessment for having a child affected by these disorders.

If your screening test is negative (normal), your odds of having a baby with the disorders listed above are very low.

If your screening test is positive (abnormal), don't freak out. Most of the time, it is just a false positive. Again, that means that although your test came back abnormal, your baby is just fine.

Here are a few reasons why you might get a positive test:

◆ Your dates are off. The test can only be done between 15 to 20 weeks, and is most accurate between 16 and 18 weeks.
◆ You are carrying multiples and didn't know it.
◆ You have higher or lower amounts of certain hormones in your blood.
◆ You actually have a baby with one of these disorders.

Your practitioner will go over your test results with you. The results specify which condition is of concern (for example, positive screen for Down syndrome, positive screen for neural tube defects, etc.). If your dates are solid and you aren't carrying multiples, you will be offered the option of doing more tests—an ultrasound and/or amniocentesis.

This test may also throw you a curveball. Although your hormones may not indicate a specific disorder, some of the individual hormone levels can suggest an increased risk of pregnancy-related complications. These include: fetal growth restriction, preterm delivery and **PREECLAMPSIA**. See Chapter 16, Complications (Complication #20, 46). Your doctor will go over what additional monitoring you and your baby might need.

Insider Tip

Carrying twins can make test results for the second trimester screening a bit tricky to interpret (because multiples will increase the levels of AFP, one of the substances tested). And the test is inaccurate if a woman is carrying a multiple pregnancy greater than twins (triplets, quads, etc).

So, it's a good idea to know if you are carrying one or more than one baby before signing up for this test.

Reality Check

It is important to realize that although the words "positive" and "negative" are typically used when discussing test results, what you actually get is a "risk assessment." For example, a positive screen may say that the risk of having a baby with Down syndrome is one in 75. Look at it this way, however: the odds of having a normal fetus are 75 times greater than having a fetus with Down syndrome.

CVS vs Amniocentesis: Which is the better test?

Unfortunately, you are going to have to decide for yourself. But we'll give you the pros and cons to make the call.

CVS

Pros

- ◆ Done between ten and 13 weeks.
- ◆ Allows decisions to be made earlier in pregnancy regarding termination.
- ◆ "FISH" test gives preliminary results in two to three days.
- ◆ Final results obtained within seven to ten days.
- ◆ Will definitively identify 99% of all chromosomal abnormalities.
- ◆ Can also test the fetus for certain diseases, such as cystic fibrosis & thalassemia.

Cons

- ◆ Invasive test (risk of miscarriage is 0.5%).
- ◆ Small amount of pain/discomfort involved with procedure.
- ◆ Expensive, although most insurance plans cover a portion or all of this procedure.
- ◆ Vaginal/cervical cultures necessary prior to the test.
- ◆ Sometimes difficult to find a well-trained physician to perform procedure.
- ◆ Need to be on bed rest for 24 to 48 hours after procedure with activity restrictions for seven days.

Amniocentesis

Pros

- ◆ Done between 15 and 20 weeks. Helpful if there is an abnormality on a second trimester ultrasound once the window for CVS has passed.
- ◆ "FISH" test gives preliminary results in two to three days.
- ◆ Final results obtained within seven to ten days.
- ◆ Will definitively identify 99% of all chromosomal abnormalities.
- ◆ Can also test the fetus for different diseases, such as cystic fibrosis & thalassemia.
- ◆ AFP levels are tested in the amniotic fluid, which help detect brain/spinal cord (neural tube) and stomach/intestine (abdominal wall) defects.

Cons

- ◆ Invasive test (risk of miscarriage is 0.2%).
- ◆ Small amount of pain/discomfort involved with procedure.
- ◆ Need to be on bed rest for 24 to 48 hours after procedure with activity restrictions for seven days.

CHROMOSOME TESTING OPTIONS

How do you decide which chromosome testing you want to do? There are basically three options:

Option #1: 1st Trimester Screening Test/2nd Trimester Screening Test
An ultrasound and blood work recalculates your risk of having a baby with one of the two most common chromosomal abnormalities early in pregnancy. The test changes your risk from a generic age-related risk to an *individual* risk for your particular pregnancy. It allows you to get more information about risks for your fetus before deciding to have a CVS or amniocentesis.

If the results show that you are at *increased* risk of having a chromosomally abnormal fetus, you'd have the option to proceed to a diagnostic test, like CVS or amniocentesis.

If the results show that you are at *decreased* risk, you may be able to wait until 15 to 20 weeks and do the second trimester screening test—which only requires more blood (you are used to that by now, anyway). The results of both first and second trimester screens combined give you a final risk assessment (called a Full Integrated Screening Test).

If the results of the second trimester screen are abnormal, there is still time to have an amniocentesis, if you desire.

Pro: Screening tests offer accuracy with no risk of miscarriage from having the tests done.

Con: These are screening tests and cannot definitively diagnose or rule out Down syndrome or other chromosomal abnormalities.

Dr. H's opinion: Even though it is optional, I definitely recommend doing the full integrated screening test.

Option #2: Chorionic Villus Sampling
This is the better choice if you want definitive testing early on in your pregnancy. Your doc may recommend it if you had a previously abnormal fetus, had multiple miscarriages, or have other risk factors that place you into the "high risk" category.

Pro: Testing provides a definitive answer, in the first trimester.

Con: There is a small risk of miscarrying from the procedure.

Option #3: Amniocentesis
Just like the CVS, you will know your fetus' exact chromosomes. The test is performed between 15 and 20 weeks (but usually between 16 and 18 weeks).

Pro: Testing provides a definitive answer. Amniocentesis also offers additional screening for certain malformations. The risk of miscarrying from the procedure is slightly lower than with CVS.

Con: There is a small risk of miscarrying from the procedure; and it is done later in your pregnancy.

2nd Trimester Tests

1st/2nd/3rd trimester, optional/additional tests
ULTRASOUNDS

Q. What is an ultrasound anyway, and how does it work?

An ultrasound is a machine that uses sound waves to form pictures of internal body structures. Denser structures (like bone) look bright white on the screen and liquids (like urine, amniotic fluid and blood) look black.

Yes, it is safe when a skilled ultrasonographer or practitioner is doing it for a medical reason. There is NO radiation risk to the baby with an ultrasound.

Ultrasounds have been used for about thirty years now, and to date, no significant health concerns have popped up. If you Google this topic, you'll see speculation that ultrasounds cause lower birth weights or left-handedness. But there's no quality research to back up these claims.

However, both ACOG and the American Institute of Ultrasound in Medicine (AIUM) only recommend ultrasounds for medical purposes. Doing an ultrasound for other reasons (keepsake pictures, for example) is not wise.

Q. What can you see on an ultrasound?

Doctors can actually see lots of things. But you'll think your doc is making it up because to the untrained eye, the images resemble fuzz on an old black and white TV!

Early in pregnancy, docs can see:
- ◆ whether the pregnancy is in the uterus.
- ◆ the number of fetuses in the uterus.
- ◆ abnormalities like an ovarian cyst.
- ◆ the length of the cervix.

By mid-pregnancy, docs can see:
- ◆ all major organs of the fetus.
- ◆ the placenta, thriving and in a good position.
- ◆ whether there is an adequate amount of amniotic fluid.
- ◆ the sex of the baby!

In late pregnancy, docs can see:
- ◆ fetal position—what direction the baby is facing in mom's pelvis.
- ◆ baby's size (give or take a little).
- ◆ volume of amniotic fluid.
- ◆ placental health.
- ◆ baby's overall well-being.

FYI: Remember…If you don't want to know the sex of your baby, tell anyone who is caring for you, has access to your chart, and gives you test results that you want to be surprised!

TESTS

? ?

Q. How accurate is the ultrasound?

When it comes to the baby's age and size, it depends on when it is done. First trimester ultrasound exams can accurately determine how far along your pregnancy is and your actual due date. It's less accurate as the pregnancy progresses. The same goes for size. An ultrasound exam can more reliably predict a baby's weight at 25 weeks than at 40 weeks.

Ultrasound is very good at detecting some major abnormalities, but it can't identify every structural birth defect. Ultrasounds are amazing, but not perfect. The humans performing the exams aren't perfect, either. For instance, an ultrasound may not always pick up a cleft lip, cleft palate, or even some heart defects. Ultrasounds also cannot screen for disorders that affect body function and not structure—like cerebral palsy, intellectual disability, or autism. But *most* of the time, ultrasounds identify *most* major structural defects.

If you only have one ultrasound exam, the ultrasound done between 20 and 22 weeks is most useful. This ultrasound is performed to see all of your baby's anatomy in detail. At this point, most problems involving the major organs are detectable.

In a few cases, however, they will be missed or will develop later on in pregnancy after most ultrasounds have already been performed. So although it is rare, it is possible to deliver a baby with a problem that wasn't detected on any of your earlier ultrasounds.

Q. How often will I have an ultrasound?

It depends on your practitioner and whether or not you have a high-risk pregnancy. If you are carrying multiples, have a history of preterm labor or diabetes, you will undoubtedly have more ultrasound exams than your low-risk preggo friends.

Some practitioners do not perform *any* ultrasounds. Some will do two to three throughout the pregnancy. Others will do more. An ultrasound is not absolutely necessary if you have a low-risk pregnancy. But ultrasounds do provide reassurance and some pretty useful information.

No matter what the frequency, you probably won't have an ultrasound at every office visit!

Here are the typical times for ultrasounds and the reasons why:

◆ *First prenatal visit:* to confirm that your pregnancy is in the uterus, that your dates are accurate and to detect the presence of a fetal heartbeat.

◆ *First trimester screening test*: to measure the fetus' neck area (see info on chromosome testing earlier in this chapter).

◆ *20 to 22 weeks*: to look at all of baby's internal/external structures.

◆ *28 to 32 weeks*: to assess fetal growth, confirm or follow-up on the location of your placenta and assure an adequate amount of amniotic fluid.

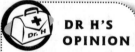

DR H'S OPINION

"I think it's help-ful to do at least two to three ultra-sounds for a low risk pregnancy. But every doc has his or her own opinion."

Insider Tip

If your doctor doesn't do ultrasounds, you can request one. ACOG policy says your doctor should honor that request and make a referral *(ACOG)*.

Q. What happens if an abnormality is found on an ultrasound?

Remember our analogy of false positives and shrimp nets? Most of the stuff an ultrasound identifies is seaweed.

In this case, the seaweed is either a normal variation in fetal development, one that resolves on its own . . . . or one that you or your baby would never know about if you didn't have an ultrasound.

So the first thing to do is relax. Second, listen carefully to everything your doctor tells you. Third—ask questions. And call your doctor the next day if you come up with 22 more questions once you have had time to absorb it all.

What happens next depends on what the abnormality is, when it is found, and where it is found. See Expecting411.com/extra for a detailed discussion. We suggest that you don't read this content before going to bed at night. Better yet, only take a look at it if an issue arises.

Partner tip

Remember at the beginning of this chapter when we said it was your job to be there to support your pregnant half? Well, here is where the rubber meets the road: if an abnormality is found on an ultrasound, you have to help calm the waters. It is your job to take notes and organize questions. Calm and cool is your mantra.

Q. All of my friends are getting 3-D and 4-D ultrasounds of their babies. My doctor only does 2-D ultrasounds. Is that OK?

Yes.

A three-dimensional (3-D) or four-dimensional (4-D) ultrasound can help rule out certain defects, like a **CLEFT LIP** or **CLEFT PALATE**. However, an experienced doc can often identify birth defects and problems in pregnancy with a conventional 2-D ultrasound.

FYI: ACOG does not find any clear advantage of using 3-D or 4-D ultrasound routinely over 2-D.

Yes, it is pretty cool to see what your baby really looks like inside your womb with one of these fancy 3-D or 4-D ultrasounds. Fun, yes. Necessary, no.

Reality Check

Your practitioner can print out some pictures (or make a CD/DVD) of your medical ultrasound if you want a keepsake for your baby book.

TESTS

? ?

DR H'S OPINION:
MALL ULTRASOUNDS

Like ACOG, I believe that ultrasounds should be done for medical reasons only. I discourage you from going to the mall and getting a Glamour Shots-style 3-D or 4-D ultrasound.

Why? First of all, you don't know whether the technician has received proper training. And you don't know if the technician's supervisor has had any medical training. Or if the mall ultrasound machine is properly maintained.

And some of these "photo shoots" can last three to four hours. It's not worth the risk of exposing your baby to several hours of sound waves and excess heat.

Bottom line: Medical ultrasounds, okay. Mall ultrasounds, not okay.

2nd trimester, Routine test
ONE HOUR GLUCOLA

Q. What is the one-hour glucola test?

The one-hour glucola screening test identifies those at risk for diabetes during pregnancy (**GESTATIONAL DIABETES**). It is usually done between 24 and 28 weeks. But women who have risk factors for gestational diabetes may have this test done as early as the first visit. It tests how efficiently your body handles sugar.

We know what you are thinking. You don't have a history of diabetes or any symptoms. No one in your family has diabetes. But despite all of that, being pregnant is a risk factor in and of itself, so everyone—yes, you too—gets screened. The only people who don't get this test are those who already have diabetes and know it.

Here's how the test works: an hour before your lab appointment, you drink eight ounces of a sugary liquid that tastes like an extra sweet, flat soda. If you're lucky, you get to pick the flavor. One tip: chill the drink. It tastes better that way.

Some docs will request you fast before drinking the cocktail; some don't.

The key part: you must drink the whole thing in about five minutes, *exactly* an hour before having blood drawn. It's best to be on the safe side and arrive a little early for your appointment. Why? If you are late, your blood can't be drawn and (yep, you guessed it) the test has to be repeat-

DR H'S OPINION:
GLUCOLA TASTE TESTS

I tried the orange glucose drink with my first pregnancy and the lemon lime with my second. I came to the following scientific conclusion: if you are a 7-Up or Sprite fan, pick the lemon-lime flavor. If you like orange soda, go for the orange one.

? ?

TESTS

ed again on another day. So if you are stuck in traffic and will be two hours late, call your doctor's office to reschedule (and get another sugar drink).

Common risk factors for gestational diabetes include:

◆ history of gestational diabetes with a previous pregnancy.

◆ family history of diabetes.

◆ obesity.

◆ ethnicity (Hispanic, African, Native American, South or East Asian, or Pacific Islands ancestry).

◆ over the age of 35.

◆ history of previous stillbirth.

◆ history of having a large baby.

◆ other endocrine problems such as thyroid disease.

Factoid: Insulin is a hormone that tells your body to process sugar (glucose) you eat and turn it into energy. Excess sugar is stored for later use.

If you *aren't* pregnant and have diabetes, your body does not make enough insulin—or does not respond to the insulin it does make.

Diabetes *during pregnancy* (gestational diabetes) is usually due to a completely different issue. The culprit: a hormone made by the placenta (human placental lactogen or hPL). This hormone impairs the mother's body's ability to use insulin.

Reality Check

If you had gestational diabetes with a previous pregnancy, you have a 33% to 50% chance of having it with any subsequent pregnancy.

Q. My glucola test was abnormal. What does that mean?

It means your blood sugar level was higher than what it should be.

According to ACOG, an abnormal test result is anything above 140.

FYI: many practitioners are being more conservative with this test, especially for moms-to-be who already have other risk factors for diabetes. In these cases, test results in the 120's or 130's may be flagged as abnormal.

Of course, there is a downside to this conservative approach: more women who *don't* have diabetes have to endure additional testing.

If the glucola test is abnormal, your practitioner will ask you to do another test to see if, in fact, you really have gestational diabetes. This is called a **THREE-HOUR GLUCOSE TOLERANCE TEST** (GTT). Personally, we think this test should be named the Glucose Torture Test . . . it's no fun.

Here's how the test works. You:

◆ Eat an unrestricted diet with at least 150 grams of carbohydrates per day for at least three days before the test (your practitioner will provide a list of good carb choices; see the box on the next page).

◆ Fast after midnight.

◆ Show up at your doctor's office or lab first thing in the morning.

◆ Get your fasting blood drawn.

◆ Drink another yummy glucose drink, one with twice the amount of sugar of the first test.

Then, here comes the really fun part. Wait for it . . .

◆ You sit in the office or lab for THREE hours and get your blood drawn each and every hour.

Sorry, you can't run errands in between. Getting up and running around affects your metabolism and how your body uses sugar (glucose)—thus ruining your test results. Bring your laptop or favorite book.

Q. My 3 hour GTT was abnormal. My doctor said I have gestational diabetes. Now what? Will my baby be okay?

An abnormal test means that at least two of the four glucose levels came back elevated. Don't panic. Most women who develop gestational diabetes control their sugar levels with diet and exercise alone. With excellent control of sugar levels, your baby will be fine.

Here is the key issue: because of the placenta and the process of diffusion, your unborn baby has the same sugar levels as you do. If your blood sugar levels are high, so are your baby's. So, you and your baby benefit from keeping your blood sugars under control.

Your practitioner may refer you to a diabetic educator or nurse. That person will teach you about your diet and optimal blood sugar levels. He also instructs you how to check your own blood sugars (yes, unfortunately, that

---

CARB LOADING BEFORE YOUR THREE-HOUR GTT

If your one-hour glucola screening test came back abnormal (that is, you might have diabetes), the natural tendency after hanging up the phone is to go into starvation mode. You'll be tempted to cut out those foods you think might worsen blood sugar. . . pastas, breads, sweets, fruits, etc.

THIS IS NOT THE RIGHT THING TO DO!

Ironically, if you skip the carb loading for at least three days prior to your next test (three-hour GTT), you are more likely to falsely *elevate* your blood sugars. Then you will get a false positive diabetes test . . . and be treated like a diabetic for the remainder of your pregnancy. You'll endure daily finger pricks to check your sugar levels upon waking in the morning and after meals. Yes, that's 200 to 400 needle pricks during the rest of your pregnancy!

Our advice: just follow your doc's directions and enjoy carb-loading prior to your three hour GTT. Your doctor typically will provide you a list of foods; we have also included one below:

Eat at least ten servings of foods each day such as bread, fruit and milk. Here is an example of ten servings:

1 cup milk	1 slice bread
1 dinner roll	1/3 cup cooked pasta
1/2 cup black beans	1 tortilla
1 cup berries	1 small apple/orange
1/2 cup corn	3 cups popcorn

---

means you need to poke your fingers a few times a day) and how to record them. Although we know it is a pain in the butt (or finger), you need to follow your diet, and monitor your sugar levels closely.

You will discuss your sugar levels with your doctor at each visit. Occasionally, glucose levels remain elevated despite a patient following a strict diet. If this is the case, you may need an oral medication and—less commonly—injectable insulin.

If you need more inspiration, read more about gestational diabetes in Chapter 16, Complications, complication #26.

End of 2nd/3rd trimester, routine test
FETAL KICK COUNTS

Q. My doctor talked to me about "fetal kick counts." What are they? Do I really have to do them everyday?

A healthy baby is a baby that moves around. Most babies have certain times during the day and night (4am is a popular time) that they are most active, and that varies from baby to baby. When you are active, you probably won't notice your baby moving until you come home and sit down at the end of the day.

Fetal kick counts are one way to make sure your baby is healthy. We usually recommend starting to do kick counts at about 26 weeks. Before this time, fetal movement is pretty random. You might go for days without feeling movement that you once noticed before.

So how do you count the kicks? If you follow the textbook method for fetal kick counts, you should sit down for one hour during each 24-hour day to count how many times your baby moves. Ten kicks during one hour is the standard for a healthy fetus.

Of course, most of us don't have an hour a day to sit there and do nothing but write down how many times our baby is moving. And what if the baby only moves eight or nine times? Should one panic? Rush off to the hospital? The answer is no.

A more realistic approach to fetal kick counts: be aware of fetal movement everyday. Do not go more than 12 hours without feeling some movement.

If you don't have a reassuring count, call your practitioner to investigate things further.

Reality Check
Most women pregnant with their first babies are aware of movement somewhere between 18 and 22 weeks. Women pregnant with their second or third child are often aware of fetal movement much earlier. At first, early fetal movement feels like little bubbles inside your belly and women often mistakenly think they have gas!

Q. I haven't felt my baby move all day. What should I do?

Here are a few tips if you notice a decrease in or absence of your baby's movement:

◆ Drink and eat something (preferably something with sugar in it).
◆ Lie on your left side.
◆ Place your hands on either side of your belly and gently "move" your baby.
◆ Count how many times your baby moves in the next hour or two.

Usually, you will feel your baby moving around and breathe a sigh of relief. If you still feel very little movement (the baby moves once in two hours, for example) or no movement at all, you should contact your practitioner immediately.

It could mean many things and most of them are nothing to panic about.

Most commonly, you have been moving around all day and although your baby has been moving too, you have been unaware of it. Sometimes babies have very long sleep cycles, lasting up to 90 minutes. If you are trying to do your kick counts during a sleep cycle, there won't be too much kicking. Sometimes babies are just resting and are lazy for lack of a better word.

In some situations, however, decreased fetal movement means that a fetus is not getting what she needs. Lower levels of amniotic fluid can cause less fetal movement. Fetuses that aren't getting enough oxygen, nutrients, or blood from the placenta often have decreased fetal movement.

Studies have shown that women often perceive decreased movement days before a fetal death. (*Fretts RC*) Obviously, this is a situation everyone wants to prevent. That's why you need to call your practitioner pronto if you notice a sudden decrease in movement.

2nd/3rd trimester, additional test
FETAL FIBRONECTIN (fFN)

Q. I am 24 weeks and starting to have some contractions. I heard there is a test to see if a baby is at risk for premature birth. Is it done routinely?

This is the Fetal Fibronection test (fFN). It isn't done routinely, but it's useful for patients between 22 and 34 weeks who are at risk of going into preterm labor.

What is fFN? It's the "glue" (really a protein) that attaches the amniotic sac (water bag) to the inner lining of the uterus.

The fFN leaks into the vagina when patients are in preterm labor or in danger of going into preterm labor. Your practitioner will collect some fluid from the back of the vagina with a long Q-tip and have it analyzed. The results are usually back in one to two hours.

If your fFN test is negative, you have a pretty low risk (about 5%) of going into preterm labor in the next ten to 14 days. But no test is 100% accurate. If you continue having contractions, you still need to call your doctor if they get more frequent or more severe. If your symptoms continue, your doctor may repeat the fFN test every two weeks until you approach 34 weeks.

If your fFN test is positive, it's *possible* that you will deliver soon. The test is actually more reliable in ruling *out* preterm labor than ruling it *in*. About 60% of women who have a positive fFN test actually deliver before 35 weeks. That means that about 40% of women with a positive fFN test will make it beyond 35 weeks—if preterm labor is a worry, this is a great goal to reach.

If your test is positive, however, you will probably stay overnight at the hospital and be monitored for uterine contractions. If you have real contractions and delivery looks imminent, see Chapter 19, Preterm Labor for what happens next.

Note: it is possible to get a false positive result from the fFN test (seaweed in the net, to use our earlier analogy). This can happen if you've had sexual intercourse in the past 24 hours. It also happens if you've had any vaginal bleeding or your doctor did an internal exam to check your cervix within 24 hours of the fFN test. The most reliable fFN test is one done at least 24 hours after sex or an internal exam, assuming you've had no vaginal bleeding.

3rd Trimester

3rd trimester, routine test
GROUP B STREP SCREEN

Q. What is Group B Strep?

Group B Streptococcus (GBS), or *Streptococcus agalactiae*, is a bacteria that normally lives in harmony in your gastrointestinal tract (the gut/bowels).

The GBS that lives in your intestinal tract can easily spread to the vagina. As women, we have three body cavity openings sitting right next to each other—the urethra, the vagina, and the rectum. That makes it pretty easy for bacteria to spread from one area to the next no matter how clean you are. This happens to about 10% to 30% of healthy women.

Usually, the GBS just hangs out in the vagina without causing any problems. Occasionally, GBS causes bladder infections, an infection of the amniotic sac (**CHORIOAMNIONITIS**), or an infection in the blood.

The key concern for pregnancy and GBS: a newborn can be infected as he passes through the birth canal. So while a mom may just be a carrier of GBS without any problems (docs call it "GBS positive"), her baby may get very sick if he gets the infection.

Your practitioner does a vaginal/rectal swab at 35 to 37 weeks and sends it to the lab for a culture. Yes, that means your vagina and rectum are swabbed. Although the thought makes you want to run and hide, the collection procedure itself takes about two seconds. And your doc will distract you by talking about baby names, or something. So it's not really as bad as it sounds.

The only time this test is NOT done is if:

◆ GBS was already found in your urine or
◆ you've already had a baby with a GBS infection. In that case, docs assume you are GBS positive and treat the condition during labor.

If you go into labor or need to be induced *before* 35 weeks and haven't had a GBS culture yet, you automatically get treated with preventive antibiotics in case you are GBS positive.

Q. What precautions are taken if I am GBS Positive?

If you are GBS positive, the goal is to give you one full dose of intravenous (IV) antibiotics during labor, at least four hours before delivery. You will also be on IV antibiotics if you have one of these issues:

◆ You have not yet had a GBS culture done before you go into labor.

◆ Your water has been broken for more than 18 hours.

◆ You go into labor earlier than 35 weeks.

◆ You have a fever greater than 100.4°.

If you have a C-section, you don't have to worry about this stuff since your baby isn't going through the birth canal... unless you go into labor or have your water bag break prior to your scheduled C-section. In those scenarios, you'd need antibiotics to treat GBS prior to your C-section.

It is standard protocol *for the newborn* to get a complete blood count and blood culture if mom is Group B Strep positive and didn't get pretreated with at least one dose of antibiotics (which happens with quick labors). Ditto when the baby is born sooner than 35 weeks gestation or if a baby starts misbehaving (temperature instability, labored breathing, stealing the car keys, etc.). These tests help tell the pediatrician if the baby may have been infected with GBS.

Q. Will it hurt the baby?

Group B Strep can cause infection in the blood, pneumonia, and meningitis in newborns. All newborns are watched closely, but those babies with moms who test positive for Group B Strep are watched even more closely. Babies born before 37 weeks are the most likely to get a GBS infection if a carrier mom is not treated.

That's why there is a standard protocol to test all pregnant women for GBS and to treat GBS positive women with antibiotics when they go into labor. FYI: routine screening and treatment of GBS during labor, in fact, has cut the rate of newborn infections by two thirds since 2002.

Reality Check

Don't be too alarmed if you carry Group B Strep. This does not mean you are Typhoid Mary. Most babies with GBS positive mothers do not get sick and do absolutely fine.

Q. I tested positive with my first pregnancy, and negative this time. Should I still be treated?

Nope. GBS comes and goes. In fact, some women who are positive in the first part of pregnancy are not near the end. The same goes for women who have been positive in previous pregnancies. Assuming your baby did not develop a GBS infection (in which case you would automatically be treated during this pregnancy), you should only be treated if you have tested positive in the current pregnancy or fit one of the other criteria mentioned earlier.

Reality Check

If you are GBS positive, you won't pass it to your husband. GBS is not a sexually transmitted infection. But (there's a butt here) if you engage in anal intercourse, you should always use a condom and should never go from the rectum to the vagina. This is a very easy way for bacteria to spread!

3rd trimester, additional test
NON-STRESS TESTS

Q. I called my doctor to tell her that my baby wasn't moving around like usual and she wants me to come into her office for a non-stress test. What is that?

A non-stress test (NST) is one of the ways to reassure both doctors and patients that the baby in question is not in any distress. It is sort of like an "EKG" for baby—specific heart rate patterns tell your doc that the placenta is doing what it's supposed to do to support a growing baby.

This is a pain-free test for you and your baby. So how does it work? First, two monitors are strapped on the outside of your belly. One monitor helps to pick up uterine contractions, while the other one tracks your baby's heartbeat. The doctor evaluates both uterine activity and fetal heart-beat on a display.

By evaluating many different aspects of your baby's heart rate, docs determine whether your baby is fine . . . or if further testing is needed. Sometimes, especially when there is little fetal movement, an ultrasound is performed to measure the amount of amniotic fluid around the baby.

NSTs are also used to monitor fetuses in women with high-risk pregnancies, such as those with high blood pressure, diabetes, certain clotting disorders and multiple pregnancies (twins, triplets, etc.).

Q. My friend starting getting NSTs at 32 weeks and now has them twice a week. I haven't had one yet. Why?

Certain women with high-risk pregnancies need NSTs once or twice a week. These are pregnancies that have a higher-than-average risk of the baby getting sick or being a stillborn. Your friend is likely getting tested frequently because she has one of a number of high-risk conditions.

If you have what your doctor considers a "low-risk" pregnancy, you may never have an NST during your pregnancy, unless you happen to go past your due date or another unforeseen condition arises.

Q. Why would I need a non-stress test?

This is a useful test for a variety of conditions. Here's a list of them:

Examples of maternal conditions requiring non-stress tests

◆ High blood pressure (**HYPERTENSION**)
◆ Diabetes
◆ Severe asthma
◆ Certain clotting disorders

TESTS

? ?

- Seizure disorders
- Poorly controlled thyroid conditions
- Certain blood diseases such as sickle cell anemia, thalassemia, hemoglobin S disease
- Chronic kidney disease
- Lupus
- Certain types of heart disease

Examples of fetal or pregnancy-related conditions requiring non-stress tests

- Small size (**FETAL GROWTH RESTRICTION**)
- Decreased fetal movement
- Too little amniotic fluid (**OLIGOHYDRAMNIOS**)
- Too much amniotic fluid (**POLYHYDRAMNIOS**)
- Post-term pregnancy
- Immune response to Rh factor (**ISOIMMUNIZATION**)
- Previous stillborn (fetal demise)
- **PREECLAMPSIA**
- **GESTATIONAL DIABETES**, poorly controlled or on insulin
- Multiples

Q. My doctor told me "everything looked great" with my NST. But he said it must be done again next week. Why?

Most of the time, it's highly reassuring to have a normal NST. A normal test means that there is less than a 0.5% chance of having a stillborn in the next seven days. This is why docs usually repeat the test once a week.

In certain very high-risk conditions, however, the test is done *twice* weekly.

3rd trimester, additional test
CONTRACTION STRESS TEST

Q. My OB wants to do a contraction stress test. Why?

A contraction stress test (CST) is similar to a non-stress test (NST)—two monitors are strapped to your belly. Your doctor will monitor both the fetal heart rate and contraction pattern.

The difference: with a CST, your doc is watching what your baby's heart rate does in the *presence* of contractions. By contrast, an NST is done in the *absence* of contractions. (Yes, there are ways to make these contractions happen—see the next question!)

What is the point of this test? Your baby gets less oxygen during a contraction. That is normal. The uterine muscle contracts and the arteries supplying the placenta are temporarily squeezed, allowing less blood to the placenta (and therefore the baby).

If a baby is not getting enough oxygen in the first place, a contraction drops the amount of oxygen delivered to the baby even further, leading to specific heart rate patterns that your doctor can interpret.

Q. How am I made to have contractions?

Are you sitting down? The most common way to induce contractions is nipple stimulation. Docs will ask you to rub your nipples vigorously. Don't worry—the medical staff will not participate in this experience!

If contractions do not occur after nipple stimulation, docs can give you a small dose of pitocin (a synthetic form of oxytocin) through an IV until adequate contractions happen.

3rd trimester, additional test
BIOPHYSICAL PROFILE

Q. What is a biophysical profile (BPP)?

This is yet another noninvasive test that docs use to gain valuable information about your baby's well-being. It involves doing an NST (as described above) in conjunction with an ultrasound. In recent years, this test has replaced the Contraction Stress Test as the most popular way to seek reassurance about your unborn baby.

The ultrasound looks at four different parameters: fetal movement, breathing, fetal tone, and the amount of amniotic fluid present. A score is given from zero to ten (you get two points for each of the components of the test). The total score helps docs determine whether:

- ◆ your baby is okay and can be observed.
- ◆ more testing is needed or
- ◆ immediate intervention is needed.

The biophysical profile (BPP) is considered more reassuring than an NST alone because it provides more information about a fetus and her environment. A normal score on a BPP indicates there is just a 0.1% chance of having a stillbirth in the next seven days.

Yep . . . that's a lot of tests. Now, let's talk about nutrition—what does your baby need? What does it really mean to be "eating for two"? The answers are next!

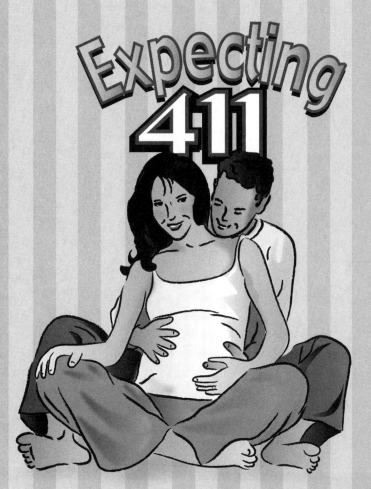

Expecting
411

section two

Life Goes On

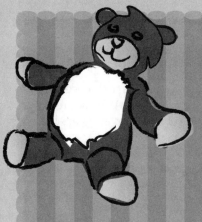

NUTRITION
Chapter 6

"The perfect lover is one who turns into a pizza at 4 AM."
—Charles Pierce

WHAT'S IN THIS CHAPTER

Stop us if you've heard this before: when pregnant, you're eating for two.

But what does that mean in the real world? How does what you eat affect your baby? Can you take herbal supplements? How much water should you be drinking?

This chapter covers everything you wanted to know about nutrition and your baby.

Yes, you are eating for two—literally. That doesn't just mean that you clean your plate and then poach what's left on your spouse's. It means that what you eat, your baby eats too.

So if you eat out regularly or routinely have the danish du jour with your grande latte in the morning on the way into work, it's probably time to make a few changes in your life.

If you've picked up some unhealthy eating habits, now is the time to begin changing your lifestyle. You have the perfect motivation. If you can't do it for yourself, do it for your baby.

We know it's hard to change your ways—but you need to create a healthy diet for your child—right now. The nutrition your baby gets in the womb actually does impact her later health. Studies suggest that good fetal nutrition reduces the risk of obesity, heart disease, and high blood pressure later in life. *(Osmond C.)*

And once the baby is born, you need to KEEP up the healthy diet that you start in pregnancy. Why? Because your child relies on you to buy the groceries. You and your child both eat what is in your pantry.

For those of you who like to count carbs or calories and squeeze into those skinny jeans, it's time to change your mindset! We're not recommending that you head to the all-you-can eat buffet for every meal, but you need to be realistic.

We are women and we know this is really hard. But for now, eat what you need to eat, and try to stop fretting about your body image. Being pregnant is a beautiful thing.

Nutritional Needs

Q. What do I need to eat during my pregnancy?

In general, you need more protein, iron, and folic acid than you did pre-pregnancy. And it wouldn't hurt to crank up your fiber intake to save you from wonderful pregnancy constipation. If you are a vegetarian, you also need a B12 supplement. Otherwise, you should be able to reach your nutritional goals with a well-balanced diet.

Here is a list of nutrients you should aim to get each day of your pregnancy (okay, *most* days because we won't count the days that all you feel like eating are Cool Ranch Doritos). *(US Dept Health & Human Services)*

VITAMINS/MINERALS	WHY?
Vitamin A	Helps with fetal growth, vision, and immune function.
Vitamin D	Helps with fetal bone and tooth development. Deficiency may increase risk of preeclampsia.
Vitamin E	Antioxidant. Note: excessive intake may lead to congenital heart defects.
B1 (Thiamin)	Helps with nerve conduction.
B2 (Riboflavin)	Supports energy metabolism.
B6	Helps with amino acid (protein) metabolism.
B12	Works with folic acid in cell formation. Deficiency causes anemia, neurologic issues.
Vitamin C	Antioxidant. Helps body use iron. Helps with connective tissue production.
Folic Acid	Deficiency causes neural tube defects in fetus (spina bifida).
Niacin	Helps with energy metabolism.
Calcium	Helps fetus bone, cartilage, tooth growth, nerve conduction. It may prevent preeclampsia.
Iodine	Helps make thyroid hormone, which regulates body growth and energy use.
Iron	Deficiency causes anemia for moms, potential prematurity and low birth weight baby.
Magnesium	Helps with energy metabolism, muscle contractions, nerve conduction.
Phosphorus	Supports bones, teeth.
Zinc	Helps with metabolism, growth, and development. Deficiency may increase risk of prematurity and low birth weight baby.

SOURCES OF NUTRIENTS YOU NEED

So now you know what nutrients you need. How do you get them in your diet? Here's a list of common foods and what you'll get out of a typical serving.

Vitamin A   **RDI* 1500 mcg**
3 oz organ meats	1500–9000 mcg
3/4 c carrot juice	1700 mcg
1 sweet potato	1000 mcg
1/2 c carrots	670 mcg

Vitamin D   **RDI 1,000 I.U.**
1 T cod liver oil	1360 IU
3.5 oz salmon	360 IU
1 c fortified milk	100 IU

Vitamin E   **RDI 15 mg**
1 oz almonds	7 mg
1 oz sunflower seeds	6 mg
1 T sunflower oil	5.6 mg
2 T peanut butter	3 mg

Thiamin (B1)   **RDI 1.4 mg**
3.5 oz pork chop	0.9 mg
1 oz sunflower seeds	0.6 mg
1 c cooked pasta	0.3 mg
2 T brewer's yeast	2.3 mg

Riboflavin (B2)   **RDI 1.4 mg**
3.5 oz beef liver	4 mg
1/2 c almonds	0.8 mg
1 c yogurt	0.5 mg

B6   **RDI 1.9 mg**
3.5 oz beef liver	1.4 mg
1 c oatmeal	0.7 mg
1 banana	0.7 mg
3.5 oz salmon	0.7 mg

B12   **RDI 2.6 mcg**
3.5 oz beef liver	112 mcg
3.5 oz steamed clams	99 mcg
3 oz crab	9 mcg
3.5 oz trout	5 mcg

Vitamin C   **RDI 85 mg**
1 c fresh orange juice	124 mg
1 c strawberries	85 mg
1 orange	70 mg
1 mango	60 mg

Folic Acid   **RDI 600 mcg**
1c breakfast cereal	100 mcg
1/2 c orange juice	100 mcg
1/2 c asparagus	130 mcg
1/2 c lentils	180 mcg

Niacin   **RDI 18 mg**
3.5 oz beef liver	14 mg
1/2 c peanuts	10.5 mg
3.5 oz salmon	8 mg
1pkt corn grits	7 mg
1 c Cheerios	5 mg

Calcium   **RDI 1000mg**
1 c yogurt	350 mg
1 c milk	300 mg
1 oz cheese	200 mg
3 oz salmon	180 mg

Iron   **RDI 27 mg**
1 c Total cereal	22 mg
3.5 oz steamed clams	22 mg
1/2 c tofu	6.7 mg
1/2 c spinach	3 mg
1/4 lb. burger	3 mg

Magnesium   **RDI 350 mg**
1/4 c pumpkin seeds	303 mg
1/2 c almonds	240 mg
1/2 c cashews	150 mg
1/2 c tofu	130 mg
1 c yogurt	40 mg

Phosphorous   **RDI 700 mg**
1/4 c pumpkin seeds	665 mg
1/4 c sunflower seeds	380 mg
1 c yogurt	350 mg
3.5 oz salmon/trout	260 mg

Zinc   **RDI 11mg**
3.5 oz cooked oysters	39 mg
3.5 oz ground beef	5.5 mg
3.5 oz turkey	4.5 mg
1 c yogurt	2 mg

* The Reference Daily Intake (RDI) is the value established by the Food and Drug Administration (FDA) for use in nutrition labeling

nutrition

NUTRITION

NUTRIENT	HOW MUCH DO I NEED OF IT?

Protein 71g

Why? Protein makes blood and energy stores for you and body tissue for your fetus.

Where to get it? Lean meats, beans, nuts, seeds, peas, soybean/tofu, eggs, dairy products.

Carbohydrates At least 50% of your daily food intake

Why? Provides both energy and fiber. You need 20 to 30g of daily fiber to help you poop!

Where to get it? Grains (whole grain bread, cereals, brown rice, pasta), fruits, vegetables.

Fat < 30% of your daily food intake

Why? Some fats needed for fetal brain and vision development.

Where to get it? Vegetable oil, nuts, eggs, fish, avocado, peanut butter, reduced fat margarine/salad dressing, olives, sunflower seeds, mayonnaise.

Q. 71 grams of protein? What does this mean in the real world?

Here is the suggested food pyramid for pregnant women (courtesy MyPyramid.gov)—it gives you a good overview of nutrition for the next nine months.

Food Group	1st Trimester	2nd and 3rd Trimesters	What counts as 1 cup or 1 ounce?
	Eat this amount from each group daily.*		
Fruits	2 cups	2 cups	1 cup fruit or juice ½ cup dried fruit
Vegetables	2½ cups	3 cups	1 cup raw or cooked vegetables or juice 2 cups raw leafy vegetables
Grains	6 ounces	8 ounces	1 slice bread 1 ounce ready-to-eat cereal ½ cup cooked pasta, rice, or cereal
Meat & Beans	5½ ounces	6½ ounces	1 ounce lean meat, poultry, or fish ¼ cup cooked dry beans ½ ounce nuts or 1 egg 1 tablespoon peanut butter
Milk	3 cups	3 cups	1 cup milk 8 ounces yogurt 1½ ounces cheese 2 ounces processed cheese

NUTRITION

Even though there are several food groups, they all boil down to three *types* of foods that your body recognizes and utilizes in different ways: proteins, carbohydrates, and fats. Here's a look at each.

1 PROTEIN. Why do we need protein? Our bodies break protein down into amino acids. These amino acids then make proteins for our body. In pregnancy, that extra protein you eat becomes the basis for your baby's cells and tissues.

Yes, you need a little more protein in your pregnancy diet. But what's the difference between 45 grams of daily protein and the 71 grams you need now? It may mean noshing on a high-protein snack and adding one glass of milk a day. Just take a look at the amount of protein in some typical foods below. It takes remarkably small amounts to meet your additional protein needs.

Protein Goal: 71 grams/day

SERVING SIZE	AMOUNT OF PROTEIN (IN GRAMS)
3 oz. chicken breast	27 grams
3 oz. fish	21
1 cup cottage cheese	28
1 cup low fat yogurt	11
1 cup skim milk	8
2 T peanut butter	8
1/2 cup black beans	7.5
3 oz. tofu	7
1 egg	6
1 oz. almonds	5
1/2 cup green peas	4.5

Bottom Line
You need 5.5 to 6.5 oz. of meats/poultry/fish (or nuts/legumes) a day and three cups or servings of milk/dairy products a day to reach your protein goal.

Old Wives Tale
Avoiding peanuts during pregnancy will keep my child from developing a food allergy. *False.*

Current pediatric research shows that infants who are exposed to high allergy foods earlier in life may actually have a lower risk of developing a food allergy. So feel free to have a PB&J while you read this chapter.

2 CARBOHYDRATES. What's so special about carbs?

Our bodies break down most carbs (with the exception of fiber) to become sugar, our main energy source.

NUTRITION

? ?

There are simple sugars, like honey, corn syrup, and fruit. And there are complex carbohydrates, like starches found in grains, legumes, and vegetables. Finally, there are indigestible complex carbohydrates (better known as fiber). These are found in vegetables, seeds, citrus fruits, oats, and barley. High-fiber foods go in and come out of our bodies virtually undigested (without breaking down into sugar).

You don't really need more carbohydrates during pregnancy. About 55% to 65% of your daily intake should be in this category. But you will do your bowels a favor if you eat more fiber. That's one reason we suggest making whole grains at least *half* of the grains you eat.

What does "55 to 65%" of your daily intake really look like? Well, that depends on how many calories you need to eat a day. And that total calorie goal depends on your pre-pregnancy weight, height, and level of activity during the day. But for simplicity sake, most pregnant women need roughly 300 to 375 grams of carbohydrates per day.

Let's take a look at serving sizes and carb content:

Carbohydrates Goal: 300–375 grams/day

SERVING SIZE	AMOUNT OF CARBS (IN GRAMS)
1 cup skim milk	12 grams
1 cup low fat yogurt	46
1/2 cup black beans	22
1 apple	32
1 banana	28
1 cup orange juice	24
1/2 cup potatoes	26
1/2 cup green beans	4
1 large bagel	48
1 cup raisin bran cereal	46
8 saltines	17
1 cup pasta	40
1 cup brown rice	45

Aim for six to eight oz. a day of grains, three cups a day of vegetables, and two cups a day of fruit. And try to have a variety of fruits and veggies to round out your diet.

Q. Why are whole grains important?

"Whole grain" means that a food product is made from the entire grain seed. Grains that get "refined" lose many of the good nutrients—fiber, vitamins, minerals—in the manufacturing process. But manufacturers often enrich these grains after refining to add back some of the lost nutrients. (*US Dept of Health and Human Services*)

Eating a diet rich in whole grains may reduce cholesterol levels, and thus, lower the risk of heart disease. Added bonus: they're loaded with fiber so they'll make you poop (the all-purpose cure for constipation).

Bottom line: *Try to make at least half of your grains whole grains.*

So where are these whole grain foods lurking? Look for products made with whole wheat flour. Or choose brown rice or wild rice instead of white. Other options include: multigrain bread, oats/oatmeal, whole grain corn, popcorn, whole rye, whole grain barley, buckwheat, triticale, bulgur, millet, quinoa, sorghum.

Yes, you now have an excuse to eat popcorn.

And some carbs are beter than others. Your body quickly digests simple carbohydrates (such as white bread, white rice), causing a rapid rise and fall of glucose and insulin. It's better for you to eat carbohydrates that your body digests more slowly, causing a more gradual rise and fall of insulin levels. Here are some examples of more complex, slow-digesting carbohydrates:

Fruit and vegetables

Lentils	Peas	Carrots
Sweet potatoes	Oranges	Grapefruit
Peaches	Pears	Plums
Apples	Cherries	Grapes
Kiwi		

Beans/legumes

Kidney beans	Baked beans	Chickpeas
Soybeans	Peanuts	

Dairy

Yogurt	Milk

Bread and grains

Pasta	Hot oatmeal (not instant)
Sour dough bread	100% stone ground whole wheat bread

HIGH FRUCTOSE CORN SYRUP 411

High fructose corn syrup (HFCS) is a simple sugar.

How is it made? Cornstarch is processed to convert glucose sugar to a combination of glucose and fructose sugar. In use since the 1960's, food makers love high fructose corn syrup because it is a) cheaper than sugar and b) extends the shelf life of processed foods.

There's nothing inherently evil about high fructose corn syrup itself. Of course, over-consumption of sugar isn't a good thing. One recent study found an association between HFCS-containing sodas and obesity. *(Ebbeling CB).* Another study found an association between fructose intake, overeating, and diabetes. *(Stanhope KL).*

While no study has shown definitive evidence that HFCS really *causes* health problems, think about the types of food that contain this stuff. Our concern: HFCS is in processed foods and sweetened beverages (such as soda and sweetened fruit drinks). Processed foods have more additives and usually more calories.

Bottom line: it's always a better health choice to opt for fresh food rather than processed. And the American Medical Association recommends consumers "limit the amount of caloric sweeteners in their diet." *(AMA)*

NUTRITION

? ?

3 **FAT.** Why do we need fat? Your body uses fat for energy, brain, and nerve function. …. and your unborn baby needs it for his developing nervous system (that includes *his* brain). Hence, contrary to popular opinion, all fat is not bad.

So which fats are better than others? Here's an overview.

Fats come in three flavors: good, bad and ugly:

Good

- *Monounsaturated fats*: These are the great fats for your heart. They lower both your *total* cholesterol and bad (LDL) cholesterol. Look for them in nuts, olives, avocados, canola oil, and olive oil.
- *Polyunsaturated fats*: These fats are good because they lower cholesterol and may reduce the risk of heart disease. They also promote your baby's overall growth as well as brain and vision development. Sources: Essential fatty acids (omega-6 and omega-3) are in corn oil, safflower oil, soybean oil, margarine, soybean oil, walnut oil, walnuts, flaxseed, salmon, mackerel, and herring. The only downside is that polyunsaturated fats also lower the body's HDL or good cholesterol. Hence, limit the amount of these fats in your diet.

Bad

- *Saturated fats*: These fats raise your body's LDL cholesterol, which can lead to strokes and heart disease. You'll find saturated fats mostly in animal products (red meat, pork, lamb, veal, eggs, butter, cream, any dairy product made from whole or 2% milk) and a few plants (coconut, coconut oil, palm oil, and palm kernel oil).

Ugly

- *Trans fats*: These are man-made fats, designed to be solid at room temperature. Manufacturers take vegetable oil and partially hydrogenate it. This process makes this synthetic fat a double whammy because it raises your bad LDL cholesterol and lowers your good HDL cholesterol. There is no data to say what effect it has on your unborn baby, but what it does to your body is probably enough to make you steer clear of it. Sources: Processed baked goods and snacks, commercially prepared fried foods. Trans fats are also cleverly disguised as "hydrogenated" or "partially hydrogenated" vegetable oil on ingredient labels. See "Cholesterol and your Pregnancy" below.

How much fat do you need? Fats should make up less than 30% of your daily food intake. However, this depends on your pre-pregnancy weight and how active you are. But in real world numbers, that's about 40 to 70 grams a day. Preferably, that's mostly from good fat, not the stuff that clogs your arteries!

The American Heart Association (AHA) recommends that less than 7% of your daily fat intake come from saturated fats and less than 1% from trans fats. The balance (92%) should be from mono and polyunsaturated fats.

Here's a shocker: Americans eat more fat than recommended. And as a pregnant woman, you can reach half your daily fat intake with just two

CHOLESTEROL AND YOUR PREGNANCY

Now that you've got the skinny on fats, what about cholesterol? Here's a little secret: your body makes its own cholesterol, so you don't *need* to eat any if you are over two years of age. The American Heart Association recommends you eat less than 300mg of cholesterol a day.

Here's the 411 on cholesterol:

Cholesterol is needed by your body to make cells and hormones. The problem: an excess of cholesterol piles up, clogging up your blood vessels. That makes your heart work extra hard to pump blood through those vessels. It also clogs the arteries that provide blood flow to the heart and the brain. Bottom line: those clogged pipes leave you at risk for a heart attack or stroke.

There are three types of cholesterol:

◆ *LDL* (Low Density Lipoprotein) is bad cholesterol. It clogs your arteries. Your body makes some LDL naturally . . . and genetics puts some folks at risk because they make too much LDL. Of course, eating fats that raise LDL levels doesn't help the situation.

◆ *HDL* (High Density Lipoprotein) is good cholesterol. Instead of allowing cholesterol to collect in your arteries, HDL carries it to your liver, where it is broken down and eliminated. That's a good thing!

◆ *Triglycerides* are fats that your body makes. People who smoke, don't exercise, drink a lot of booze, and over-eat carbs tend to have high triglycerides. High triglycerides usually go hand in hand with high LDL and low HDL (a recipe for a heart attack).

tablespoons of oil.

The following chart gives you an idea of how little fat you need to reach the recommended levels: *(Northwestern University)*

Fat Goal: 40-70 grams/day

SERVING SIZE	TOTAL FAT (IN GRAMS)	TYPE OF FAT
1 T butter	11.5 grams	mostly saturated
1 T margarine	11.4	monounsaturated, polyunsaturated, trans fat
1 T canola oil	13.6	monounsaturated
1 T corn oil	13.6	mostly polyunsaturated
1 cup ice cream	24	mostly saturated, 90 mg cholesterol
1 oz. cheese	9.4	mostly saturated, 30 mg cholesterol
1 cup skim milk	0	none

1 cup whole milk	8.2	mostly saturated, 30 mg cholesterol
1/4 pounder burger	21	saturated and monounsaturated, 80 mg cholesterol
3 oz. chicken breast	3.8	saturated and monounsaturated, 70 mg cholesterol
1 egg	1.6	saturated, 200 mg cholesterol
1 oz. peanuts	14	mostly monounsaturated
1 oz. almonds	16	mostly monounsaturated
2 T avocado	5	mostly monounsaturated
1 Danish pastry	26	mostly saturated
1 doughnut	3.2	trans fat
1 order French fries	6.8	trans fat

Reality Check

Which is better, butter or margarine? Butter contains saturated fats and cholesterol (bad). Margarine contains trans fats (also bad). So which is the lesser of two evils?

First, we suggest limiting use of both butter and margarine. If you like margarine, choose a soft or liquid margarine with the lowest amount of trans fats. These types of margarines are better than stick margarine.

Helpful Hint: What is a serving size?

Just take a look at your hand.

A 3 oz. serving of meat or fish is about the size of your palm.

A 1/2 cup serving of rice or pasta is what you could place in your rounded hand. A serving of fruit or vegetable is the size of your closed fist.

Q. Are there any other nutrients I need to be certain to get while pregnant?

1. *Calcium.* Technically you don't need *more* calcium during pregnancy. But most Americans don't consume enough calcium, pregnant or not. You need 1000mg a day in divided doses—three cups of milk would do it. If you are pregnant and younger than 18 years of age, you need 1200 to 1300mg/day (four cups of milk).

2. *Folic acid.* This key nutrient prevents brain and spinal cord (neural tube) defects. Since 1998, all fortified cereals and grains in the U.S. are enriched with folic acid (folate). Most prenatal vitamins have 1000 micrograms (1 milligram)—which covers your daily dietary needs.

3. *Iron:* You need almost 40% *more* iron in your pregnancy diet. Here are a few practical tips:

◆ Eat more meat—if you're not a vegan! Your body absorbs iron from animal sources (like meat) the best. It absorbs iron from plant sources (like spinach) the least.

NUTRITION

◆ But don't have a glass of milk with your steak. Calcium prevents the absorption of iron–so avoid eating iron-rich foods or taking your iron supplements with calcium rich-foods (dairy products, milk).

◆ Do eat iron-containing foods or supplements with Vitamin C (fruit, orange juice). Vitamin C helps the body absorb iron.

Insider Secret

Odds are, you have started this book after you got pregnant. If you are planning a future pregnancy, however, it is a good idea to maintain a healthy weight and take a folic acid supplement before getting pregnant. Folic acid helps the brain and spinal cord (neural tube) form properly.

Fifty percent of pregnancies are unplanned. By the time you know you are pregnant, your baby's future brain and spine (neural tube) have already developed. Note: obese–especially severely obese–women have a greater risk of having a baby with a neural tube defect (for example, spina bifida). *(Rasmussen SA)*

Q. How much water do I need to drink?

Water is the ideal beverage for everyone, but it's especially perfect for pregnant women. Staying well hydrated helps decrease your risk of bladder infections, dehydration, preterm contractions, and feelings of dizziness. Water also ensures that your baby is cushioned by an adequate amount of amniotic fluid.

Do you really need to drink at least 64 ounces (eight full glasses) of water a day? Not only should you, but you will want to. You will be thirstier as your body requires more water throughout pregnancy.

This extra water creates amniotic fluid, increases your blood volume to be twice the amount of normal, and helps ensure breast milk production.

If that isn't enough, water helps prevent constipation. By the end of the first trimester, you'll be willing to drink an ocean to prevent that!

Q. What about salt? Do I need to be more cautious about my intake?

Salt is not your friend when you are pregnant.

You don't have to cut it out completely, but you should watch your intake. That means you need to be aware of how many chips you are inhaling at your favorite Mexican food joint. Or how much soy sauce you are putting on your rice and tempura at the Japanese restaurant.

A higher intake of salt can lead to some serious swelling during pregnancy. You may have already noticed this. A word to the wise: don't overdo the salt!

Vitamins and Supplements

Will your diet alone be enough to fulfill your body's nutritional needs? For many nutrients, the answer is yes. But all pregnant women need prenatal vitamins, almost all need calcium supplements, and some need additional supplements to sustain a healthy pregnancy.

Prenatal vitamins

Q. What type of vitamins do I need?

You need a daily prenatal vitamin (a multivitamin made especially for pregnancy) and most likely, a 500 or 600mg calcium supplement—even if you are a healthy person who actually eats from all the food groups! Your body has a lot of work to do to grow that baby.

You will also need to take an iron supplement if you begin pregnancy anemic, or become anemic during pregnancy.

Women with pre-existing medical conditions, such as celiac disease or a history of weight-loss (bariatric) surgery, often need additional supplements (such as vitamin B12). Women who follow vegetarian diets also need a B12 supplement.

Insider Tip

Most women need the additional calcium supplement beyond what's found in a prenatal vitamin because they don't drink enough milk or eat dairy products to achieve their daily needs. It is best to take that calcium supplement at a different time of day than your prenatal vitamin. Your body can't absorb all the calcium at once.

Q. Are prenatal vitamins and iron supplements available over-the-counter? Or do I need a prescription?

Yes, you can buy over-the-counter prenatal vitamins (as well as calcium and iron supplements) and these are often less expensive than the prescription options. Consult with your practitioner to be sure the supplement has the right amount of nutrients.

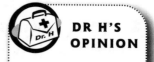

DR H'S OPINION

"Many over-the-counter prenatal vitamins contain too much Vitamin A. As of today, prescription prenatal vitamins no longer contain or have decreased amounts of Vitamin A. That's because too much Vitamin A can be associated with birth defects."

Q. I'm at the drug store and there are SEVERAL types of prenatal vitamins. Is there any major difference among them?

Most prenatal vitamins are created equal. These pills vary in size—although none of those pills would ever be classified as "small"!

Some over-the-counter vitamins contain more iron than others and some contain a stool softener (which is usually a welcome treat in the first trimester as constipation is a frequent side effect of pregnancy). Many prenatal vitamins also contain DHA (an omega-3 fatty acid), which is a good idea—we'll discuss that later in this section.

There are also prenatal vitamins available by prescription. Most prescription prenatal vitamins now have lower amounts of Vitamin A, and some have none at all. The reason? Most women get enough Vitamin A in their diet and too much Vitamin A in pregnancy is not a good thing.

Until your first visit with your practitioner, take any over-the-counter prenatal vitamin that looks appealing. Most are just fine, assuming there is at least 400 mcg of folic acid and the Vitamin A level is less than 5,000 IU (International Units). When you get to that first appointment, ask your practitioner what she recommends.

Q. My prenatal vitamins nauseate me. Any suggestions?

You're not alone. This is a VERY common complaint.

Here's our advice: don't follow the instructions that tell you to take them on an empty stomach—unless, of course, you want to vomit. It's best to take them with some food. We suggest taking your prenatal vitamin on a full stomach, with your biggest meal of the day.

You can also crush your vitamin into a powder form and mix it with a spoonful of peanut butter or applesauce. This is easier said than done and you may actually need a mortar and pestle to accomplish this task. There are also some chewable prenatal vitamins on the market.

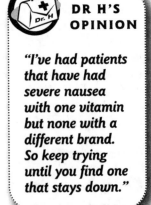

DR H'S OPINION

"I've had patients that have had severe nausea with one vitamin but none with a different brand. So keep trying until you find one that stays down."

And yes, many prenatal vitamins leave a terrible "vitamin taste" in your mouth which may make you nauseated just thinking about taking another one. There are some newer vanilla-coated prenatal vitamins just for those of you with a discriminating palate.

Finally, if nothing else works and you are so sick you just can't stand it, ask your practitioner about the option of taking individual supplements (folic acid, iron and calcium in particular) or taking two children's vitamins (gummy or Flintstone vitamins). Do be sure to let your practitioner know if you plan to take children's vitamins because they do NOT contain iron and you'll need to take an additional iron supplement.

Q. I'm a vegetarian. Are there any prenatal vitamins that do not contain animal products?

All prenatal vitamins are animal-product free, except those that contain DHA, which is often derived from fish. Gesticare sells prenatal vitamins, and one variety has DHA from a plant source. Pronexa also contains DHA from a plant source. So, if you don't do fish, these may be the vitamins for you.

FYI: Both of these vitamins contain gelatin, however—since gelatin comes from animals, they are not completely vegetarian. If you want to take a prenatal vitamin that does not contain animal products, you will need to take a prenatal vitamin and then a separate DHA supplement that is animal-product free (Whole Foods carries these, as you might imagine).

DHA supplements

Q. What are omega-3's and do I need them?

Omega-3's are unsaturated fatty acids which provide essential nutrients for heart health, as well as brain, eye and nervous system development. There are three types of omega-3's used by the human body: DHA, ALA, and EPA. DHA is the most common—we'll discuss this next. Yes, you need them.

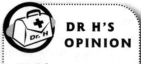

DR H'S OPINION

"With so many potential health benefits, there's really no downside to taking a DHA supplement...except for those occasional fish flavored burps."

Q. Do you recommend I take DHA supplements?

Yes.

DHA (docosahexaenoic acid) is an omega-3 fatty acid that helps in fetal brain and eye development. In fact, in some studies, moms-to-be who consumed higher levels of DHA (in their diets or by taking supplements) had children with slightly higher IQ's when tested at four years of age. (*Helland IB*)

Here's the catch, however (pun intended): fatty fish is the most common source of DHA in our diets. And because of the high levels of mercury in certain types of fish, pregnant and nursing women are told to limit their intake of some fish. As a result, the average American woman consumes less than 100 mg/day of DHA. Although the Food and Drug Administration (FDA) has not yet established a recommended daily amount for DHA, most experts recommend 300 mg/day for pregnant and nursing women.

So it makes sense to pick a prenatal vitamin that contains DHA. It's unlikely that you will get that much in your diet.

Q. How much DHA do I need a day? How do I get this in my diet?

Nutrition experts recommend 300 mg of DHA per day.

Foods that contain DHA naturally are mostly fatty fish (see chart below). Bottom line: *you can probably get enough DHA if you eat fatty fish two to three times a week.* Here's a look at the fish with the most DHA:

How much DHA?

FISH (PER 3 OZ. SERVING)	DHA (IN MILLIGRAMS)
Salmon, Atlantic	1825 mg
Herring, Atlantic	1700
Salmon, pink, canned	1400
Whitefish	1400
Tuna, bluefin	1300
Trout, rainbow	1000
Sardines, oil-canned	800
Tuna, water-canned, white	700

NUTRITION

Q. What about omega-3 fortified foods?

This is the latest rage in the grocery aisle: food makers are adding omega-3's to a wide variety of foods. But they are adding ALA, not DHA. And unfortunately, ALA does not have the same health benefits. Foods that naturally contain ALA are plant-based: flaxseed oil, soybean oil, canola oil, and walnuts. Food makers are adding these oils into foods to tout omega-3 benefits.

But take a look at the chart below: most omega-3-enriched foods have just a fraction of the good stuff that fatty fish has. That's why it's better to eat fish than relying on omega-3-enriched mayo to reach your DHA goals!

FOOD	OMEGA-3 CONTENT
Smart Balance Omega Plus Buttery Spread (1T)	160 mg
Land O Lakes "Omega-3" Eggs (1 egg)	150
Breyers Smart DHA Yogurt (6 oz)	30
Horizon Organic DHA Milk (1 cup)	30

Feedback from the Real World

Which DHA supplements are the least "fishy" tasting? Our readers suggest Gummy Omega-3 Naturals from Costco and Nordic Naturals, sold in natural foods stores (nordicnaturals.com).

Reality Check

Is there mercury in fish oil supplements? No. Consumer advocate groups tested the top 40 brands of fish oil supplements and have found no significant levels of mercury. This is most likely because mercury collects in fish meat and not the oil, and the fish used to produce oil are lower on the predator fish food chain.

If you are really nervous about mercury levels in fish oil supplements, find a brand that lists "pharmaceutical grade" on the packaging. It means that the fish oil has been processed and contains no other substances.

Old Wives Tale

Fatty acid supplements like DHA increase your risk of bleeding during pregnancy. *False.* There is no valid evidence to support this theory. Hence, you can take DHA supplements all the way up to delivery.

Vitamin D supplements

Q. I've heard a lot about women not getting enough Vitamin D. Is there any risk to me or the baby if I have a deficiency?

Yes, you need Vitamin D. It works with calcium to build both your and your baby's bones during pregnancy and breastfeeding.

A few recent studies have found a link between Vitamin D deficiency and a type of high blood pressure (**PREECLAMPSIA**) that can occur during pregnancy *(August P.)*

Vitamin D deficiency is more common than you would think, even for women who eat a healthy diet. Our bodies make most of our Vitamin D

when our skin is exposed to the sun. But since many of us avoid sun exposure to prevent skin cancer (hats, sunglasses, sun block and shade), we
aren't letting our skin manufacture Vitamin D! So it's a Catch 22.

Unfortunately, most adults don't get enough Vitamin D from a typical
diet either. Milk is an obvious source, since it is fortified with Vitamin D. You
can get most of your daily Vitamin D needs if you drink three cups a day,
but most women don't drink that much milk.

You can also get quite a bit of Vitamin D from a teaspoon or two of
cod liver oil, but, seriously, very few of us would guzzle this stuff. Salmon,
mackerel, and tuna are about the only other foods that contain high levels
of Vitamin D.

Although more studies are needed, it's a great idea to get your Vitamin
D level checked prior to getting pregnant. If it is low, begin supplementa-
tion. Most calcium supplements include Vitamin D. You can take 400 I.U.
(International Units) in the morning and 400 I.U. in the evening. *(Bodnar LM)*

Another option: Nature Made sells a small Vitamin D gelcap that contains
1,000 I.U. (of mostly D_3, the form of Vitamin D that is best) per capsule.

Insider Secret

Your newborn also needs a Vitamin D supplement. The
American Academy of Pediatrics recommends that all infants
get 400 IU of Vitamin D a day.

Iron supplements

Q. My iron supplement makes me constipated. Any sug-
gestions?

You have a few options.

Over-the-counter, slow release iron supplements (like Slow Fe) are often
less constipating. You can also ask your pharmacist to make a liquid iron

---

TOO MUCH OF A GOOD THING

Vitamin supplements are good for you and your baby. But going
above and beyond the standard recommended intake is NOT a
good thing. In fact, it may even do some harm. Here are some ugly
examples of why more is not necessarily better:

◆ **Vitamin A:** High doses of Vitamin A (greater than 10,000
IU/day) can cause birth defects. This is why many vitamin companies have removed Vitamin A from their prenatal vitamins
altogether.

◆ **Vitamin E:** Excessive Vitamin E levels are associated with congenital heart defects. *(Smedts HP)*

◆ **Folic Acid:** Most prenatal vitamins contain one milligram (more
than double the dose needed to prevent neural tube defects).
In higher doses, it can hide the symptoms of a rare type of
anemia in mom and thus, delay treatment.

NUTRITION

formula, which may help.

Make a goal to get more iron from food in your diet. This iron is more easily absorbed. Foods such as dried apricots, raisins, lentils, eggs, chicken, red meat, liver, kale and spinach are high in iron. Remember that your body absorbs iron from animal sources most effectively.

If you have tried it all, nothing is working, and you still need to take an iron supplement, eat a ton of fiber and take a stool softener.

Herbal supplements

Q. Can I take herbal supplements?

With all the supplements stocked at your local natural food store, it may be tempting to sneak one of these into your diet. But are they safe?

Short answer: there is little scientific research on most supplements. That means we have *no idea* how they may affect pregnancy and breastfeeding.

We'll discuss the most common supplements in Expecting411.com/extra.

Bottom line: ask your practitioner about particular supplements *before* taking them. Don't take anything on the sly!

Protein supplements

Q. Are protein drinks okay?

Yes.

Just read the nutrition facts to see how much protein is in your drink. During pregnancy, you need 60 to 70 grams of protein each day. If you aren't getting enough in your diet, protein shakes are an excellent way of getting more. Inadequate protein intake in pregnancy is linked to growth problems in the fetus—so try to meet your body's needs. *(Kramer MS)*

Probiotics

Q. What about probiotics? Are they safe? Is there any benefit in taking them?

Yes, probiotics are safe to take during pregnancy. Known to promote healthy digestion, probiotics are also touted to boost immune function, inhibit the growth of harmful bacteria and increase resistance to certain infections and disease-causing bacteria. While the jury is still out on some of these claims, there is enough scientific evidence on probiotics to say they are helpful.

Pregnant women have more digestive issues than any other group of people on the planet (the nausea, vomiting, heartburn, belching, gas, constipation—need we continue?) Probiotics help keep your gastrointestinal tract functioning normally. They also prevent recurrent vaginal infections, such as candida (yeast) and gardnerella (bacterial vaginosis).

Despite all the good things we can say about probiotics, always check with your practitioner first before adding any new supplement to your diet during pregnancy.

PRObiotics and PREbiotics

Probiotics and prebiotics are popping up at natural and conventional grocery stores alike, thanks to the potential health benefits. But what are they?

What are PRObiotics?

These are "good germs" (bacteria or yeast) that help the body digest food. They are found naturally in yogurt, kefir, kombucha, tea, miso tempeh and sauerkraut. You can also buy them in capsules or powder form. Note: the good germs are only present when you ingest them. So once a person stops taking them, the benefits go away.

What are PREbiotics?

These are complex starches or polysaccharides in food that help the gut grow the good bacteria mentioned above. This is what sustains the healthy gut environment. Prebiotics are found naturally in whole grains, honey, bananas, garlic, onions, leeks, and artichokes. Other food and beverage products are fortified with them. Note: prebiotics basically provide the nesting ground for good germs. So, even if someone doesn't take prebiotics everyday, the benefits have longer lasting effects.

Counting Calories

Q. How much weight should I gain?

The amount of weight you should gain during pregnancy depends upon your pre-pregnancy weight. Check with your doctor to help you determine if you are staring out at a healthy weight, underweight or overweight.

Once you have figured this out, you can see how much weight you will need to gain to have a healthy pregnancy. The Institute of Medicine established new pregnancy weight gain guidelines in 2009, based on women's pre-pregnancy Body Mass Index (BMI). Here's the scoop:

BMI*		ESTIMATED WEIGHT GAIN
BMI < 18.5	(underweight)	30-40 lbs.
BMI 18.5–24.9	(healthy weight)	25-35 lbs.
BMI 25–29.9	(overweight)	15-25 lbs.
BMI > 30	(obese)	11-20 lbs.

* To calculate your BMI, go to nhlbisupport.com/bmi and plug in your height and pre-pregnancy weight. It's confidential, so no cheating! We also have a BMI chart on our web site at Expecting411.com (bonus).

Reality Check

55% of American women of childbearing age are overweight.

NUTRITION

FYI: counting calories. Carbohydrates have four calories per gram. Proteins have four calories per gram. Fats have nine calories per gram.

Q. How much weight should I gain in each trimester?

This is a tough question to answer because all of us are different.

We will give you a rough guideline of average weight gain by trimester, but remember this is ONLY A GUIDELINE. It is not something to obsess over.

Ok, that's easy for us to say. We realize it is common to get freaked out after seeing your weight at your practitioner's office–is it too much? Too little? Again, take a deep breath–remember your practitioner is tracking your weight and will let you know if there are any concerns. If your doc isn't worried, you shouldn't be!

Here is the rough guideline of how much weight you should gain:

Healthy Weight Before Pregnancy

First Trimester:	3-5 lbs.
Second Trimester:	1 lb. per week
Third Trimester:	1 lb. per week

Underweight Before Pregnancy (talk to your doctor)

First Trimester:	5-8 lbs. depending on your starting weight
Second Trimester:	1-2 lbs. per week
Third Trimester:	1-2 lbs. per week

Overweight or Obese Before Pregnancy

First Trimester:	1-2 lbs.
Second Trimester:	< 1 lb. per week
Third Trimester:	< 1 lb. per week

Reality Check

If you are getting really depressed about how much weight you are gaining, don't look at the weigh in!

Partner Tip

If you value your life, don't talk about your partner's weight gain. Remember, you are also at risk for gaining a few extra pounds during pregnancy.

Q. How many extra calories do I need?

Fewer than you think.

Even though you are growing a baby and the accessories that go with him or her, you only need about 300 to 350 extra calories a day. That's the equivalent of some peanut butter crackers and a one ounce bag of almonds. Or, it's one milkshake indulgence.

So you don't need to clean your plate and your partner's to meet your calorie needs. It may just mean you add in a couple of healthy snacks throughout the day.

NUTRITION

Bottom Line

Don't go overboard on counting calories and checking your weight on a daily basis. Just make wise food choices.

Q. What happens if I don't gain enough weight?

Your practitioner keeps an eye on your overall weight gain. That's why you have to suffer through a weigh-in at every visit. There are two key reasons your doc tracks weight gain:

◆ You need enough calories to maintain your changing body. Your organs get bigger and your nutrient stores decline.

◆ If you don't eat, neither does your baby. Your fetus may not grow properly if you don't gain enough weight.

If your weight gain is not what it should be, your practitioner will probably tell you to do some of the following:

◆ Keep a food diary to make sure you are eating enough.
◆ Eat whole milk dairy products instead of low-fat options.
◆ Add snacks in between meals.
◆ Have a protein shake or smoothie instead of lower calorie snacks.
◆ Add nuts to your diet.

Q. I've been a chronic dieter for most of my adult life. I am currently on a low-carb diet. Will this be safe to continue during my pregnancy?

Short answer: NO.

Long answer: A growing fetus requires a constant supply of glucose (from carbohydrates) to grow normally. Low carb diets don't provide enough carbs for a growing baby.

Glucose is the fuel for developing the brain and nervous system. If a pregnant woman's diet does not provide carbohydrates for her fetus, her body tries to use fats and protein for energy. Fat cannot be broken down into glucose. Instead, it breaks down into something called *ketones*.

Normally, a small amount of ketones float around in the blood. But if a pregnant woman continually deprives herself of carbohydrates, large amounts of ketones accumulate. Ketones can and do cross the placenta. This can result in fetal **KETOACIDOSIS**, which can lower the baby's blood pressure and increase the baby's heart rate.

Low carb diets also promote water loss. When the body breaks down

DR H'S OPINION:
STRESSING ABOUT WEIGHT

I have seen so many women come in and really stress over the fact that they have gained six pounds in a month . . . or lament that they have only gained two pounds during that same time period. It is okay. As your practitioners, we keep a close watch on overall trends and will let you know if you are gaining too much or too little.

? ?

NUTRITION

WEIGHT GAIN 411: WHERE DOES IT GO?

The good news is that if you gain between 25 to 35 lbs. during your pregnancy, only about seven to eight pounds is actually fat tissue. In general, the rest is as follows:

Baby	7-8 lbs.
Uterus	2 lbs.
Placenta	1-2 lbs.
Amniotic Fluid	2 lbs.*
Extra Blood Volume	4 lbs.
Increase in the size of your organs	1-2 lbs.
Maternal breast tissue	2 lbs.
Extra fluid in maternal tissue	4 lbs.

*This is why your doctor is covered in waterproof attire at the time of your delivery!

proteins instead of carbs, water is lost. Important body electrolytes, like sodium and potassium, are lost with the water.

This all spells danger for the fetus. Many studies show elevated ketone levels stress the fetus (changing fetal vital signs) and put the baby at risk for health problems later in life, such as high blood pressure, heart disease and diabetes. (Gabbe SG)

DR H'S OPINION

"This is the one time in your life that you need to put your dieting aside and do what is best for your little one."

Q. What happens if I gain too much weight?

If you gain too much weight (but had a normal BMI prior to pregnancy), your practitioner will watch you a little more closely, looking for any potential health risks. Examples: gestational diabetes and high blood pressure (**PREECLAMPSIA**). See Chapter 16, Complications, #26 and 20). It may also make delivery a bit more difficult as increased weight gain in mom is often associated with bigger babies—and bigger babies are tougher to get out!

If all goes well with pregnancy and delivery, you've just got a few extra pounds to work off afterwards.

Q. I have battled obesity all my life. I am now eight weeks pregnant—what risks do I face?

If you are already overweight and then you gain more than you need to during pregnancy, there are some potential health risks to both you and your baby. Your job is to do the best you have EVER done in your life to watch what you eat, how much you eat, and be physically active.

The key health concerns for you: potential gestational diabetes, high blood pressure (**PREECLAMPSIA**), impaired immunity to fight infections, and an increased risk of having a Cesarean delivery. The key health concerns for your baby: potential birth defects, increased risk of miscarriage/stillbirth, bigger birth weight (increasing risk of complications and Cesarean delivery), future risk of diabetes, obesity, and heart disease. *(Stothard KJ)* Scary, we know. Be assured that your practitioner is looking out for all these issues to try to prevent them or treat them early if they arise.

Reality Check

About one-third of overweight women end up having a C-section.

Real World Tip: Banish the 4C's

Sometimes it's hard to resist temptation because it's simply too easy to access junk food. Don't get us wrong, we need our

EAT WELL AND SPARE THE CALORIES

It's easy to avoid gaining too much weight during pregnancy. This chart shows you how simply picking low-fat options makes it easy: *(US Dept of Health and Human Services)*

FOOD	PORTION	FAT CONTENT	CALORIES
Cheese			
Regular	1 oz.	6 grams	114
Lowfat	1 oz.	1.2 g	49
Ground beef			
Regular (25% fat)	3 oz. cooked	6.1 g	236
Extra lean (5% fat)	3 oz. cooked	2.6 g	148
Milk			
Whole (3.2%)	1 cup	4.6 g	146
1% milk	1 cup	1.5 g	102
Desserts			
Ice Cream	1/2 cup	4.9 g	145
Frozen yogurt	1/2 cup	2.0 g	110
Table spreads			
Butter	1 tsp	2.4 g	34
Margarine	1 tsp (no trans fat)	0.7 g	25
Meat			
Fried chicken leg	3 oz.	3.3 g	212
Roasted chicken breast (no skin)	3 oz.	0.9 g	140
Fish			
Fried fish	3 oz.	2.8 g	195
Baked fish	3 oz.	1.5 g	129

TAKE HOME TIPS: WEIGHT GAIN

3 tips for women who were overweight before they got pregnant

◆ See a nutritionist when you realize you are pregnant.

◆ You still need to gain weight during pregnancy. But it should be no more than 15 to 20 lbs.

◆ Incorporate exercise into your daily routine (always check with your practitioner first before beginning any exercise program).

3 tips for women who were underweight before they got pregnant

◆ You need to gain between 30 to 40 lbs. during your pregnancy.

◆ Remember, don't get freaked out by those large numbers on the doctor's scale—your baby needs that extra weight.

◆ Make sure you are eating a balanced diet with enough caloric intake. Keeping a food diary is helpful.

nutrition

chocolate fix, too, every once in a while.

Our point: if it's not in your pantry, it's much more likely to be a treat. If it's in your pantry, it's a staple. So consider banishing the Four C's: cola, candy, chips, and cookies. These are empty calorie foods. Just eliminating the temptation to snack on this food/drink will go miles in helping you maintain a healthy pregnancy weight.

Partner Tip

Got to have those potato chips but your pregnant other half has banned them from the house? Our advice: man up! Be supportive and suffer along with her. You both will be healthier as a result!

Factoid: One-third of the added sugar in the American diet comes from soft drinks.

Bottom Line

To limit calories, just switch to some of the alternatives mentioned earlier. Pick lean meats, low fat milk and cheese, and start baking/broiling instead of frying. And once you see how easy this is to do while you are pregnant, it will be a cinch to make this a lifelong change.

Q. How quickly will I lose my pregnancy weight?

You will lose ten to 13 lbs. shortly after birth, but you won't see it on the scales until a week or two later. That's because you will initially have quite a bit of fluid retention.Here's an important fact: *only 28% of women are back to their pre-pregnancy weight within six weeks.*

So don't compare yourself to celebrity newbie moms flaunting their post-pregnancy bikini bodies on the cover of *People*. Most normal women (without 24 hour chefs and trainers on call) lose their weight in three to six months after delivery.

NUTRITION

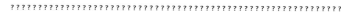
? ?

DOES FOOD "PROGRAM" YOUR BABY'S HEALTH?

Does what you eat during pregnancy set up your baby for a life-long health? Or chronic disease?

There is a scientific theory (the "thrifty gene" or Barker Hypothesis) that suggests poor pregnancy and newborn nutrition permanently changes a child's metabolism. In other words, mom's nutrition "programs" her baby's metabolism for life. This alteration can lead to obesity and diabetes, which can cause heart disease.

While science has yet to confirm this theory with overwhelming evidence, it's a good enough reason to eat healthy during pregnancy!

Bariatric Surgery

Bariatric surgery refers to the surgical procedures used to aid in weight loss. There are two primary types:

Gastric Banding places a fluid-filled band around the stomach to reduce its volume. This makes patients feel full faster and decreases total food intake.

Roux-en-Y gastric bypass uses a loop of your intestine to "by-pass" the lower portion of your stomach and upper intestine. This decreases stomach capacity and food absorption.

Q. I have had the gastric banding procedure and want to get pregnant. How long do I have to wait to conceive?

Most experts recommend waiting 12 to 24 months after bariatric surgery before conceiving. The reasons: to avoid exposing the fetus to all of the metabolic changes that occur when rapid weight loss happens; and to allow patients to achieve their full weight loss goals before becoming pregnant.

Q. I had gastric bypass surgery 18 months ago and am pregnant. Am I at risk for any additional complications?

Yes.

Many patients remain obese after undergoing bariatric surgery. If you haven't reached your maximum weight loss goal, you may still be obese. Hence, you will be at risk for all of the complications mentioned above.

With bariatric surgery, your risk of needing a C-section increases by 62%, according to the latest research. *(Weintraub AY)*

Also: you should be watched closely for complications due to the bariatric surgery itself (bowel obstruction and severe bleeding from your stomach or intestines). Tell your practitioner if you have any abdominal pain during your pregnancy.

Reality Check

If you have lost the excess weight after bariatric surgery, terrific! Then you have lowered your risk of gestational diabetes and high blood pressure (**PREECLAMPSIA**).

Q. Is my baby at risk if I've had bariatric surgery?

If you have lost weight after having your procedure, then your baby is actually much better off. Fetuses born to women who have had this procedure are more likely to be of normal weight. The risk of stillbirth and birth defects also decreases.

Q. Are there any special tests or consultants needed during my pregnancy because of my history of bariatric surgery?

Yes.

Your pregnancy medical team should include an OB, a perinatologist (maternal fetal medicine or high-risk pregnancy specialist) as well as the surgeon who performed your bariatric surgery.

Women who are followed by their bariatric team during pregnancy are able to manage their weight much better than those who are followed by an OB alone. *(Karmon A)*

You also have some special nutritional issues. If you had a Roux-en-Y procedure, there is an increased risk of protein, iron, Vitamin B12, folate, Vitamin D and calcium deficiencies. Your practitioner will check for these and will recommend supplementation if necessary.

If you had a gastric bypass procedure, you won't be able to do the standard glucola screening test for gestational diabetes. You may have a severe reaction if you take 50 grams of glucose. So, you may need to have your fasting blood sugar checked and pass these numbers on to your doc for review.

Lastly, if you are still obese, you may need non-stress tests (NSTs) in your last month of pregnancy to assess the well-being of your fetus.

Special Diets

Q. I am a vegetarian. What should I add to my diet to be sure my baby gets what she needs?

If you eat eggs, legumes (beans, lentils), tofu and milk, you have a variety of options for your protein needs. However, you will need a source of iron and B12. Ask your practitioner if you need to take a B12 supplement.

Q. I am a vegan. Any special precautions?

If you don't eat any meat, milk, or eggs, it may be challenging to meet your protein needs. Nuts and legumes are great sources of protein, so load up! But your pregnant body also needs a variety of protein sources, not just a particular amount.

You will also need to be creative on finding a food source for iron, calcium, and Vitamin D. You will likely be asked to take a calcium supplement during both pregnancy and breastfeeding (lactation), so find one with vita-min D in it as well. And you will probably need a B12 supplement, as that vitamin is only plentiful in animal food sources.

Talk to your practitioner about your dietary restrictions. You may also want to consult a nutritionist.

Q. I am lactose intolerant. What should I eat to replace what I am missing in milk and dairy products?

A quick primer on lactose intolerance: this means that you have trouble digesting the sugar that is found naturally in milk, called lactose. It does NOT mean you are allergic to milk. People with a true milk allergy are aller-gic to milk *protein*, not sugar.

In this case, you can eat dairy products that are lactose-free (there are many lactose-free milks, cheeses, and yogurts). Or you can take a lactaid digestive enzyme supplement before eating dairy.

Bottom line: you need the calcium and Vitamin D in milk products dur-ing your pregnancy.

As a side note, some people who are lactose-intolerant find that they can eat cheese or yogurt, but cannot tolerate drinking straight milk. If you have never tried this, it might be worth it to do a little experiment.

FYI: Are you looking for the answers to burning questions on the safe-ty of caffeine, artificial sweeteners, fish, cheese, lunchmeat, or alcohol? Read the next chapter, Chapter 7, The Environment for the low down.

Now that we have tackled the kitchen, let's take a look at how the envi-ronment you live in affects your baby—and how you can limit potentially dangerous exposures.

THE ENVIRONMENT & YOUR BABY

Chapter 7

"The only way to keep your health is to eat what you don't want, drink what you don't like, and do what you'd druther not."
—Mark Twain

Your baby's placenta acts as a great barrier to the outside world—but it doesn't block the passage of *everything* to your unborn baby. Germs (viruses, bacteria), drugs, and certain toxins that circulate in your bloodstream can go right to your developing baby. Some of these items have well-known adverse health effects. For others, the jury is still out.

This chapter will cover things you may never have considered before—how the air you breathe, the food you eat, the house you keep, and some of the bad habits you have, affect you and your unborn baby.

Scary fact: over 100 environmental chemicals are found in umbilical cord blood. That means your developing baby is exposed to the same daily toxins you are.

Here's the take-home message: don't let this chapter alarm you. The goal is to open up your eyes to the world you live in.

No book or expert has all the answers on what is "safe" or "acceptable" exposure, because environmental health is an emerging science. Compared to other fields, scientists have only just started to look at the effects of natural and man-made environmental exposures. Until we have more answers, it makes sense to limit or avoid potential environmental hazards when it is practical to do so.

ENVIRO

HAZARDOUS TO YOUR HEALTH?

Enviro toxins can be broken into six basic categories:

◆ *Carcinogens*: Known to cause cancer. Examples: arsenic, tobacco, solvents like benzene.

◆ *Mutagens*: Increase the rate of change ("mutation") in genetic material, leading to possible defective cells and cancer. Example: radiation.

◆ *Teratogens*: Alter a fetus during development in the womb. Abnormalities are present at birth. Example: alcohol.

◆ *Neurotoxins:* Damage or interfere with nerve/brain function (example: lead, methylmercury, Polychlorinated Biphenyls or PCB's, organophosphate pesticides). Severely affected people will have obvious symptoms. Lower amounts of exposure may cause more subtle symptoms such as a shorter attention span or slightly lower IQ.

◆ *Endocrine disruptors:* Mimic the body's natural chemical messengers (hormones) and can potentially interfere with body responses in the reproductive system and thyroid gland. Examples: phytoestrogens and Bisphenol-A or BPA.

◆ *Irritants and allergens:* These agents cause allergic responses in the airway and/or the skin. Example: Volatile Organic Compounds or VOC's.

How do these toxins affect a fetus developing in the womb? It depends on the toxin . . . and when the exposure occurs. For instance, a significant toxin exposure in the first two weeks of pregnancy might result in miscarriage. The same exposure during the fifth or six week might cause a birth defect. Exposures after the first trimester might result in low birth weight.

An important caveat: the brain is sensitive to injury during the *entire* pregnancy.

So, let's sum the potential effects of toxins on a fetus:

◆ Miscarriage, stillbirth, infant death.
◆ Birth defects (congenital malformations).
◆ Low birth weight.
◆ Developmental delays.
◆ Childhood cancer.

Reality Check

Most of the evidence we have about toxins and their potential damage comes from animal studies—the effects on humans are guesswork. There simply isn't enough research on many of these issues to tell which toxins are most dangerous to humans. That said, it makes sense to reduce exposures to the top toxins when you can. Up next: specific advice on how to do this!

ENVIRO

Food & Drink

ALCOHOL

Q. Can I drink at all during my pregnancy?

The most recent studies say no. Even small amounts of alcohol during pregnancy can affect your unborn baby. Bottom line: if you are drinking, so is your baby.

FETAL ALCOHOL SYNDROME DISORDERS (FASD) is the fancy name for health effects from alcohol exposure in the womb. These disorders share common issues: behavioral, learning, and physical problems. *Fetal alcohol syndrome (FAS)* is the most severe form. Children with FAS have lifelong neurological and physical disabilities.

We know that 40% to 60% of women who binge drink or have chronic alcohol intake (five to seven drinks per day) have babies with FAS. But the latest research shows that much smaller amounts (one to two drinks a day) may adversely affect a child's birth weight, attention, behavior, and IQ.

Bottom line: don't drink. Good news: most women actually lose their taste for alcohol during pregnancy, so you probably won't be craving a margarita with Mexican food anyway.

Q. I had some drinks before I realized I was pregnant. Is this going to harm my baby?

This is one of the Top 10 most-asked pregnancy questions.

In a perfect world, women would abstain from alcohol while attempting to become pregnant. In reality, however, most have a few alcoholic drinks before they know they are pregnant.

If you discover you are pregnant after being late for a period and doing a home pregnancy test, four or more weeks may have gone by while you were pregnant, didn't know it . . . and visited the local happy hour.

So, should you be freaking out now? Answer: no.

It may sound harsh, but there is an "all or nothing effect" for alcohol (as well as other toxin) exposure in the early part of the first trimester. If enough damage is done to a growing fetus, a miscarriage happens. If your pregnancy continues, most of the time, your baby will be just fine.

Bottom line: once you know you are pregnant, stop drinking. Your baby should be fine as long as you do this.

Q. Why is alcohol risky for baby?

Let's be blunt: alcohol affects the brain. Exposing a rapidly growing brain to alcohol is just a bad idea.

Fetal alcohol syndrome is the number one *preventable* cause of intellectual disability (formerly known as mental retardation). A child with FAS has a misshapen face, a small head, poor growth, kidney and heart problems, hearing and vision problems, as well as behavioral and learning issues.

Although FAS is the most severe end of the spectrum, *any* alcohol-related birth defect is devastating . . . and avoidable.

ENVIRO

? ?

Q. What about the amount of alcohol in cough and cold meds?

There is a negligible amount of alcohol in some cough and cold medications. Don't worry unless you are downing large amounts of the stuff for days on end. If you have specific concerns, check with your practitioner.

CAFFEINE

Q. I admit it. I have to have my coffee in the morning. Can I have any caffeine during my pregnancy?

Caffeine is a stimulant that increases heart rate and blood pressure. Caffeine is also a diuretic, causing your body to lose water.

When caffeine crosses the placenta, your baby's developing metabolism can't quite handle the caffeine jolt the way you do.

So what does the science say on caffeine and pregnancy? There are no conclusive studies in humans showing that caffeine consumed during pregnancy causes birth defects. Some studies in animals, however, have shown decreased fertility, birth defects, preterm delivery, and an increased risk of low-birth weight babies. *(Gillen-Goldstein J)*.

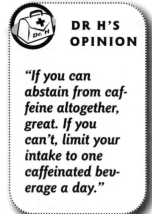

DR H'S OPINION

"If you can abstain from caffeine altogether, great. If you can't, limit your intake to one caffeinated beverage a day."

Despite the lack of clear-cut science on this issue, the general consensus among OB/GYN's is to limit caffeine intake during pregnancy.

What does that mean in the real world? Well, unfortunately, there is no science that says 200mg is safe, more than 300mg is dangerous, etc. Despite the lack of evidence, March of Dimes, Health Canada, and UK Food Standards Agency all recommend limiting caffeine intake to 200mg a day during pregnancy.

Our advice: no more than one (or on rare occasion, two) caffeinated drinks a day. By one beverage, we are referring to an average eight-ounce cup of coffee (sorry, that venti Starbucks counts as nearly three drinks). And if you are having some caffeine, make sure you stay well hydrated (with water or fluid-replacement drinks such as Gatorade) to prevent dehydration.

CAFFEINE & PREGNANCY: WHAT STUDIES SAY

When researchers study caffeine's effects on pregnancy, they are looking at "high levels" which generally mean more than 300mg/day. As you can tell from the chart on the next page, one Starbucks can put you over that limit.

A few studies show an association between high levels of caffeine intake and delayed fertility (taking a long time to get pregnant), miscarriage, and preterm labor/low-birth weight babies. *(Norman RJ.)*

ENVIRO

The Daily BUZZ

Remember that caffeine isn't just in coffees and teas, but also in sodas, chocolate and some over-the-counter headache medicine (such as Excedrin).

	AMOUNT OF CAFFEINE (MG)
Starbucks Venti Coffee, 20 oz	415 milligrams
Starbucks Grande Coffee, 16 oz	330
Starbucks Tall Coffee, 8 oz	260
Coffee, 8 oz	150
Red Bull	80
Coffee ice cream, 1 cup	60–75
Excedrin, 1 capsule	65
Black tea, 8 oz	50
Coke, 12 oz	34
Green tea, 8 oz	30
Candy bar	10

HERBAL AND NON-HERBAL TEAS

Q. What is the difference between herbal and non-herbal teas?

Non-herbal teas come from leaves of tea plants and there are three types: black, green and oolong. They contain different amounts of anti-oxidants, as well as caffeine. Types of black tea include English breakfast, Earl Grey and Orange Pekoe. Oolong teas are a combination of black and green tea.

Herbal teas are made from seeds, berries, roots, flowers and a variety of other plant parts, not from actual tea leaves. True herbal teas do not contain caffeine. These teas often claim to have medicinal uses.

Q. Can I have non-herbal tea during my pregnancy?

Yes. Non-herbal teas may offer health benefits, thanks to anti-oxidants found in the tea leaves.

But remember that the average cup of non-herbal tea contains between 40 to 50 mg of caffeine. Caffeine crosses the placenta and enters your baby's circulation. So drink it in moderation.

Q. Can I have herbal tea during my pregnancy?

Yes, if you stick to commercially-made herbal teas.

Commercially-made herbal tea (such as Celestial Seasoning) are regulated by the FDA and are presumed safe.

Of course, there are many other herbal teas, sold online and in health food stores. Some folks make their own herbal teas from herbs they collect from a garden or farmer's market.

Non-commercial herbal teas may have varying (sometimes excessive) amounts of herbs or herbs known to be dangerous during pregnancy (such as Nettle). And there isn't much research or safety data on these teas and developing fetuses.

ENVIRO

Our advice: avoid non-commercially made herbal tea products, unless you are using them under the supervision of your doctor or midwife. Some herbal teas, like red raspberry leaf, are probably safe in pregnancy. Midwives often use this tea to decrease the length of labor, help with blood loss after delivery, increase milk production and decrease nausea.

Herbal teas are naturally caffeine free.

Reality Check

While we are on the subject of herbs…many herbal supplements are off limits during pregnancy. But it is certainly fine to cook with herbs like garlic, nutmeg and cinnamon.

ARTIFICIAL SWEETENERS

Q. What are artificial sweeteners and can I use them during pregnancy?

Artificial sweeteners are sugar substitutes. They add sweetness to different foods and drinks, such as sodas, juices, desserts, chewing gum, certain candies and pastries. They are also used as table-top sweeteners for coffee and tea, taking the place of sugar.

Yes. It's fine to eat or drink limited amounts of Equal, NutraSweet, Sunett, Truvia and Splenda. There is some data to show that these are safe. What's a "limited" amount, you ask? Well, a packet of artificial sweetener in your tea or one diet soda is no problem. Drinking ten diet sodas a day, however, is not a good idea!

Just avoid Sweet N Low. It contains saccharin, which crosses the placenta. Studies show that saccharin remains in fetal tissues for long periods of time, so it is probably safer to use one of the above-mentioned alternatives during pregnancy. The FDA still considers saccharin safe for non-pregnant people.

CHEESE

Q. My friend has completely freaked me out—she said I shouldn't have eaten brie at that dinner party last night! Is this true? Why? Are there other cheeses I should avoid?

Here's the basic rule: avoid unpasteurized cheese and dairy products during pregnancy. Why? In a word, Listeria.

Listeria is a bacteria that's found in certain imported, *unpasteurized* soft cheeses. Listeria can cross the placenta and may cause an infection in your fetus, which can sometimes lead to miscarriage.

Here's a list of soft cheeses that raise red flags:

- Brie
- Camembert
- Roquefort
- Feta
- Gorgonzola
- Blue-veined cheeses
- Mexican cheeses (such as queso blanco and queso fresco)

Avoid these cheeses unless they clearly state that they have been pasteurized or made with pasteurized milk. This advice goes for all dairy prod-

ENVIRO

ucts. Unpasteurized products are commercially available in the U.S., so don't assume cheese is pasteurized because it is sold at the grocery store or natural foods mart. When in doubt, ask.

If you are out at a restaurant, check with the waiter or kitchen before ordering any dish with soft cheese. For more info on Listeria, check out Chapter 17, Infections.

FISH AND SHELLFISH

Q. I am dying for sushi. Why is my doctor telling me I shouldn't have any?

Two words: food poisoning.

Don't get us wrong, we are both huge sushi fans. However, when pregnant, you need to think of yourself as "immune-compromised." This means that you and your partner can eat the same food, but you are the only one who gets sick.

As an OB/GYN, I see this all the time—patients who end up with severe food poisoning from eating just one piece of sushi, a medium rare steak or that seared (but still rare) ahi tuna.

As we've discussed before, your immune system is temporarily suppressed during pregnancy (so you don't reject that foreign DNA growing in your uterus). Bottom line: you are much more susceptible to getting sick from both viruses and bacteria.

Most sushi contains raw fish or fish eggs (smelt). Raw or undercooked fish (just like any other meat) may be contaminated with multiple types of bacteria including Salmonella, Shigella, and toxoplasmosis. Not only can you get extremely sick from these germs, but your baby can get infected too. Infection can cause miscarriage as well as multiple birth defects including intellectual disability.

Have some celebratory sushi on your first date night with your partner *after* the baby is born. For now, you'll have to get your sushi fix by eating vegetable sushi or sushi with cooked fish such as imitation crab or shrimp tempura. Just be certain that the chef doesn't prepare it on the same cutting board with the same knife that is being used for all of the other uncooked sushi.

Q. Which fish are safe to eat during pregnancy? How much can I eat?

Fish is good for you and your developing baby. You just have to choose the *right* fish. The big concern with some fish: mercury contamination.

Developing fetuses whose moms eat diets high in fish contaminated with mercury are at risk for developmental delays, intellectual disability, learning issues, and attention problems.

Predator fish (example: swordfish) have the highest levels of mercury, so those are the ones to avoid. See the handy table below for more info. Also: check out gotmercury.org.

If you want a handy wallet card to take to the grocery store with you, check this out: nrdc.org/health/effects/mercury/walletcard.PDF

Enviro

? ?

HIGHEST MERCURY LEVELS: AVOID

Grouper	Mackerel
Marlin	Orange roughy
Tilefish	Swordfish
Shark	

HIGH MERCURY LEVELS: STEER CLEAR

Bass	Bluefish
Croaker	Halibut
Lobster (American/Maine)	Tuna (canned, white albacore)
Tuna (fresh bluefin and ahi)	Sea trout

MEDIUM MERCURY: HAVE LESS THAN THREE 6 OZ SERVINGS/MONTH

Carp	Cod
Crab (blue and snow)	Herring
Mahi Mahi	Monkfish
Perch (seawater)	Skate
Snapper	Tuna (canned, chunk light)
Tuna (fresh Pacific albacore)	

LOW MERCURY: HAVE TWO 6 OZ SERVINGS PER WEEK

Anchovies	Butterfish
Calamari (squid)	Catfish
Caviar (farmed)	Clams
Crab (king)	Crawfish/Crayfish
Flounder	Haddock
Hake	Herring
Lobster (spiny/rock)	Oysters
Perch (ocean)	Pollock
Salmon	Sardines
Scallops	Shad
Shrimp	Sole
Sturgeon (farmed)	Tilapia
Trout (freshwater)	Whitefish

Q. **I'm confused about tuna. I've heard that some is safe and some is not. Is that true?**

Yes. Mercury levels vary in tuna based on the *type* of tuna and where it was caught.

Because of this confusion, the Natural Resources Defense Council developed guidelines to help families decide how much and what kind of tuna can be eaten by children, women wanting to conceive, and pregnant and lactating women (see below). The chart is based on weight. *(FDA)*

ENVIRO

IF YOU WEIGH:	WHITE ALBACORE	CHUNK LIGHT
	DON'T EAT MORE THAN ONE CAN EVERY:	
20 lbs	10 weeks	3 weeks
30 lbs	6 weeks	2 weeks
40 lbs	5 weeks	11 days
50 lbs	4 weeks	9 days
60 lbs	3 weeks	7 days
70 lbs	3 weeks	6 days
80 lbs	2 weeks	6 days
90 lbs	2 weeks	5 days
100 lbs	2 weeks	5 days
110 lbs	12 days	4 days
120 lbs	11 days	4 days
130 lbs	10 days	4 days
140 lbs	10 days	3 days
150+ lbs	9 days	3 days

Q. What about smoked seafood?

It's a no-no.

Even refrigerated, smoked seafood (such as lox, nova scotia style or jerky) may contain public enemy number one, Listeria.

On the bright side, it's okay to eat if this type of seafood is an ingredient in a *cooked* dish like a casserole.

Q. I am on a camping trip with my family. Is it okay to eat the fish we catch?

Nope.

Unfortunately, some of our lakes and rivers are contaminated with industrial pollutants that may be a health hazard to developing fetuses. You can contact your local health department or the EPA (epa.gov) to figure out which lakes/streams/rivers are polluted.

Even if a local river or lake is deemed safe, we'd still err on the side of caution and not eat any fish caught during a camping trip.

Q. What about raw shellfish?

Sorry, you can't eat uncooked oysters, clams, or mussels. Even if you're not pregnant, these are high-risk items for food-borne illnesses. You are welcome to eat shellfish if you cook it. But save the oyster shooter for that glass of champagne you will have after delivery.

MEAT

Q. Can I eat deli meat?

No, unless it is heated or cooked. Since deli meat can be contaminated with Listeria, either avoid it altogether or reheat the meat until it is steaming to kill off any potential bacteria.

So, if you crave a pastrami sandwich on rye, just order it *hot*.

environment

Q. What about raw or seared meat?

No—for the same reason you can't eat sushi. Again, you are temporarily immune-compromised. Undercooked or uncooked meat/poultry/seafood may contain Salmonella, toxoplasmosis, and other bacteria (like E. coli) that can make you sick. Cook all meat thoroughly before you eat it.

EGGS

Q. I love eating cookie dough. Is it okay to eat raw eggs while pregnant?

No.

Salmonella is the big risk with any food containing raw eggs. Examples include:

◆ Homemade ice cream
◆ Custard
◆ Freshly made Caesar salad dressing
◆ Hollandaise sauce
◆ Homemade mayonnaise
◆ Homemade eggnog

Commercially made ice creams, dressings, and mayonnaise are safe because they use pasteurized eggs. Typically restaurants use pasteurized eggs, but ask if there is any doubt. The eggnog you buy in the grocery store has so many preservatives it's probably safe to drink until next Christmas!

DR H'S OPINION

"I commiserate with you. I would rather eat an entire batch of cookie dough than eat the actual baked cookies! But this is a dangerous thing to do, especially while you're pregnant."

OTHER FOOD AND DRINK

Q. Are freshly squeezed juices ok?

Yes, if you are the one freshly squeezing them. Unpasteurized fruit or vegetable juices, or even ones that are "flash" pasteurized and sold at natural food stores may contain bacteria you and your baby don't want to encounter.

Reality check: Skip the sprouts
Raw bean sprouts and alfalfa spouts can also be a source of food-borne infections.

FYI: We will cover the debate on pesticides in foods (organic vs. conventional produce and milk) in the Household Exposures section later in this chapter.

ENVIRO

Bad Habits

SMOKING

Q. I was smoking before I knew I was pregnant. Is this going to harm the baby?

Probably not—if you find out that you are pregnant between four and nine weeks *and* you quit smoking right then and there.

Truth is, many folks indulge in bad habits (alcohol consumption, tobacco) before they know they are pregnant. The key is to stop once you know you are expecting.

New Parent 411

Moms who smoke are more likely to have children with asthma, but we have never known why. New research shows that smoking in the first trimester may alter the genes of the fetus, which puts the baby at risk. *(Breton C.)*

Q. I am still smoking. Is this going to harm the baby?

Short answer—yes.

A mom who smokes has less circulating oxygen in her body and thus, so does her unborn baby. This is called **FETAL HYPOXIA.** There is also less blood flow to the uterus and placenta, and therefore to the baby. Lastly, nicotine goes right through the placenta and circulates in the bloodstream of the fetus.

So how do all of these things affect your baby? There's an increased risk of:

◆ Having a small fetus who doesn't grow properly.
◆ A placenta that implants over the cervix (**PLACENTA PREVIA**).
◆ A placenta that pulls off the wall of the uterus prematurely (**PLACENTAL ABRUPTION**).
◆ Breaking your water bag early (**PREMATURE RUPTURE OF MEMBRANES**).
◆ Preterm delivery.
◆ Low birth weight (less than five lbs.).
◆ Stillbirth and newborn death.
◆ Sudden Infant Death Syndrome in infancy.
◆ Asthma, colic, and obesity in infancy and childhood.

We know it sounds grim, but it's the truth. There has really never been a better time to quit.

Q. I am smoking, but I want to quit. I've tried before and have been unsuccessful. What should I do?

Good news: there are many options. The best advice is to have a detailed conversation with your practitioner. You can create a plan that works best for you, discussing what symptoms you may have during withdrawal and how to cope with them.

To get started, figure out what situations increase your desire to smoke. Do you smoke with meals? After meals? At the end of the day? Before bed? While driving? Once you identify your triggers, change or eliminate them.

Next, create a "smoke-free" home. It really helps to have a "quitting buddy." If your partner smokes, this is a great time for *both* of you to stop. Having other people in your home that smoke can make the process of quitting extremely challenging, to say the least.

Your practitioner should have a list of resources to help educate you about the risks of smoking and most importantly, strategies on quitting. But here are a few great places to start:

- HelpPregnantSmokersQuit.org
- American Legacy Foundation's Great Start. (866) 66START
- SmokeFreeFamilies.org
- SmokeFree.gov
- National Quitline Network (800-QUITNOW) has local services in your state.

Although quitting in the first trimester is the best thing for your baby, it's beneficial to quit at any point. Even if you quit before the third trimester, you will greatly lower the risk of harm to your baby.

You can do this…for you and your baby.

Q. Is it safe to use a nicotine patch or gum?

Ideally, the safest way to quit is to . . . just quit. There is zero health risk in support groups, counseling, or group therapy. All of these things can help you change your behavior.

Docs can't say with 100% certainty that nicotine replacement products (like gum, lozenges, patches and inhalers) are safe during pregnancy or in breastfeeding women. But the American Congress of Obstetricians and Gynecologists says if you have failed at quitting, the benefit of stopping smoking outweighs the risks potentially associated with these the products.

If going cold turkey doesn't work, trying a nicotine replacement product is the next step. Most OBs (me included) recommend trying nicotine gum or an inhaler first. These products offer nicotine in intermittent doses. Nicotine patches are the last choice because they administer nicotine continuously. If you must resort to the patch, remove it at night to decrease nicotine exposure to your fetus.

Q. My doctor is recommending an anti-depressant to help me quit. Is that okay?

DR B'S OPINION: SMOKING AND SIDS

I am going to play the guilt card here, so be warned. As a mom myself, I could never knowingly put my child in harm's way. I know that having a nicotine addiction is extremely hard to kick—but if you can't do it for yourself, do it for your child!

Yes. Some medications have multiple uses, so don't worry—your doc doesn't think you are depressed!

Bupropion (Wellbutrin) is an anti-depressant, which in certain doses, helps reduce withdrawal symptoms in people trying to quit smoking. Taking this medication is almost certainly safer than smoking. See Expecting411.com/extra for more info.

Q. If I smoke after I give birth, are there any risks to the baby?

YES. *A mother's smoking habit is one of the key risk factors for* Sudden Infant Death Syndrome (SIDS).

If the risk of SIDS isn't enough to convince you to stop smoking, children born to women who smoke also have an increased risk of asthma, ear infections, infantile colic and childhood obesity.

If you weren't able to quit during your pregnancy, it's never too late to try.

Factoid: Babies whose moms smoke and breastfeed sleep 30% *less* than their baby friends whose moms don't smoke. When you realize how little sleep you get as a new parent, this may also inspire you to quit smoking!

Illicit drugs

MARIJUANA

Q. I smoked marijuana before I knew I was pregnant. Have I done anything to harm the baby? Is it a problem if I continue to smoke during pregnancy?

There's not much research on this issue. But marijuana use in the first trimester may increase your risk of miscarriage.

Regular marijuana use in pregnancy (loosely defined as four to six times a week) increases chances of preterm delivery. And since marijuana crosses the placenta, your baby is also getting high. Babies born to women smoking marijuana regularly are at risk for withdrawal-like symptoms, including excessive crying, trembling, and irritability.

What we don't know is how your marijuana use affects your baby in the long-term. Some studies show no long-term problems in children, and others have found an association between marijuana exposure in the womb and learning and attention problems. *(Chang G)*

The most important thing to do (as with all other drug use) is to quit now. If you have trouble quitting, ask your practitioner for a referral to an addiction medicine specialist, a substance abuse treatment center or a counseling group.

COCAINE

Q. I used cocaine before I knew I was pregnant. Have I done any harm to the baby? Are there any health risks if I continue to use it occasionally during pregnancy?

ENVIRO

? ?

Possibly.

Cocaine is a powerful stimulant that, without any doubt, affects most major organ systems in developing fetuses. Cocaine has the biggest impact on the developing nervous system, including the brain. So even if a woman only uses cocaine before discovering she is pregnant, damage to the fetus has most likely already happened. Cocaine-exposed babies have higher risks of learning disabilities, attention-deficit disorders and emotional problems in childhood.

If you continue to use cocaine, your health risks include a greater chance of miscarriage, preterm labor and preterm delivery, placental abruption, high blood pressure (hypertension), and stroke.

Experts don't know the exact amount of cocaine that triggers the above problems. But even if an adult uses cocaine *once*, she can have a heart attack or stroke. The same is probably true for your baby.

The safest thing to do is to stop using cocaine once you find out you are pregnant. If you need help, ask your practitioner or contact the National Drug Help Hotline (1-800-662-4357) or the National Alcohol and Drug Dependence Hopeline (1-800-662-2255).

METHAMPHETAMINES

Q. **I have been using methamphetamine prior to pregnancy. I am now pregnant and just can't stop. What are the risks to me and my baby?**

Methamphetamine is a stimulant that elevates your heart rate, as well as your baby's. Meth causes problems similar to cocaine when used during pregnancy. Risks include miscarriage, preterm delivery, low-birth weight babies and placental abruption.

Methamphetamine crosses the placenta into your unborn baby's bloodstream. So babies that are born to women using methamphetamine are also likely to suffer withdrawal symptoms including tremors, sleeplessness, feeding difficulties, bonding issues, and muscle spasms.

Children who were exposed in the womb may have behavioral issues and learning disabilities.

HEROIN

Q. **What about heroin? Can my addiction be treated during pregnancy?**

PRENATAL SUBSTANCE ABUSE AND THE LAW

Drug abuse is not only unhealthy during pregnancy, but it's also considered child abuse or a criminal act in some states. The Child Abuse Prevention and Treatment Act requires Child Protective Services (CPS) to investigate when a newborn tests positive for exposure to drugs, alcohol, or controlled substances. In some cases, parents could lose custody of a baby exposed to drugs. *(Child Welfare Information Gateway)*

Heroin is an extremely addictive drug and like other drugs, it crosses the placenta. Your baby may be born premature, with low birth weight, low blood sugar (that can lead to seizures), breathing problems, and bleeding into the brain. And some heroin-exposed babies die.

Heroin is so addictive that even an unborn baby can become dependent on the drug and suffer severe withdrawal symptoms at birth. Newborn withdrawal symptoms are similar and often just as severe as those seen in adult heroin addicts. They include irritability, convulsions, diarrhea, fever, joint stiffness, and sleeping difficulties. FYI: a mom who uses IV drugs also puts herself *and* her unborn child at risk for HIV and Hepatitis B and C infections.

This is a very tough addiction to treat. Start by talking to your practitioner. He/she will likely refer you to an addiction medicine specialist for help. You may need to take methadone as part of the treatment program. While not an ideal medication, methadone is much better for you and your baby than the ongoing use of heroin, especially if you are injecting it.

The best thing you can do is quit, no matter how far along you are in your pregnancy.

PRESCRIPTION PAIN MEDICATION

Q. **I am addicted to prescription pain medication (Vicodin, Vicoprofen, Percocet, Darvocet, Tylenol with codeine). What are the health risks to me and my baby during my pregnancy?**

Prescription pain medications are among the most commonly abused substances. Examples include Oxycontin (oxycodone), Vicodin (hydrocodone), morphine, codeine and Demerol (meperidine).

You can take some of these medications safely during pregnancy if the need arises—like when you need a root canal or some equally unpleasant medical procedure.

But there is a difference between appropriate use . . . and abuse. Taking these medications in larger doses than prescribed, at more frequent intervals than prescribed and for reasons other than what it was prescribed for, is considered abuse of the drug and is *not* safe for your developing fetus.

These medications cross the placenta and impact your baby. They can lead to preterm delivery, low birth weight babies, withdrawal symptoms, and difficulty breathing.

Other Exposures

HEAT

Q. **Is it okay to sit in a hot tub or sauna?**

A *warm* tub is okay. A *hot* tub is not.

Saunas, Jacuzzis, and steam rooms all fit into the hot category. The concern here is two-fold:

1. *Neural tube defects*. Neural tube refers to the beginnings of your

ENVIRO

? ?

baby's spine, skull, and brain. In the early part of pregnancy (usually before six weeks), high heat exposures that increase your body temperature over 101 to 102°F can disrupt development of your baby's neural tube. That can cause birth defects called **NEURAL TUBE DEFECTS** (**SPINA BIFIDA, MENINGOCELE** and **MYELOMENINGOCELE**). FYI: the neural tube closes after four weeks, so the concern over hot tubs in the second or third trimesters focuses on risks to mom (see #2 below).

2.   *Dehydration.* You are more likely to get dehydrated, which can lead to dizziness, fainting, and preterm contractions. Anything lukewarm is fine (under 99°F). We know it's not fun to take a lukewarm bath, but it's better than passing out in the tub.

Q. Can I take hot showers?

Absolutely, as long as you limit your time. Your body isn't submerged in water when you're in a shower, so you are less likely to overheat. Just limit your shower time or turn down the water temperature after a few minutes.

Q. Can I use a heating pad?

Yes. It's just wise to avoid placing a heating pad directly on your belly. Using one for low back pain and to help ease the muscle pain in your calf after that excruciating middle-of-the-night charley horse is okay.

Q. Are hair dryers safe?

Yes. But it's best to dry your hair in a well-ventilated place so you don't get too hot.

Q. Can I lay in the sun during my pregnancy?

Yes, with caution.

Good news: there's no direct damage to your baby from sunbathing. Bad news: there's potential of skin damage for you. You are more likely to develop **MELASMA,** a darkening of your skin. It happens on your face and it can be permanent. So if you must get your sun time in, shade your face with a hat and use lots of sunscreen.

You can also get overheated and dehydrated by lying in the sun too long. Make sure you are drinking lots of water. Avoid the sun when it is at its hottest, between the hours of 10am and 4pm.

MICROWAVES AND AIRPORT SCREENING

Q. Can I use a microwave?

Yes, it is absolutely safe to use a microwave during pregnancy. Just move away from the microwave while it is on and don't open the door until the microwave has completely stopped.

FYI: Other radiation sources. The National Academy of Sciences has concluded many non-ionizing radiation exposures are safe for preg-

ENVIRO

nant women. Electromagnetic Fields (EMF's) are invisible lines of force that electric charges create. Power lines, electric appliances (blowdryers, heating pads, warming blankets, microwave oven), cell phones (and towers), airport screening devices, the earth's magnetic field, and even humans, emit these fields. *(Goldman RH)*

Low frequency fields don't have enough energy to cause damage to you or your developing baby's DNA or body organs. *(National Institute of Environmental Health Services)* But researchers continue to look at possible connections between EMF's (including cell phone use) and brain tumors and certain types of leukemia. The greatest concern here is the distance of the body organ (for example, the brain) from the EMF source (a cell phone). A major study to date has found no connection, though. *(Deltour I).* Even so, it's not a bad idea to use a Bluetooth headset instead of holding a cell phone to your ear for hours on end.

Q. How about the X-ray machine at the airport?

It's safe. For starters, you actually don't walk through an X-ray machine. It's a glorified metal detector and the machine can't hurt your baby, no matter how far along you are in your pregnancy.

Q. I see those full body scanners at the airport. Are they safe?

Yes. These scanners use non-ionizing radiation to see under your clothes. Since the scanners use low-dose X-rays that don't penetrate the body's organs, experts say they are safe. To get a harmful dose from a full-body scanner at an airport, you'd need to be screened 2500 times in a year. *(TSA)*

Or, you can opt for the pat down by airport security instead! Good times.

X-RAYS, CT SCANS, MRI IMAGING

Q. Why do they always ask if you are pregnant before an X-ray?

There are two concerns with X-rays: developmental abnormalities (**TERATOGENIC EFFECTS**) and cancer risk (**CARCINOGENESIS**).

Developmental abnormalities

High levels of ionizing radiation early in pregnancy can lead to miscarriage, growth restriction, small head size, and intellectual disability. Fetuses between eight and 25 weeks (especially eight to 15 weeks) are the most susceptible.

Before you worry, let's discuss how experts come up with these risks . . . and what defines "high levels" of radiation (that's at least 20 to 50 rad). The studies on this issue are all from animals and pregnant women unlucky enough to be present and survive an atomic bomb explosion. Even if you have multiple diagnostic X-ray procedures, you still won't reach these levels of exposure.

A pregnant woman needs to be exposed to a large dose of radiation (more than five rads) to have an increased risk of having a miscarriage, a baby with birth defects, intellectual disability, or growth restriction. No diagnostic procedure has this much radiation (see chart below).

environment

Cancer risks

The average risk of getting leukemia in the general population is about one in 3000. With limited data, we estimate children exposed to radiation (at least one to two rad) while in the womb have about one in 2000 risk. That's a small increase in risk, but it's why ultrasound and MRI are safer choices than standard X-rays or CT scans during pregnancy.

But there are certain situations when these tests are necessary (for example, when a pregnant women is injured in a car accident).

BOTTOM LINE: If you have an X-ray done only to find out later that you were pregnant, don't sweat it. Better yet, if there is chance you may be pregnant, take a home pregnancy test the day before your procedure. If it is positive, notify your practitioner and radiologist immediately.

IMAGING STUDY	AMOUNT OF RADIATION IN RAD OR MILLIRAD*
Chest x-ray	0.02–0.07 mrad
Abdominal x-ray	100 mrad
Intravenous pyelogram	> 1 rad
Hysterosalpingogram	1 rad
Hip x-ray	200 mrad
Mammogram	7–20 mrad
Barium enema	2–4 rad
CT scan (head or chest)	< 1 rad
CT scan (abdomen or spine)	3.5 rad
CT scan (pelvis)	3.5 rad

*Note: "rad" stands for radiation absorbed dose, "mrad" stands for millirad which is 1/1000 of one rad. (ACOG)

Q. Is it okay to get X-rays or dental X-rays?

It's best to avoid all X-rays if possible.

Of course, it is extremely important to take care of your teeth during pregnancy. You need regular visits and regular cleanings. And if necessary, you can have fillings or even a root canal.

If your dentist feels that X-rays must be done, try to postpone them until after the first trimester. Make sure your belly is completely covered with a lead apron.

As for X-rays of other body parts, avoid them as well. But if you are in a car accident and need an X-ray to rule out a broken bone, do it and have a lead apron draped over your belly.

If there is ever a question, get your OB on the phone. The dentist, orthopedist or any other medical personnel taking care of you can discuss a plan of care with your practitioner. Getting one or two diagnostic X-rays during pregnancy does not pose a significant risk to your fetus, in our opinion (we'll discuss this more below).

Reality Check

Try to wait until after your first trimester to have a routine dental cleaning. Your gag reflex is at an all-time high and watching your breakfast land on the lap of the hygienist is not fun!

ENVIRO

Q. Is it okay to have a CT scan during pregnancy?

Only if you absolutely have to (which is rare).

CT scans (computerized tomography) emit ionizing radiation, which has potential risks for you and your developing fetus. In most cases, a safer MRI (magnetic resonance imaging) would work just as well (see below for details).

There are rare situations that require a CT scan instead of an MRI, such as assessing for a blood clot in the lungs. And some trauma centers do not have an MRI scanner immediately available.

CT scans emit differing amounts of radiation, depending on what body part is involved (see the chart earlier).

Q. Is an MRI safe?

Yes. An MRI uses a magnetic field and radio waves instead of ionizing radiation to produce the images and can usually provide your medical provider the information he needs.

An MRI can help rule out appendicitis, or make the diagnosis when a pregnant woman has chronic, severe abdominal pain or severe headaches.

People who are claustrophobic (even those who aren't) may be scared of the very narrow tunnel and the loud buzzing of the machine as it takes pictures. But from a pregnancy standpoint, you don't have to worry. They are safe and there are no concerns for adverse effects on a fetus.

So … if you need an MRI, do it.

Q. Is it safe to use radio-opaque dye and contrast agents during pregnancy?

It's best to avoid both if you can.

In the little research done on *contrast agents* and pregnancy, there is some concern about risks of miscarriage, bone defects, and other birth defects. The studies were done on animals that received two to seven times the normal dose of contrast agents given to humans. So you should only have an imaging study with a contrast agent if the potential benefit out-weighs the risks to the fetus. *(ACOG)*

Radioactive dyes (like radioactive iodine) easily cross the placenta and can affect the fetal thyroid gland, particularly after ten weeks. These are absolute no-no's during pregnancy. If you require diagnostic imaging of your thyroid during pregnancy, ask your doctor and radiologist about using Technetium Tc 99m instead of radioactive iodine.

Q. Is it okay to have ultrasounds done?

Short answer: yes. See Chapter 5, Tests for a detailed discussion

Q. Is it safe to work at a radiology office while I am pregnant?

Yes, just take some minor precautions.

Previously, many workplaces just reassigned a pregnant woman's duties to avoid any possible exposure. Workplaces feared legal action if the

environment

employed woman delivered a baby with any sort of a birth defect.

Today, medical offices now use the "Principle of ALARA (as low as reasonably achievable)" to devise radiation protection measures for pregnant workers. Bottom line: the levels of radiation are so low that experts conclude there is no significant risk to the fetus. Otherwise, there wouldn't be women of childbearing age ever working in radiology offices!

If you are a radiology tech, radiology nurse, physician-in-training, or radiologist, the easiest way to decrease exposure to your fetus is to restrict the type of work you are doing and to limit the number of times you perform a particular task. Tell your employer that you are pregnant as soon as you find out so that the two of you can review your exposure history and discuss possible new work assignments.

Procedures involving fluoroscopy and portable X-rays do not put your fetus at an increased risk. Radiology techs and radiologists can continue their work in stationary radiography, portable radiography, fluoroscopy and other special procedures throughout pregnancy. You should wear a lead apron during all procedures and monitor your film-badge readings.

SURGERY

Q. If I need a surgical procedure done, can anesthesia be used? Or do I need to wait on the operation until after I am no longer pregnant?

Yes, for emergency surgery. No, for elective or cosmetic surgery.

Docs would rather not expose your fetus to general anesthesia unless it's necessary. Appendicitis and broken bones that poke through the skin are examples of surgical emergencies that simply won't wait. When the benefit outweighs the risk, you need the operation and the general anesthesia.

The "best" time to operate on a pregnant woman is in the second trimester because it puts her fetus in the least danger of miscarriage (first trimester) or preterm delivery (third trimester). For urgent, but not emergency situations, it's optimal to delay surgery until the second trimester if possible.

Q. My dentist says I need a root canal. Is it safe?

Short answer: Yes.

However, your dentist and your practitioner need to chat with each other. They can discuss the procedure as well as pain medications and antibiotics that are safe to use in pregnancy.

It's common to have dental problems during pregnancy. Pregnant women are more likely to suffer from cavities and oral infections than non-pregnant women. Be sure to take care of all dental problems!

MEDICATIONS

We'll cover common concerns in Appendix A, Medications and in detail at Expecting411.com/extra.

? ?

ENVIRO

Household Exposures

INSECTICIDES/PESTICIDES

Q. Is it okay to use insect repellant while I am pregnant?

Yes!

All Environmental Protection Agency-registered insect repellants are safe to use at recommended doses during pregnancy. That includes products containing these active ingredients: DEET (N, N-diethyl-m-toluamide or m-DET), picaridin (KBR 3023), and oil of lemon eucalyptus.

Studies of insect repellant (even in toxic doses) and pregnancy showed no increase in birth defects, preterm labor, stillborn or growth restriction. So bug spray is safe.

Insider Secret

Pregnant women are mosquito magnets. Mosquitoes like things that put out heat. We don't need to tell you that pregnant women emit more heat than other people because you know how hot you are right now! You also exhale more carbon dioxide with each breath, which makes you very attractive to a mosquito.

It's never fun getting a thousand mosquito bites, especially when you are pregnant, itchy, and uncomfortable anyway . . . so spray up!

Q. I live in an agricultural area and I constantly smell pesticides as they are sprayed on neighboring crops. What should I do now that I am pregnant?

If possible, avoid agricultural pesticide exposure during your first trimester.

During this time, your baby's nervous system is rapidly developing so you definitely want to avoid *any* type of contact with pesticides that can lead to brain/spinal cord defects.

Numerous studies have looked at pesticide/insecticide exposure during pregnancy and there are definite associations between *agricultural* pesticides and miscarriage as well as birth defects (particularly cleft lip/palate, brain/spinal cord, heart and limb defects). Women living within a quarter mile of agricultural crops seem to be at highest risk. *(Frazier LM)*

Before you decide to move to Antarctica, most experts believe that you need *prolonged* and/or *intense* exposure to be at risk. Unless you are the one flying the crop duster, you should be fine.

To err on the side of safety, however, we'd advise leaving an agricultural area with heavy pesticide use, particularly during the first trimester if you can. We know this is much easier said than done.

Q. Is it okay to have the bug guy come over to spray the perimeter of my home?

Try to wait until after your first trimester.

The greatest risk to the fetus from home pesticide use may be during the first three to eight weeks while the brain is developing. *(Weiss B)*

ENVIRO

? ?

If necessary, it's probably safe to have the perimeter of your home sprayed during the second and third trimesters. Just take a few precautions. Stay out of the area for at least 24 hours (a good excuse to take a spa retreat!) and avoid direct contact with anything that has been sprayed outside your home.

Q. What about indoor pesticides? Can I bomb my house to get rid of pests?

According to a recent scientific report, fetuses who are exposed to "higher levels" of indoor pesticides have a higher risk of developing leukemia in childhood. *(Turner MC)*

The highest risk appears to be exposure during the first trimester or when a professional pest control service is used.

Pregnant women exposed to household gardening pesticides have an increased risk of delivering babies with cleft palates, neural tube, heart, and limb defects.

So, you may be wondering, what exactly is a "higher level" of pesticide? Unfortunately, researchers didn't quantify that. Bottom line: although occasional or small exposures are probably okay, it is best to avoid all household, pet, and garden pesticides and/or insecticides during pregnancy.

Here are some suggestions to safely deal with your insect issues:

1. Try bug killers such as Raid roach paper/traps that you can direct at a specific area.
2. Make sure you are not the one doing the spraying.
3. Keep the room well-ventilated and if possible, stay away for 12 to 24 hours after spraying.
4. Try home remedies such as using salt and vinegar to ward off ants and cockroaches.
5. If you must bomb your house (we understand, we wouldn't want to be living in a bug-infested house either), consider these tips:

   ◆ Go away for the weekend (or longer, if possible) and have it done while you are away.
   ◆ When you return, make sure you are not the first one in the house. Have someone ventilate the house (open windows and turn on fans for a while) before you enter.
   ◆ Make sure that all sheets, towels, exposed dishes/cups/utensils are washed after the treatment.
   ◆ Remove and throw away all food that could have been exposed and thoroughly clean any surfaces where food preparation occurs.

Q. What about organic or natural pesticides during pregnancy?

Almost all chemicals used in pesticides are compounds that are naturally present in plants. Although they may sound healthier, the terms "organic" and "natural" do not mean "better" or "safer." All of these chemicals, including natural chemicals, are toxins and have the potential to cause harm if you don't handle them properly.

ENVIRO

Read the warning labels on all pesticide and insecticide packages before handling them.

Bottom Line
It is best to avoid all pesticides/insecticides (conventional or organic) during pregnancy.

Reality Check
Once your baby is born, it's still a good idea to limit pesticide exposure and skip "routine" home pesticide treatments. According to the Centers for Disease Control, "home pesticide use overall has been linked to childhood cancers such as soft tissue sarcomas, leukemias, and cancer of the brain." *(Centers for Disease Control)*

Q. Should I eat organic fruits and vegetables to reduce my exposure (and my baby's) to pesticides?

Well, let's look at the data and then you can decide. Recently published studies found that children who were exposed to higher levels of a pesticide (organophosphates) in the womb scored slightly lower on IQ tests than less exposed peers. (Note: Only trace amounts of organophosphates are found in your typical grocery store produce. Higher levels were common in indoor pesticides when these studies were conducted.) *(Bouchard MF, Engel SM.)*

We agree that it is a good idea to limit your exposure to pesticides in general. But your exposures both inside and around the outside of your home are much more significant, compared to the amount you ingest in food. And remember, "organic" does not mean a product is pesticide-free.

Our opinion: You don't need to spend your entire paycheck on organic foods. To reduce pesticides in your fruit and veggies, it is a good idea to buy produce in season. And you should wash all produce thoroughly—even if you peel off the skin before eating.

Q. Should I drink organic milk?

Well, it is really a personal choice because there is no significant evidence that says conventional milk is dangerous. Thus, no major medical organization recommends organic milk over the regular stuff.

Q. I love to garden but my roses need spraying. What should I do?

Avoid gardening for seven to ten days after the pesticide was applied. When you do resume gardening, wear protective clothing to help avoid contact with plants that have been sprayed.

FYI: Whether you use pesticides or not, you should always wear gloves when gardening. Gloves help reduce your risk of toxoplasmosis exposure, which can be present in soil.

Q. My husband didn't tell me he just treated our dog for fleas and I have been playing with her all afternoon. I'm

environment

panicked, what should I do?

First of all, don't panic. The real risk here is *long-term* or *intense* exposure to chemicals. Your dog's flea bath presents a *very* small risk to your unborn baby—especially if you are out of the first trimester.

FYI: Call your poison center at (800) 222-1222 and OB immediately if you inhale or swallow a pesticide, or your skin comes in direct contact with a pesticide. The poison control experts will want to know the specific ingredients, so have the pesticide container nearby to reference when you call.

HOUSEHOLD CLEANING PRODUCTS

Q. I'm worried about using cleaning products during pregnancy. Should I have someone else clean my house?

Household cleaning products are safe . . . but accept help if anyone volunteers for the job!

Pregnancy is an excellent excuse to call in a cleaning crew. Between the awkward positions that leave your back aching and fumes that only worsen your nausea, cleaning is not an easy task. Unfortunately, many of us get hit with that "nesting phenomenon" and cleaning is not just a necessity, but an obsession.

If you can call in help (your husband, partner, a cleaning service), do so. If you are going to do all the dirty work yourself, rest easy since most cleaning products are thought to be safe to use during pregnancy.

Here are a few suggestions:

◆ Minimize contact with chemicals: wear long sleeves, gloves and a mask (particularly for cleaning small spaces like ovens).
◆ Read all instruction labels.
◆ NEVER mix cleaning products with each other or with other chemicals.
◆ Try to keep the area you are cleaning well-ventilated with open windows and/or a fan.
◆ Have your partner do some/most/ALL of the cleaning if possible.

Q. I just can't bring myself to use my normal cleaning products while pregnant. Is there anything else I can use?

If you are uncomfortable using your regular cleaning products, you have a few options. You can water-down many products to decrease the intensity of fumes. You can use more natural products, such as those sold at organic grocery stores. You can also use baking soda or vinegar to clean most things. Check out Earth Easy (eartheasy.com) for an extensive list of options and homemade recipes.

FUMES

Q. Is it okay to paint the house?

Yes, with a few precautions.

Like many eco hazards, there isn't much research on this subject to suggest what the health hazards are for you or your fetus. But here are some common sense suggestions:

◆ If possible, get someone else to do the painting for you and remove yourself from the area until the project is complete.
◆ Do not use oil-based paints. They contain organic solvents whose fumes can be irritating.
◆ *GOOD NEWS:* You can't buy any lead or mercury based paints. Since 1978, the Consumer Product Safety Commission has required paints to have less than 0.06% lead. The Environmental Protection Agency banned mercury levels above 0.06% in latex paint in 1990.
◆ *BAD NEWS:* Lead-based paint was commonly used before 1978. If you live in a house built before 1978, *do not* scrape or remove the old paint (or perform any other do-it-yourself home renovation projects)! Consult with your local health department for a list of certified professional lead remediators. See the box "Get the lead out" later in this section for more details.
◆ Minimize exposure to paints that contain ethylene glycol ethers and biocides (pesticides/anti-microbials). Ethylene glycol ethers are associated with miscarriage.
◆ Consider using paints labeled "zero-VOC." VOC stands for Volatile Organic Compounds. VOC's can cause nasal congestion, eye irritation, headache, nausea, and vomiting. They are also possible carcinogens (cancer-causing agents). Zero-VOC is the same paint, without the toxic smell. Many paint stores such as Dunn Edwards and Benjamin Moore carry this type of paint. Sherwin Williams offers a "Green Sure" emblem on its low-VOC (Duration Home) and zero-VOC (Harmony) products. Dutch Boy, sold at Walmart, also offers a low-VOC version.

If you must paint the nursery yourself, there are a few precautions that we suggest:

◆ Talk to your practitioner before beginning a project.
◆ Protect yourself by wearing long sleeves, long pants, gloves and a mask.
◆ Make sure the room is well-ventilated with open windows and/or a fan.

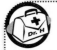

DR H TRUE STORY: PAINTING THE NURSERY

Painting the nursery is often a rite of passage for new parents—myself included. The hardest part: picking the right color. It took me, my husband, four grandparents, and three neighbors to select the perfect hue for my first child's nursery . . . the nursery color for our second child took less than two minutes at the hardware store while my husband was looking at power tools.

ENVIRO

? ?

◆ Absolutely avoid scraping and sanding old paint. This releases chemicals into the air, which increases the risk of inhaling chemicals.

◆ Work in small bursts of time and take frequent breaks to go outside and get fresh air.

◆ Keep all food and drinks away from the area you are painting.

◆ Avoid spray paints as the mist increases the amount of chemicals that you might inhale.

◆ STOP painting if you begin to feel light-headed, nauseated, dizzy, short of breath, or experience chest pain. Contact your practitioner.

Q. What if I have already been exposed to paint/paint fumes when I didn't realize I was pregnant?

Don't sweat it. There are no studies that indicate any harm to a fetus from accidental paint exposure during pregnancy.

However, recreational use of paint (yes, there are people who sniff or inhale paint solvents to get high) exposes fetuses to much higher levels of chemicals and there is definite potential for miscarriage, birth defects, and intellectual disability.

Q. Can I get new carpeting installed in my home?

Yes, but we recommend that you leave the house while installation is going on. And get someone to open the windows and run the fans before you return home.

New carpeting, as well as the padding and adhesive that goes under it can release VOC's (Volatile Organic Compounds). VOC's can cause eye/nose/throat irritation as well as coughing or trouble breathing. The health risks of VOC's depend on the type of VOC, the duration of the exposure, and the amount of exposure. Currently, there aren't any specific health risks associated with typical exposure in the womb to new carpet fumes.

FYI: Other sources of VOC exposures include: dry cleaning fluid, hobby and craft supplies, photographic solutions, permanent markers, printer ink, and smog. The best you can do is limit exposures where possible.

HEAVY METALS

Q. I'm worried about mercury exposure during pregnancy. How can I limit exposure?

Short answer: limit your intake of high-mercury containing fish (as discussed earlier in this chapter).

Long answer: Some flu shots contain an "ethyl" based mercury-preservative. This is a very different compound than "methyl" mercury that is in fish. And yes, it is safe to get it during pregnancy.

Certain compounds have completely different properties even though they may be related. For instance, take the alcohol family. *Methanol* is antifreeze; *ethanol* is a Bud Light. Methyl mercury is a small molecule that can get into the brain—it takes almost two months to break down in the body. *Ethyl* mercury is a large molecule that cannot enter the brain and is rapidly eliminated from the body within a week.

ENVIRO

The information known about mercury poisoning comes from unfortunate communities that have experienced it. Children, especially those exposed as fetuses during their mothers' pregnancy, have lower scores on memory, attention, and language tests than their unexposed peers. (They were *not* diagnosed with autism or Attention Deficit Disorder, however.) *(American Academy of Pediatrics)*

Chronic exposure to liquid methyl mercury causes Mad Hatter's Disease, named for hat makers who used liquid mercury in the hat-making process. The disease consists of psychiatric problems, insomnia, poor memory, sweating, tremors, red palms, and impaired kidney function.

However, if you have concerns, ask your practitioner for a mercury-free (preservative-free) version of the flu vaccine. Either way, get your flu shot— your immune system is weakened and you're at high risk for serious complications of the flu.

You may also hear that dental fillings (amalgams) contain mercury. Yes, that is true. However, if you already have amalgams in your mouth, they do NOT need to be removed. If you have a cavity that needs to be filled during pregnancy, talk to your dentist about your options (there are several mercury-free alternatives). The FDA is reviewing the safety of dental amalgams, so stay tuned to Expecting411.com for updates.

Q. I'm worried about lead exposure. Is there any way to reduce my exposure?

Good question. We know a great deal about lead exposure during pregnancy and early childhood—and what we know is scary.

Pregnant women exposed to lead have:

◆ a greater risk of preterm labor.
◆ low birth weight babies.
◆ babies with brain/spinal cord defects.

The risk of preterm labor is three times greater even with mild exposure to lead (officially, that is a lead level over five microgram per deciliter).

Babies of mothers who have lead levels over ten mcg/dl during pregnancy have lower IQ's than their unleaded peers. In fact, *any* level of lead exposure can have subtle, but permanent effects on the brain. *(Canfield RL)*

So what can you do to reduce your lead exposure? Here are five tips:

1. Do not eat out of lead-glazed ceramics.
2. Do not drink out of lead-crystal glassware (it is particularly important not to store liquids like juice in lead-crystal containers as more lead is able to leach into the beverage when it sits).
3. Avoid DIY home improvements if you live in a home built before 1978. (more on this in the box below).
4. If you live in a home built before 1986, run your tap water for two minutes in the morning before drinking. Older homes have lead solder in the water pipes.
5. Get tested if you work in a job where you might be exposed to lead (lead refiner, automobile finisher, typesetter, spray painter, printer, pottery, ceramics, rubber/plastic products maker, brass/bronze products maker, etc).

environment

GET THE LEAD OUT

If you live in a home built before 1978 and want to do some home repairs or painting, don't pick up a Bob Vila video and think you can tackle this project yourself. You can inhale a significant amount of lead dust by tearing up the house or even just scraping off old paint. Here is our advice:

Call in an expert. Your local or state health department should have a list of certified home lead inspectors and contractors who specialize in lead renovation work.

If the old lead-based paint is in good condition, you should paint over it. Do *not* scrape it or sand it off.

The biggest problem areas are windows and other areas that rub and create dust.

Yes, there are DIY home lead test kits, but each kit only tests one small area. They aren't going to save much money because you'll end up buying several test kits.

If it is necessary to do a lead remediation, you should leave the house and not return until both the job and the cleanup is done.

For more info, contact the Environmental Protection Agency (EPA) at epa.gov/lead/pubs/nlic.htm or 1-800-424-LEAD.

ENDOCRINE DISRUPTORS

Q. I've heard about certain plastics causing health problems in babies. What should I know and do I need to avoid exposure to them?

There are two commonly used chemicals found in plastics that have potential health risks: Bisphenol-A (BPA) and phthalates. Both of them are "endocrine disrupters." These chemicals can mimic the actions of actual hormones found in our body, even in low doses. Despite much speculation, we don't exactly know how our bodies respond when exposed.

Let's take a look at each of these chemicals:

Bisphenol-A. Prior to 2009, most clear, hard plastic water bottles were made of polycarbonate, which contained a chemical called Bisphenol A (BPA). It is the BPA that makes the hard, clear plastic bottles . . . well, hard and clear. BPA is also used in plastic containers, the linings of metal cans for liquid foods, and soda cans.

BPA's chemical bond with polycarbonate breaks down over time, especially with repeated washing or heating. As a result, BPA leaches out of the plastic and ends up in the food or liquid you are ingesting.

BPA can mimic the natural female sex hormone, estradiol. While most data about BPA comes from animal research, these studies show even low level exposure of BPA may be linked to everything from early puberty and breast cancer, to attention and developmental problems. Although research is evolving, an independent panel from the National Institutes of Health/National Toxicology Program has "some concern" that exposure to

ENVIRO

BPA affects brain and neurologic development in fetuses, infants and young children.

As a result, all major baby bottle manufacturers reformulated their plastic bottles to drop BPA. And many BPA-free products hit the market. (But off-brand bottles sold in discount or dollar stores may still contain BPA. Remember, BPA has not been officially banned in the U.S.)

So how do you lower exposure to BPA to protect yourself and your unborn baby? The National Toxicology Program has these recommendations to reduce BPA exposure:

- Avoid plastic containers with #7 on the bottom (some—but not all—that have a #7 recycling number may have BPA).
- If you own polycarbonate plastic containers, do not wash them in the dishwasher with harsh detergents.
- Do not microwave polycarbonate plastic food containers. BPA may break down from repeated use at high temperatures.
- Eat less canned food. Opt for fresh or frozen foods.
- Use glass, porcelain, or stainless steel containers, particularly for hot food or liquids.

Phthalates. Phthalates are plasticizers that make plastic soft and durable. Phthalates mimic our natural estrogen and androgen-blocking hormones. They are also animal carcinogens. While there is much controversy about phthalates, there is still no scientific consensus that they are dangerous to humans.

Phthalates are widely used in everyday items. For example, you'll find them in plastic cooking wrap, plastic food packaging, and personal care products. You can ingest them or absorb them through your skin.

Our advice: If you want to reduce phthalate exposure, use a napkin or paper towel to cover food when you heat it up in the microwave.

PETS

Q. I have a cat. I've heard they can carry a disease that can be harmful to the fetus. Can I still play with her?

The concern with cats is toxoplasmosis.

This is a parasite that lives in the soil and can also live in cat poop. Cats don't usually have any symptoms when they are carriers of the parasite, although sometimes they have soft poop or diarrhea. Outdoor cats and kittens are more likely to be carriers than indoor cats.

You can be exposed with a cat bite, scratch, or just by cleaning the litter box.

About 15% of American women are immune to toxoplasmosis, and it's more likely if you are a long-time cat owner.

If you are immune to toxoplasmosis before pregnancy (determined by a simple blood test), then the baby is safe. If you are not immune, you can play with your cat, but be careful. Contact your doctor if you are scratched or bitten. And don't change the litter box!

For a more detailed discussion of toxoplasmosis, check out Chapter 17, Infections.

ENVIRO

Q. Why do I have to avoid changing the litter box?

The parasite is in the cat poop. And even stirring up some dust while you are cleaning the litter box can expose you to it.

Ask, barter, or pay your spouse, partner, or friend to do the dirty work. If you live alone and absolutely must do it yourself, move the litter box outside while cleaning it, wear a mask and gloves and wash your hands thoroughly afterwards.

Q. I was cleaning the litter box during my first trimester before I knew I was pregnant. Is that okay?

The best advice is to stop cleaning the litter box once you know you are pregnant.

DR H'S OPINION

"I test all of my cat-owning patients (either attempting conception or at the first prenatal visit) to see if they are already immune to toxoplasmosis. If you have an outdoor cat, ask your practitioner about being tested."

There is a chance that you are already immune. So relax.

If you get infected for the first time between ten to 24 weeks, your newborn has a 5% chance of having serious problems. See Chapter 17, Infections, for the details.

If you get infected during the third trimester, your fetus can still get sick, but the risk of damage is much less since most of your baby's organ development has already occurred.

TOXOPLASMOSIS RECAP

Where do you get it?

1. Cats are symptom-free (usually) carriers of the parasite.
2. Unwashed/poorly washed fruits and vegetables from contaminated soil.
3. Undercooked meats (beef, poultry, pork).

How to prevent it:

1. Don't clean the cat litter box.
2. Feed your cat her cat food (not undercooked meat).
3. Wash all fruits and vegetables thoroughly.
4. Cook meat thoroughly—use a food thermometer to measure the internal temperature of cooked meat.
5. Beef, lamb, veal roasts and steaks should be cooked to at least 145°F throughout.
6. Pork, ground meat, and wild game should be cooked to 160°F.
7. Whole poultry should be cooked to 180°F in the thigh.
8. Freezing the meat for several days before cooking it is another way to greatly reduce the chance of infection.

For more details, see Chapter 17, Infections.

ENVIRO

If you think you may have been exposed to toxoplasmosis, ask your practitioner to test you. The blood test will tell if you already have immunity or if you have had a recent infection.

Q. Do I have to give up my cat while I am pregnant?

No, you don't. Follow the safety guidelines listed below and talk to your practitioner if you have any questions or concerns:

- ◆ Avoid changing the litter box if possible.
- ◆ Have your cat's litter box changed daily.
- ◆ Do not feed your cat raw or undercooked meat, only commercial cat food (dry or canned).
- ◆ Do not get a new cat during your pregnancy and avoid stray cats and kittens (as cute as they may be).
- ◆ Speak to your veterinarian about whether your cat can be tested for toxoplasmosis.

Q. My friend's cat just scratched me. What should I do?

Contact your practitioner so you can be tested for immunity or to see if you've had a recent infection. Clean the area well to prevent infection.

Feedback from the Real World

How do you keep your cat out of your baby's crib? Cats love warm spots and a crib is a cozy place. Simple advice: keep your nursery room door closed when baby is sleeping or the room is unoccupied. That will keep your cat from converting your baby's crib into his favorite nap spot.

Q. I have a dog. Is there anything I have to worry about during my pregnancy?

Dogs pose no significant infection risk to you or your unborn baby.

If you have a big dog, just keep him from jumping on your belly. And exercise extreme caution if you are the one who walks the dog. As your belly gets bigger and your center of gravity begins to shift, you are much more likely to fall after getting twisted in the leash or after man's best friend goes chasing after the neighborhood cat. Falling when you are pregnant can be dangerous for your baby, so take care to avoid it.

Q. Will my baby be prone to allergies if we have a cat or dog in the house?

Actually, the opposite is true.

Early exposure in the first year of life to cats and dogs may prevent allergies. It's called the Hygiene Hypothesis. It goes like this: if your body is busy fighting off germs (like the ones the cat or dog carries), it doesn't have the desire to mount an allergic response to things (like cat dander).

Kids who grow up on farms have significantly fewer problems with allergies, presumably because they have constant exposure to animals and the germs they carry. (Ownby D.)

ENVIRO

Q. I live on a farm. What concerns should I be aware of?

Farm animals carry certain germs (Salmonella, Listeria, Campylobacter and Cryptosporidium) that can pose a risk to you and your fetus. Since you can't exactly vacate the farm for nine months, here are a few things you can do to help prevent infection:

◆ Never drink untreated water. If you have well water, have it tested for nitrates and bacteria, as well as other possible contaminants.

◆ Only eat or drink pasteurized dairy products.

◆ Do not handle stillborn animals.

◆ You should not be present when animals are fed with food stored in a silo.

◆ Wear gloves if possible when feeding or handling the animals.

◆ Always wash your hands with soap and water after any contact with animals or their living quarters.

◆ If you believe you have come in contact with an infected animal, contact your OB.

INTRODUCING FIDO TO THE NEW FAMILY MEMBER

Many couples get a dog as their first test of parenthood. If your dog is your first child, how do you introduce him to the first human baby of the house?

Here are some things you can do to help make the transition easier:

◆ Prepare your dog for the baby ahead of time. Do routines that will be commonplace after the baby arrives. You can even pretend using a baby doll.

◆ Once the baby is born, bring home an article worn by your baby (hat, shirt) for your dog to sniff before the baby arrives.

◆ Teach your dog the difference between his toys and the baby's toys.

◆ Always keep an eye on your baby/child when she is with your dog and never leave the two of them alone.

◆ Remember that your dog may act like an older child and become jealous of all the attention lavished on a new baby. Make sure you pay extra attention to your dog and if appropriate, include your dog in play with the new baby.

◆ Keep the dog's food bowl away from the baby. Once your baby is crawling, he may either a) try to eat it, or b) get into a fight with your dog who wants to defend his territory.

◆ Ask your OB, pediatrician, and veterinarian for more suggestions!

Note: babies and young children are the most frequent victims of dog bites. Children are curious and will poke, pull hair, and scare dogs. Sometimes this innocent play can lead to a dangerous bite by a startled dog.

ENVIRO

Q. I have a pet turtle (lizard, iguana, frog, snake, etc). Any health risks to worry about?

Although pet turtles (as well as other reptiles and amphibians) are fun, they can pose a health risk for you during pregnancy. The problem: Salmonella.

These animals may carry the bacteria Salmonella which comes out (guess where)... in their poop. (We aren't afraid to talk about anything in this book, including turtle poop!)

Direct or indirect contact with your pet's poop can lead to infection in you and your baby.

Our advice: it's probably best to give up Mr. Turtle (or any other reptile or amphibian pet) when you learn you are pregnant. Even after delivery, your baby is at risk becoming ill from a Salmonella infection.

If you and your little guy are inseparable, take these precautions to reduce the risk of infection with pet turtles, lizards and the like:

◆ Wear gloves when handling the turtle or its cage.
◆ Wash your hands with warm water and soap after handling the animal.
◆ Do not have your pet on or near any area where food preparation may occur.
◆ Do not wash the pet or its cage in the kitchen sink. Ideally, have someone else do it and do it outside your house.
◆ Do not let your pet roam freely in your house.

Q. I have a pet bird. Is it okay to keep it during my pregnancy?

Birds may carry germs that can infect humans, including Salmonella, Campylobacter, some protozoal infections, and chlamydiosis (we know what you are thinking, not the same as the sexually transmitted chlamydia!).

Our advice: a healthy bird is fine to keep around during pregnancy. Take your bird to see a veterinarian for a well-bird visit and make sure.

Here are some bird safety tips:

Always wash your hands with soap and water after handling your bird or bird cage.

Some birds (especially cockatoos) are very dusty. You may want to consider getting an air filter. This may be especially helpful when the new baby comes home.

DR B TRUE STORY: PET IGUANAS

I have had more than one baby patient get a Salmonella infection long before she was old enough to eat steak tartare. Example: one baby got sick after her uncle's pet iguana roamed freely on the kitchen counter (near washed baby bottles). Another baby was infected after his grandmother prepared chitterlings (pig intestine) in the kitchen sink before he took a bath there. Truth is sometimes stranger than fiction!

environment

Q. I was bitten by a_____ (fill in the blank). Are there any health risks?

No matter what bites you, call your practitioner. Some animal bites are only dangerous because of the risk of skin infection (like most dog bites, assuming there is no rabies).

Other bites, however, can be much more dangerous such as those from a cat infected with toxoplasmosis or a wild animal, like a squirrel or raccoon.

Wash the area immediately with soap and water, then seek medical advice.

NOISE

Q. Can I go to a rock concert during my pregnancy?

Yes. Just make sure you are not in the front row.

At about 16 weeks, your developing baby can hear noises and by 27 to 30 weeks, his ears are fully formed and he will begin to respond to many sounds.

These sounds include blood rushing through the vessels in your body, the sound of food moving through your intestines as well as the sound of your voice.

Your baby doesn't hear sounds as clearly as we do. The amniotic fluid, uterus and your body act as barriers that help muffle external sounds and noises. Additionally, the baby's eardrum and middle ear can't amplify sounds like ours do, so loud sounds to us aren't quite as loud to them.

However, we still don't want to expose fetuses to really loud noises for prolonged or repeated intervals. Babies can suffer hearing loss in the womb, but that typically results from conditions such as working an eight-to-ten hour workday next to a chainsaw or lawnmower (85 to 100 decibels). Extremely intense sounds (over 140 decibels) such as a jet engine or rock concert speaker, can also cause similar problems.

Loud noises to avoid during pregnancy:

- ◆ Standing near jet engines.
- ◆ Being at a firing range or firing guns yourself.
- ◆ Being in the front few rows of a rock concert.
- ◆ Working at a job that subjects you to constant, loud noise (above 80 decibels for many hours a day, day after day)

Q. What about my hair dryer?

Using a hair dryer during pregnancy is fine.

Resources For More Info. The National Birth Defects Center offers a free pregnancy exposure hotline: 800-322-5014. The National Library of Medicine also provides great information on environmental exposures and pregnancy. Go to their website at toxnet.nlm.nih.gov.

Hope this chapter didn't induce contractions! We'll move on to more uplifting subjects now: exercising, traveling, and making love.

LIFESTYLES

Chapter 8

"Note for new mama:
Falling asleep during sex?
It's forgivable."

—Haiku Mama, Kari Anne Roy

Your life still goes on, despite being pregnant. You want to feel like you are a normal human being and we'd like you to feel that way as much as possible!

This chapter will walk you through activities of daily living and adventures along the way. We cover both work and play in this chapter—exercise, sex, travel and more.

Exercise

We know, we know—you are nauseated, bloated, and so exhausted that there is no way in the world you are gonna get off that cozy sofa and go work out. But your mind, your body, and your developing baby need to get through the next nine months together—and exercising helps all of these aspects of pregnancy. Yes, it is *that* important to make exercise part of your *daily* routine.

Here are some reasons if you need convincing (or sheer motivation) to take off your fuzzy slippers and put on running shoes.

Overall, exercise helps decrease weight gain, improve body image, decrease stress, and reduce your chances of having low back and pelvic pain. Exercise throughout pregnancy helps to reduce labor and delivery time, as well as delivery complications.

In the first trimester, exercise can

reduce nausea and fatigue. As exhausted as you are, that 30-minute walk outside is worth the effort. You will feel better in the long run and also have *more* energy than your non-exercising preggo friends.

In the second and third trimesters, exercise helps decrease the risk of gestational diabetes. If you do have diabetes, it can help treat it.

Exercise also benefits your baby. Babies born to moms who exercised moderately during pregnancy tolerate the stress of labor better, and are more alert and less irritable as newborns.

One added bonus: Over 90% of women who exercise during pregnancy will continue to do so afterwards—leading to a healthier lifestyle and quicker weight loss after pregnancy ends.

Bottom line: we recommend daily exercise even if you didn't do this prior to getting pregnant. But be sure to talk with your practitioner before beginning any exercise regimen. *(ACOG)*

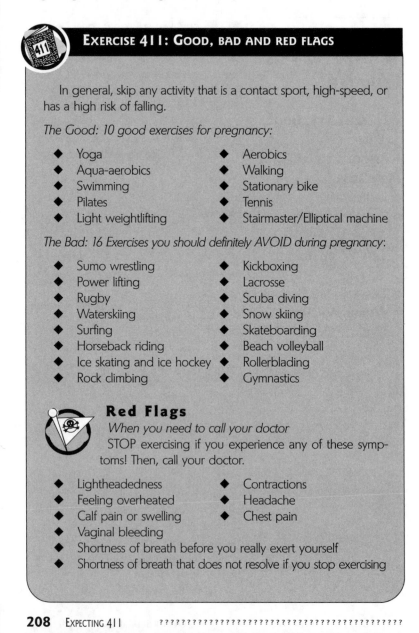

EXERCISE 411: GOOD, BAD AND RED FLAGS

In general, skip any activity that is a contact sport, high-speed, or has a high risk of falling.

The Good: 10 good exercises for pregnancy:

- Yoga
- Aqua-aerobics
- Swimming
- Pilates
- Light weightlifting
- Aerobics
- Walking
- Stationary bike
- Tennis
- Stairmaster/Elliptical machine

The Bad: 16 Exercises you should definitely AVOID during pregnancy:

- Sumo wrestling
- Power lifting
- Rugby
- Waterskiing
- Surfing
- Horseback riding
- Ice skating and ice hockey
- Rock climbing
- Kickboxing
- Lacrosse
- Scuba diving
- Snow skiing
- Skateboarding
- Beach volleyball
- Rollerblading
- Gymnastics

Red Flags
When you need to call your doctor
STOP exercising if you experience any of these symptoms! Then, call your doctor.

- Lightheadedness
- Feeling overheated
- Calf pain or swelling
- Vaginal bleeding
- Shortness of breath before you really exert yourself
- Shortness of breath that does not resolve if you stop exercising
- Contractions
- Headache
- Chest pain

Partner Tip
Want to do something to help your baby-carrying mate? Exercise with her. Find an activity you both can do and enjoy (okay, you may need to make some concessions here) and spend some healthy, quality time together.

Factoid: *ACOG recommends 30 minutes of exercise a day.* If you have no medical reasons or pregnancy complications (see below), your goal should be 30 minutes a day of aerobic exercise.

Reasons NOT to exercise

Note: this list does not include "I just did my hair" or "American Idol is on tonight." These are legitimate medical reasons to avoid aerobic exercise, not excuses:

- Heart disease that alters blood circulation.
- Lung disease limiting the air volume breathed in.
- Incompetent cervix (**CERVICAL INSUFFICIENCY**) with or without a **CERCLAGE**.
- Multiple babies at risk for preterm labor.
- Persistent second or third trimester bleeding.
- **PLACENTA PREVIA** after 26 weeks gestation.
- Premature labor.
- Ruptured membranes.
- **PREECLAMPSIA** or pregnancy-induced hypertension (**GESTATIONAL HYPERTENSION**).

We discuss all of these medical conditions in Chapter 16, Complications.

Other good reasons to skip aerobic exercise *(ACOG)*

- Severe anemia.
- Abnormal heart rhythm that has never been evaluated (cardiac arrhythmia).
- Chronic bronchitis.
- Poorly controlled pre-existing diabetes.
- Extreme obesity.
- Extremely underweight (BMI < 12).
- History of extremely sedentary lifestyle.
- Fetal (intrauterine) growth restriction.
- Pre-existing bone, joint, or soft tissue problem.
- Poorly controlled high blood pressure.
- Poorly controlled seizure disorder.
- Poorly controlled thyroid disorder.
- Heavy smoker.
- Your practitioner has placed you on bedrest.

Q. I've heard I shouldn't be flat on my back during my exercise regimen. Is that true? Why?

That's true—for pregnant women after about 20 weeks. Why? Because this position lowers your blood pressure, which can lead to dizziness and fainting.

Your uterus lies on top of your major blood vessels (the vena cava and aorta) that take blood to and from your heart. After 20 weeks, when lying on your back, the increased size and weight of the uterus can cause a relative blockage of blood flow. Less blood returns to your heart and so less blood leaves your heart, hence, lower blood pressure.

What does that mean for your baby? Less blood goes to your uterus and to him. What does that mean for you? Less blood goes to your head. You feel dizzy or faint.

The take-home message: don't lie on your back during exercise after 20 weeks.

Q. We are going on vacation to the mountains. Can I exercise at higher altitudes?

Yes, up to certain altitudes.

Altitudes up to 6,000 feet above sea level appear to be safe. But even at these altitudes, you may feel out of breath faster. You may need to shorten the length of your workout and stop if you have any of the Red Flag symptoms mentioned above.

Above 6,000 feet in altitude, exercise can lead to altitude sickness, dizziness/fainting, shortness of breath, and chest pain. So it is best to avoid exercise at these altitudes.

If you live at elevations above 6,000 feet, check with your practitioner before beginning any exercise regimen.

Q. Can I swim in a chlorinated pool?

Yes.

Don't let the prospect of wearing a pregnancy bathing suit scare you away. Swimming is a great form of exercise during pregnancy, even if you weren't a swimmer beforehand.

Chlorine kills germs, and that's a good thing. An adequately chlorinated pool will prevent the spread of viruses (like enterovirus and Hepatitis A). So yes, you *want* to swim in a chlorinated pool.

Q. Can I swim in a fresh water lake or stream?

Sorry, but the germ factor makes fresh water lakes and streams off limits.

Everyone (including non-pregnant swimmers) faces *some* risk when they swim in fresh bodies of water. But as you become an infectious disease expert with this book, you know that germs and pregnant women are often risky business.

Here are the three bugs (bacteria and parasites) that can bug you when swimming in fresh water lakes/streams—Giardia, leptospirosis, and amebiasis. All of them can cause horrible cramps, diarrhea, and potentially, miscarriage and preterm labor.

So the safest thing to do when you are pregnant is to use the pool or sit in the shade and enjoy some alone time reading while everyone else is in the water!

Q. Can I go waterskiing or scuba diving?

No. These are two activities that are better left for days without a baby in your belly.

Waterskiing can be dangerous, particularly during a fall. The impact of a fall can cause extreme jolting, which may lead to a separation of the placenta from the wall of the uterus (**PLACENTAL ABRUPTION**).

Scuba diving is another activity that's not recommended. First, you have to strap on some serious gear. This can be uncomfortable, especially as you get bigger. Second, you descend to depths that can decrease oxygen levels in your bloodstream and therefore, baby's bloodstream. Finally, divers have to decompress as they return to the surface. Developing babies may have difficulty decompressing.

While there is no solid scientific evidence, there is a concern for potential birth defects and preterm delivery among women who go scuba diving during pregnancy. *(Camporesi EM)*

So although we know we are taking all of your fun away, stick with a virgin daiquiri on the beach while the rest of the crew heads down below. You can return to all these activities about six weeks after having the baby, with your doctor's blessing.

FYI: Placental abruption can even happen with low-impact falls or accidents. That's why it's a good idea to avoid any activities that cause sudden or abrupt jolts.

Q. I went diving during my last vacation and didn't know that I was pregnant at the time. Is that a problem?

Probably not.

There's no evidence that diving around the time of conception leads to miscarriage. Pregnant women were diving for years before docs started advising against it. And there was no significant health impact to mother or the developing baby.

Experts don't recommend it anymore because of the theoretical risk and some research that suggests concern.

Q. Will exercising really make my labor and delivery go more smoothly?

It would be nice to say that exercise would shorten labor and make delivery smoother . . . but there are no guarantees.

What we can tell you is that it reduces your overall weight gain and chances of gestational diabetes—both of which can complicate labor and delivery.

And continuing the exercise routine that you start during pregnancy will help you lose those pregnancy pounds afterwards and improve your overall health. Daily exercise also gives you more muscle tone and stamina to endure labor and delivery.

Q. I am an avid runner. Can I still run a marathon while I am pregnant?

Can you continue to run? Yes. Should you run a marathon? No.

LIFESTYLES

? ?

Studies show that runners who continue exercising during pregnancy gain less weight, have leaner babies, and shorter labors. Running a marathon, however, is a tremendous strain on a non-pregnant body, let alone a pregnant one.

If you have any pregnancy complications, your practitioner will probably tell you to stop jogging. Otherwise, keep up the jogging, with a few precautions:

◆ Stay well hydrated.
◆ Exercise for a maximum of 60 minutes.
◆ You should base your workouts on something called Rate of Perceived Exertion (RPE). RPE is how hard you feel your body is working. This means that you can continue exercising as long as you aren't experiencing any physical symptoms such as chest pain, shortness of breath or dizziness.

Ask your practitioner about specific advice for you.

Truthfully, most runners stop running in the second trimester as the weight of their belly becomes uncomfortable when bouncing up and down. They usually trade in running for the elliptical machine, swimming, hiking, or something less jarring.

Reality Check

Pregnant women get all sorts of advice about what exercise is kosher—and what to avoid.

The problem: it's impossible to do a study that shows exercise X leads to birth defect Y. Or that exercising with a target heart rate of 140 is more dangerous than 130. That's why most practitioners follow the precautionary principle—better to be safe than sorry, even in the absence of scientific proof.

Here is the concern: when a person is exercising, blood flow is diverted away from the abdominal organs (intestines, spleen, and in pregnancy, the uterus) and diverted towards the skeletal muscles. Decreased blood flow to the uterus means less oxygen goes to the fetus. But does this significantly impact a growing fetus? Studies show conflicting results. There is

---

7 RULES FOR EXERCISING WHILE PREGNANT

1. Wear comfortable clothing.
2. Consume lots of water to keep well hydrated.
3. Walk with a friend or bring a cell phone.
4. Take frequent breaks. (Some of you will feel like you aren't even breaking a sweat with all the restrictions, but now is not the time to train for a marathon.)
5. If you are new to an exercise regimen, periodically check your pulse and if it is persistently over 140 beats/minute, slow down (see "How to Check Your Pulse" below).
6. Do not lie flat on your back for long periods of time after 20 weeks.
7. Do notify your trainer or gym that you are pregnant.

? ?

LIFESTYLES

also a risk of the mother's core body temperature increasing as her heart rate goes up. We know that a pregnant woman's body temperature above 101.5 in the first trimester can be associated with birth defects.

Bottom line: ask your practitioner for specific advice on exercise options. Your exercise regimen should be tailored to your physical conditioning and general health. There is not one target heart rate for everyone. While her opinion may vary a bit from your friend's OB, they will both probably tell you not to run the New York Marathon or swim the English Channel (although pregnant women have accomplished both of these feats!).

Q. After I deliver, when can I start exercising again?

The textbook answer is six weeks, if you had an uncomplicated pregnancy and delivery.

Occasionally, practitioners might give the green light a little earlier to a patient who had an uncomplicated vaginal delivery. But "green light" means she can do some light walking before six weeks—not a triathlon.

Always check with your practitioner first before starting or resuming any exercise program after delivery. We know six weeks seems like a really long time but it's really important to listen to your practitioner and to your body.

Q. I have a high-risk pregnancy. Am I still able to exercise?

It depends on what makes your pregnancy high-risk.

For example, if you have gestational diabetes, then yes, you can and should exercise during your pregnancy.

But if you have a **PLACENTA PREVIA** and have had two episodes of vaginal bleeding, then the answer is no, you should not exercise during your pregnancy.

Again, always check with your practitioner about what is right for you.

Helpful Hint

How to check your pulse: The easiest places to find your pulse are your neck (just under your jaw bone on either side) or the inner part of your wrist. Count how many times you feel a beat in 15 seconds and then multiply that by four. That equals your pulse (how many times your heart beats in a minute).

DR H'S TRUE STORY: EXERCISING TOO SOON

I had a patient who was determined to get back on her treadmill after a C-section. I told her that *after* her six-week postpartum visit, we would decide when she could go back to exercising.

She decided that she felt great at two and a half weeks. She returned to my office with her previously closed surgical incision now gaping open. She had to wait another month to have the wound surgically repaired!

Sexuality

Here's the section you (and your partner) have been waiting for. Do you have the green light to continue your sexual relations? Will you want to? Will your partner want to? And what do you do if only one member of your party is ready to party? Read on.

Q. Will I die if I have oral sex?

No. Oral sex is considered safe during pregnancy.

A popular pregnancy book warns women about fatal oral sex, so we are here to allay your fears.

Medical journals from decades ago reported on a few extremely rare cases of fatal air embolism in pregnancy from forcefully blowing a lot of air into a woman's vagina during oral sex. *(Ashai S, Aronson ME.)*

How could this happen? Well, pregnant women have engorged, enlarged blood vessels in their pelvis. When pushed forcefully, those vessels are more likely to allow water or air to enter.

If you look at the millions of women enjoying oral sex during pregnancy (okay, that's an optimistic assumption, but quite possibly true) and you compare that to a few fascinating cases in the medical literature, having a fatal air embolism is far-fetched. In fact, you are 1000 times more likely to get into a car accident during your pregnancy than die from oral sex. And most people don't forcefully blow air into the vagina during oral sex anyway—so the risk here seems very remote. (If this is something you practice, please write to us and explain why this would be a desirable thing to experience.)

In fact, the medical journals indicated you have to force so much air into a vagina to cause a problem there probably isn't a concern here . . . unless your partner is a professional balloon animal artist.

Bottom line: oral sex is safe during pregnancy, and many pregnant women find it more pleasurable than vaginal intercourse.

Q. Is it normal to not be in the mood?

Absolutely, and you are not alone.

Although some women have an increased sexual desire (see below), most do not. You have tender breasts, you are exhausted, your hormones are running amuck and you are most likely self-conscious about your weight gain (not to mention the fact that in the later stages of pregnancy you can't see your legs, let alone shave them).

Even if you are not in the mood, make sure to take some time for intimacy during your pregnancy. Being intimate does not always mean having intercourse. Kissing, holding hands, bathing together, massaging each other, and hugging are all forms of intimacy.

We cannot overemphasize the importance of talking to your partner about this issue. Lack of communication can lead to dysfunction and hurtful feelings in your relationship.

Partner Tip:
When you're up and your partner isn't

Yes, you may resort to masturbation. That may take the stress off of both of you! By the way, it is safe for your baby-carrying partner to perform oral sex on you and yes, it is safe to swallow, if she is so inclined. Although beware, her gag reflex is at an all time high.

Q. Is it normal to be excessively horny?

For some women, yes.

The physiologic changes happening to your body may increase your sexual desire. Your breasts are larger, your nipples are more sensitive, and you have more blood flow to your vagina and vulva. These changes often lead to increased desire.

You'll also be naturally lubricated (with all that lovely vaginal discharge), which enhances the intercourse experience. In fact, some women experience orgasms for the very first time during pregnancy.

If you are one of the lucky ones experiencing an increase in sexual desire (and you have your doctor's blessing), go for it!

Q. What will happen to my sexual desire, trimester by trimester?

All women are different—but here is a rough guideline on what may happen to your sexual desire as your body changes throughout pregnancy:

◆ *First trimester:* Most women are fatigued beyond belief and most experience some degree of "morning sickness" or really, "all-day sickness." Even if you aren't truly nauseated, you may feel queasy or have an upset stom-

---

5 TIPS TO STAY CONNECTED

Yes, it might be stating the obvious, but you probably won't have intercourse as often as usual during pregnancy (and even beyond that). Maybe you're not in the mood as often as your partner is. Or, maybe you have a high-risk pregnancy that requires you to temporarily stop sexual relations. And maybe (okay, more than maybe), you are apathetic about sex for a while *after* you deliver, too (while your body heals and you have to deal with newborn parent sleep deprivation).

Whatever the case may be, it's mission critical to maintain your loving relationship beyond friendship and just being roommates. So make a plan together to keep your relationship on course. Here are a few suggestions:

1. Communicate with your partner.
2. Give each other a massage.
3. Foreplay. Remember what that was?
4. Oral sex. Yes, it's safe.
5. Take a bath together (as long as it's not over 99 degrees).

LIFESTYLES

? ?

ach, which usually doesn't make anyone feel sexy. Breast sensitivity is worst in the first trimester—to the point where some women can't even tolerate a sheet or water in the shower touching their nipples and breasts. You may find this very uncomfortable and may not want your breasts touched during intercourse. Or like other women, you may find extreme pleasure in your larger and more sensitive breasts during foreplay and lovemaking.

◆ *Second trimester:* Good news, you are over the fatigue and nausea. But you'll probably be more uncomfortable with low back pain and continued soreness around the breasts and nipples. You may continue to have low libido, or you may have a peak in sexual desire. This is due to increased blood flow that causes the vulva and vagina to swell.

◆ *Third trimester:* The third trimester is tough, no matter how you look at it. You are bigger, more uncomfortable, and you may feel your baby move around after having an orgasm. (This is not a problem, but it might be a real mental leap for you to overcome.) As the baby's head moves lower into the pelvis, you may also be more uncomfortable with vaginal intercourse. For most women, and their partners, the third trimester is a time when sexual desire is at an all time low. (Yes, there will be a point when your partner doesn't want to have sex with you, either.)

Q. My clitoris seems to be more sensitive now. Is this permanent?

You now have a super-sized clitoris! And no, it's not permanent.

Because of that increased blood flow, your entire pelvic region is completely engorged and swollen—especially during the second and third trimesters.

This can be good or bad. Some women find that it heightens their sensation and so they have really easy, great orgasms. Others find this sensation rather uncomfortable.

This is not a permanent change and the size of your clitoris will go back to normal after delivery. So either enjoy it now or relax knowing you will have your regular body back soon.

Q. Is it normal for my partner to be uninterested in sex?

Yes.

Some partners are less interested in sex for a number of reasons. . . they may feel extra stress from the impending birth and becoming a parent. Or there may be fear in potentially harming you or the baby during intercourse. (You can assure a male partner that having vaginal intercourse will not poke the baby's head!).

Again, it is extremely important to talk with your partner about his or her fears and concerns. Don't be shy about bringing up this topic at one of your prenatal visits. You and your partner will have a sense of relief if you discuss this subject with your practitioner. She/he can reassure you that all is normal and offer helpful suggestions.

Q. Is it normal for my partner to have an increased sex drive during my pregnancy?

Yes.

Some partners may be more aroused by your fuller breasts and rounded figure, the chance to try new positions, and the fact that contraception is a non-issue.

And believe it or not, impending parenthood can be a turn on! The concept of becoming parents together often strengthens the relationship bond and increases sexual desire between two people.

FYI: Your doctor may put you on bed rest or pelvic rest during pregnancy. Here's a brief description of each:

◆ **Bed Rest:** Resting and reclining 24/7, likely with brief bathroom breaks and trips to the shower and kitchen.
◆ **PELVIC REST:** No sexual intercourse, no tampons, no douching . . . nothing in the vagina.

Q. What happens if I go on bed rest? Can I still have an orgasm, even if we can't have intercourse?

It all depends on why you are on bed rest.

Orgasms can cause uterine contractions. Although contractions usually don't put normal women into labor, they can worsen preterm labor or increase bleeding if there is a **PLACENTA PREVIA**.

If your OB sidelines you for the remainder of your pregnancy, ask for detailed instructions on sexual restrictions.

Q. Can an orgasm cause a miscarriage or hurt my baby?

No.

An orgasm will make you have a contraction, though, and you will feel it. Your uterus is simply flexing its muscles for a moment. This will not hurt the baby.

Once intercourse and your orgasm are over, the contraction should stop. If you feel like you are continuing to have contractions for more than 60 minutes following an orgasm, contact your practitioner.

Q. Can my partner hurt my baby?

Nope. Your baby is well protected.

In fact, she has several layers of protection. She sits inside an amniotic sac, which sits inside the thick, muscular walls of your uterus . . . which sits within the bones of the pelvic cavity. The cervix, and the **MUCOUS PLUG** within the cervix are also barriers between your baby and the outside world of the vagina.

The penis does not come into contact with the fetus during sex. This could only happen if your cervix was dilated or you were having intercourse during labor, which you shouldn't be doing anyway!

Q. Why does my baby move so much during and after sex?

Some couples feel weird about having their unborn baby participate in their lovemaking. Don't let this get to you!

Think about it. Babies are human beings, albeit tiny ones. They are simply responding to stimulation and touch. When his little home (your uterus) starts rocking and rolling with an orgasm-induced contraction, it's going to make him move around.

And because you have an adrenaline rush when you have an orgasm, so does your baby. Medically speaking, your body releases a large volume of adrenaline into your bloodstream and a little bit of that also goes into your baby's system.

Don't worry about any of this, because it is safe (assuming you have your doctor's blessing). Your developing baby has no idea what the two of you are doing. When he is old enough to understand, make sure you have a lock on your bedroom door!

Q. I've heard that sex can trigger labor. Is that true?

This falls into the "I'll try anything to go into labor" category. People hear that spicy food or long walks will induce labor. Unlike those myths, this one actually has some truth behind it. Yes, sex can make you go into labor if your body is ready to go.

When a man has an orgasm, he releases *semen* (also called seminal fluid). That fluid contains sperm as well as the hormone *prostaglandin*. And prostaglandin is the same ingredient in many of the medications docs use to help soften the cervix and help start labor. So, your partner's "natural" prostaglandin has the potential to do the same thing.

Before you tie your husband up and demand that he make love to you, know that there probably isn't enough prostaglandin in his semen to induce labor (no matter how virile he thinks he is). The odds go up slightly if you were ready to go into labor even without his contribution. Most women will just have a few contractions after intercourse and that's it.

If you are at high risk of going into labor early, however, your doctor may want to restrict any activity that increases the motion of your uterus. That may mean no orgasms, nipple stimulation, or sexual intercourse at all. Be sure to get details from your doctor.

Reality Check

If you do decide to tie your husband up and demand he make love to you when you are nine months pregnant, he may not be as excited as you'd like (or need him to be). It's a lot of pressure! You may want to inform him that you will be off limits for six weeks after delivery, so his chance to enjoy it is now!

Q. What happens if my partner has herpes? Do I need to take special precautions?

Yes, you do need to take special precautions if your partner has herpes and you don't.

The reason? You really don't want to get herpes while you are pregnant. It's miserable for you and dangerous for your unborn baby (see more info on herpes infections in Chapter 17, Infections).

Here are your options:

◆ Abstain from all intercourse.
◆ Have intercourse, but make your partner always wear a condom.
◆ Abstain from all intercourse if your partner feels like an outbreak is imminent or there are visible lesions.

Talk to your doctor about a preventive medication for your partner. Your partner can take a daily anti-viral medicine (such as acyclovir) that reduces the chance of shedding the herpes virus and spreading it to you.

FYI: Herpes. Even if your partner does not have any visible lesions, there's a 1% chance on any given day that he or she is shedding the herpes virus without any symptoms. And that means there is a 1% chance that you can get it from him or her. Having your partner take anti-viral medication reduces those chances.

Q. Are there any positions that are more comfortable than others?

That's a trick question because *no* position will be really comfortable towards the end of your pregnancy. You will be uncomfortable just sitting or standing, let alone twisting like a pretzel during intercourse.

But if you are still game, we have some suggestions for you. We'll start with the old standby, the missionary position. But you will probably find that options two, three and four below are more comfortable for you.

◆ *Missionary position.* Lying on your back with your partner on top. After about 20 weeks, you should not by lying flat on your back for long periods of time. But if this is the most comfortable intercourse position for you, put a small pillow under your pelvis to tilt yourself to the left a bit. This will take most of the weight of the uterus and the baby off of your major blood vessels.

◆ *Doggie Style.* You bend over and lean on your hands and knees, with your partner behind you. If you have never tried this position, now may be the time. It allows easier access without your belly coming between the two of you.

7 REASONS WHY YOUR DOC WON'T LET YOU HAVE SEX

1. History of premature labor or birth.
2. Ruptured membranes.
3. Unexplained vaginal bleeding.
4. **PLACENTA PREVIA** or low-lying placenta.
5. Incompetent cervix (**CERVICAL INSUFFICIENCY**) with or without **CERCLAGE.**
6. Dilated cervix.
7. Sexually transmitted disease in you or your partner.

◆ *Spooning.* You lie on your left side and your partner enters behind you. This is a popular pregnancy lovemaking position for the same reasons as the doggie style. It requires less energy than doggie style, since you are lying down.

◆ *You on top.* You straddle yourself on top of your partner, who lies beneath you. This gives you more control over your belly and how your bodies move together.

Q. Can I have anal sex during pregnancy?

Yes, but we don't recommend it.

If you decide to give it a try, you should always use a condom, lubrication, and have your partner be very careful.

Hemorrhoids are common during pregnancy. You may have internal hemorrhoids even if you can't see any on the outside of your anus. Anal sex can flare up hemorrhoids and cause them to bleed. Proceed with caution!

Q. Can I use sex toys during pregnancy?

Yes, as long as you are careful.

It's safe to use a vibrator externally on the clitoris. You need to be very careful using other toys *in* the vagina. Any high-risk condition that makes sexual intercourse off limits means these toys are off limits, too.

Make sure you clean all toys appropriately after using them.

Q. Are there any other sexual behaviors that are not safe during pregnancy?

Yes.

Do *not* have intercourse with anyone who has a known STD (sexually transmitted disease) or HIV (the AIDS virus), or with anyone whose sexual history is unknown to you.

You and your unborn baby can both get sexually transmitted infections such as HIV, Hepatitis B or C.

Red Flags: When to call your doctor
◆ If you aren't sure if sex is safe for you.
◆ If you experience unusual symptoms after intercourse such as severe or persistent pain, vaginal bleeding or abnormal discharge.
◆ If you have contractions that continue after sex.

Travel

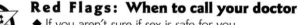

Many people have a last fling before they take on the rigors of having a newborn in the house. This is a good idea, because you won't get another vacation without kids for a very long time (unless you can persuade the grandparents to babysit). We want you to have fun, but here are a few precautions:

- Tell your practitioner about your plans.
- Take your prenatal medical records with you.
- Make sure you get up and stretch your legs regularly during flights.
- Stay hydrated.
- Have an obstetrician and hospital lined up at your destination, just in case.
- Purchase travel insurance and in the case of a boat/cruise, evacuation insurance (like MedJet Assist).

Q. How far along in my pregnancy can I continue to travel by car?

There are no restrictions, except that you probably don't want to be more than 45 to 60 minutes away from your practitioner and delivery/birthing center in the final weeks of your pregnancy.

Sitting around for long periods of time in a car puts you at risk for forming a blood clot in your legs (deep venous thrombosis or DVT). Long flights carry the same risk. So be sure to take frequent breaks to walk around (you'll probably need to take several potty breaks anyway). Always clear travel with your doctor.

Q. My husband doesn't want me driving anymore. Is it okay for me to drive up until the end of my pregnancy?

Yes. We understand his concern, but tell him not to worry.

You can get behind the wheel up until the end of your pregnancy. Just adjust your seat so that you are comfortable and there is some distance between your belly and the steering wheel. That way, the airbag can properly deploy in an emergency. Note: the bottom portion of your seatbelt should go *under* your belly, not across it.

Feedback From The Real World

We should point out that it's okay to drive assuming you are *not* on bed rest! True story: a fellow OB colleague was placed on bed rest at 20 weeks for preterm labor with her first child and was bored out of her mind. While her husband (also an OB) was at work, she snuck out of the house to run a few errands. When she ended up in a car accident and went to the nearest hospital for evaluation, she sheepishly called him and said, "Hi honey, I'm being taken to the hospital because I got into a car accident." His response was, "You must have mistaken me for someone else because my wife is on strict bed rest so its absolutely impossible for her to have been in a car accident!"

I don't think we really need to point out the moral of the story here!

Q. How far along in my pregnancy can I travel by plane?

ACOG says 36 weeks. Your doc may say something different.

Barring any medical complications, it is safe to fly in the first 28 weeks of your pregnancy. It gets riskier with each subsequent week after that. Your practitioner may tell you to stop flying at 28 weeks or 32 weeks, even though ACOG's cut off is 36 weeks. And if you have a high-risk pregnancy (such as carrying multiples), your practitioner will have his or her own set of rules. Ask before you book those non-refundable tickets to Hawaii.

Airlines vary with their own policies—especially with international carriers, so you'll need to check that as well. You may need a letter from your doctor in order to travel by air on some carriers late in pregnancy; check this in advance. *(ACOG)*

Reality check

Here's what one airline (American Airlines) says about pregnancy travel restrictions. "For international travel or any flights over the water, travel is not advised within 30 days of the due date, unless the passenger is examined by an obstetrician within 48 hours of outbound departure and certified in writing as medically stable for flight. Travel within ten days of the due date for international travel must have clearance from our Special Assistance Coordinators."

Helpful Hint

This may be the one time that it is worth it to purchase travel insurance for your trip. You may be a low-risk pregnancy when you book the trip and confined to bed rest when it comes time to travel.

Q. I have a high-risk pregnancy. Can I still fly?

No.

You should not be flying on a plane if you have pre-existing medical or obstetric complications. Emergency situations happen without warning in obstetrics and being on a plane over the Atlantic is one of the last places you want to be. You do NOT want to be in preterm labor as the captain asks via the overhead speaker if there is a doctor on the plane and the only person who raises his hand is a podiatrist.

Here are just a few examples of pregnancy conditions where you should avoid air travel: preterm labor, high blood pressure, poorly controlled diabetes, and sickle cell disease or trait (which can flare up with high altitude).

Always check with your practitioner first.

Travel 411:
7 Tips For Travel During Pregnancy

1 **GO GAS-FREE.** Don't drink or eat any gas-producing items (carbonated beverages, refried beans, etc) before or during your flight. Entrapped gas expands at higher altitudes and can give you a stomachache. Avoiding these foods also prevents burping and gas passing next to a stranger who can't escape!

2 **PREVENT AIR SICKNESS.** If you are still in the morning sickness phase of pregnancy, air travel may make things worse. Consider asking your practitioner for an anti-nausea medication to take with you.

3 **TAKE A WALK.** You should not be immobilized for long periods of time. Being pregnant means you are at higher risk of developing a blood clot in your leg (DVT), which can potentially travel to your lungs.

Stretch your calves periodically while you are seated and walk the aisle once an hour if you are on a long flight.

4 **BOOK AN AISLE SEAT.** It's easier access for your hourly walks and trips to the restroom.

5 **TED HOSE.** Some practitioners recommend that you wear support stockings to increase circulation and help prevent a blood clot from developing in your leg.

6 **DRINK WATER.** You'll feel better by being well hydrated. It also helps prevent those blood clots. Take an empty water bottle with you in carry-on luggage and fill it up after you get through security.

7 **WEAR YOUR SEATBELT.** Since air turbulence is unpredictable, it's wise to wear your seatbelt when you are seated. The seatbelt should rest as low as possible under your belly, not across the top.

Old Wives Tale:
I've heard that I shouldn't fly because of radiation risk?
False. All available data says that the amount of cosmic radiation is negligible and not a health concern for pregnant air travelers.

Q. How far along in my pregnancy can I take a cruise?

The cut off varies between 23 to 27 weeks.

Just like the airlines, every cruise line has its own policy. Many require your doctor to fax a note prior to the day you board. Even if it isn't required, we recommend that you take a note from your doctor and a copy of your prenatal medical records with you.

Some cruise lines do not have a doctor on board. That may impact

SEASICKNESS AND MORNING SICKNESS

If you are already suffering from morning sickness or get seasick even when you aren't pregnant, be prepared for motion sickness. If you are prone to puking, you might want to wait on that cruise vacation until after the first trimester.

Here are a few things you can try to avoid getting green around the gills:

◆ Book a cabin in the middle of the ship.
◆ Book a cruise on a larger ship with better stabilizers (you'll appreciate it on rough seas).
◆ Spend more time outside on the deck.
◆ Exercise.
◆ Eat frequently (that's easy). Choose non-greasy meals or bread and crackers.
◆ Pack an emergency supply of acupressure wristbands, or medication prescribed by your doctor.

which cruise line you decide to take—check this before booking. As long as you have a low risk pregnancy, it perfectly safe to take a cruise vacation. Just chat with your practitioner before you set sail. And consider purchasing medical evacuation insurance (example: MedJet Assist; medjetassist.com)

Helpful Hint

Vacationstogo.com has a specific section on cruises for pregnant women and infants, listing the restrictions of each individual cruise line. This is a great place to start before booking a cruise.

Q. Are there any special things I should bring on my cruise?

Yes. Remember to bring enough of any medication you are currently taking as well as prenatal vitamins. Ship pharmacies may not carry everything you need.

Wear a hat and lots of sunscreen, especially on your face to help prevent **MELASMA**.

And if there is any chance you may become seasick, talk to your doctor about possible medication. It's better to have it with you, just in case.

Q. Will the ship have a life preserver that will fit me correctly?

Yes.

Since most cruise lines do not allow you to travel after 24 weeks, you are still small enough to have a life preserver fit you correctly (just think about all the old men on the ship who eat five meals a day and don't miss the nightly midnight buffet!).

If you actually need a life preserver beyond the routine drill on the first day, ask for assistance.

Q. What are the restrictions on amusement park rides?

Basically, any ride that causes a jarring motion or abnormal force is off limits for you.

Most amusement parks, including Busch Gardens, Disney, Six Flags and even local fairs and carnivals have warning signs directed at pregnant women.

Admittedly, we don't have any studies showing that they are dangerous, but we also don't have any demonstrating they are safe. The big concern is the potential for damage to the uterus, placenta, and fetus. Rigorous movements (similar to a car accident) can cause a separation of the placenta from the uterine wall, which compromises the fetus' blood flow and oxygen supply (**PLACENTAL ABRUPTION**).

Although plenty of women have ridden on roller coasters and other thrill rides without serious complications, it's wise to avoid them.

Q. If I go camping, can I use insect repellant?

Yes! You can and should use bug spray. See Chapter 7, The Environment & Your Baby for detailed information.

Work

If you work outside the home, it's really important to discuss it with your practitioner—what your job entails, exposure to any chemicals, radiation or other concerns.

If you work inside the home (the hardest job of all in our opinion!), you should discuss possible infections your little rug rats may share with you. It's helpful to know if you are immune to say, chickenpox or parvovirus, before your older child comes home with it.

Q. When do I need to stop working?

It depends. There are no hard and fast rules here.

Certain occupations and workplaces set their own restrictions (examples: pilots and flight attendants). Most employers, however, will let you continue to work as long as you are low-risk, comfortable and have the okay of your practitioner.

Some women work up until the day before they deliver (it's not easy, let us tell you), whereas others need to stop at some point in the third trimester due to severe low back pain, sciatic pain, or pregnancy complications.

Q. I have a high-risk pregnancy. Do I need to stop working?

This depends on the nature of your high-risk pregnancy as well as the nature of your job. If, for example, you are a tennis instructor and you are a gestational diabetic, you can continue working. But if you are a tennis instructor and are in preterm labor, you've gotta stop running around the courts.

Sometimes practitioners limit what a woman can do at work without needing her to stop working altogether. Talk to your doc about possible accommodations instead of having to completely stop work.

Old Wives Tale
Heavy lifting causes miscarriages. *False.* While heavy lifting is not recommended for any pregnant woman, it doesn't cause miscarriages.

DR H'S TRUE STORY:
WORKING DURING PREGNANCY

Working during pregnancy certainly is not a walk in the park. I almost fainted twice in the operating room and got such severe backaches from delivering babies (the last one I delivered was two days before I had my first child!) that I almost requested an epidural for myself. But the beauty of working up until the end was that I wasn't at home lamenting about all of my discomfort. I was distracted and in the good company of many other pregnant women who were experiencing the same things as me!

LIFESTYLES

? ?

Q. My job requires me to do some heavy lifting. What are my restrictions?

You should avoid all heavy lifting.

The curvature of your spine changes during pregnancy and you are much more likely to strain the muscles of your back and create a serious injury.

So what is heavy lifting? That's anything over 15 to 20 pounds. If you need to lift items at work that weigh less than this, wear a maternity belt and stop lifting altogether if you experience back pain.

Astute readers may notice the 15 to 20 pound limit above and wonder about lifting a toddler that weighs that much—after all, if this is your second pregnancy, odds are you are also lugging around a toddler who tips the scales at more than 20 pounds. Is this safe? The answer: the same advice goes for lifting a toddler as for work-related lifting: avoid it if you can, wear a maternity belt if you can't and stop if you experience pain.

If you have a high-risk pregnancy, consult with your OB first regarding any lifting.

Q. My job requires quite a bit of walking. What are my restrictions?

None.

Walking during pregnancy is not only okay, but it is good for you! Again, consult with your doctor first, but if you are a low-risk pregnancy, it is fine for you to walk during work all the way up until the time you deliver.

Q. My job is very stressful. Do I need to quit?

Probably not.

It takes extreme amounts of stress to affect your pregnancy. By extreme, we mean divorce, death of a family member, loss of income or loss of home by fire. The day-to-day stresses of a job or home life that most of us experience is not enough to worry about.

However, we all process stressful situations differently and there is a growing body of evidence that women under stressful situations (at work or at home) are at risk for preterm birth and low-birth weight babies. So if you have a highly stressful job, it's worth discussing it with your practitioner. You two can come up with a plan to help decrease your stress.

5 Ways to Help Decrease Stress During Pregnancy

◆ Exercise.
◆ Get regular massages (your partner should be a pro by now).
◆ Consider acupuncture.
◆ Get enough sleep.
◆ Have a good support system around you . . . family, friends, neighbors, health care providers, pregnancy and new mommy groups.

Q. I work as a pilot/flight attendant. How long can I continue to work?

Most airlines restrict pregnant workers from flying after 20 weeks.

Some commercial airlines even restrict pilots from flying once pregnancy is diagnosed, even though there is no increased risk of miscarriage or pregnancy complications.

Q. When should I spill the beans to my employer?

To answer this question, we asked Matt Thompson, CEO of Medical Management Solutions, and a guru on employee rights. He offered these suggestions to make your pregnancy life at work at bit smoother:

1. *Give your employer a head's up.* Tell your employer about a pregnancy at the same time you announce it to friends and family.

YOUR RIGHTS REGARDING WORK DURING PREGNANCY

Here's a look at the law and pregnancy when it comes to work. This may become an issue if you end up on bed rest or cannot perform certain functions at work due to your pregnancy. Find out what your state laws are, as well as your individual company's disability policy. Here are the basics: *(US Dept of Labor)*

◆ You should be able to continue performing your job if you are able to.

◆ If you are unable to perform your job due to pregnancy, your employer must treat you like any other partially-disabled employee.

◆ If a partially-disabled employee is able to take leave with or without pay, that is the same option you have.

◆ If you have to discontinue work for a period of time due to a pregnancy-related issue and you recover, you should be able to return to work.

◆ There should be no predetermined length of maternity leave that requires you to stay out of work for that period of time.

◆ Employers must hold your job open during your maternity leave for the same period of time as employees out on sick or disability leave.

◆ The Family and Medical Leave Act entitles you to a maximum of 12 weeks off for certain medical or family reasons within a 12 month period. It only guarantees *unpaid* leave. If you have a difficult pregnancy (for example, bed rest), that time can be counted towards the 12 weeks. To qualify for this legal benefit, you must have worked at the employment site for at least 12 months for 1250 hours, and there must be at least 50 employees of the company within 75 miles.

For more information, go to the web sites of the U.S. Equal Employment Opportunity Commission (eeoc.gov/types/pregnancy.html) or the U.S. Department of Labor (dol.gov/esa/whd/fmla).

lifestyles

2. **Be honest.** Most employers understand that there may be times in which it is difficult for you to work. They will appreciate it if you communicate openly.

3. **Offer solutions.** If you are not able to work on a day, make suggestions for ways in which you can complete your work. Employers prefer to hear solutions to issues rather than problems.

4. **Find out about FMLA.** Not all employees are eligible for Family Medical Leave Act (FMLA—see box above for details); however, most companies are willing to allow for some time off for childbirth and recovery.

5. **Stay in touch during maternity leave.** Communicate to your employer during your time off. It's especially important if an issue arises requiring more time off than you planned.

6. **Make a financial plan.** If you qualify for FMLA, you are eligible for 12 weeks of time off, but it does not guarantee that the time off will be paid. In fact, most employers will allow you to take as much accumulated vacation or sick time as needed, but the remaining time will be unpaid.

7. **Inquire about short-term disability.** Check with your employer to see if you have a Short Term Disability Plan. Most of these plans will enable you to receive a portion of regular pay during your time off. This is a good way to supplement your finances until you return to work. Note: the paperwork required for a claim is extensive. Get going on this paperwork early in your pregnancy.

8. **Give your practitioner a head's up.** Usually, you need your practitioner to complete a portion of disability paperwork. Give him or her ample time to complete it.

9. **Be kind about quitting.** Many women decide not to return to work after the birth of a child. If you decide that you are not going to return to work, the more notice that you can give to your employer, the easier it will be to find a replacement.

Bottom Line

The birth of a child is a special moment, and most employers will share in this joy with you. However, your employer needs to do some planning in order to make it work. Communicate honestly throughout your pregnancy and maternity leave.

We've covered work and play, now let's move on to your maintenance. You know, we're talking about what you do every morning before you face the world. Are all these activities safe while you're with child? You're about to find out....

SPA TREATMENT
Chapter 9

"Maintenance is what you have to do just so you can walk out the door knowing that if you go to the market and bump into a guy who once rejected you, you won't have to hide behind a stack of canned food."
—Nora Ephron

You are beautiful, and we hope your partner tells you that every day–because it's true. But we know you won't look at your pregnant body and always feel that way. As fellow women, we know you may be tempted to try some "spa treatments" to feel better about looking in the mirror and watching that waistline disappear (as well as your chin). Admit it, your body deserves to be pampered right now!

A nice massage may be just the cure for those aches and pains, or you may want to treat yourself to a pedicure (since you can't see, much less reach your toenails towards the end of your pregnancy).

This chapter will walk you through a variety of special treatments and daily care products that you may be tempted to try. We'll discuss whether they are safe, not safe or questionable, based on the latest research.

We'll cover these topics head to toe, and point out safety concerns (if any) during certain stages of pregnancy. Check out the handy table at the end of the chapter for a recap of the thumbs up or down for each treatment.

Hair

Q. Can I color my hair while I am pregnant?

Short answer: Highlights are fine in all

trimesters. After the first trimester, hair dying is ok.

Long answer: you can highlight your hair at any point during your pregnancy because the chemicals don't touch the scalp. However, hair dye (that is, applying color to the roots of your hair) is more controversial. That's because product placed directly on the scalp has the potential to get absorbed into your body (and thus, into your baby's body through the placenta).

Of course, there are no credible scientific studies that show hair dye is harmful to babies. That's because researchers can't find 100 pregnant woman to volunteer to see if this (or any) chemical causes birth defects . . . as you might guess.

Since there is lots of blood flowing to the scalp (just think about how much it bleeds when cut!), doctors are concerned the chemicals in hair dye (ammonia, peroxide) may be absorbed through the scalp. So it's probably safest to wait until after the first trimester to dye your hair. We know this may be hard medicine to swallow because many of us are having children in our 30's and 40's and gray hair is no stranger to our heads.

Our advice: if you must dye those roots in the first trimester, use a vegetable-based dye that doesn't contain ammonia or peroxides. You can also use a Henna product, since it is completely plant based. Better yet, wait to dye your hair until after the 14th week (the end of the first trimester).

Q. Can I get a perm, relaxer, or Brazilian Blowout?

Nope, save your money for now.

Most of these hair products are applied directly to the scalp, which raises the same red flags discussed above—absorbed through the scalp, these chemicals can get into your bloodstream, the placenta, and your developing fetus. If these procedures are an absolute must for you, try to wait until after the first trimester.

From a practical standpoint, many expecting moms report a less than satisfactory result from these treatments. Why? Your hair, just like your skin, is a different animal during pregnancy. Don't expect the same results you got pre-pregnancy.

Helpful Hint
Here's one more reason to avoid hair chemicals in the first trimester: they stink! Many expecting moms are sensitive to odors (and get queasy) in the first trimester. Have a trash can nearby if you are that determined to sit in your hair stylist's chair for a couple of hours.

Reality Check
A lot of new moms wake up to find "I have hair where?!" Increased hair growth on the head is a welcome side effect of pregnancy for most moms. However, many new moms also find hair growing in other not-so-welcome areas, such as the face, around the nipples, lower belly, and the ever-expanding bikini area.

Q. What's the safest way to get rid of unwanted hair while I'm pregnant?

Shaving.

Yes, we know that trying to reach your legs may be difficult, but it is the safest strategy that won't bother your skin or potentially affect your baby. This may sound like a no-brainer here, but we recommend that you sit down while shaving your legs during pregnancy. Standing like a flamingo with a new center of gravity, on a wet tile floor is not an acrobatic feat you should attempt.

Feedback from the Real World

Many spas now cater to pregnant women—from pregnancy massages to pedicures. Ask your local spa if they have a special menu for moms-to-be.

Q. Can I use wax to remove unwanted hair?

Yes . . . but your skin will be much more sensitive during pregnancy, making waxing more painful than usual.

Q. Can I use hair removal or bleaching creams?

No.

We don't recommend using these products because they can be absorbed through your skin and into your body. Again, we don't have solid research to prove that these products are harmful to the baby, but the theoretical risk is there.

Q. Can I do laser hair removal while I'm pregnant?

No. Laser hair removal is not recommended during any trimester.

Pregnant skin is much more sensitive and responds differently than non-pregnant skin. Laser hair removal is not only extremely painful, but it can cause pigmentation changes (dark spots called **HYPERPIGMENTATION** or light spots called **HYPOPIGMENTATION**) on the skin where the hair is removed.

Our advice: Wait until after pregnancy to start or continue laser hair removal.

Q. What about electrolysis?

No. It's not recommended during pregnancy.

There are two types of electrolysis: galvanic and thermolysis.

◆ Galvanic electrolysis uses an electrical current passed down a needle to the unwanted hair follicle. The current sets off a chemical reaction to destroy it. Because your unborn baby is surrounded by amniotic fluid that can potentially conduct electrical current, having a procedure done with galvanic current is a bad idea.

◆ Thermolysis electrolysis uses an alternating current that produces heat to cauterize an unwanted hair follicle. We don't recommend this method either because a) there isn't enough safety info on this procedure and b) it may leave a dark discoloration on your sensitive pregnant skin, just like laser hair removal. Bottom line: we think it's better to be temporarily hairy than permanently blotchy!

SPA

? ?

Q. Can I dye my eyebrows or eyelashes?

Yes, after the first trimester.

Only a small amount of dye is placed over a small segment of skin for a very short amount of time. So, it's fairly safe to do.

Teeth

Q. Is it okay to get my teeth whitened?

No.

There's no proof that these products are safe during pregnancy. The American Academy of Cosmetic Dentistry currently recommends waiting to whiten your teeth until you're done with pregnancy and lactation.

Elevated hormone levels during pregnancy increase tooth sensitivity and can cause gum swelling. The bleach in teeth whiteners can aggravate this condition.

Face

Q. Can I get a facial?

Yes. But tell your technician that you are pregnant. Your skin may be more sensitive now and may react differently to previously used products. All new products should be tested on a small area of skin (such as behind the ear) prior to use. Absolutely avoid products containing:

◆ Retinol or Retin A.
◆ Accutane.
◆ Large amounts of salicylic acid.

Retinol/Retin A contains a large amount of Vitamin A. Research shows that more than 10,000 IU per day of Vitamin A can cause birth defects. And we just don't know how much of these products gets absorbed through the skin. Small amounts of substances containing retinol are theoretically safe, but most OBs agree that it is best to steer clear of these products during pregnancy.

Salicylic acid is a potential problem because it is related to aspirin. Aspirin should not be routinely used during pregnancy. In LARGE doses, it can cause early miscarriage, problems with the placenta, and heart problems for the baby.

That said, don't panic if your practitioner prescribes low dose baby aspirin for a specific medical reason. Doctors usually discontinue aspirin therapy at 28 weeks of pregnancy to avoid problems with your baby's heart. Ask your doctor if you have any concerns.

We'll talk about using small amounts of products containing salicylic acid in the section on acne later in this chapter.

Q. Can I have extractions or chemical peels done with my facial?

Yes, with a few exceptions.

Your pregnancy skin may revolt if you have an extraction-happy technician. Heavy-duty pore extractions can traumatize your sensitive skin. Just ask your aesthetician to be kind to you.

Superficial peels that use glycolic acid, TCA or lactic acid are fine during pregnancy. Test out a small area first before trying it out on your entire face. However, you should steer clear of *salicylic acid* peels for the reasons discussed above.

Q. I've got acne. Help!

Yep.

We know, we know, you thought you were done with acne years ago. Instead of that healthy pregnancy glow you hear about, you've got zits.

You can treat the affected areas with products containing salicylic acid, benzoyl peroxide and finacea. They are all safe to use in SMALL amounts. However, slathering them on can potentially lead to absorption into your bloodstream. So limit your application to small areas.

As discussed previously, you need to avoid products that contain large amounts of salicylic acid because they can cause complications for you and your baby. But, it's okay to use these products sparingly when you are spot treating a zit or two.

Q. Is it safe to use Proactiv?

Yes.

If you believe Katy Perry and Justin Bieber, this product is the miracle answer to your acne woes. The main ingredient in Proactiv is benzoyl peroxide. Because there have never been any reports of birth defects with benzoyl peroxide use, Proactiv is safe to use during your entire pregnancy.

However, if you have never used it before, now may not be the time to make your maiden voyage. Because of that darn sensitive skin you've got right now, Proactiv might irritate it.

Q. Are prescription antibiotics safe to use for my acne?

It depends on the medication.

We'll give you the full run down on medications in at Expecting411. com/extra. But in general, clindamycin taken by mouth or applied to the skin is okay to use. Erythromycin-based creams and gels are also safe.

However, tetracycline, doxycycline, and minocycline are off limits, because they can adversely affect your unborn baby's teeth. Because these antibiotics interfere with calcification, exposed fetuses can end up with discolored teeth, cavities, and poor enamel development.

Q. Okay, nothing is working and I still have acne. HELP!

You can try using a steroid cream.

Steroid creams are safe to use while you're pregnant, and they might help reduce the redness and irritation surrounding a resilient pimple. You can try over the counter 1% hydrocortisone cream. Or your doctor can prescribe a slightly higher strength cream.

? ?

SPA

Q. Can I still use my anti-wrinkle cream?

Look at the ingredients and then make the call.

Most anti-wrinkle creams contain Vitamin A, or one of its derivatives like retinol. Since these are off limits during pregnancy, so are most anti-wrinkle creams.

Q. Can I do BOTOX?

Skip it during pregnancy and wait until you are done breastfeeding.

First, let's talk about what BOTOX actually is. The key ingredient of BOTOX is a protein product (botulinum toxin type A) from the bacteria, Clostridium botulinum. The toxin blocks nerve signals in tense facial muscles responsible for those unwanted wrinkles. Injecting the toxin into the muscle makes those little wrinkles relax for about four months (until you have to do it again). *(Botoxcosmetics.com)*

That's the positive about BOTOX. The negative: Clostridium botulinum is also the same player that causes botulism (horrible food poisoning). We know we are starting to sound like a broken record, but there just aren't studies on this stuff and pregnant women.

What we do know is based on animal research, however, and it's not pretty. There is a risk of low-birth weight, delayed bone development, other malformations, and miscarriage. *(Basow DS.)* So we can't recommend using BOTOX during pregnancy for cosmetic reasons.

There are a few cases of pregnant women exposed to botulinum toxin with no ill effects to their fetuses. So if you happened to get BOTOX before you realized you were pregnant, just relax (and you can since that little worry line between your eyes is banished for a few months), and put your next appointment on hold.

You'll need to wait until you are done breastfeeding to resume your BOTOX sessions. With any BOTOX treatment, a tiny amount of botulinum toxin passes through the bloodstream, which can potentially enter breastmilk. For this reason, it's wise to avoid it while breastfeeding.

After saying all this, there are some women who need BOTOX injections for medical reasons. For example, if BOTOX is the one thing that helps you with debilitating migraine headaches, the benefit may outweigh the potential risk. Just have the doctor administering the BOTOX discuss it with your practitioner first.

Q. Can I use facial fillers?

Nope.

Restalyne and other facial fillers have warning labels advising against use by pregnant and nursing women. No studies. No green light.

Body & Skin

Q. Is it safe to get a massage? I could really use one right now!

Yes.

SPA

A massage is a welcome and often needed treat during pregnancy. It is important, however, to have a few ground rules:

Select a massage therapist who is comfortable with and has experience in prenatal massage. After about 18-20 weeks, pregnant women should not be flat on their backs for prolonged periods of time (the weight of the uterus can compress the blood vessels in the body) preventing adequate blood flow to both mom and baby.

Most therapists have either table cut-outs to allow room for a pregnant belly or know how to position a woman on her side with pillows. Also, it is very important to stay hydrated when at the spa or even if just getting an hour massage at home.

Absolute no-no's during a massage:

- ◆ NO warming or electric blankets.
- ◆ NO massage of the inner or outer ankle bones or the webbing between the thumb and index finger as these are acupuncture points that might lead to stimulation of the uterine muscle.
- ◆ NO essential oils (cedar wood, chamomile, eucalyptus, juniper, rosemary, frankincense). These oils may have the potential to cause bleeding.

Q. Is it safe to have acupuncture done?

Yes. Just be sure you use an acupuncturist who is comfortable treating pregnant gals.

Your acupuncturist needs to avoid areas that might trigger uterine contractions. Those are the inner or outer ankle bones or the webbing between the thumb and index finger.

I recommend acupuncture to many of my patients who suffer from chronic headaches, low back pain, and discomfort in their pelvic bones. And anecdotally, some have found great relief.

Helpful Hint

Acupuncture may be useful to help turn breech babies into the normal "head-down" position needed for a vaginal delivery.

Q. Can I have a mud bath, seaweed wrap, or paraffin treatment?

No.

As tempting as mud baths, seaweed wraps, paraffin treatments and hot baths sound, they should ALL be avoided during pregnancy as they can

DR H'S TRUE STORY: THE PREGNANT NOSE

Some of the wonderful fragrances a therapist uses may not smell so wonderful to your pregnant nose in the first trimester. I still can't bring myself to smell lavender, a fragrance used by many massage therapists and one that threw me for a loop during my first pregnancy.

significantly raise core body temperature. See our FYI on this below.

FYI: Keeping your cool. When a pregnant woman's core body temperature rises over 101-102° F, there are health risks to both mother and baby. Moms have an increased risk of dehydration and fainting. Fetuses are also vulnerable, mostly in the first trimester. Overheating can lead to malformation of the spine and skull (**NEURAL TUBE DEFECTS**) in the first six weeks of pregnancy. There's also a greater risk of miscarriage in the first trimester.

Q. Can I take a bubble bath?

Yes, with a few caveats.

If you are going to treat yourself to a warm bath, make sure the water temperature is under 100° F to avoid potentially overheating yourself and your baby (see discussion above).

And bubble bath solutions often irritate the vagina and vulva (your outer genitalia). Many women have learned this lesson in their own childhood. Although it looks like fun to immerse yourself in bubbles, it's not fun later when you have an itchy vagina.

Our advice: take a warm bath with candles, dial up a little Michael Bublé on the stereo, and skip the bubbles.

Q. Can I sit in a hot tub or sauna?

No.

These violate the overheating rule. But if you can control the temperature of the hot tub and keep it under 100° F, go for it.

Q. Can I spend time outside in the sun?

Yes.

While it is important to avoid direct sunlight on your face, this shouldn't prevent you, however, from enjoying a day at the beach. Being pregnant is about being smart, not crazy. Just use good judgment. Wear sunblock, and a hat or visor to protect your face.

Reality Check

Keep your face out of direct sunlight during pregnancy. It helps prevent **MELASMA**, a pregnancy related discoloration of the face. (More on this in Chapter, 4, Is This Normal?) However, be sure to get your Vitamin D from food sources or multivitamins, since you won't be absorbing it through your skin.

Old Wives Tale

Sunscreen is dangerous, especially for pregnant women. *The truth: this is more of an urban legend than an actual health concern.*

Here's what the science says: oxybenzone and avobenzone are found in most sunscreens and are absorbed into the bloodstream. And from pregnant animal studies, we know oxybenzone isn't terribly toxic. *(Hayden CGJ)* Environmental health groups claim it causes low birth weight. However, there are not enough high quality research studies to date to confirm this. As a result, ACOG says sunblock is safe to use during pregnancy—and you should use it.

If that isn't enough to ease your fears, you do have an alternative. Use a sunscreen containing zinc oxide instead. Or, just wear a coverup!

Q. Can I use any tanning alternatives, like spray on tans or tanning beds?

Yes to the sprays and creams. No to the tanning bed.

Spray-on tans use a sugar-based product called DHA (dihydroxyacetone). It acts by temporarily staining the surface of your skin (and any clothing you wear afterwards). This is safe.

Self-tanners are also safe to use. Just do a patch test first on your inner thigh or wrist since your pregnancy skin may react differently than your expectations.

We don't recommend tanning beds—whether you are pregnant or not. During pregnancy it's a particularly bad idea because, like the sun, UV rays can cause skin discoloration (**MELASMA/CHOLASMA**; more in Chapter 4, Is This Normal?).

Even if you aren't pregnant, tanning beds are still a bad idea, as recent studies have linked their use to skin cancer. *(El Ghissani)*

Factoid: Melanoma is the most aggressive form of skin cancer. It's also one of the few cancers that can spread across the placenta to an unborn baby.

Q. Is there anything I can use to prevent stretch marks?

No, because you can't select your own mom.

The likelihood of getting stretch marks is based on whether or not your mom did. (If you have never seen your own mother's belly to find out what you are in for, there's a decent chance it's because she has them and she hasn't met Dr. 90210 yet.)

Here's the skinny on stretch marks. During pregnancy or whenever someone loses or gains weight quickly, the skin stretches and can disrupt one of the layers of skin called the dermis. In pregnancy, stretch marks may appear over the lower part of your belly, your breasts, and inner thighs.

There is really only one thing you can do to reduce your chances of stretch marks: watch your diet. There are many reasons to eat healthfully during pregnancy, and this is one of them. If you don't gain weight rapidly, you may be able to fool Mother Nature's destiny for you. We make no guarantees, mind you, but it doesn't hurt to try.

You may hear that creams and oils prevent stretch marks. They definitely keep the skin moist, which may prevent *some* stretch marks. And asking your spouse do a nightly massage to apply them certainly has its benefit. But there are no guarantees here either!

Q. Can I get a tattoo while I'm pregnant?

No. It's not recommended due to both health and cosmetic reasons.

First of all, remember that your pregnant skin is more sensitive. So, getting a tattoo may be much more painful. There are also cases of people contracting Hepatitis B, Hepatitis C, and HIV from tattoo parlors that don't take sterile precautions. Those aren't diseases you want during pregnancy (or ever!).

Also, you may not be pleased with the results. Most women gain at least 25 pounds during pregnancy and certain areas of your body will change dramatically (particularly your belly, breasts, and buttocks). Your cute butterfly ink may end up looking like an eggplant after it has been stretched out.

Bottom line: It's not worth taking the health risk for you and your unborn baby. And who wants an eggplant on her butt?

Q. What about permanent makeup. Is that okay?

No.

Although it would be amazing to wake-up from just a few hours of sleep looking like a million bucks with eyeliner and pink lips, there isn't enough data to indicate whether permanent make-up is safe. Therefore, just like most of the other things in this chapter, if there isn't any data on safety, we have to recommend waiting until pregnancy and breastfeeding are over.

Q. Can I have a body piercing done while I am pregnant?

No.

Body piercing is not recommended for women who are trying to conceive or are already pregnant. Again, the skin is more sensitive, so this equals more pain. Second, as the skin stretches with the pregnancy, incomplete healing can occur leading to larger holes, infection and scarring. Last, and probably most importantly, although most places are clean and use sterilized equipment, there is always a risk of localized skin infection, as well as more serious infections such as Hepatitis B, Hepatitis C, and HIV.

Q. What about the piercings that I had prior to getting pregnant? Do I need to take any special precautions?

Short answer: yes.

If you have a piercing in your nipple, navel, or genitals, the smartest thing to do is to remove the jewelry. Why? It can catch on clothing more

---

DR H'S OPINION
BIKINI LINE TATTOOS

A popular place to put tattoos is below the belt/above the bikini line (like L.A. Ink's Kate Von D). However, this makes doing a C-section (if one is needed) a real cosmetic challenge for your doc. I remember a case where a patient of mine had a huge sunflower right in the spot where the incision for her C-section had to be made. It took a really long time to put that incision back together as I painstakingly matched up each petal and leaf on the top to it's counterpart on the bottom!

We realize you are probably not thinking of the potential of having a C-section (much less being pregnant) when you got that tattoo there. However, having a misshapen tattoo may be one of the many sacrifices you make as a parent.

often as pregnancy advances and leave you at risk of injury. Replace any jewelry with either a flexible bar made of Teflon or a flexible "space holder" made of PTFE (polytetrafluoroethylene).

For specific piercings, here are our suggestions:

◆ **Nipple Piercings.** As you might expect, there is a risk of getting a breast infection (**MASTITIS**) if you've got a pierced nipple. The good news is that most women with piercings can breastfeed. Obviously, you'll need to remove any jewelry before you nurse. Jewelry can potentially injure the baby's mouth or worse, create a choking hazard, should it become dislodged!

◆ **Navel Piercings.** As your inny becomes an outy, your piercing may get uncomfortable and it will certainly look and fit differently. Although it's not absolutely necessary, you may want to remove it for a few reasons. As we've already mentioned, it may catch and pull more on clothing. Also, as your skin stretches (I know, this is a scary thought), it may pull your piercing so that the hole stretches and enlarges. If you need a C-section, the piercing definitely has to be removed. No, not because your incision is up by your navel. The reason: an electrocautery device is used to clot off blood vessels during surgery. Any metal in its vicinity can redirect the electrical current and burn the skin. (That's probably more than you wanted to know.)

◆ **Genital Piercings.** Yes, the **CLITORAL HOOD** (see graphic in Chapter 4) is a new popular place to pierce. If you've got one of these, you should remove the jewelry once your pregnancy test comes back positive. This shouldn't be a newsflash, but you have many pelvic exams and pelvic ultrasounds in your future. Besides potential discomfort for you, the jewelry (or even a space filler) may get in the way. Your entire genital area (**VULVA**) will also get swollen as your pregnancy progresses. And some women are unlucky enough to get varicose veins in their genital area during pregnancy. Having clitoral jewelry through this experience is extremely painful and that's why it's a bad idea. But if you choose to keep it around through your pregnancy, it definitely needs to go before you go into labor.

FYI: While tongue piercings do not interfere with your growing body parts, they are potentially a problem if you needed to have a surgical procedure (electrocautery) to clot off blood vessels during surgery. Hence you may need to remove any tongue piercing during labor and delivery.

Nails

Q. Can I have a manicure or a pedicure?

Yes, just take a few precautions.

During your pregnancy, you'll notice that your hair and nails grow at a freakishly fast rate. That's normal, as you are in metabolic overdrive. And you may want to treat yourself to a manicure or pedicure. Go ahead, you deserve it. Tell your spouse or partner we said so.

Here are a few helpful tips to do it safely:

◆ **Make sure the room is well-ventilated.** Other customers who are getting services done like silk wraps or china fills can create pretty strong fumes that you shouldn't be inhaling.

◆ *Go to a licensed salon.* While having a current license from a state health department doesn't guarantee a risk-free experience, it helps.

◆ *Use sterile instruments.* Look for a clean salon that uses sterilized instruments . . . or better yet, bring your own. Dirty instruments or wash basins can put you at risk for dangerous (even life-threatening) infections. Infections in the nail beds can be more difficult to fight off during pregnancy—especially in women with chronic medical conditions, like diabetes.

◆ *If you've got open cuts or wounds, skip it.* Again, don't put yourself at risk for an infection.

◆ *Don't shave your legs the day before.* That is, if you can reach them. Shaving may cause microscopic cuts in your skin that can leave you at risk for infection.

◆ *Consider using phthalate-free nail polish.* As with just about every other environmental health concern, we don't really know if phthalates (a chemical plasticizer that makes nail polish flexible) can affect your unborn baby. But our mantra is, if there is an easy, inexpensive alternative to limit environmental exposures—why not use it? That's the situation here. If you are concerned about phthalates, choose a P-free alternative, like Loreal Jet Set enamel or Urban Decay.

Reality Check: Fungus among us

Do you have toenail fungus? Nails infected with this fungus turn white or yellow, and appear thick and hard, with white debris. Whether you are pregnant or not, it can be a real challenge to treat. But during pregnancy, many of the medications docs typically use are off limits due to potential side effects. So, your only treatment option for now (and through breastfeeding) is to use a topical prescription lotion called terbinafine (Lamisil). Alternatively, you can just wait until pregnancy and breastfeeding are over with to treat your toenails. Trust us, the fungus will still be there waiting for you. And so will your dermatologist, who can then treat it with an oral medication.

Q. Can I have acrylic nails applied?

Yes.

The nails themselves are okay. It's the really intense fumes that can be problematic. Get your nails done in a well-ventilated area.

Other Assorted Body Parts

Q. Can I douche?

No.

Douche is French, meaning "to wash" or "to soak." Women take a mixture of fluids—usually water with vinegar, baking soda, or iodine—and squirt it up their vagina with a spray bottle or tube.

It's no longer trendy for women to douche after having sex or having their periods to "clean" themselves, but some women still do it.

OB-GYN's do not recommend douching for most women. Douching can alter the normal balance of good germs that live in your vagina—which then lead to various vaginal infections.

Douching can also potentially cause pelvic infections by pushing bacteria from the vagina through the cervix and into the uterus and fallopian tubes. Contrary to what other pregnancy books may say, douching won't cause a fatal air bubble to enter your bloodstream and kill you. However, because of infection risk, douching is just a bad idea—pregnant or not.

Q. Can I have a colonic?

No. A better question is, do you really want one?

Colonic irrigation or colon hydrotherapy is an alternative medicine practice that involves flushing the colon with warm water. The colonic supposedly removes a buildup of waste, which supporters of the practice believe is harmful for digestive and general health.

A colon hydrotherapist inserts a sterile, single use speculum (attached to tubing) into the patient's anus. The colon is gently flushed repeatedly with warmed water, which loosens feces stuck in the colon and filters it out through a tube. This practice, when done occasionally, is supposedly not harmful to healthy people.

In pregnant women, there are a few reasons to avoid this practice. First of all, it's really uncomfortable . . . even if you don't have hemorrhoids the size of Texas, which most of us do at some point. Second, the elevated progesterone levels during pregnancy slow down the entire intestinal tract (leading to all the fun GI symptoms of pregnancy, like nausea, vomiting, heartburn, excessive belching, gas and constipation). This means, doing a colonic probably won't solve your preggo-related gas. And your body and your colon may respond differently to this procedure while you're pregnant.

Finally, there have been complications during these procedures leading to excessive bleeding, infection, and surgery. Bottom line: avoid colonics during pregnancy.

Q. After delivery, is vaginal rejuvenation something I might need?

Short answer: it depends on what kind of delivery you had, what size baby you had, and if you plan on having any more children.

For the long answer, check out Chapter 14, Postpartum and Beyond.

Here's a recap of this chapter:

Is it safe for	Pregnancy?	Breastfeeding?
Hair		
Highlights	Yes, all trimesters	Yes
Dying	Yes, 2nd and 3rd trimester	Yes
Perms	No	Yes
Relaxers	No	Yes
Laser hair removal	No	Yes
Waxing	Yes, but painful	Yes

SPA

???

Is it safe for	Pregnancy?	Breastfeeding?
Hair removal cream	No	Yes
Electrolysis	No	Yes
Brow/eyelid dye	Yes, 2nd and 3rd trimester	Yes

Teeth

Whitening	No	No

Face

Facial	Yes* *but no Retinol or Accutane*	Yes
Proactiv	Yes	Yes
Anti-wrinkle cream	Mostly no, check ingredients	No
BOTOX	No	No
Facial fillers	No	No

Body

Massage	Yes	Yes
Acupuncture	Yes	Yes
Mudbath	No	Yes
Seaweed	No	Yes
Paraffin treatment	No	Yes
Bubble bath	Yes, *but skip the bubbles/stay under 100° F*	Yes
Hot tub	No	Yes
Sauna	No	Yes
Sun exposure	Yes, *but avoid direct sun on face*	Yes
Sunblock	Yes	Yes
Sunless tanners	Yes	Yes
Tanning beds	No	Yes
Tattoos	No new ones	No
Permanent makeup	No	No
Body piercings	No new ones	Yes, *but not on nipples*

Nails

Manicure/pedicure	Yes	Yes
Acrylic nails	Yes	Yes

Other

Douching	No	Yes, if you must
Colonics	No	Yes, if you must

Next up, getting ready for baby—what do you need to do as a parent-to-be to prepare for your new arrival?

242   EXPECTING 411   ???

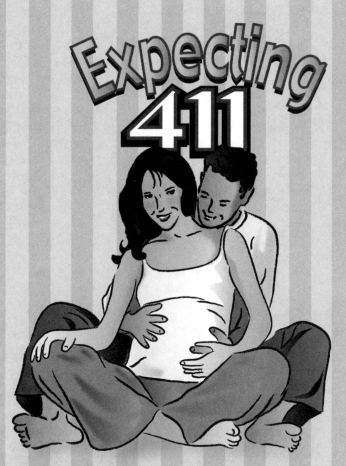

section three

*Getting ready
for the big event*

PARENTHOOD PREP

Chapter 10

*"Diaper backward spells repaid.
Think about it."*
—Marshall McLuhan

WHAT'S IN THIS CHAPTER

- ◆ **CORD BLOOD BANKING**
- ◆ **CIRCUMCISION**
- ◆ **EXPANDED NEWBORN SCREENING**
- ◆ **PICKING A PEDIATRICIAN**
- ◆ **CHILDCARE OPTIONS**
- ◆ **BREASTFEEDING & FORMULA**
- ◆ **VACCINES 411**

As your pregnancy days near an end, it's time to start thinking about your baby's life outside the womb. Pregnancy is really just the beginning of the enormous number of responsibilities and decisions you have as a parent.

Many pregnant women focus all of their energy on labor and delivery. Here's a little secret: it's just one day (albeit a very long and important day). No matter how much time you spend thinking about it, you cannot control what will occur that day. Just know that it will happen, and then it will be over.

Instead of ruminating about something you can't do anything about (while you are up at all hours of the night trying to get comfortable), you might as well make good use of your time. Start thinking about what you will do with your baby after he arrives because that encompasses Day 1 until eternity.

This chapter covers topics you are certain to have questions about like cord blood banking, circumcision, newborn screening, picking a pediatrician (baby doctor), maternity and paternity leave, childcare, breast milk and formula, vaccines, and basic stuff you've got to have in the house with a newborn. We have lots of ground to cover, so let's go!

 Partner Tip
It's okay to admit that you are scared to death of becoming a parent. So is your partner.

Helpful Hint

The topics discussed in this chapter often overlap with our other book, *Baby 411* (see the back of this book for details). Since a detailed discussion of these topics is beyond the scope of this book, you can often find a more expanded discussion in *Baby 411*.

We aren't saying this just to promote sales of that book (okay, truth be told, we'd love for you to buy all our books and recommend them to your friends)! Our point is there is only so much room here—and it makes more sense to talk in-depth about topics like infant formula in a book dedicated to infants!

Cord blood banking

Q. What is cord blood banking?

This is the saving and storing of the blood from your baby's umbilical cord.

Why is this cool? Well, that blood is loaded with the "seeds" (hematopoietic stem cells) that later grow into white and red blood cells. These very special cells are also found in the bone marrow of all humans.

As a result, umbilical cord blood can be used like a bone marrow transplant. These cells are currently used to treat some genetic and blood disorders and certain types of cancer. One of the advantages of using a cord blood transplant as opposed to getting a bone marrow transplant is that you don't need a perfect genetic match to use it and there may be less transplant rejection.

Q. Does cord blood contain "embryonic stem cells"?

No.

The stem cells in cord blood come from your baby's blood after he is born, not from an embryo. So there is no moral controversy involved!

The only similarity is that "stem cells" from anywhere (embryo, cord blood, bone marrow) are special—they can develop into white and red blood cells and other specialized types of cells.

Q. What can they be used for?

Cord blood transplant is now standard therapy for over 20 diseases—see Expecting411.com/extra for a list. And there are many more diseases where cord blood transplant is in the research or experimental trial phase.

Important point: your baby may not be able to use his own stem cells for certain diseases. For example, if your baby ends up having leukemia, his frozen stem cells cannot be used to treat it. Those stem cells may already have pre-cancerous changes in them.

But your healthy baby's stem cells could be used for another family member (sibling, parent, etc) who has a disease treatable with cord blood.

Q. I've heard you can store a piece of the umbilical cord, too. Is there additional value in doing that?

Maybe. The cord tissue is not used routinely to treat any disease—yet.

PARENTHOOD

The advantage of umbilical cord tissue over the blood itself is that the tissue contains *mesenchymal stem cells*. What's that, you say? These cells can be used for "tissue engineering"—converting them into bone cells, fat cells, or even cells that work in the pancreas, for instance. It's possible someday they could be used to treat multiple sclerosis or stroke victims.

Q. Wow, this sounds amazing. Does everyone bank their baby's cord blood? What are the bank options?

There are two options for banking your baby's cord blood: private and public. With a private bank, you pay a company to store your baby's cord blood for future personal use. Public banks are donation programs, where families contribute cord blood for use by the general public.

Does everyone bank their baby's cord blood? No. It is an *option* for all parents, but it is not currently part of routine delivery care.

Obviously, the perfect solution would be a national cord blood bank, where everyone could donate and all Americans could utilize one of these donations.

Unfortunately, a public cord blood donation program is only in an infancy stage as of this writing. There are currently 200 participating hospital programs in the U.S. You can find out if your hospital is one of them by going to the National Marrow Donor website at marrow.org or parentsguidecordblood.org.

If your delivery hospital doesn't participate, Cryobanks International (800-869-8608 or cryo-intl.com) accepts donations anywhere in the continental U.S. and sends them to the national donor bank.

If you want your baby's cord blood to go to the public donor program, you just need to pass some screening questions before the program accepts the donation. You should contact these folks before 34 weeks gestation if you want to donate.

We'll discuss private cord blood banking next.

Insider Secret

If you have twins (or more), you cannot donate to the National Donor Program. Why? With two or more umbilical cords, there is a potential to mix up the blood, making it too risky.

Q. Can I bank my baby's cord blood for our own personal use?

Yes. This is called private cord blood banking.

The current odds that your baby or a family member will actually use the blood varies from one in 400 to one in 200,000. Why is there such a big gap? Well, no one can predict the *future* uses of these stem cells—which could be huge. But if you already have a family member who has a disease known to be treatable with a cord blood transplant, your odds of utilizing it go way up.

Here's a quick way to make this decision. Look at the cord blood usage list at Expecting411.com/extra for ways cord blood stems are already used. Then look at your family medical history. This can help you decide if private banking is worth it.

Q. How much does it cost to privately bank cord blood?

There is an initial enrollment fee ranging from about $1500 to $2000. Then there is a storage fee of $100 to $150 per year. Some banks charge a one-time, lump sum fee to store the cord blood "forever."

If you opt to store umbilical cord tissue as well, expect to pay another $600 up front and twice the annual fee.

How long can cord blood be banked? With current technology, banks can freeze and utilize cord blood for at least 15 years.

Insider Tip

Some companies offer discounts to families serving in the military, repeat customers, and those having twins or who have a first or second-degree relative with an existing disease treatable with cord blood. So do your homework and ask questions.

Q. What happens to cord blood if it isn't saved or banked?

It clots in the umbilical cord and gets sent to the pathology lab with the placenta. Ultimately, it gets disposed of in a biohazard bag.

If you don't authorize it to be publicly or privately banked, the blood is discarded.

Q. If I want to privately bank my baby's cord blood, which company should I choose?

There isn't one company we recommend over all others—we advise you to check out ParentsGuideCordBlood.org. This is an excellent non-profit website with tips and advice on evaluating cord banks. They offer an easy, up-to-date comparison of private cord blood banks that are accredited by the American Association of Blood Banks (AABB.org).

Tip: Make sure the bank you select follows the standards set by the Foundation for the Accreditation of Cellular Therapy (factwebsite.org).

Q. What's the difference between public and private banking?

If you donate cord blood to the public bank, *anyone* who needs it can use it. Every day, 6000 patients worldwide are looking for a match in the national donor registry to treat their leukemia, lymphoma, or other disease with a bone marrow or cord blood transplant.

If you bank your blood privately, *only* your family or loved ones who need it and are an acceptable match can use it.

DR B'S OPINION

"Don't let potentially life-saving cells go to waste. Donate them or bank them privately."

Q. Are there any official recommendations?

The American Academy of Pediatrics (AAP) supports donating umbilical cord blood to the national donor bank.

The American Congress of Obstetricians and Gynecologists (ACOG)

? ?

PARENTHOOD

advises its physicians to provide balanced and accurate information about both public and private cord blood banking. That includes informing parents that the odds of using this blood for a child or family member is quite low (see discussion earlier). They suggest considering private banking of cord blood "when there is a specific diagnosis known to be treatable by...[cord blood transplant]...for an immediate family member." *(AAP, ACOG)*

Q. How is the cord blood collected?

After your baby is born, two clamps are placed on the umbilical cord and then it is cut. Your practitioner then places a needle into the umbilical cord vein (the part of the cord still attached to the placenta—not your baby) and draws blood into a collection bag or syringe. An adequate specimen volume is a minimum of two oz., or even better, about one-half to one cup.

If you are privately banking the cord blood, you will need to call a toll-free number on the side of the box to tell the bank your specimen is ready (your labor and delivery nurse will usually package everything up and remind you to make the call). Then someone will magically appear at your birthing facility to ship the blood to the processing and storage facility.

Q. What if there isn't enough blood in the specimen? That happened to a friend of mine.

It happens. Sometimes in certain conditions (**PLACENTAL ABRUPTION**, for example) the placenta detaches early and very little blood can be collected.

Some private blood banks offer a service called "cell amplification" in hopes of using the reduced specimen volume someday. No one can promise that those cells will be viable should the need ever arise. But the scientific research is encouraging. You'll just have to make your own call on this one.

Bottom Line
Do your homework. It's expensive to privately bank cord blood. You should know your options before investing.

Circumcision

Before we delve into this hot topic, we have a major disclaimer: our goal for this section is to let parents hear both sides of the argument so you can make an informed decision on your own. We are not here to persuade, just to educate patients on the pros and cons of circumcision. What you decide to do with your son's penis is your business.

Q. What is a circumcision anyway?

It's the term used to describe surgical removal of the foreskin of the penis. It became extremely popular in the U.S. in the late 1800's for hygienic reasons, as well as a proposed way to eliminate masturbation. (Ha! That obviously didn't work!).

Although the use of circumcision has declined in recent years, more American boys are circumcised than not. Other countries and cultures have varying viewpoints on circumcision.

Q. When do I need to make this decision?

If you want to make the decision without your child's input, you should make a decision now. Doctors typically perform the procedure before a baby goes home from the hospital, or within the first week or two of life in the doctor's office.

When a circumcision is part of a Jewish religious ceremony, it is done at eight days of life.

Alternatively, you can wait and let your son decide the fate of his penis. However, circumcision for an older child or adult is a much bigger ordeal. And there are some advantages to performing it earlier in life (see info below).

Q. What are the arguments FOR circumcision?

1 **BETTER HYGIENE.** An uncircumcised little boy has a tight, un-retractable foreskin that covers his penis. But as he gets older, the foreskin loosens up and must be pulled back to clean the head of the penis (glans). If not cleaned, the foreskin can get infected and swell (**BALANITIS**). The foreskin can also get stuck in a pulled back position (**PARAPHIMOSIS**)—OUCH! Both conditions are rare, but very painful.

2 **FEWER BLADDER INFECTIONS.** Bladder infections (**URINARY TRACT INFEC-TION-UTI**) in boys are fairly rare. But due to hygiene, uncircumcised boys have a four to eight times greater risk of infection than their circum-cised buddies. (*Shaikh N*)

3 **REDUCED RISK OF HIV.** Uncircumcised men are more likely to get HIV and AIDS. Why? Because the area under the foreskin makes a nice spot for the virus to camp out. In South Africa, circumcised men are 60% less like-ly to be infected with HIV compared to their uncircumcised peers. (*Weiss H*)

4 **LESS RISK OF PENILE CANCER.** Cancer of the penis is rare. A man's life-time risk of getting penile cancer is one in 100,000 (compared to breast cancer affecting one in eight women). But yes, it happens more fre-quently in uncircumcised men.

5 **REDUCTION IN CERVICAL CANCER.** Women involved with uncircumcised "high risk" partners (more than six previous sexual partners) have a five-times greater risk of getting cancer of the cervix compared to women whose sex partners were circumcised. The reason? *Human papillo-mavirus–HPV* (a sexually transmitted virus) loves to live under the foreskin. HPV causes 99% of all cervical cancer. So, your decision to circumcise your son may affect your daughter-in-law's health someday.

Reality Check

Even though the HPV vaccine protects against 70% of HPV-related cervical cancers, the argument for circumcision is rele-vant for the other 30%.

Q. What are the arguments AGAINST circumcision?

1 **LACK OF MEDICAL NECESSITY.** While circumcision lowers the risk of HIV infection in men, and transmission of HPV to female partners, so does abstinence and safe sexual activity (using a condom every time, etc.). So, if we could wave a magic wand and eliminate risky sexual behavior, there would be fewer medical arguments supporting circumcision.

2 **SURGICAL RISKS.** Circumcision, like any other surgical procedure, carries a small chance of bleeding (one in 3000) or infection (one in 1000). It's also possible to need a second procedure later (circumcision revision) if the results are not satisfactory. See our other book *Baby 411* for details on the "Hidden Penis" and penile adhesions. Bottom line: If your son is circumcised, learn how to clean it properly afterwards.

3 **REDUCED SEXUAL PLEASURE.** Does circumcision remove sensitive nerve fibers in the foreskin? Studies report conflicting results. Some studies show a decrease in sexual pleasure; others show no difference. The data is based on men who were circumcised as adults who subjectively rated their sexual pleasure before and after circumcision. *(Collins, Masood, Kim)*

Q. What do medical organizations say about this subject?

Not much.

While OB/GYN's do not take care of male patients, they do have skin in this game (sorry, bad pun). Their female patients' health may be affected by their partners' sexual health.

ACOG and the AAP agree that there is insufficient evidence to support routine newborn circumcision. However, parents should get accurate and impartial information to make an informed decision. And a baby should receive medication to reduce discomfort during the procedure. *(ACOG)*

However, the World Health Organization supports adult circumcision to reduce the risk of HIV in men, based on significant research findings in 2007.

Q. We've decided to have our newborn son circumcised. When is this done?

In most cases, a newborn boy has his circumcision done after he is at least 24 hours old and his pediatrician has examined him. It is performed before the mother and baby are discharged home.

The doctor needs to make sure all the boy parts formed correctly before doing a circumcision. Boys with an abnormally formed penis (**HYPOSPADIAS**) need surgery later on that utilizes the foreskin in the repair, so the circumcision is delayed and performed at that time. A pediatric urologist typically does this surgery.

Babies who are premature or ill may need to delay having a routine circumcision until they are healthy.

Ceremonial/religious circumcisions are done on the eighth day of life, unless there are medical issues.

PARENTHOOD

? ?

Q. Where is it done?

When a physician performs a routine circumcision, it is usually done at the delivery hospital before discharge home. Some physicians will perform them in their offices. For Jewish families, a mohel performs a Brit milah either in the family's home or place of worship.

Beyond the newborn period, it is a day surgery procedure that is done with general anesthesia in an outpatient surgery center.

Q. Who performs the circumcision?

It really depends on where you live and where you deliver. If you are Jewish, you will hire a mohel and you should have that person lined up before delivery. Everyone else has a physician perform the procedure.

But which doctor does it? Truth be told, it doesn't matter what his or her specialty is as long as the doctor is trained to do the procedure. It is usually the OB, pediatrician, or family practitioner you have a relationship with who does it.

If your baby has an anatomic abnormality, then a pediatric urologist performs the circumcision. The urologists don't usually do routine circumcisions, even though that is the specialist who deals with penises the most.

If you want your son to have a circumcision, ask your OB and your baby's doctor who is able and willing to do it.

Q. Does the baby feel any pain?

Anytime the skin is cut, it hurts. That's why almost all doctors use medication that numbs the area and makes your baby comfortable. Every doc has his or her own approach, so feel free to ask about it.

Q. Will my baby be fussy afterwards?

Actually, most babies just want to sleep it off for a few hours. It is their way of responding to stress. When they awaken, they are in a pretty good mood, unless you muck around with the surgical dressing on the penis. Be gentle with that area for a day or so, and your baby should be very comfortable.

Bottom Line
The whole procedure takes only a few minutes. Yes, it hurts—but using pain medication is now the standard of care. Most babies go to sleep for a few hours and wake up happy to see you.

Q. Is circumcision covered by insurance?

If the procedure is done at the hospital before discharge and IF the doctor doing the procedure is a participating provider, then at least a portion of the bill should be covered by insurance.

Because insurance companies have so many restrictions on individual policies, contact your plan to see if it covers a routine circumcision.

Check out our companion book, Baby 411, for details on how to care for a healing circumcision.

Bottom Line

Talk to your doctor. Get educated. But in the end, you have to make the call. Circumcisions are done more for social, cultural, and religious reasons than for medical necessity.

Expanded newborn screening

Once your baby is born, the testing begins. Your state health department requires some blood tests, but others are optional. Here's the scoop.

Q. What is the "newborn screening" test?

In 1961, Dr. Robert Guthrie figured out that he could diagnose a newborn with a genetic metabolic disorder called phenylketonuria (PKU) using a little dried blood on some filter paper.

This was a huge deal because babies with PKU weren't ordinarily diagnosed until at least six months of age . . . after permanent neurological impairment occured.

That one test evolved into an entire panel of tests called "newborn screening", which has come a long way in 50 years. Every state health department in the U.S. now screens for 28 to over 50 disorders with just a few drops of a newborn's blood.

Most tests screen for the inability of the body to break down certain nutrients (called metabolic disorders). Delayed detection can lead to heart enlargement, intellectual disability, and even death. Other tests screen for hormone abnormalities, blood disorders, and cystic fibrosis.

Every state tests for the standard 28 disorders. Some states also include 25 additional screening tests—these other diseases are very rare and there's no treatment, even if a diagnosis is made in the first weeks of life.

Find out what your own state tests for at the National Newborn Screening & Genetics Resource Center (genes-r-us.uthscsa.edu).

Q. Can I get my baby tested for more disorders than my state requires?

Yes. Many private labs and academic institutions offer low cost "expanded" newborn screening for up to 60 metabolic disorders. The cost: about $25.

Note: if you opt for private cord blood banking, some companies throw in a free expanded newborn screening test. Ask about it.

Bottom Line

Although most metabolic diseases are rare, early detection is critical to the health of an affected baby.

DR B'S OPINION

"Even if your state tests for the bare minimum number of disorders (or you have a family history of these disorders), expanded newborn screening is worth the cost."

Picking a pediatrician

While you have bonded with your OB/GYN by now, it's time to start thinking about a new doctor in your life: your baby's pediatrician. You'll be spending some serious quality time with this person over the next several years, so it's important to find the right one. Here is a brief summary of our advice. For a detailed Q&A on finding a pediatrician, go to Expecting411.com/extra.

You'll want to begin your selection process in your third trimester, since you never know exactly when you will deliver! The pediatrician performs your baby's first physical within 24 hours of delivery, so you want that person lined up now. An early start also gives you time to ask your baby's doctor about decisions you will make prior to delivery or just afterwards (such as breastfeeding, cord blood banking, and circumcision to name a few).

Ask your OB and your friends for recommendations and definitely contact the baby's doctor before delivery to make sure he/she is accepting new patients and your insurance plan. Some pediatric practices offer prenatal classes or "meet the doctor" consultations, so it pays to plan ahead.

We'll give you all the questions to ask your baby's potential doc in our special online content—go to Expecting411.com/extra.

Going back to work/childcare options

If this is your first pregnancy, you are probably working outside the home while you are pregnant. Your office might have set up a "baby pool" to see who correctly guesses your baby's birthday. Odds are, there is also a private baby pool you don't know about to see who correctly guesses whether you are returning to work after your maternity leave!

Assuming you will choose to (or need to) go back to work, here are some things you may want to think about now!

Q. Why do I need to sign my unborn baby up for childcare now? That's crazy.

Yes, we agree that it is a nutty world. But your pals in your prenatal class are also looking for childcare and the highest quality programs fill up fast. Many daycares will ask for your baby's due date (instead of his birth date) on the waiting list application.

Some programs require a deposit, others don't. Even if you aren't sure of your work plans (and childcare needs) after your delivery, get on waiting lists that don't require a deposit.

Q. What are my options for childcare?

Your childcare decision is an important one. In the first three years of life, your child will learn to trust others, function independently, problem solve, and learn the boundaries of acceptable behavior. Be very selective of the person/people you choose to care for your baby.

Here are the five basic choices for childcare:

? ?

PARENTHOOD

1 **PARENT AT HOME.** A mom or dad caring for a baby at home is certainly preferable. But you may not be able to afford the cost–the loss of one parent's salary. Full time parenting is hard work, and an admirable profession. (We have great respect for stay at home parents! Our jobs as doctors are much easier than our jobs at home.)

2 **FAMILY CARETAKER.** This is when a grandparent or another family member cares for your baby while you go to work. It's a win-win if you have someone who is able and willing. It lets you pay the bills while your baby is at home with someone you trust. Not only is family childcare free, but your child develops a special relationship with a family member.

3 **NANNY/AU PAIR.** Hiring a professional or someone who just enjoys being with kids is the most expensive childcare option. The upside: when your baby gets sick, there's always someone there to take of him. It's also a good option for families who work odd or long hours.

4 **IN HOME DAYCARE.** Some parents form neighborhood co-ops or get a license to care for a few children in their homes. Moms-for-hire may be a great option and less expensive than a licensed daycare facility. Just make sure you and the mom have similar parenting styles.

5 **LICENSED DAYCARE FACILITY.** This is the option chosen by many working families. You may have a sense of security knowing that providers are licensed professionals (and you can catch a glimpse of your kiddo during your workday on their webcams). It's one of the least expensive options for childcare, but there is a hidden cost that centers don't put in their promotional brochures–increased sickness. Factor several missed workdays and doctor bills into your budget equation.

FYI: Obviously, there is much more to the above choices than this brief overview. We have an expanded discussion of childcare options in *Baby 411* (see back of this book for details).

Insider Secret
You don't need a nanny-cam to check on your childcare employee. Your baby will tell you loud and clear if he or she likes this person. Just watch them interact together.

Q. How much will it cost?

Below is a table with stats to help in your decision making process.

Q. What are my legal rights under the Family Medical Leave Act (FMLA)?

See Chapter 8, Lifestyles for information on your rights in the workplace.

Reality Check
Find out what you can use to piece together a decent maternity leave. You may be able to use vacation time, personal

parenthood prep

COSTS: CHILD CARE OPTIONS

CHILD CARE	COST	MORE INFO
Au Pair	$15,000 per year or $290 per week	AuPairAmerica.com or AuPairCare.com
Nanny	$17,500 to $50,000 per year or $340 to $970 per week	Nanny.org
Day Care	$4500 to $16,000 per year or $90 to $320 per week	Naeyc.org

days, sick leave, or even short-term disability. FMLA only guarantees that you will have a job after taking 12 weeks off. It doesn't guarantee any income while you are out. Find out what your state laws say.

Q. Can my doctor sign off on disability or FMLA forms?

Yes. And you have to submit these forms in writing to your employer 30 days in advance of your leave. Talk to your boss/company regarding employee leave benefits. Sometimes there is A LOT of paper work. It's nice to fill in as much as you can for your practitioner, so she only has to do her part.

Drop the paperwork off well in advance of when it is due because it often can't be filled out in full at the time of your visit. Ask your practitioner to have everything ready in a few days—then you can come back to pick it up or have it mailed to you.

In addition to the forms you may receive from your work, there are also state disability forms that can be filled out and sent in depending on your occupation. Check with your practitioner for details. Most OB practitioners have them in the office to hand out to patients.

Q. What are my partner's rights for parental or paternity leave?

Parental leave is an employee benefit, not a federally mandated law. With some employers, a parent may take up to 12 weeks leave after a baby is born or after an adoption is formalized. But the parent is not eligible to

DR B'S OPINION: WORK VS. FAMILY

You can do it all, but you can't do it all at the same time. You will have to make some sacrifices/delays with your career path to accommodate your new full time job as a parent. But I promise you that you won't ever regret the time you spend with your baby or child.

DR H'S OPINION
WORK VS. FAMILY

People often say to me that I must be really proud of the fact that I have accomplished so much in my career, spending all those years in school and now having the privilege of taking care of women. They are right. But no matter how much I love my job (and I do!), the best thing I have ever done with my life is being a mommy to my kids.

receive insurance during the leave.

In contrast, *paternity* leave is part of the Family Medical Leave Act. A father is eligible if he is employed for at least one year, has worked over 1250 hours, and works in a U.S. company that employs at least 50 people. A dad has the same rights to leave as a mom who delivered that baby.

Factoid: We know there is always "mommy guilt" when it comes to going back to work after having a baby. A key point to consider: *quality* time is more important than the sheer number of hours you spend with your child. Research shows that children do best when their moms focus their attention, engage, and respond to them. *(Huston, AC)*

Breastfeeding vs. Formula

You've got questions. We've got answers. We will cover the majority of breastfeeding questions in Chapter 11, Breastfeeding. But we address the basics on formula here.

Q. Is it really true that breast milk is better for my baby than formula?

Yes. There isn't really anything to debate here. It just makes sense that human milk is more suitable for a human baby than any artificially prepared product made from cow's milk or soy. But you can find the entire list of advantages for both mother and baby in Chapter 11, Breastfeeding.

Q. Is it okay to feed my baby formula?

Yes. Infant formula is an acceptable substitute for breast milk for a baby's first year of life. Be forewarned that it is an expensive option, though. Expect to pay $500 just for the first six months (that is, if your baby tolerates the least expensive cow's milk-based product on the market). Hypoallergenic formula costs twice as much.

DR B'S OPINION

"While I recommend breastfeeding for all the numerous health benefits, your baby will be fine if he is formula-fed."

Q. What formula do you recommend using?

Generic, cow's milk based formula with iron, in powder form. That's as cheap as it's gonna get, with all the nutrients your baby needs.

Here's the Cliffs Notes version on baby formula. Yep, you guessed it— *Baby 411* has an expanded discussion of this topic.

There are four basic types of formula:

1 **COW'S MILK BASED FORMULA WITH IRON.** This is the formula tolerated by most babies and recommended first by most doctors.

2 **SOY PROTEIN FORMULA WITH IRON.** This formula is for babies who can't tolerate cow's milk based formula. Intolerance is a vague term used to describe a baby who is really gassy or pukey with cow's milk formula. Vegetarian families also choose this option.

3 **PROTEIN HYDROLYSATE FORMULA WITH IRON.** This formula is reserved for babies who truly have a *milk protein allergy*, not merely an intolerance to regular milk-based formula. If your baby's doctor diagnoses him with a milk protein allergy, this is the formula of choice for six months to a year. (Many babies with milk protein allergy also have a soy protein allergy, making this expensive—and smelly—formula the best option.)

4 **"GOURMET" FORMULAS.** These are formulas that are for special situations such as premature babies or those with acid reflux, or for parents seeking an organic formula option.

Bottom Line

All formulas sold in the U.S. must contain minimum levels of 29 nutrients according to law (the Infant Formula Act of 1986). So, despite the hype, any formula—brand name or generic—is acceptable.

Q. How much will my baby need to eat?

In the first two or three days of life, your baby will probably drink about an ounce or two every two to four hours. By day three or four, he or she will take about two to three ounces every three to four hours and will keep up that pace for the first couple of weeks of life.

If you plan to feed your newborn formula, the hospital will supply you with ready-to-feed formula. But once you get home, you are the one picking up the tab. Buy a can or two before you deliver, so you will be cov-

**DR B'S OPINION:
WHICH FORMULA BRAND IS BEST?**

There are a HUGE number of formula choices out there, and many companies tout their products as being superior for this or that . . . but in 16 years of practice, I've yet to see that proven or else I would recommend one brand over the other!

ered for a week or so after you come home. Once you know your baby is tolerating your formula choice, go to a warehouse club or big box discount store and stock up!

Vaccines 411

If you think the topic of circumcision is controversial, just Google "vaccines" in your spare time.

Better yet, don't.

When it comes to vaccines, the web is full of info that is both good, bad . . . and ugly. For example, you'll find some very accurate information on vaccines and the diseases they protect against if you go to a site like CDC.gov.

However, surf into some dark corners of the web and you'll find enough scary stories about vaccines to keep you awake for weeks. Produced by anti-vaccine groups, these web sites purport to "educate" parents about vaccine risks. They use scare tactics, outright lies and worse. To get an idea of the agenda of these groups, you'll note the sites include handy links to personal injury lawyers (for the "vaccine-injured").

And the web is just the beginning. Whether in a line at the grocery store or at a local playground, your baby bump will attract those folks who think it is their duty to warn you of the evils of vaccines. Of course, these are the same people who want to tell you how painful labor will be. It's probably best to offer these folks a polite smile and get outta there.

Given all the mis-information both online and offline about vaccines, let's take a second to set the record straight. Our goal with this section is to tell you the truth about vaccines—both the benefits and risks.

First, let's discuss the key truth about vaccines:

Vaccines are one of the most important things you can do to protect your child from serious and life-threatening infections.

There are many myths and misunderstandings about vaccines—we'll discuss these next, as well as the most common questions and concerns about immunization. While this section is meant as a short primer on the topic, you may want to read the expanded section on vaccinations in *Baby 411*. Reputable sites like cdc.gov and aap.org also have helpful info.

And, of course, please talk with your baby's doctor BEFORE making any decision on this topic. *Your child's life is too precious to base vaccine decisions on bad information.*

Q. What is the standard vaccination schedule?

The routine childhood immunization schedule is listed in the chart below. *(Immunization Action Coalition)* Don't worry

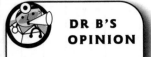

DR B'S OPINION

As a parent and a pediatrician, I want what's best for my child and my patients. That's why I recommend vaccinations. My kids are vaccinated. I wouldn't recommend you do anything I wasn't willing to do with my own children.

??

if you don't understand it right now. It's here to give you the big picture. You can read all the details about the diseases and vaccines in *Baby 411*.

If you have concerns, discuss them with your baby's doctor *before* your child is born (the pre-delivery visit is best). That's because the first round of shots is usually administered at birth and two months of age.

Bottom Line

Many experts who are tops in their fields created this vaccination schedule. And there is a specific reason for the timing, spacing, and offering of certain vaccines.

Age	HepB Hepatitis B	DTaP/Tdap Diphtheria, tetanus, pertussis	Hib Haemophilus influenzae type b	Polio	PCV Pneumococcal conjugate	RV Rotavirus	MMR Measles, mumps, rubella	Varicella Chickenpox	HepA Hepatitis A	HPV Human papillomavirus	MCV4 Meningococcal conjugate	Influenza
Birth	✓											
2 months	✓ (1–2 mos)	✓	✓	✓	✓	✓						
4 months	✓[1]	✓	✓	✓	✓	✓						
6 months		✓	✓[2]	✓ (6–18 mos)	✓	✓[2]						
12 months	✓ (6–18 mos)	✓[4] (15–18 mos)	✓ (12–15 mos)		✓ (12–15 mos)		✓ (12–15 mos)	✓ (12–15 mos)	✓✓ (2 doses given 6 mos apart at age 12–23 mos)			
15 months												
18 months												
19–23 months		Catch-up[5]	Catch-up[5] (to 5 years)	Catch-up[5]	Catch-up[5] (to 5 years)		Catch-up[5]	Catch-up[5]				✓[3] (given each fall or winter to children ages 6 mos–18 yrs)
4–6 years		✓		✓			✓	✓				
7–10 years	Catch-up[5]	Catch-up[5]							Catch-up[5]			
11–12 years		✓ Tdap		Catch-up[5]			Catch-up[5]	Catch-up[5]		✓✓✓[6]	✓	
13–18 years		Catch-up[5] (Tdap/Td)								Catch-up[5,6]	Catch-up[5,7]	

??

PARENTHOOD

Q. Is it safer to separate or delay shots?

Easy answer: no.

The routine immunization schedule was not created out of thin air. It is designed to protect babies as soon as it is safe and effective to do so.

What is guaranteed is that you are leaving your baby at risk the longer you wait to protect him or her. Delaying shots is like playing Russian Roulette with your child, at a time when he or she is the most vulnerable.

Our suggestion: do not walk into your pediatrician's office dead set on using a staggered or alternative vaccination schedule. That says to the doc, "I don't really care what you think about children's health, even though you are, ahem, a pediatrician." It's a real flashpoint. You will find that 99.9% of pediatricians are very passionate about vaccinating their patients in a timely manner. That's because we have all seen, at one point or another, what some of these horrible diseases can actually do.

If this is something you are thinking about, set up a consultation to get advice and come up with a plan together.

DR B'S OPINION:
DR. BOB'S SCHEDULE

The most vocal proponent of alternative vaccine schedules is Dr. Bob Sears. Through both his web site and books, he suggests you shouldn't follow the standard immunization schedule. Instead, he's prepared his own alternative schedule.

So who is Dr. Bob Sears? Sears is a general pediatrician in a private practice, not an infectious disease expert or vaccinologist. Hence, he is making up this vaccine schedule all by himself. There's no science behind it.

Don't take our word for this, however. Here is Dr. Bob in his own words about his schedule: "My schedule doesn't have any research behind it. No one has ever studied a big group of kids using my schedule to determine if it's safe or if it has any benefits." *(Ramnarance, C)*

I'd much rather follow a schedule that has been extensively researched for both safety and effectiveness by multiple people who are truly experts in the field of vaccines.

Q. Why do we have so many shots now?

Because for many diseases (particularly viruses), vaccines are the only way to prevent some really serious illnesses for which there is no treatment. And we have the advanced medical technology today to safely make vaccines.

It's true that we did not get nearly as many shots when we were kids. But let's take a look at some of the vaccines we have now.

Three of them protect against forms of bacterial meningitis (HIB, Strep, and Neisseria). One of them protects against a virus, which, prior to the vaccine, hospitalized over 10,000 Americans and killed about 100 every year—that would be chickenpox. Surprised?

And although the number of shots has gone up, the shots today are much "smarter." They are engineered to have LESS impact on the body than the old shots. Hence, the immune load of the entire vaccination series has gone down. In fact, the *total* number of immunologic agents in today's vaccinations is less than what we got in just two vaccines in 1980. Our children get smarter, safer vaccines today and better protection than we ever got as kids.

Q. Do vaccines cause autism?

No.

How can we be so certain, you ask? First, consider the valid scientific research disproving a link (and yes, there is plenty of it).

As a primary care pediatrician for 16 years now, I can tell you from my professional experience that a baby is born with autism and the signs become apparent over time. Kids don't come in to get their shots and come back the next week with autism. It just doesn't happen that way.

There have been anti-vaccine groups since the smallpox vaccine was created in 1798. Of course, back in those days, you could be burned at the stake for refusing to vaccinate. Now you get a national talk show. Modern day anti-vaccine folk have teamed up with a small, vocal group of

---

FIVE VACCINE MYTHS

Too many vaccines, too soon. Thank goodness we have so many vaccines! Nine of the shots in the routine vaccination series today protect against three different forms of bacterial meningitis (HIB, Strep, and Neisseria). No, you didn't get those shots as a child. But these are NOT diseases you want your child to get naturally. We are lucky to live in today's world where far fewer kids suffer or die from infectious diseases. And we give vaccines as soon as it is safe and effective to do so to protect those who are the most vulnerable—our babies.

We need to green our vaccines. While it's clever to play the environmental green card, vaccines are cleaner than the air our kids breathe, the water/breast milk/formula they drink, and the food they eat. Mercury-based preservatives are no longer in routine childhood vaccines, and breast milk contains more aluminum salt than what is in vaccines.

Vaccines cause autism. While anti-vaccinationists love to make this argument, the research and clinical evidence simply does not support it. Autism has a strong genetic basis and kids with autism are born with autism—long before they get any shots. There are readers who will tune us out at this point, we know, but science is science and facts are facts. Period.

You can't trust doctors—they make money on vaccines. Pediatricians would make a heck of a lot more money if our patients WEREN'T vaccinated. The outbreaks of whooping cough alone could pay for our own kids to go to college or a nice Bentley. The truth: docs go into pediatrics to help kids grow up healthy.

It's all a government conspiracy to protect Big Pharma. This would be the largest worldwide conspiracy in history. Just ask your pediatrician if she vaccinated her kids.

---

parents who believe their kids have autism due to vaccines. And together, they are making lots of noise.

Medicine has not ignored these cries. Vaccines have received intense scrutiny over the past ten years in the search for the cause of autism. Numerous studies have been done and no link has been found.

Alison Singer, Executive Director of the Autism Science Foundation and mother of a child with autism spectrum disorder has said it best: "The question has been asked and answered and it's time to move on...we need to be able to say, 'Yes, we are now satisfied that the earth is round.'"

Reality Check

While parents are asking more questions about vaccines, they are still choosing to vaccinate their kids. The most recent CDC survey showed 99% of U.S. children aged 19 to 35 months get their shots. *(MMWR)* Yes, 99%. Despite what you might think based on media hype, only a tiny fraction of parents opt out of shots.

Q. When is the first vaccine given?

The Hepatitis B vaccine is recommended for all newborns as part of the routine vaccination series. Infants can get the first of a series of three doses between birth and two months of age.

However, if a mother is Hepatitis B positive (a "chronic carrier" of the disease), it's essential that her newborn get that Hepatitis B vaccine and a dose of immunoglobulin within 12 hours of life to prevent the spread of infection. Without the shots, that newborn has a 90% chance of having a chronic, lifelong Hepatitis B infection (which potentially can lead to liver failure and liver cancer).

Factoid. Since we began vaccinating all children in 1991 for Hepatitis B, the rates of new cases in the U.S. are down by 82%. In children, the rates are down by 94%. *(CDC)* But there are still about one million Americans walking around with a chronic Hepatitis B infection.

Q. Can we delay giving the Hepatitis B shot?

Yes, but there are very rational reasons to give it to all newborns after birth.

You might think that babies whose moms have Hepatitis B are the only ones who really need that birth dose. Here's why that's not the case.

◆ *The blood test isn't perfect.* Women who receive prenatal care get tested for evidence of Hepatitis B infection. However, the blood test isn't 100% accurate (it can fail to detect some cases) and some women acquire Hepatitis B after the test has been done and before delivery. Couldn't you just retest every mom when they arrive in labor? Nope. There just isn't enough time to get those test results back.

◆ *Slipping through the cracks.* We know you are the ideal patient who shows up to all her prenatal visits and even brings her prenatal lab work with her to the hospital! However, some women

PARENTHOOD

? ?

(believe it or not) get no prenatal care or actually claim they did not know they were pregnant when they arrive in the ER in labor. No one knows if that woman has Hepatitis B or not. Couldn't you just test that mom on the spot and find out? No. Again, we would not get the results back soon enough. A baby needs to get Hepatitis B vaccine within a 12-hour window to prevent the spread of the disease. Picking and choosing which baby absolutely needs that Hepatitis B shot based on mom's lab work allows some of those at-risk babies to slip through the cracks of a busy maternity ward. So, there is less of a chance of this happening if all babies get this shot.

◆ *Early exposure of newborns is the worst kind of exposure.* Newborns who are infected between birth and one month of age have the greatest risk of having chronic, lifelong Hepatitis B. They have a 90% chance of having this disease for life.

◆ *Babies develop the best immunity.* You may view your newborn as a fragile little thing, but his or her immune system works extremely well! Babies mount a better response to the Hepatitis B vaccine than their parents do, with about 95% lifelong protection from the disease. They have about 85% protection after just the first dose.

◆ *You don't have to have sex to get it.* Hepatitis B spreads through both blood and sexual contact. So you might think the only people at risk are IV drug users, prostitutes, and healthcare providers. But 50% of kids under age ten who get Hepatitis B don't get it from their moms, sex, IV drugs, or tattoos. Someone can get Hepatitis B from sharing a toothbrush, being in contact with a child with a bloody nose on the playground, or contact with a childcare provider with an open cut on her hand. Since you aren't going to check the Hepatitis B status of all humans your baby is exposed to on a daily basis, it is safer to protect your baby before he spends time out in the world.

**DR B'S OPINION:
HEP B VACCINE**

If a mom has Hepatitis B, there is no choice. Her newborn needs Hepatitis B preventive treatment (the vaccine and immunoglobulin) within 12 hours of life. If a mom doesn't have Hepatitis B, it is still smart to give that shot before your baby enters the real world.

Wow. That covered a lot of ground! Hope you sleep better now that you are more prepared for your baby's life outside the womb. Onwards to breastfeeding!

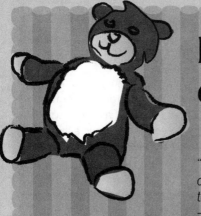

BREASTFEEDING
Chapter 11

"My opinion is that anybody offended by breastfeeding is staring too hard."
—David Allen

I t's one of the key decisions you must make for baby right away: how will you feed him?

Right now, he's getting all his nutrition through his umbilical cord lifeline to you. Once that cord is cut at delivery, he's going to be looking around for something to eat!

For your baby's first year of life, he has one of three food options: breast milk, infant formula, or a combination of both. (You'll add solid food to the menu between four and six months.)

What you decide to feed your baby is your choice. But believe us, the forces of human nature (albeit, well meaning) will try to influence that decision. Every woman you meet while pregnant (from your mother-in-law to the saleswoman at the maternity store) will add in her two cents.

This chapter helps you make an informed decision. But we are very open about our bias: we—like every major medical organization in the world—recommend that all babies be breastfed. So we are going to do our best to convince you to give it a try. And we'll give you tons of practical tips to be successful!

However, ·unlike some experts, authors, or so-called friends you may encounter, we won't make you feel guilty if you decide on formula or can't make a go of breastfeeding. We just hope you will give it your best effort, because *any*

? ?

BREASTFEEDING

breast milk you feed your baby is a gift.

Why? Human breast milk is the ideal nutrition for human babies. No matter how much formula companies tinker with their products, formula is only a close approximation of the real thing. Breast milk has living ingredients (including all those antibodies you've been making your entire life). But, if there are reasons you cannot breastfeed, don't beat yourself up about it—know that your baby can and will thrive on infant formula.

NEW PARENT 411: BREASTFEEDING LINGO

Breastfeeding has a language all its own. Here is a quick overview:

◆ **Colostrum.** The first milk that your breasts produce. Some women start making (and leaking) it before the baby is even born. It is a high-protein drink, filled with mom's antibodies that boost the immunity of a newborn. It has fewer calories than mature milk because of a lower fat content.

◆ **Mature Milk.** The milk that arrives on the third or fourth day after birth. It is about 50% fat.

◆ **Foremilk.** The milk that comes out in the first several minutes of feeding. In general, it contains slightly less fat. Babies who "snack" end up getting mostly foremilk, leading to more frequent feedings (and possibly, fussiness).

◆ **Hindmilk.** The milk that comes out in the later part of a feeding. It is slightly higher in fat than foremilk. Babies who drain a whole breast in a feeding tend to be more satisfied, for good reason.

◆ **Let down.** When your milk rushes into the milk ducts as your baby suckles or as you pump. Most women feel this "let-down."

◆ **Engorgement.** In the first days when you make mature milk, your breasts may feel full, tender, lumpy, and hard.

◆ **Plugged ducts.** An area of the breast has obstructed milk flow, creating a hard, tender lumpy area. These areas are at risk of getting infected (mastitis—ouch!). See tips below for more info.

◆ **Inverted nipples.** Your nipples have an indentation in the center. It can make it more difficult for your baby to latch on.

◆ **Flat nipples.** Your nipples are flush against your breast tissue. Like inverted nipples, flat nipples can make it difficult for baby to latch.

◆ **Breast shells.** Plastic devices that pull out inverted nipples. They can also be worn to protect sore nipples from rubbing against your bra.

◆ **Nipple shields.** Plastic devices that protect sore or cracked nipples. These are also used for moms with flat or inverted nipples. Unfortunately, they can sometimes limit the amount of milk that flows to the baby's mouth.

◆ **Lanolin.** A thick emollient that helps heal cracked nipples. Brand names: Lansinoh, Pur-lan. Available at breastfeeding boutiques and even Wal-Mart.

The best advice we can give you is to think about (and prepare for) breastfeeding now. Remember when you took driver's ed? Breastfeeding education is similar in that you won't really know how to do it until you get behind the wheel. But if you have the general concepts down, you'll feel much better about your first test drive.

See Expecting411.com/extra for more info on surviving the early days of breastfeeding and our companion book *Baby 411* for details for your baby's first year.

Time for an introduction: We'd like to give a shout out to Linda Hill, a registered nurse and certified lactation consultant. She is our go to source on breastfeeding (Linda works with Dr. B) and she shares her wisdom and practical tips to help you become a nursing pro. Look for Linda's tips scattered throughout this chapter and at Expecting411.com/extra

Breast Milk

Q. I have heard that breastfeeding is best for babies, but what are the real advantages?

There are advantages for both baby and mom. Let's take a look at each:

Breastfeeding Advantages for Baby
Mother's milk:

◆ Has the ideal ingredients for a human body. Breast milk is living food.

◆ Carries the mother's antibodies to protect baby from various infections.

◆ Reduces the severity of certain infections, like stomach viruses and the common cold.

◆ Is hypoallergenic. It is rare to be allergic to human milk.

◆ Is brain food. Breast milk naturally contains nutrients (DHA and ARA) that stimulate brain and vision development.

◆ Reduces risk of diabetes, inflammatory bowel disease, asthma, and some forms of cancer later in life.

◆ Reduces your baby's risk of Sudden Infant Death Syndrome (SIDS).

Breastfeeding Advantages for Mom

◆ It may be the easiest way to lose those pregnancy pounds and still eat like you are a professional wrestler. You will continue to have higher calorie needs, but your body will use them up while nursing.

◆ It is always ready to serve, at the perfect temperature. That's convenient in the middle of the night . . . or at the mall.

◆ It is free. Formula can cost $1200 or more for the entire first year of life.

◆ It reduces your risk of breast cancer. Any amount or duration of breastfeeding lowers your risk of developing breast cancer before menopause. Currently, one in eight women will get breast cancer. (Stuebe AM)

BREASTFEEDING

? ?

◆ It may lower your risk of osteoporosis, diabetes, high blood pressure, heart disease and rheumatoid arthritis. You can lower your risk of high blood pressure, heart disease, and diabetes by nursing for at least a year of your life (not necessarily with just one baby). You can lower your risk of having a heart attack or stroke after menopause by 10% if you nurse for at least one month.

◆ It can be a form of birth control, but don't rely on it exclusively (unless you want a toddler and a newborn in the same house!).

BOTTOM LINE: Breastfeeding is worth the effort!

Reality Check

Women in some countries nurse their babies longer than American women. Those same countries have lower rates of breast cancer.

Q. How long should I breastfeed?

This may come as a surprise to you, but the American Academy of Pediatrics recommends breastfeeding for the entire first year of life (and beyond that, if you desire).

But despite all the benefits and recommendations from major medical organizations, very few American babies are breastfed for the first year. About 75% of American newborn are breastfed, but only 30% are still breastfeeding at six months of life (and fewer than that actually nurse until their first birthdays).

Q. If breast milk is important for a year, why do most American moms stop before then?

Great question, but more importantly, how can you help change those statistics?

Most of the time, women stop nursing because breastfeeding can be a real pain (literally and figuratively) for the first couple of weeks. No matter how many breastfeeding books you read or classes you take, you have to learn how to do it as you go along.

Breastfeeding is not as natural as you might think. Your baby knows how to suck and your body knows how to make milk—but the technique of getting the baby latched on appropriately requires some real patience, persistence, and perseverance. Add in your hormonal roller-coaster, discomfort as your body heals, and sheer exhaustion and you'll understand why a mom might consider stopping nursing.

To make breastfeeding even more undesirable, it can be painful! That is, if you and your baby start off with a poor technique. It takes some real cajones to continue breastfeeding when your nipples are raw, cracked, and bleeding.

If that's not enough to cause moms to give up, your mother or mother-in-law probably won't help. She'll watch you struggling and will tell you how much easier it was just to feed her babies formula. (Kindly ask her to cook you dinner if she really wants to help.)

In truth, breastfeeding is like running a race with the hardest hurdles up front. Most women don't make it past those hurdles to realize it's a straight shot to the finish line. And if you don't think you can make it over those hurdles…ASK FOR HELP!

Q. If I have trouble breastfeeding, whom should I turn to for help?

You already have relationships with people (practitioners) who can help–your obstetrician, family practitioner, midwife, doula, and pediatrician. All of us have some experience handling common breastfeeding issues.

However, if you feel like you are a dog paddling in the middle of the ocean, your best bet is to call in another expert. Enter the lactation consultant.

Certified lactation consultants (IBCLC's) are individuals who are specifically trained and certified to handle breastfeeding challenges and can be the difference between

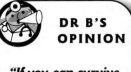

DR B'S OPINION

"If you can survive the first couple of weeks, breastfeeding is as easy and natural as you think it should be!"

breastfeeding failure and success. There are other professionals who are "breastfeeding educators," but we prefer certified IBCLC's because they go through a formal training and certification process. Ask your practitioner for a recommendation.

Unfortunately, most insurance companies do not cover the services offered by a lactation consultant (even though breast milk can reduce a child's risk of illness and thus, his healthcare costs–but perhaps someday insurance companies will realize that!).

You'll probably have to pay out of pocket for a consultation and then submit the bill to insurance. However, a skilled lactation consultant is worth every penny and costs less than buying a couple of week's worth of formula!

6 reasons why women stop breastfeeding—and our solutions

1 **IT HURTS.** Yes, nursing hurts . . . if your technique is bad. It's painless if you do it right. Get professional help to learn how to get the baby latched on appropriately. If your baby has a tongue tie (short frenulum), have it clipped. Use a *nipple shield* (see info on page 266) and/or pump until your nipples heal and your technique improves.

2 **YOU ARE EXHAUSTED AND NO ONE ELSE CAN FEED THE BABY.** That's true, but only for the first few weeks while you stabilize your milk supply to meet your baby's demands. Then, you can start pumping and let your partner (and anyone else who is willing) take a turn feeding your baby with a bottle of expressed breast milk.

3 **YOU GET A BREAST INFECTION (MASTITIS** or yeast infection). Ouch! It's possible to get both bacterial infections (mastitis) and yeast infections of the breast when you nurse. Neither are fun and both are often the straw that breaks the camel's back when it comes to nursing. But both are also temporary and treatable. Read through this chapter and additional content at Expecting411.com/extra so you don't end up in this situation.

4 **YOU DON'T HAVE ENOUGH MILK.** This is rare, but it happens. And watching your baby screaming for more food after being at the breast can make a mom want to just throw in the towel. Women of a "certain age" (over 35) and those who have had certain types of breast surgery may never make enough breast milk to nurse their babies exclusively. Other under-producing women may be able to rev up their supply by nursing often, pumping in between nursing sessions, and taking medications that increase milk production. But remember, any breast milk is a gift. You don't have to breastfeed exclusively for your baby to benefit from it.

5 **YOU RETURN TO WORK.** Ideally, a woman should pump (express her breast milk) as often as her baby eats. That ensures adequate milk production and a stash of expressed milk to feed the baby. But that means taking a pumping break at work about every three hours. Some workplaces are very progressive and allow this schedule. But many working/nursing moms find this goal nearly impossible. Figure out what works for you. Even if you cannot breastfeed exclusively, some breast milk is better than none at all. Some moms can only pump once at work and continue to nurse at home. Do what you can to continue some level of breastfeeding even after you head back to work.

6 **YOUR BABY HAS A PROBLEM THAT MAKES BREASTFEEDING DIFFICULT—PREMATURITY, MILK PROTEIN ALLERGY, ACID REFLUX (GERD).** These are often the most challenging breastfeeding situations to overcome.

Bottom Line

Yes, breastfeeding can be a real test of wills. But you can overcome most challenges with a little guidance and a lot of support.

DR B'S OPINION

"Breastfeeding is not an 'all or nothing' situation. Some breast milk is better than none at all. Every ounce counts."

Partner Tips

1. Be supportive of breastfeeding.
2. Become an honorary lactation consultant.
3. Pick up the slack.

Breastfeeding can be an emotionally charged experience (especially if your nursing partner encounters problems). You need to be there to support the decision to breastfeed. And although you may feel awkward about it, yes, you should accompany her to a breastfeeding class.

Breastfeeding takes a lot of patience and often four hands. (To let you in on a little secret, your expert author, Dr. H, needed three people and 12 towels rolled into various shapes to properly position her and her first baby for breastfeeding!).

You will become the honorary lactation consultant since you will have a bird's eye view of the way your baby latches on to your nursing partner. Watch how the lactation consultant does it and take notes.

Until the nursing mother and baby get the hang of it, you may need to place your baby open-mouthed onto the breast as your partner holds the baby and her breast upwards. So, don't think you are off the hook because your partner is the one actually nursing!

By the way, it's also helpful if you take charge of all other baby needs (soothing, diaper changes, etc.) as well as household needs (laundry, meal preparation, etc) so your exhausted nursing partner can catch some much needed shut-eye between feedings.

Q. If I stop breastfeeding before my baby is one, what do I offer him instead?

Commercial-brand formula is the acceptable substitute for breast milk in the first year of life. If you think selecting a crib is mind numbing, wait until you see your options for formula! Check out our companion book *Baby 411* to help you navigate the formula aisle at the grocery store.

Note: whole milk, soymilk, goat's milk, and rice milk are NOT substitutes for breast milk in the first year of life.

Q. If I decide not to breastfeed, will my body make milk? Do I need to take a medication to stop it?

Yes, your body will naturally make milk. And no, you don't need medication to stop it.

After delivery, your hormones will tell your body to produce milk for your newborn. But your body will only continue to make milk if it is regularly encouraged to do so. That encouragement comes either naturally, with a baby nursing at the breast or artificially, using a breast pump.

If neither of those things happen, your body will quickly stop producing milk in a week or so. You can wear a tight sports bra and apply ice packs for ten minutes once every hour to accelerate this process. You also might want to wear some nursing pads for a few days to conceal any leakage.

FYI: medication is no longer used to "dry up" breast milk. The risks outweigh the benefits, therefore it is no longer recommended.

Getting Ready

Q. Should I take a breastfeeding class?

Yes, if you have never nursed before. And your partner should go with you. As we mentioned earlier, it really is like taking driver's ed. You will get the big picture idea in a class, but you will learn the finer nuances once you really do it. Nursing is also a team sport. And you are taking the class without your key player (your baby). You will have to teach him or her the game plan as you go along.

Certified lactation specialists (IBCLC's) usually teach these classes, so get the instructor's contact information if you like her—you might need to track her down later!

Q. My breasts started leaking already. Is this a good sign?

Yes.

While it's no guarantee that you will have enough milk, it does mean that your body is getting ready to go.

Q. I have flat/ inverted nipples. Will this be a problem with nursing?

It might be.

Babies need an easy target to transfer milk out of the breast . . . and into their mouths. A newborn may get frustrated at the breast because she has difficulty latching on and, subsequently, eating.

But there are a few solutions to this problem. First, you can manually draw out your nipples by pulling on them before you go to nurse. The other option is to use *nipple shells*. You can start wearing these little accessories before you even deliver to help draw out your nipples. You can also use them after delivery.

Note: NOT every women with inverted nipples has a problem with nursing. But it's good to take a peek at your nipples right now, so you can prepare yourself for this potential issue.

FYI: Yes, there is even a web site that can help you do your own nipple assessment (007b.com/nipple_gallery.php). As Dave Barry would say, we are not making this up!

Q. I have small breasts. Will I make enough milk?

Probably. Size doesn't matter. It's what's inside that counts.

You should have enough milk if you have normal breast anatomy (milk ducts, nipples), make hormones that trigger milk production, and have the right amount of stimulation (from your baby naturally suckling or using a breast pump).

Old Wives Tale

Women who are flat chested can't nurse. *False.* While there are some women who do not make enough milk to exclusively nurse their babies, it is not because they have small breasts.

FLAT AND INVERTED NIPPLES

When a woman gets physically cold, it's normal for her nipples to harden and stick out like that famous Farrah Fawcett poster. If this doesn't happen to you, you might have flat or inverted nipples.

Flat nipples: Is your breast perfectly smooth? Try pinching the pigmented area (**AREOLA**) just beneath the nipple to help your baby find it. Avoid baby bottles and pacifiers in the beginning, as your baby will prefer them since they are easier to latch on to.

Inverted nipples: Do you see an indentation in the center of your nipple? Try pinching your nipple. Does it stick out or go in? If it goes in, pull your nipple out before offering it to your baby. If it "hides," then you may want to wear *nipple shells* during your pregnancy. You can also use a breast pump after you deliver to help bring out your nipple. *Nipple shields* are useful if the baby can pull the nipple into the shield.

? ?

BREASTFEEDING

Insider Secret:
No two breasts are created equally.

One of your breasts may produce more than the other. In fact, it's quite common. And your baby will figure that out and may develop a preference for the better-producing breast. Some babies will even refuse the breast that has slower flow or less volume.

If your baby doesn't get too frustrated, offer the slower flow breast first because he will nurse more aggressively at the beginning and that helps increase your supply. And try pumping the lower-producing breast after nursing to improve production.

Does your baby completely refuse one breast? No worries. It's possible to make enough from one breast to completely satisfy your baby. So, nutrition isn't a problem. You'll just start to look rather lopsided if you only nurse on one side!

Q. I have very large breasts/nipples. Is this good for nursing?

It can be good or bad.

If you have large pendulous breasts, you may have more difficulty getting your baby correctly latched. You may want to try the "football hold" or lying on your side while nursing so you don't have to hold up the weight of your breast. Or, you may want to use a nursing pillow that supports both your breast and your baby.

If the entire dark pigmented area including the nipple (**AREOLA**) is so large that your baby cannot latch on, you may need to pump until he and his mouth get bigger.

Q. I've had a breast reduction. Will this be a problem?

Possibly.

Certain types of breast reduction surgery disrupt the milk duct superhighway. If this is your situation, you may not have enough breast milk to breast feed exclusively. You may not even make more than a drop or two at each nursing session. This may be a situation where formula feeding is the most reasonable choice for your baby.

But we can't predict whether you will be able to nurse or not before you *try*. And even if you cannot nurse for the long haul, it's great to offer your first milk (**COLOSTRUM**) to your newborn. Give it a try. And we highly recommend you work with a lactation consultant.

Q. I've had a mastectomy. Can I nurse with only one breast?

Yes, in fact I (Dr. B) had a patient whose mother successfully breastfed with one breast for a whole year. So, it can be done! Each breast is capable of providing enough milk to meet a baby's nutritional needs.

Q. I have implants. Can I still nurse?

Yes, you can nurse even if you have breast implants. However, certain types of reconstructive surgery may interfere with your ability to breastfeed exclusively. Get professional help from a lactation consultant.

First days

Right from the start, we want you to have good nursing technique. That prevents those raw, bleeding nipples you've been warned about! It all boils down to good positioning and a good latch.

There are four basic positions to hold your baby while you nurse.

Head over to the Expecting411.com/extra for details on breastfeeding positions and tips for a comfortable latch.

Linda's tips for positioning

◆ Mom should be comfortable with her arms and back supported.

◆ Mom should not lean over the baby. Instead, use a breastfeeding pillow—a firm pillow that wraps around Mom's waist and allows baby to rest supported.

◆ Baby should directly face the breast without having to turn his head.

◆ Baby's stomach should be pulled in close to Mom.

◆ Baby's ear, shoulder, and hip should be in a straight line.

The other critical issue is making sure your baby's bottom lip latches well below the nipple and not at the base of the nipple. His bottom lip should be on the areola and not the nipple.

Q. When is the first time I should nurse my baby?

Shortly after delivery. But be patient—baby needs to learn how to breathe first!

As long as there are no emergency medical issues for you or your baby, you will have a chance to nurse your baby in his first hour of life. He will be awake, alert, and interested in suckling. Take advantage of this moment to bond and start breastfeeding.

After that golden wakeful hour, your baby will want to sleep for the next few hours and will want nothing to do with the breast.

Q. Is it okay to supplement with formula until my mature milk comes in?

Yes, it's okay, but it's usually not necessary.

Mother Nature has an elaborate plan for babies and breast milk. Newborns arrive with some extra nutritional baggage to carry them through the first few days of life. That's good because they'd rather sleep than eat. It's also good because your body is making early milk (**COLOSTRUM**) that is antibody-rich, but calorie-poor (it has fewer calories in it than mature milk, which shows up around day three or four).

In fact, we pediatricians expect most newborns to *lose* about 10% of their birth weight by the third or fourth day. That's supposed to happen.

At about 48 hours of life (at precisely the moment most of you are heading home from the hospital), your baby suddenly says, "Hey, I'm starving, what have you got to eat around here?!"

He'll act completely differently than his first two days and want to nurse non-stop. That demand drives your milk supply up. Although that can be pretty nerve-wracking for about 24 hours or so, it's what gets your milk production going.

Bottom Line

You don't need to tinker with Mother Nature's grand scheme by offering formula. Unless there is a medical reason to give formula (your baby's doc will tell you), let nature take its course.

Q. Can my baby use a pacifier if I am nursing?

Yes.

Your baby won't be confused about where his next meal is coming from. If he is hungry, a pacifier just won't do.

But pacifiers can be very useful for a baby whose tummy is full and is just looking for a way to settle down. Babies have very few strategies to soothe themselves when they are first born. Sucking is one of them (they have been doing that in the womb already).

A few notes of caution, however.

◆ Not all pacifiers are the same shape. If you plan to nurse, choose one that has a nipple shaped more like a human one—lactation consultants prefer the Soothie Brand (soothie-pacifier.com) for that reason. If your baby sucks a certain way on a pacifier, he may resort to that strategy at your breast and it might result in some discomfort for you.

◆ Wait until your baby is a proficient nurser before offering that binky. That way, you will be an expert at deciphering your baby's hunger cues versus grumpy cues. And your baby will be an expert at suckling. For most babies, that's at about a week or two of life.

◆ Know when to stop. Babies learn other soothing strategies quickly. Your baby won't need a pacifier after he is six months old. Trust us on this one.

◆ Alternatively, you can let your newborn suck on your clean finger to be soothed.

Old Wives Tale
Pacifiers interfere with breastfeeding.

False. Babies who use pacifiers tend to breastfeed for a shorter period of time than those who don't. But it's not *because* of the binky. Moms who opt to use binkies are the same ones who opt out of breastfeeding. It's just a coincidence—one doesn't cause the other. *(O'Connor NR)*

FYI: Rooming in. Breastfeeding friendly hospitals will encourage mother and baby to "room-in" together. This means that your baby will stay in your hospital room virtually 24 hours a day. She will only go to the newborn nursery if she needs to have a blood test, physical exam with good lighting, or a procedure. This helps you learn your baby's hunger cues and feed her when she needs to be fed.

Q. What do I need to know about my baby's first few days of breastfeeding?

Let's break this down, day by day...

First Day of Life (0-24 hours old):

1. Nurse your baby for the first time within an hour or so of his birth. He will be awake, alert, and interested.
2. At two hours of life, he will be exhausted and hard to arouse for several (three to four) hours. Don't get too worked up about trying to nurse right now. Take a nap yourself.
3. Aim for six to eight feedings in the first 24 hours of life.
4. Your baby will probably fall asleep at the breast after a few minutes of nursing. An acceptable feeding session for today is five to ten minutes per breast.

Second Day of Life (24-48 hours old):

1. Today's goal: work on your technique. It may take a second set of hands to position the baby while you hold your breast. (Your partner can help here.) You will fly solo eventually.
2. Aim for eight feedings in 24 hours. Do not let your baby sleep more than three hours during the day or four hours at night at a stretch . . . or you will have trouble meeting this goal.
3. Length of feedings goal: at least five to ten minutes per breast. Do not take baby off the breast at ten minutes if he is still actively sucking.
4. If your nipples are cracked and bleeding, you need help with your technique.

Third Day of Life (48-72 hours old):

1. Your baby is suddenly awake and sometimes, insatiable. As long as your baby has lost less than 10% of his birth weight (and has no other medical issues), keep your chin up and resist the temptation to supplement with formula. Your baby's demand is precisely what your body needs to create the supply of milk.
2. Make sure your technique is okay and you are comfortable when your baby latches on.
3. Frequency goal: eight feedings in 24 hours (it should be an easy goal to reach today!)
4. Length of feedings goal: at least ten minutes per breast.
5. You may feel that your baby is on your breast non-stop. If that is the case and your nipples are sore, take a break if you have nursed for more than 45 minutes. Let someone else have a chance to soothe your baby. (Letting baby suck on someone's finger may be helpful.)

Fourth Day of Life (72-96 hours old):

1. Hello milk! There is usually little question of whether or not your milk has arrived. How will you know? Your breasts will be much larger, heavier, and tender. You should feel full before you nurse, and softer after you nurse. You should also see milk when you burp your baby (and sometimes when you shower). The change in your baby's poop will also tell you the milkman has arrived.
2. If your breasts are rock hard and your areola (the darker colored area including your nipple) are flattened against them, you are officially engorged. This lasts for a day or two. See Expecting411.com/extra for tips.
3. Frequency goal: eight feedings in 24 hours. Do not let your baby sleep for more than a four hour stretch.

4. Length of feedings goal: at least ten to 15 minutes per breast. Once your milk supply is well established (around four weeks of life), some women prefer to nurse with one breast per feeding. For now, use both at each feeding as it stimulates your milk production.

5. You should be on your way now. Your baby should be gaining about an ounce a day.

Helpful Hint

When you are told that babies feed every two to three hours, time is measured from the BEGINNING of one feeding until the beginning of the next. If the feeding session itself lasts 45 minutes or an hour, that may leave less than an hour before it's time to nurse again.

Your goal is to nurse at least EIGHT TIMES a day. This may be every two to three hours or it may be a series of cluster feedings every 90 minutes, followed by a four-hour stretch. As long as the number of feedings add up to at least eight in a 24-hour period, it is fine.

Red Flags

Check in with your baby's doctor if:

◆ You don't have a dramatic change in your breasts by the fifth day of life.

◆ You don't hear your baby swallowing ("cuh" or "ca-ca" sound) when he is at the breast.

◆ Your baby's poops have not changed from black tar (meconium) to a greenish–yellowish color by the fourth day.

◆ Your baby does not have at least four wet diapers on the fourth day.

◆ Your baby is sleepy and hard to arouse for feedings.

◆ Your baby is nursing non-stop.

Troubleshooting For The First Week

Running a fever? Worried you might have a breast infection (**MASTITIS**)? Struggling with engorgement or cracked nipples (OUCH!)? Head over to Expecting411.com/extra for all the answers.

4 Breastfeeding Concerns: True or False?

Wondering if you can go on a diet while you are breastfeeding? Worried that you can't have ice cream, coffee, sushi, wine, or your favorite peanut butter cookies while nursing? Will you need to use birth control? Check out Expecting411.com/extra for more info.

But here are a few myths you may wonder about:

YOUR BOOBS WILL SAG IF YOU BREASTFEED.

Technically true. But your boobs will also sag even if you don't breastfeed. It's one of the joys of going through pregnancy and motherhood. If you are really bothered by your new appearance, we can suggest some nice plastic surgeons in LA and Austin who will be happy to help you regain your perky, pre-motherhood breasts!

2 YOU CAN'T GET PREGNANT WHILE YOU ARE BREASTFEEDING.

False. It is true that many women do not *menstruate* while they are nursing. But it's still possible to ovulate (produce a mature egg) and conceive without menstruating. The odds of becoming pregnant while nursing are lowest during the first six months of breastfeeding if you have no vaginal bleeding after 56 days post delivery and are breastfeeding exclusively. *(Lawrence RA)* But you can lower those odds even more if you use an additional form of birth control!

3 YOU NEED TO AVOID GASSY FOODS LIKE BEANS BECAUSE IT WILL MAKE THE BABY GASSY.

False. Your baby will be gassy no matter what you eat. All newborns are gassy in the first six to eight weeks of life. You don't need to restrict your diet unless you see a real correlation between what you ate and your baby's level of discomfort (it takes four to 24 hours to see a problem). Potential problem foods include cabbage, turnips, broccoli, rhubarb, apricots, prunes, melons, and peaches. *(Lawrence RA)*

4 DRINKING ALCOHOL IMPROVES YOUR MILK SUPPLY.

False. Drinking may be relaxing, but it does not encourage milk production. It can help with milk let down if a mom is having trouble relaxing.

Ok, now you have a handle on this breastfeeding thing. Next, let's talk about the home stretch before labor!

HOME STRETCH

Chapter 12

"Can I just spray a little PAM down there right before the baby comes out?"
—Baby Mama

Most pregnant women spend their entire pregnancy preparing for the big day. As you get closer to this becoming an actuality, we know you have many questions about the nuts and bolts of the whole experience. This chapter will cover common concerns at the end of your pregnancy and all the things you should think about *before* you go into labor.

The next chapter (Labor Day) walks you through what really happens at the big show. We recommend you read both of these chapters before those first contractions start.

View this chapter as the dress rehearsal.

Labor Lingo

Bookmark the next two pages. We'll refer to these terms in both this chapter and the next one.

◆ *Dilation*: The cervix begins to open to let the baby out. Your practitioner measures it with his/her fingertips on an internal pelvic exam. Docs measure the diameter of the cervix opening in centimeters. It ranges from zero to ten. When a cervix is not open at all, it is "closed" or "zero centimeters dilated." When the cervix is completely dilated it is called "complete" or "ten centimeters dilated." See graphic on next page.

HOME STRETCH

Dilation

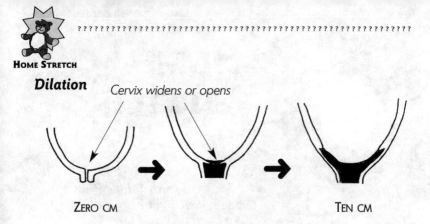

Cervix widens or opens

ZERO CM   TEN CM

◆ **Engaged:** This term refers to the process of the baby's presenting body part (usually the head) moving down and settling into the pelvic cavity. This often occurs in the last month of pregnancy, but it may happen earlier if this is your second or third baby. People refer to it as "dropping" or "**LIGHTENING**" and you may see that your belly changes shape and you can breathe easier. But if you didn't have to pee enough already, you will now feel like you should set up shop on the potty.

◆ **Lightening:** This is the lay term for **ENGAGED**. See above.

◆ **Station:** This measurement compares where your baby's head is in relation to the location of specific bones in your pelvis (the ischial spines). It tracks your baby's descent into the birth canal. See graphic below.
   The most commonly used system (yes, there's more than one) ranges from -5 to +5, where -5 means the baby's head is 5 cm above your pelvic bones (ischial spines) and +5 means the baby's head is at the opening of your vagina. Your practitioner determines the station by an internal pelvic exam.

Station

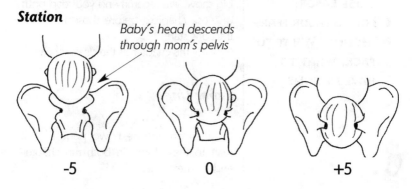

Baby's head descends
through mom's pelvis

-5   0   +5

◆ **Bloody Show:** This is blood-tinged mucous discharge from the vagina, which often signals the onset of labor.

◆ **Effacement:** The cervix also starts to thin out as it prepares for birth. Again, your practitioner can determine this from an internal pelvic exam. Docs measure effacement in percentages. So, for example, you will be "0% effaced" when the cervix is at its longest and hasn't started to thin yet (most of your pregnancy). And you will be 100% effaced when you begin pushing.

◆ **Ripe Cervix:** The term used to describe your cervix as it thins and softens, in preparation for delivery.

Effacement

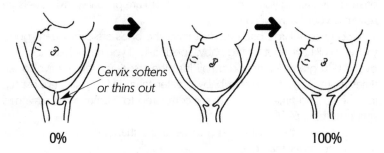

Cervix softens or thins out

0%   100%

◆ *Mucous Plug*: A yellowish, pinkish thick substance that acts as a plug (hence the name) by blocking the cervix during pregnancy. You may lose your mucous plug as the cervix starts to open up. This is often a sign that labor will begin soon. Some women actually see a big blob of mucous. But most don't notice anything until they are in the heat of labor and bloody show begins.

◆ *Presentation:* As the end of your pregnancy nears, your practitioner will check to see if your baby plans to exit the birth canal going head first (called cephalic or "**VERTEX**")—the safest and least complicated way. The head, in this case, is the "presenting part," which means it is the first body part to emerge. 95% of babies are vertex.

Occasionally, babies make their exit a bit more challenging by sitting in a **BREECH** position. That means that the baby's butt (or foot in some cases) is the presenting part.

And a few indecisive babies lie sideways (**TRANSVERSE LIE**) or diagonally (**OBLIQUE LIE**).

It's helpful to know what your baby's plans are, so your practitioner can make plans of her own for your delivery. OB's get that information by doing a physical exam and using an ultrasound.

Late stage pregnancy issues

Q. When does the baby "drop" in preparation for delivery?

The fetus is basically swimming around until about 33 weeks, when he moves to a head-down position (**VERTEX**).

But even once he moves into this position, his head may still be "floating" in the pelvis, meaning that it has not dropped. Your girlfriends (who are intensely watching your belly) may tell you that once the baby drops, your labor is imminent. That's not necessarily true.

Some babies may not drop until actual labor begins, especially with second and third pregnancies. Other babies may start heading into the pelvis as early as 35 weeks.

Q. I had a very large baby with my first pregnancy. What are the odds that I'll have another big kid with this pregnancy?

You and your practitioner are visiting on a weekly basis now. Since he or she is measuring you every week, you both are probably taking bets on how big your baby will be.

If you had a large baby the first time, the odds are pretty darn good that you will have another big baby. Specifically, if you had a baby that was over 4,000 grams (eight and a half lbs.) the first time, you are five to ten times more likely to deliver a baby greater than 4,500 grams (almost ten lbs) the second time around. This is compared to women who have had smaller babies. *(ACOG)*

Second and third babies tend to be larger than first babies, and boys tend to be larger than girls.

Finally, your own birth weight is a predictor of your newborn's birth weight. If you were a big baby, there's not a whole lot you can do to change your baby's fate.

Q. This is my second baby, I'm at 37 weeks, and already dilated 3 cm. Will I go into labor before 40 weeks?

It's pretty common for women who have already had a baby before to be sitting around with a dilated cervix. Your body knows what to do and that is one of the reasons that second and third labors are so much quicker, on average.

You do not need to race home, pack a bag, and head over to the hospital if your practitioner tells you that you are three or four centimeters. In fact, many women with prior deliveries and even a few women who haven't had a baby before, walk around for weeks at three to four centimeters without having regular contractions.

Q. Should my partner come to my appointments in the final weeks?

Your partner can join you at any and all office visits. Ask your practitioner if he or she feels there are any "not-to-be-missed" appointments on the horizon.

Dr H's Opinion: Preparing for Delivery!

In my practice, I strongly recommend that partners are present for the 32 to 33 week visit because after the routine exam, I take couples into my office and go over what they need to know about labor and delivery.

This includes: when to call, where to call, what labor feels like, when to go to the hospital (and where to park!), when I show up, my philosophies on fetal monitoring, augmenting labor with pitocin, epidural/pain control, vacuum/forceps delivery, and C-sections. We also discuss episiotomy, at which point my patients' and their partners' faces begin to grimace.

This visit also gives my patients a chance to ask other questions about what they may or may not want in labor, what to pack in their bag, how many family members/friends can be in the room, etc. And it's my chance to remind them about choosing a pediatrician, cord blood banking if they choose to do so, making a decision on circumcision and having a properly installed car seat ready to go.

Q. I've heard that massaging my genital area (perineum) once a week in the last month of my pregnancy will help prevent tearing or the need for an episiotomy. Is this true?

Although some people suggest this, there is no evidence that it works. But you are welcome to test out this theory since there's no risk in doing it.

Childbirth Classes

Q. There are a variety of childbirth classes available in our community. Which one should I take and when should I take it?

If this is your first baby, it's a good idea to take a childbirth education class. Most hospitals that have maternity services offer classes in childbirth, parenting, breastfeeding, and infant CPR. Some even offer C-section classes for women who know in advance that they will have this procedure.

But do not feel like you are wedded to take a class at the hospital at which you will deliver. Your practitioner may be able to recommend a particular class or a childbirth educator who does private home classes for one, two, or more expecting couples.

Reality Check

If you go on bed rest or simply cannot find a course that works for your schedule, there are plenty of educational DVD's or online childbirth courses you can take.

Bradley vs. Lamaze

The *Bradley Method* of childbirth is named after Dr. Robert Bradley (an American obstetrician) who developed this technique in the 1940's. The goal: natural, drug-free childbirth.

It is now taught as a 12-week course that educates a couple on how to cope with the pain of childbirth by using deep breathing and relaxation techniques. The Bradley method was one of the first to involve fathers in the birthing process (instead of keeping them pacing in the waiting room, which was typical at that time).

The father or partner takes the role of coach, helps to keep mom focused on the delivery, aids with breathing exercises, and gives constant reassurance. He/she also provides different forms of massage to help ease the discomfort. (Our tip: don't buy a whistle, even if you are playing the coach.)

Bradley classes prepare patients for possible unexpected outcomes, but argue against the use of pain medication and C-section unless absolutely necessary.

The *Lamaze method* of childbirth is named after Dr. Fernand Lamaze (a French obstetrician) who also debuted this method in the 1940's. Lamaze gained acceptance in the US and is now the most popular of all childbirth techniques.

The Lamaze technique also teaches breathing exercises during labor (this is the one most of us know as "hee-hee-hoooo"—that is, taking a short, quick inhalation before uttering each "hee" and a longer inhalation before each "hoooo").

Unlike the Bradley method, Lamaze teaches various distraction techniques to help cope with the pain of labor, such as concentrating on a pleasant memory like a vacation or an older child. Lamaze techniques also include using a "birthing ball," hot and cold packs, and changing positions to help ease the pain of labor.

The Lamaze method is not as strict or regimented as Bradley and holds a neutral position on pain medication, as well as other forms of intervention during labor (such as pitocin to stimulate labor, vacuum/forceps delivery, and C-section).

If you are unsure on what is best for you, do some research to learn about these two techniques. Many women choose to use a little from each method to help cope with labor. For example, you could use the Lamaze method of breathing during a painful contraction, then try the Bradley method of long, deep, relaxing breaths in between contractions.

Bottom line: the Bradley method teaches women to FOCUS on their pain in order to help control it and the Lamaze method teaches DISTRACTION from pain. For more information, check out Bradleybirth.com (800-422-4784) and Lamaze.org (800-368-4404).

Q. What is hypnobirthing?

Hypnobirthing is having a baby while you are under hypnosis.

Classes on this technique teach expectant mothers and birth companions how to deal with anxiety, fear, and pain while in labor. The concept: create harmony between the mind and the body, remove bad thoughts

DR H'S OPINION: BIRTHING CLASSES

If you plan to attempt labor without an epidural or any type of pain medication, I absolutely recommend two things: 1) take a birthing class (see above on Bradley and Lamaze) and 2) seriously consider having a doula at your side. Among their many roles, doulas are a great resource for childbirth education and many offer prenatal classes as part of their global fee/package.

If you plan to have an epidural, taking a general childbirth class should be just right for you. You do not necessarily need to take a Lamaze and Bradley class. Here are the things you should find out:

1. Does the class teach a particular birthing philosophy or method? Or, is it broad-based, offering up several suggestions? (Think about what is best for you.)
2. What is the class size? (Small groups of five or fewer couples make it more individualized.)
3. Is the instructor certified? (You want to know what credentials the person has to teach the class.)

(fear or anxiety), and let the body function as nature intended.

Obstetrician Dr. Grantly Dick-Read came up with this concept in the 1930's, but several techniques have popped up since the 1980's. Hypnotherapist Marie Mongan developed the most popular one used today.

Hypnotherapists who specialize in childbirth hypnosis can offer a tailored approach towards individual women. If you have other phobias about childbirth—like being in a hospital or being poked with needles, this may be especially helpful for you.

Insider Secret

Many hospitals offer sibling classes and tours for the expectant big brother or sister. This may be useful so your toddler or pre-schooler isn't completely freaked out by the birth.

If this is your first baby, now may also be a good time to take an infant CPR class. You'll have very little spare time for classes once the baby is actually born.

Q. Do you recommend that I have a birth plan?

Do you need to have a written birth plan? No. Should you talk to your doctor about your vision for labor and delivery? Absolutely.

This advice has become *de rigueur* from some pregnancy books—the notion that you need a detailed written plan covering your labor and delivery.

In reality, you don't need a notarized document to use a birthing ball, dimmed lights, or play your iPod. Nor is a written request required to avoid using pain medication. No one is going to sneak an epidural into your back! Practitioners want you to have the most amazing experience possible, with a healthy mom and baby as the end result.

That said, you should talk to your practitioner about your wishes so he or she has an idea of how you see your labor and delivery. Do you want a natural childbirth? Do you want an epidural as soon as it is humanly possible? Discuss this with your doctor.

If you want to bring in a five-foot plastic ficus tree to decorate your

DR B'S TRUE STORY:
THE EIGHT HOUR BIRTHING CLASS

There are a variety of scheduling options for birthing classes . . . hour-long classes offered over several weeks, a full-day class, and even some weekend retreats held at swanky resorts so you can combine a babymoon and education.

Before you pay your course fee, I highly recommend you get an endorsement from your practitioner or even a friend. And take a class that fits both your schedule *and* your philosophy.

Because of our schedules, my husband and I chose an eight-hour marathon course at our delivery hospital. The course was almost more agonizing than my labor! We got up and left after a couple of hours. I figured I would just follow directions when I was told to push, which I did.

home stretch

delivery suite (Dr. B had a patient do this), it may be best to check with your practitioner first.

At the same time, it's important to remain flexible. Let's put that into bold caps: **REMAIN FLEXIBLE**. No one knows what lies ahead during labor and sometimes in-the-moment medical decisions must be made if unforeseen circumstances arise. Everyone's goal is to have you and your baby make it safely through delivery.

7 Things YOU can control during labor

1. Music. You can pick any genre you like, or decide you want complete silence!

2. Support. You can decide who is by your side and who sits in the waiting room (or flies out to see you *after* you get home).

3. Mobility. You choose whether you prefer to move around or remain in one place during labor. (The type of pain medication you receive may affect this decision.)

4. Lighting. During labor, you can do whatever you like. Your practitioner will need good lighting during delivery, however.

5. Use of pain medication. It's your call. It's also possible to change your mind during the experience (most, but not all, of the time).

6. IV Fluid. Depending on your individual situation, you may be able to decide if you want a capped IV ("Hep locked") or if you don't mind an IV that runs fluid and keeps you hydrated during childbirth.

7. Birthing position. If you opt out of an epidural for pain control, you can squat, use a birthing bar, or select a variety of other positions to get through your contractions as labor progresses.

Old Wives Tale
You'll get an enema when you go into labor. *False.*
Some women think they need a birth plan so they can avoid getting an enema when they are in labor. Truth is, enemas are not part of routine delivery protocol anymore—this went out of style about the same time as leisure suits.

It's true, though, that most women will have some sort of a bowel movement during the pushing phase of labor. It is almost inevitable: you use the same muscles to push the baby out as you do to poop.

The pressure of the baby's head pushes down on your rectum as he descends through the vagina. We know, it's embarrassing, but you can't control this and from the practitioner's end, this is as natural as breathing. The only one who has to know is your practitioner (and trust me, we don't care). She will quickly move it out of sight. We are so quick in fact, that one of my patients even dubbed me "Poo-dini" for the speed at which I cleaned her up and magically "hid" her poop from her hubby.

Q. What are my options for where I can deliver? How do I decide what is the best fit for me?

The three main options are a hospital, birthing center or at home.

Other options such as the car, back of an ambulance or on a stretcher in the elevator happen on occasion but obviously no one plans this!

Let's look at the different options. And why the type of delivery you want will influence this decision:

Hospitals. If you are strongly considering an epidural, then you should deliver at a hospital. And if you are a high-risk pregnancy, it is safest to deliver at a hospital.

If you want to have a physician deliver your baby, you will most likely need to deliver at a hospital as well. If your OB delivers at more than one hospital, you may consider choosing the one that is closest to you or take a tour to see which you like best. Here are some things to consider when you assess potential delivery hospitals:

◆ How many delivery rooms are there?
◆ Is there a neonatal intensive care unit (NICU)?
◆ Is there a specialist in the care of premature or sick newborns (**NEONATOLOGIST**) in the hospital 24/7? What happens if you need one and there isn't one on staff?
◆ Are there residents (doctors in specialty training) working in the hospital?
◆ Is there an **ANESTHESIOLOGIST** (the doc who performs that epidural/spinal) in the hospital at all times? What happens if there isn't one?
◆ How far is the hospital from your home?

Birthing centers, home birth. If you have a low-risk pregnancy and plan to have a natural childbirth, then you have several options (birthing center, home, etc). Of course, you may still choose to have a natural childbirth in a hospital too.

If you plan to have a midwife deliver your baby, find out whether she delivers at a hospital, birthing center, or at home. If you have your heart set on a home birth, don't just assume your midwife will be able to accommodate your request. It pays to ask!

And remember, if you choose a birthing center or home birth, find out what the back up plan is should an emergency arise. You'll want to know how a facility and practitioner outside of a hospital handle medical emergencies. This may help you decide where you feel the most comfortable.

Talk to your friends, do some research and talk to your provider to discuss what option is best for you.

Inductions

Q. My doctor has offered to do an induction. What is it? Is this a good idea?

An induction is the use of medication or other methods intended to bring on labor. Whether or not it is a good idea depends on the reason for the induction.

There are many medical and obstetrical reasons for recommending an induction, such as **PREECLAMPSIA**, , spontaneous rupture of membranes without labor, and going considerably past your due date (**POSTDATES**) to name a few. If your doctor recommends an induction for a medical reason,

home stretch

it's probably the safest plan for you and your baby.

If you are contemplating an *elective* induction or one for non-medical reasons—like your doctor will be out of town on your due date, you want your child to be a Virgo with Pisces as a rising sign, or you really want your baby to be born on a date other than your mother-in-law's birthday—you should carefully weigh the pros and the cons.

Although inducing a woman's labor is a safe procedure when done in a hospital, there are still inherent risks in using induction medication (Cervidil, misoprostol and/or pitocin). You have a slightly increased risk of needing a Cesarean section if your labor is induced, particularly if you are beginning your induction with an **UNFAVORABLE CERVIX** (this means a cervix that is not particularly "ready"). That being said, inducing someone on her second or third child is much easier and less likely to lead to a C-section compared to someone pregnant with her first child.

Doctors actually rate your cervix prior to induction to see how ready or "favorable" it is. This is expressed as a **BISHOP SCORE**, an equation that takes many variables into account—where the baby's head is in relation to certain bones in your pelvis, the dilation and effacement of your cervix, etc. (See more details on the Bishop Score in the box below). The greater the number on the Bishop score, the more likely you will have a successful vaginal delivery.

Bottom line: discuss your concerns with your OB. If you want an elective induction, you should decide together with your OB that this is the right thing for you and your baby.

Reality Check

To give you some perspective, here is a good example of when an elective induction just makes sense. I had a patient who was pregnant with her third child. She had fast labors with her other babies and her second child came after only three hours of labor.

She was here from a foreign country, didn't speak much English, and lived a good 60 minutes from the hospital where I perform my deliveries. Setting a date for an induction gave her time to set up a sitter for her two older children and the security of knowing she would deliver in the hospital . . . instead of in a car in the middle of a freeway during rush hour.

It also gave me time to line up a labor and delivery nurse who spoke fluent Russian to help translate and make her more comfortable.

Induction 411:
What does ACOG say about inductions?

Unless there is a good medical reason, your labor shouldn't be induced before 39 weeks. Why? Sometimes due dates aren't exact and your 38 3/7 week baby might really be a 36 or 37 week baby who is technically a premature or "**LATE PRETERM**" infant. These babies still have risks of having immature lungs, poor sucking technique, low blood sugar, and jaundice. This is not the way to start life if you can avoid it.

Q. What are the reasons that I might get induced?

There is a long list of both medical and obstetrical reasons for induction. For some women, having the baby is safer than continuing the pregnancy. You may be induced if you haven't gone into labor on your own before 41 or 42

HOME STRETCH

NEW PARENT 411: YOUR BISHOP SCORE

Want to know if you have a "favorable cervix" for being induced? Here's how the pros do it. Docs use a scoring system created in 1964 by Dr. E. Bishop—hence, the Bishop Score. It's extremely good at predicting if a woman is likely to have a successful vaginal delivery should she be induced.

A doctor examines a woman's cervix for the following measurements:

◆ Cervical consistency. (Is the cervix soft, medium or firm?)
◆ Position of the cervix as it relates to the vagina. (Is it way the heck in the back or can it be easily reached?)
◆ Amount of cervical dilation and effacement. (How thin is it?)
◆ Station of the presenting part. (Where is the baby's head in relation to specific bones in your pelvis?)

Here's how the scoring works:

SCORE	DILATATION	EFFACEMENT	STATION	POSITION	CONSISTENCY
0	closed	0 – 30%	-3	posterior	firm
1	1-2 cm	40 -50%	-2	mid-position	moderately firm
2	3-4 cm	60 -70%	-1,0	anterior	soft
3	5+ cm	80+%	+1,+2		

A point is added to your score for:

◆ Preeclampsia
◆ Each prior vaginal delivery

A point is subtracted from the score for:

◆ Postdate pregnancy
◆ Nulliparity (never having had a baby before)
◆ Premature or prolonged rupture of membranes

That is probably more than you ever wanted or needed to know about the Bishop Score. But here's the key part. Below is the percentage of moms who end up with a C-section, given a certain Bishop score:

C Section Rate, based on Bishop score

BISHOP SCORE	FIRST TIME MOTHERS	WOMEN WITH PREVIOUS VAGINAL DELIVERIES
Scores of 0–3:	45%	7.7%
Scores of 4–6:	10%	4%
Scores of 7–10:	1.4%	1%

Unless there is an emergency, practitioners generally only attempt induction when a mother has a favorable Bishop's score. What is favorable versus unfavorable?

Unfavorable (a score of 5 or less): If you have this score and you need an induction, you would qualify for medication to ripen your cervix (a prostaglandin-based product, such as Cervidil or misoprostol). This helps improve the Bishop Score and decreases your risk of needing a C-section.

Favorable (a score of 7 or more): Your cervix is very ripe or "favorable" and there is a high likelihood of having a successful vaginal delivery. *(Bishop EH)*

home stretch

weeks (**POSTDATES**). You may also be induced if you have a certain medical problem that puts you or your baby at risk if the pregnancy continues.

Here is a list of possible reasons to induce labor. While we haven't included every last possibility, here are the big ones:

Medical Reasons

◆ Lupus.

◆ Pre-existing diabetes.

◆ Pre-existing maternal kidney disease.

◆ Pre-existing maternal high blood pressure.

◆ Pre-existing chronic lung disease.

◆ Severe depression, anxiety or other psychiatric conditions.

Obstetrical Reasons

◆ Too little amniotic fluid (**OLIGOHYDRAMNIOS**).

◆ High blood pressure of pregnancy (**PREECLAMPSIA** and **ECLAMPSIA**).

◆ Syndrome of high blood pressure, blood cell and liver abnormalities (**HELLP SYNDROME**).

◆ Certain types of gestational diabetes.

◆ Pregnancy goes beyond 41-42 weeks (**POSTDATES** or postterm).

◆ Water bag breaks prematurely (**PREMATURE RUPTURE OF MEMBRANES**).

◆ Some cases where the placenta has begun to separate from the wall of the uterus (**PLACENTAL ABRUPTION**).

◆ Certain maternal infections (for example, **CHORIOAMNIONITIS**).

◆ Severe fetal growth restriction.

◆ Complications due to Rh blood type incompatibility (**RH ISOIMMUNIZATION**).

◆ Non-reassuring Non Stress Test (docs are concerned about abnormalities of the baby's heart rate detected on a monitor).

◆ Placental malfunction

◆ Pregnancy related liver problems (**CHOLESTASIS OF PREGNANCY** and **ACUTE FATTY LIVER**).

◆ Severe pregnancy related skin problem (**PUPPS**).

Other Reasons

◆ You live a far distance from the hospital.

◆ You have had rapid labor before.

Remember to check the glossary in the back of the book for an explanation of all these technical terms.

Helpful hint

Unless there is a good medical reason, your labor shouldn't be induced before 39 weeks. Are there any exceptions? Yes, if you have an amniocentesis to document that your baby's lungs are mature (able to hold oxygen and function normally), you might be induced and delivered before 39 weeks.

Q. What does it mean when someone gets "induced"?

It means you put someone into labor who previously was not in labor.

If you and your practitioner decide that it is time to schedule an induction, you set up an appointment at the hospital.

Yep, it's just like scheduling a haircut, except that the times may not be quite so ideal.

Occasionally, your practitioner detects something at an office visit that requires immediate induction (like severe high blood pressure or too little amniotic fluid). You might have to head straight over to the hospital or you may get the green light to run home quickly to grab your stuff first. Unlike your hairdresser, the hospital *will* take you if there is an emergency!

You will get admitted to the hospital and be evaluated in the same manner as if you went into labor on your own. Then, if your cervix is not ready or ripe (see earlier box on the Bishop Score), you will get medication to ripen it.

Next, you get another medication called oxytocin (Pitocin) through an IV to get labor started. We'll cover the details on how this all works in Chapter 13, Labor Day.

Factoid: In the United States, up to 18% of all labors are induced.

Q. What medications are used to induce labor?

Doctors use two different types of medications:

1. ***Acts on cervix.*** Prostaglandin is a natural agent your body makes that softens the cervix during labor. (If you recall from Chapter 8, Lifestyles, men also secrete prostaglandins with their sperm in their ejaculate.) For an induction, docs will use prostaglandin medication placed directly near the cervix to achieve the same results. Note: This is used for women with an unfavorable or unripe cervix.

   ◆ Cytotec (misoprostol) is a prostaglandin made into a pill form. It is placed near the cervix via a vaginal exam and dissolves over time.

   ◆ Cervidil is a prostaglandin in a mesh-like preparation that is placed near the cervix (also with a vaginal exam—let the good times roll!) and removed after 12 hours.

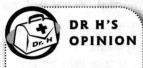

DR H'S OPINION

"At the hospital where I practice, induction times are as follows: 8 am, 10 am, 4 pm, 8 pm, 10 pm, midnight, 2 am, 4 am. You can imagine how the woman getting induced at 2 or 4 am feels!"

2. ***Acts on uterus.*** Oxytocin is a naturally occurring hormone made in the pituitary gland of your brain that causes uterine contractions and starts labor. (We give you this information in case you have a know-it-all brother-in-law who has a law degree but is trying to one up you on medical knowledge!) Pitocin is the brand name of the lab-made form of oxytocin used to stimulate contractions if your cervix is ripe.

You get this medication through an IV. Your practitioner controls the amount of medication you get because the IV is connected to a pump. You usually start off with a small dose, then your practitioner increases the amount gradually until you reach a desired contraction pattern (usually that means until you are having contractions two to three and a half minutes apart).

The amount you will need and for how long you will need it depends on how responsive your uterus is to the drug, what your Bishop score is prior to needing it, and how well your baby is tolerating labor. Some women need very little, and others need a lot.

The goal here is to give you just enough so that you have a contraction pattern that allows your cervix to dilate and your baby's head to descend. Likewise, docs want to avoid giving you too much to avoid contractions that are too frequent or last too long.

While you are on oxytocin, you are continuously monitored so that your practitioner can keep tabs on both your contraction pattern and the well-being of your little one.

Q. Will my doctor break my water bag during an induction?

Probably.

In addition to medication, your practitioner may also decide to perform an **AMNIOTOMY** (that's a fancy word for breaking your water bag).

Docs use a nifty little instrument that looks a lot like a crochet hook. We sneak it up along our fingers, which are sitting in the cervix, hook the amniotic sac, and rupture it. It doesn't hurt you any more than the discomfort of having your cervix examined. And it doesn't hurt the baby at all.

This will release prostaglandins that help ripen the cervix. Most women notice a dramatic change in the intensity of their contractions after their water bag breaks.

Q. My doctor said he could "strip my membranes" to help get me into labor. I'm not sure if that sounds sexy or painful. What will he do?

That term is just awful, isn't it? It is also sometimes referred to as "sweeping the membranes," but that doesn't sound much better.

Despite the inelegant word choice, it definitely describes what doctors do. Yes, it hurts. And yes, it might jumpstart your labor.

Stripping the membranes is done in term or post-term pregnancies, usually in your practitioner's office. To strip your membranes, your practitioner checks your cervix with a gloved finger. Next, he will place his finger through your cervix and sweep it between your amniotic sac (water bag) and the wall of your uterus. You may feel some intense cramping like period cramps.

This causes your body to release prostaglandins, which soften the cervix and may cause contractions. There is no guarantee, though, that stripping your membranes will lead to labor. It's common to have spotting for up to a day or two afterwards. If bleeding becomes heavier than this, call your doctor.

Q. I've heard inductions hurt a lot more. Is that true?

Yes and no.

The main difference between an induction and going into labor on your own is how rapidly your contractions start.

If you go into labor on your own, your body may start having irregular contractions over a period of days that slowly get stronger and closer together. You have some time to get used to the pain of the contractions as they slowly increase in intensity.

With an induction, those same contractions occur, but your doc is making them come on more quickly. So, the strength of each contraction is not necessarily stronger with Pitocin versus the natural oxytocin that your body makes, but you will experience the contractions in a much more condensed time frame.

Q. What are the risks involved with inducing labor?

The most common problem (which is rare) is that the medication used for an induction over-stimulates the uterus, causing it to contract too frequently.

Overall, the risk of anything happening from the use of Pitocin is very low. But over-stimulation of the uterus means that too many contractions occur at intervals that are too close together. The uterine muscle has no time to relax between contractions and this can cause problems for baby.

In short, this can decrease the amount of blood flow to baby, causing a drop in baby's heart rate. If this happens, your practitioner can lower the dose or stop the Pitocin and the effects wear off very quickly. If the baby recovers well, your practitioner will restart the Pitocin at a lower dose.

If the baby cannot tolerate the stress of the contractions and his heart rate pattern becomes concerning, a Cesarean section is in order. Note: your practitioner should be knowledgeable about Pitocin and should be monitoring you closely during the induction to modify the dosing, if necessary.

Like any other medication, misuse of Pitocin can cause some pretty nasty complications—which is why you want a skilled practitioner using it. But diligent and judicious use of Pitocin is a safe and effective way of inducing and augmenting labor.

Old Wives Tale: Self-induced labor?

You've probably heard it all by now, those wacky off the wall ideas to induce labor. Eating Thai food, taking an invigorating walk, having a salad drenched in balsamic vinegar. Or standing on your head while chewing the root of a rare lemongrass found only in the Himalayas (okay, kidding on the last one).

Can anything actually make you go into labor besides Mother Nature? Answer: nothing is a sure thing, but you can certainly try.

If you are a heterosexual couple, you have a source of natural prostaglandin—in your spouse's semen. Prostaglandin is the ingredient in many of our induction agents and when it comes in contact with a cervix that's ready, may induce labor (that's the reason that "pelvic rest" is recommended for women who are at risk for preterm labor).

We don't recommend trying to induce labor, unless you are at least 39 weeks along.

Nipple stimulation is another technique that almost always causes uterine contractions. It releases oxytocin, the body's natural Pitocin and stimulant of uterine contractions. In fact, prior to the widespread use of Pitocin,

? ?

HOME STRETCH

doctors used nipple stimulation to induce labor and evaluate a baby's heart rate pattern during these contractions. Today, however, nipple stimulation is NEVER recommended as a way to put yourself into labor.

The bottom line is that as uncomfortable as you are (and we've been there, trust us), you should wait for your labor to begin naturally or talk to your practitioner about an induction.

Old Wives Tale: More deliveries happen during a full moon or changes in barometric pressure. *FALSE!*

Does a full moon's gravitational pull affect amniotic fluid in much the same way it affects ocean tides? There have never been any studies on whether this is true or not, but it's hard to believe that the moon affects the small amount of water surrounding the baby in the same way as tides in the Atlantic Ocean.

There certainly are more visits to labor and delivery units during a full moon—but it's unclear why this happens. And these visits do not translate into more babies being born under a full moon. Many women are sent home after their contractions subside without any dilation of the cervix.

C-Sections

Q. **I'd love to have a C-section and get this all over with. How do you feel about elective C-sections?**

The official name for this is *primary elective Cesarean section*. It means this will be your first C-section and you are requesting one without a real medical or obstetric reason.

Elective C-sections have been trendy in the U.S. for the past five to ten years. In fact, 2% to 4% of all U.S. deliveries are primary elective C-sections. Some countries, like Brazil, deliver more than 50% of their babies by elective C-section for "perineal preservation" (keeping the vagina and surrounding tissues intact).

Why would you want one? Some women are afraid of labor and a vaginal delivery. There is fear of pain . . . or that your genital area will never be the same . . . or that you'll be incontinent as a result and need Depends forever. Others just fear being in labor for hours and then needing a C-section anyway.

And elective C-sections are certainly convenient. They can be scheduled on a specific date and you can have everything taken care of at home. It's also true that there is no risk of vaginal or anal tearing.

However, let's be clear here—it is *major* surgery and there are risks. As with any surgery, you face a risk of infection. Additionally, you're at risk for excessive bleeding and possible injury to surrounding body organs like the bladder and bowel during surgery.

On top of that, your baby faces the small risk of having difficulty breathing at birth, which sometimes requires admission to the neonatal intensive care unit (NICU). When a baby is delivered by C-section and does not squeeze through the birth canal, he may have some residual amniotic fluid in his lungs at birth that needs to be cleared out (**TRANSIENT TACHYPNEA**

OF THE NEWBORN or TTN).

We don't point these things out to scare you, but the truth is C-sections are not risk-free and the decision to perform one shouldn't be taken lightly. See more in the box below.

Here are some things to keep in mind if you are considering an elective C-section:

◆ Sit down with your partner and your doctor and make a list of all the potential risks and benefits so that you can make the best decision for you.

◆ Your doctor will consider your age, body mass index, accuracy of estimated gestational age, future reproductive plans, personal values, and cultural context before advising you.

◆ If you understand all the risks and benefits of each mode of delivery, and there are no absolute reasons not to have a C-section, most American doctors will perform elective C-sections.

Your baby should not be delivered electively prior to 39 weeks unless you make sure that your provider documents the baby's lungs are mature via amniocentesis (called *fetal lung maturity*).

Q. My doctor said she will do an elective C-section. How will this affect any future pregnancies I may have?

If you decide to have an elective C-section this time around, odds are any future babies you have will also be delivered by C-section.

Each C-section that you have increases the risk of having a **PLACENTA PREVIA, PLACENTA ACCRETA/INCRETA/PERCRETA**, and **UTERINE RUPTURE** (see Chapter 16, Complications, #37, 39). It also increases the possibility of a postpartum hysterectomy. Because of this, no one recommends elective C-sections for women who plan to have many children ("many" is hard to quantify but certainly more than three). *(ACOG)*

Risks and Benefits of Primary Elective C-sections

Interestingly, a panel of medical experts recently compared the risks and benefits of primary elective C-sections and normal vaginal deliveries and concluded that the information to date "does not provide the basis for a recommendation for either mode of delivery." *(National Institutes of Health.)*

DR H'S OPINION: ELECTIVE C-SECTIONS

I think that primary elective C-sections can and should be performed for patients upon request in certain circumstances. I say that with a caveat: they should *only* be performed if the patient is well informed. What is well informed? This means that the practitioner has discussed the potential risks, benefits and alternatives with the patient and her partner, there was ample opportunity for questions to be asked and answered, and the patient still desires to proceed.

And surprisingly, there was *no difference* in complication rates between the two types of delivery.

As OB/GYN's, we recognize that more research needs to be done. But what do we know about primary elective C-sections from the limited studies that we have? Here are the risks and benefits to both mom and baby:

Maternal Risks
◆ Longer hospital stay.
◆ Higher risk of anesthetic complications.
◆ Greater complications in future deliveries.
◆ Increased risk of inadvertent injury to adjacent organs such as the bladder and bowel.
◆ Increased need for **HYSTERECTOMY** to stop excessive bleeding (surgical removal of the uterus).
◆ Increased risk of significant blood accumulation in the wound.
◆ Increased risk of blood clots that can lead to death. *(Liu S)*
◆ Increased risk of heart attack after delivery.

Maternal Benefits
◆ Decreased risk of significant bleeding after delivery (**POSTPARTUM HEMORRHAGE**) that might require a blood transfusion.
◆ Fewer wetting "accidents" (**URINARY INCONTINENCE**) during the first year after surgery.

Fetal Risks
◆ If your baby has breathing problems at birth, he may need to stay longer in the hospital.
◆ Increased risk of breathing difficulties at birth if delivery is earlier than 39–40 weeks of gestation.
◆ For infants delivered before 39 weeks of gestation: increased rate of prematurity complications such as breathing difficulties, low blood sugar, and difficulty maintaining body temperature that require admission to the neonatal ICU (NICU).
◆ Risk of accidentally cutting the baby (fetal laceration). Although it only happens 0.8% of the time, yes, it's possible to accidentally superficially cut part of the baby when making the incision on the uterus.

Fetal Benefits
◆ Lower risk of fetal death.
◆ Lower newborn infection rate.
◆ Reduced risk of bleeding inside the skull.
◆ Reduced risk of lack of oxygen at birth and brain damage.
◆ Fewer birth injuries, such as injury to the nerves supplying the shoulder, arm, and hand (**BRACHIAL PLEXUS INJURIES**).

Q. I'd really like to deliver vaginally and NOT have a C-section. Is there anything I can do to prevent this from happening?

This is how most women feel. Although a few women would prefer to have an elective C-section, most would rather avoid it if possible.

There are a few cases where a C-section is planned for a medical or obstetric reason. For instance, you need a C-section if your baby is positioned to exit butt or foot first (**BREECH**) or your placenta is lying directly over your cervix (**PLACENTA PREVIA**).

Of course, even if you don't *plan* for a C-section, one might be recommended during delivery. Hence, you go into labor expecting to have a vaginal delivery and some situation arises where your doctor recommends a C-section (see box on next page). These are most often unpreventable.

Occasionally, a baby is too big to fit through a mom's pelvis—this happens sometimes because baby's head to too big or mom's pelvis is too small. The size of a baby can be hereditary (if you were a large baby, you will likely have a large baby), but it can also be due to excessive weight gain during pregnancy or uncontrolled diabetes.

Here's what you can do to lower your chances of having a C-section: keep your weight gain in the appropriate range and keep your blood sugar under control, if you are diabetic.

Your doctor doesn't want to do a C-section, either, if she can avoid it. But docs cannot always predict what happens during labor. If your doctor says the baby won't fit or is concerned about the baby's heart rate (and therefore is concerned about the amount of oxygen reaching the baby's brain), then a Cesarean delivery is the best thing for you and your baby.

The take-home message: be an informed patient. Ask questions and make sure you understand your practitioner's recommendations, including current and future implications.

Q. What's the difference between a planned or scheduled C-section versus an unplanned or emergency C-section?

A scheduled C-section occurs when you know in advance that there is a mother or baby issue requiring a C-section. Or you are deciding to have an elective C-section. In most cases, you will have adequate time to talk with your doctor about everything it entails and to go over the risks, benefits, and alternatives.

Unplanned or emergency C-sections happen when a vaginal delivery was otherwise planned for or was already in progress. Some condition then arises (see list below) requiring a C-section for a safe delivery. These are often heat of the moment decisions and depending on the condition may involve quick movement into the operating room (like what you see in the movies).

Reality Check: Emergency C-section

This can often be very scary for a laboring woman and her partner. While this is a RARE event, we want you to be prepared—so that's why you are reading it here before you go into labor.

Here is an emergency C-section scenario: monitors detect that the fetal heart rate is dropping. Many nurses and doctors and other hospital personnel enter the delivery room, attempting to help increase the fetal heart rate. This may include changing your position, turning off your Pitocin (if you are receiving some), placing an oxygen mask over your face (it will smell like plastic), giving you intravenous medication (if indicated) and performing a vaginal exam.

If they are unsuccessful, all of these people (and about 20 more!) rush

23 REASONS YOU MIGHT NEED A C-SECTION

Planned/Scheduled C-Sections

1. Baby is in a position that is dangerous to deliver vaginally (**BREECH** or **TRANSVERSE**).
2. Some types of twins (if one or both twins are in breech or transverse position).
3. Triplets or anything greater.
4. Certain fetal abnormalities/birth defects.
5. Placenta lies over the cervix (**PLACENTA PREVIA**).
6. Abnormal placenta (**PLACENTA ACCRETA, PLACENTA INCRETA, PLACENTA PERCRETA**).
7. Abnormal uterus (**BICORNUATE UTERUS, UTERINE DIDELPHYS**).
8. Previous C-section with a vertical uterine incision (often done when delivering preterm babies).
9. Previous surgery performed to remove uterine fibroids (some, but not all require future C-sections).
10. Estimated baby weight over ten lbs.
11. Significant tear in the genital area (fourth degree laceration) during previous delivery.
12. History of a baby's shoulder getting severely stuck (**SHOULDER DYSTOCIA**) during a previous delivery.
13. Mother has a medical condition that makes vaginal delivery too risky.

Unplanned/Emergency Section

14. Baby is too big to get through the birth canal (**CEPHALOPELVIC DISPROPORTION**).
15. Fetal Distress/Non-reassuring fetal heart rate. If your baby is at risk and you are not close to delivering, a C-section is needed.
16. Labor stops. Either you stop dilating or your baby's head stops descending through the birth canal (**FAILURE TO PROGRESS**).
17. Severely elevated blood pressure with or without seizures or blood cell/liver abnormalities (**PREECLAMPSIA, ECLAMPSIA, HELLP SYNDROME**) and delivery is not imminent.
18. Failed attempt at a vaginal delivery using a vacuum or forceps.
19. Placenta starts to tear away from the wall of the uterus before delivery (**PLACENTAL ABRUPTION**).
20. Umbilical cord slips out of the vagina after the water breaks and before delivery (**UMBILICAL CORD PROLAPSE**).
21. **UTERINE RUPTURE**.
22. Umbilical cord vessels or placental blood vessels lie over the cervix (**VASA PREVIA**).
23. Baby is breech, but it was not diagnosed before labor. Yes, it happens.

See Chapter 16, Complications for details on all of these situations.

you into the operating room. Many monitors are placed on your arms and chest, people are moving around at lightening speed and yelling orders left and right—there's a lot of commotion! I warn my patients that it will be a zoo and it will be scary. I ask them to try to keep calm, trust us and let us do what we need to do to get their baby out as quickly as possible.

Remember, no one can predict what will happen in labor. Although this situation rarely arises, it is important to trust the decisions made by your delivery team to ensure the delivery of a healthy baby.

Insider Secret: Scheduled C-sections

As with an induction, the magic number for having a scheduled C-section is 39 weeks. At any point before 39 weeks, you should first have an amniocentesis to confirm that your baby's lungs are mature.

A baby born between 37 and 38 weeks has between a ten and 26 times greater risk of immature lungs at birth compared to babies born between 39 and 41 weeks. *(Bakr AF)*

We should point out here that you DO NOT need to have an amniocentesis to deliver prior to 39 weeks if you are being delivered for a serious medical or obstetrical reason, such as severe preeclampsia at 35 weeks. The risk to the mom and baby are greater if the baby stays in versus coming out a little premature.

VBAC (Vaginal Birth After Cesarean)

Q. I had a C-section with my first pregnancy. Will I be able to deliver vaginally this time?

The answer is not straightforward. It depends on whether your doctor performs **VBAC's** (Vaginal Birth After Cesarean), whether the hospital where she delivers allows them, and what type of uterine scar you have.

There are two main types of C-section incisions: *low-transverse* and *vertical (also known as classical)*. The names describe the type of incision that is made on the uterus (not the outer cut on your skin, but the one on *inside* on your uterus).

Most C-sections (over 95%) are of the low-transverse type. Classical or large vertical incisions are rare and are mostly done to deliver a very premature infant.

If you used a different practitioner with your previous delivery, you'll need your medical records since the doctor's operative notes describe which type of incision you had.

If you had a vertical incision, you cannot have a subsequent vaginal birth. That's because you have a 4% to 9% risk of **UTERINE RUPTURE** (where the scar bursts open during labor). This is a risk that obstetricians and ACOG are not willing to take.

If you had a low-transverse incision, it may be possible for you to have a VBAC. The risk of uterine rupture after only *one* previous low-transverse C-section is much lower—between 0.7 and 0.8%.

Factoid: The C-section rate in the United States increased dramatically from 5% in 1970 to 34% in 2009. *(HealthGrades)*

Factoid: Many hospitals and physicians stopped allowing VBAC's in 2002.

Q. I'm worried that even if I decide to have a VBAC the second time, I will end up with a C-section again anyway. What are my chances of having the baby vaginally?

If you look at the studies, you have a 60% to 80% chance of success.

The problem is that we cannot reliably predict how any one individual patient will do.

In general, if you had your first C-section for a specific reason that tends not to re-occur with a subsequent pregnancy (such as a breech baby or a non-reassuring fetal heart pattern), you're more likely to have a successful vaginal delivery (between 75% to 86%).

If you had your first C-section because you stopped dilating or your baby's head was too big to fit through your pelvis, your success rate is lower (50% to 80%). *(ACOG)* Talk to your doctor about your wishes and to get her recommendation.

No VBAC's ALLOWED

There are certain women who should absolutely NOT have a vaginal delivery because of the high risk for uterine rupture.

You are a high-risk person if you have a previous classical or T-shaped uterine scar, previous uterine rupture, or two or more previous uterine scars.

Also, you can only have a VBAC delivery at a hospital—no home births, birthing centers, etc. That's because if you run into any complications, you need immediate access to an operating room and personnel capable of performing an emergency C-section. That's why home births are a no go in this scenario.

VBACs are also off the table if a complication arises that requires a C-section—like a placenta previa or a breech baby.

General Concerns

Q. I am delivering at a teaching hospital and I don't want an intern examining me, while 20 other folks look on. Is there a way to ensure crowd control?

Every teaching hospital is different.

If this is an important issue, you should discuss your concerns with your OB early on in your pregnancy. And remember that this is YOUR birth experience. If you absolutely do not want medical students or residents in the room, it is your right to say so.

You can decide how many people are in there (you won't care at a certain point—trust us)—just one additional intern or enough to require stadium seating.

Talk to your doctor about the kind of hospital she practices in, teaching or non-teaching, and discuss your concerns.

Q. How will I know I am really in labor versus having false contractions?

Braxton Hicks refer to "practice contractions" and they occur at various times during pregnancy, but can increase in intensity during your last month.

They happen at random, often in the middle of the night, and are associated with a hardening or tightening of your belly. Some women do experience mild menstrual-like cramping associated with Braxton Hicks (BH), but typically, they are not very painful.

The most important difference between Braxton Hicks contractions and real labor contractions is that BH contractions do not dilate the cervix and real contractions do.

Real labor contractions are *painful*. They often have a pattern to them, so for example, they will begin at intervals of 20 minutes apart and gradually shorten—becoming ten, seven, and then five minutes apart. They are often, but not always, accompanied by an increase in mucous discharge and sometimes, bloody show.

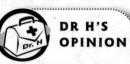

DR H'S OPINION

"Real contractions hurt. I have only had one patient in 12 years who felt like she was having some mild stomach discomfort and was actually nine centimeters dilated! We all want to be that woman (believe me, I prayed for it every night starting at about 26 weeks), but in reality, 99.9% of us will feel labor when it happens.

home stretch

Q. When do I call my doctor?

All physicians do things a little differently. Find out what *your* doctor wants you to do and when he or she wants to be called. As an OB, here is what I tell my patients:

◆ *If you are beyond 35 weeks*:
Call when contractions are consistently five minutes apart for two hours.

◆ *If you are less than 35 weeks*:
Call if you have more than four to six contractions in an hour and they do not resolve with rest and drinking lots of water.

◆ *If your water breaks*:
This is not usually the first sign of labor. Your water bag most often breaks after you have been contracting for a while. Alternatively, your doctor might break it for you at the hospital. If it does break, it's not always like the movies, where you are mulling over peas in the frozen foods aisle and suddenly you are standing in Niagara Falls. Often it's just a leak that doesn't stop or a constant sense of wetness. Call your practitioner for this one, no matter how far along you are in your pregnancy.

◆ *If you have vaginal bleeding*:
A little bit of spotting (pinkish, reddish, brownish discharge) is OK as

TRUE LABOR VS. FALSE LABOR: BOOKMARK THIS PAGE

True Labor
- ◆ Contractions occur at regular intervals.
- ◆ Contraction intensity and discomfort gradually increases.
- ◆ Intervals between contractions gradually decrease.
- ◆ Discomfort occurs in the lower back and abdomen.
- ◆ May be accompanied by increased vaginal discharge or bloody show.
- ◆ Contractions cause cervical dilation.
- ◆ Contractions do not stop with rest, hydration or medication.

False Labor
- ◆ Contractions occur at irregular intervals.
- ◆ Contraction intensity and discomfort remain unchanged.
- ◆ Intervals between contractions remain long.
- ◆ Discomfort is mainly in the lower abdomen, or no discomfort other than tightening.
- ◆ No accompanying bloody show.
- ◆ The cervix does not dilate.
- ◆ Discomfort from contractions is relieved by rest and medication.

your pregnancy comes to an end, especially if you have had recent intercourse or your practitioner has recently checked your cervix. Anything more than spotting deserves a phone call to your doc. And any bleeding during a high-risk pregnancy (preterm labor or placenta previa, for example) should be discussed with your practitioner as well.

◆ Decreased fetal movement:

Monitor your baby's daily movements. In the final weeks of pregnancy, your baby's movements will be smoother and less noticeable than those jolting kicks in the second trimester (because your baby has less space to move around). But you still need to feel them. Call your practitioner if you detect fewer movements.

Partner tip: Just the facts, ma'am

When you call the OB (you are likely making the call because your partner is so uncomfortable she wants to die), keep your cool and stick to the facts. We know you haven't been sleeping and you're nervous/excited/full of adrenaline about what's to come.

I'll be very honest here. When docs get that phone call in the middle of the night, it often wakes us out of a deep sleep. It takes us a few moments to get focused. It's hard to follow someone talking at an auctioneer's pace and going into excruciating detail about how the new chair is ruined because of the bloody show all over it.

Or, my personal favorite is a patient's husband (who I love dearly after going through two pregnancies with him) who gave me an in depth run down on the contraction pattern like a football game commentary. I listened patiently (at 4am) for over four minutes as he told me about the timing and length of each contraction from start to finish, the intensity of each, what his wife was doing during each contraction, what she ate for dinner and finally what she threw up! I still give him a hard time about this and we always have a good laugh.

Bottom line: keep it simple. Here's an example: "Hi Dr. H, it's Paul Smith, Sarah's husband. She has been contracting every five minutes for about three hours, is having some bloody discharge and is really uncomfortable. We'd like to go to the hospital now." That's perfect. It's easy for us to understand, sticks to the facts, and allows our sleepy brains to get a handle on the situation.

Q. My mother had very quick deliveries. I don't want to deliver on the highway. Are my chances any greater with my mom's history?

Let's start with a definition of "very quick deliveries" or in technical terms, a "**PRECIPITOUS LABOR.**" That's a labor that lasts less than three hours from start to finish.

While there aren't any firm stats on this, it happens in about two in every 100 births.

It's more likely to naturally happen if you have delivered a baby before because your first baby paves the way for the next one. Or you've had a prior precipitous delivery. Or you have a large pelvis. Or you have a well-positioned and smaller than average baby. It can also happen artificially if you receive too much pitocin or use cocaine.

I hate to disappoint you, but it's an old wives tale that labor patterns run in families. (Especially if your mom told you she had quick, easy deliveries!) It's true, though, that you may inherit the shape of your pelvis (a.k.a. "good birthing hips") from your mom, which may be a positive.

But you have to factor several other variables that affect the ease or difficulty of labor and delivery. For instance, you might want to see if your hubbie has a big head (literally)—and then pray, for delivery sake, your baby doesn't inherit that trait!

Factoid: Women who have given birth before start having contractions earlier in their subsequent pregnancies and have them more often than those who've never given birth. By the time you are on your third or fourth pregnancy (if you are one of the brave), you are having so many Braxton Hicks that you feel like you will be delivering in your kitchen!

Q. Do tall women have easier deliveries than short women?

Yes. Women less than five feet tall (especially those who have never given birth before) have twice the risk of having a C-section. Why? That's often due to the baby's head being too big to fit through mom's pelvic bones (**CEPHALOPELVIC DISPROPORTION**).

The C-section rate *increases* as mom's height *decreases*—maxing out at 30% of women who are under four feet, six inches tall.

If you have normal stature or are just slightly smaller than average, you don't have any higher risk of a complicated delivery. And if you were teased in high school for being head and shoulders above your classmates, you can now thank (instead of curse) your parents' genes. They may just make your labor easier. *(Cnattinguis R, McGuinness BJ).*

HOME STRETCH

? ?

Top 13 fears about labor—and how to defeat them

From the home office in Beverly Hills, California, we present the top 13 fears about labor:

13. I want a natural childbirth and I'll end up with a C-section.
12. I'll be in pain and it will be too late to get pain medication.
11. Something bad will happen to the baby.
10. Something bad will happen to me.
9. There will be horrible traffic on the highway and I'll deliver in my car.
8. I won't know what contractions will feel like or when I'm really in labor.
7. I'll never deliver and I'll be pregnant forever.
6. My body will never be the same after this.
5. I'll never want to have another baby after I deliver this one.
4. My doctor will be in Jamaica when I go into labor.
3. If my husband sees anything down below he will never want to be intimate with me again.
2. My epidural won't work, I will have chronic back pain or be paralyzed after receiving one.
1. I will poop during my delivery.

How can you ease your fears? Educate yourself! Read books, watch DVDs, take a childbirth class, and talk to your doctor/midwife/doula.

You have to feel comfortable asking your practitioner about your concerns

OTHER PEOPLE'S WAR STORIES

You may not know this, but there's a sorority for women who've given birth before. And like all sororities, the initiation ceremony is a secret ritual that's only known to those in the club.

Most of us in the club won't tell you the nitty gritty details of our labor and delivery experience (a.k.a. the initiation ritual). We only share it with other members who are already in the sorority.

This unwritten rule is usually followed. We abide by it because we don't want to scare the living daylights out of you. And Mother Nature has a way of erasing those memories with the amazing joy of holding a newborn afterwards.

If it's your mother we're talking about, she won't tell you because she was either completely knocked out with laughing gas when she gave birth to you . . . or she wants more grandchildren.

However, there are a few sorority girls who break the rules. A few chatty Cathy's want to relive their labor experience with you, even if you don't ask them to share these personal details.

We suggest finding a good exit strategy if you encounter one of these women at the summer office party or in line at Costco. Hearing these stories are not helpful to your mental state, nor terribly useful to your prenatal education.

After you deliver, welcome to the club. And remember, mum's the word.

and anxieties. This is the whole reason for choosing a practitioner that you love.

Of course, it's normal to have these thoughts run through your head in the middle of the night when you get up to pee, keeping you from going back to sleep. Your brain will rest easier if you get these questions answered (of course, the disrupted sleep patterns are still out of our control).

FYI: *Wondering about your pain medication options?* We discuss all pain medications in Chapter 13, Labor Day. It will help you know what your options are.

Q. When should I pack a bag for the hospital, and what should go in it?

Pack it up at 33 to 34 weeks.

And keep it light—it's not like you're going to summer camp for a month. Your partner (or whoever is staying with you at the hospital) should pack a bag, too.

Yes, this seems early, but if you pack now, you won't have to panic if you break your water bag at 2am when you are 35 weeks.

Keep items you will need during labor separate from things you'll need while you recover. Here's a packing list:

♦ *Your own toiletries*—toothbrush, toothpaste, shampoo, conditioner, face soap, face lotion and lip balm (this is a lifesaver during labor!).

♦ *A robe.* You can also bring your own PJs to sleep in after delivery is over. You'll wear a hospital gown during labor.

♦ *Hair ties.*

♦ *Socks for labor and slippers or flip-flops for afterwards.*

♦ *An outfit to go home in.* Select a comfy maternity outfit because your baby bump won't disappear for several weeks.

♦ *An outfit for the baby to go home in.* Note: a two-piece outfit is better since the baby will have his umbilical stump for a couple of weeks or so. One-piece outfits or "onesies" can rub on the stump.

♦ *Food and drink.* Check with your doc regarding hospital policy on eating/drinking during labor. If allowed, you may want to bring things to sip on or hard candy to suck on.

♦ *BYOP. (P is for Pillow)* Some women like to bring their own pillows. If you do, be forewarned that it may go home a little bloody as deliveries can be a messy sport.

♦ *Camera/Video camera.* Some people also bring in their laptops and download baby pictures shortly after delivery. You probably shouldn't stream the birth live on Skype unless your partner is deployed in the military.

♦ *Cord blood collection kit if you are using one.*

♦ *List of relatives/friends to be notified once baby is born.*

◆ Insurance card and Driver's License or another form of picture I.D.

◆ If you are a second or third time parent, pictures of your older child/ren to put in the room when they come to visit.

◆ If allowed, bring your own music/iPod.

◆ If allowed, whatever else you need that provides comfort to you or you feel will aid you in the labor/delivery experience.

◆ The baby's car seat, properly installed. The hospital will only release the baby home in a vehicle that contains an infant car seat. And no, the nurses won't give you a car seat demonstration at checkout. You are responsible for doing this before you use it for the first time. (See helpful hint below)

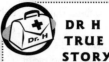

DR H TRUE STORY

"I've had patients bring anything from an old sweater knitted by her grandmother to a baby blanket that was hers when she was a baby."

Helpful hint: Car seats

Installing an infant car seat isn't as easy as it should be—and this vexes many first-time parents. Yet correct installation is crucial to protect your newborn.

If you need help, contact a local baby gear store. And getting your car seat installation safety checked is another wise move—fire stations, car dealers and other local groups do these checks for free. Go online to Children's Hospital of Philadelphia at chop.edu/carseat for a demonstration or the National Highway Traffic Safety Administration at nhtsa.gov for more details.

Our sister book *Baby Bargains* rates and reviews the best infant and convertible car seats, along with advice on how to make sure you get a rock solid install. See the back of this book for details.

Nesting

In the final weeks before delivery, your nesting instinct will kick in. Just like a momma bird, you too will have an overwhelming urge to prepare your nest for your little one. If you want to use all that energy in a productive way (instead of rearranging your kitchen cabinets, which is what Dr. H did), here are our suggestions:

Have these items for YOU when you return home

◆ *Lots of BIG sanitary pads.* I mean the BIG ones, like you used in high school before you discovered the beauty of tampons.
◆ *Nursing bras.*
◆ *Nursing pads.*
◆ *Lanolin ointment.* If you are nursing, this is a lifesaver for cracked nipples. It also works well for your baby's diaper rash!

- *Ibuprofen.* Brand names: Advil or Motrin
- *Comfortable sleepwear.* Not that you will actually be sleeping!
- *Breast pump and all of its paraphernalia if you plan to use one.* You can also research renting a hospital-grade breast pump from a local hospital, nursing supply store, or lactation consultant.
- *Nursing pillow.* Dr B's favorite is "My Brest Friend" for comfort and best positioning.
- *Soothies.* Gel pads for soothing nipples.

Have these items for BABY when you return home

- *Diapers.* If you are doing disposable diapers, you won't need the newborn size for too long, so don't buy a box full of them. Babies quickly go to "Stage 1".
- *Diaper rash cream.* Anything that's zinc oxide or petroleum based will do. Aquaphor is a personal favorite.
- *Baby wipes.* Yes, they are safe to use.
- *A bassinet or crib for baby to sleep in.*
- *Baby clothes.* If you didn't get an entire wardrobe at your baby shower, steer clear of buying expensive newborn outfits that are outgrown in a matter of weeks. No name onesies are more practical, cheaper and easier to clean after spit up happens!
- *Sleeper pajamas.* Pick the right fabric for the season your baby is born. Light cotton works for summer, and fleece is fine for winter.
- *Swaddle blankets.* Learn how to do the baby burrito wrap from the nurses at the hospital! You may also want to check out the Miracle Blanket–very popular with newborns.
- *Burp cloths.* You'll need lots of those. Cloth diapers make great burp cloths.
- *Pacifiers if you plan to use them.* If you are breastfeeding, I suggest the Soothie brand which is more similar to mom's nipple.
- *Bottles if you plan to use them.* You never know what might happen, so get at least one for emergency use.
- *Formula if you plan to use it.* Pediatricians usually recommend a cow's milk based formula with iron, but ask your baby doc for advice if you have specific health concerns.
- *Digital rectal thermometer.* Yes, this is how you need to take your baby's temperature. Fancy ear thermometers, pacifier thermometers, etc. are not accurate enough for a newborn.
- *Perfume and dye free bathing soap.* Brand names: Aveeno, Cetaphil, Dove.
- *Perfume and dye free laundry detergent.* Brand names: Tide Free, All Free and Clear.
- *Distilled, bottled water* to prepare formula.
- *Breast pump* if you are nursing.
- *2 x 2 or 3 x 3 gauze pads* if your son has a circumcision in his future.
- *Big tub of petroleum jelly* (Vaseline). Good for when you need to use the rectal thermometer, circumcision care, and as diaper rash cream.
- *Emory board/Nail file.* Newborns are too young for nail clippers.

- *Saline nose drops.* Good for stuffy noses.
- *Vitamin D Drops* (D-vi-sol or Tri-vi-sol). Your baby will need a Vitamin D supplement.

Partner tip: Do hospital reconnaissance

If you don't take a childbirth class at the hospital where you are delivering, be sure to know where to go when your partner goes into labor. Arrange to take a tour or do a practice run, so you know where to park and where to go at 2am.

Partner Tip

Want to score bonus points? Line up a babysitter and/or pet-sitter now, for the big day. You may be out of your home for 24 hours or more and Fido can't cross his legs for that long! Your partner will be relieved to not have to worry about this item.

Now you are really ready to go. The next chapter will walk you through the day you've been waiting for.

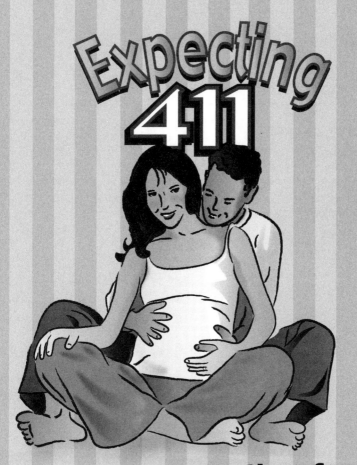

Expecting 411

section four

The Big Event

LABOR DAY

Chapter 13

"I like trying [to get pregnant]. I'm not so sure about childbirth."
—Mary Ann Evans

L et's pretend that you, indeed, are in labor and there is no turning back. Of course, you'll want to read this chapter before this day actually happens (you won't want to read it in between contractions). This chapter will give you all the details you will need to prepare for the big day (or night!).

First, we'll discuss giving birth at a hospital—what to expect, who will be helping with the birth and so on. Next we'll discuss the labor process at a birthing center and at home.

Factoid: Most women go into spontaneous labor (inductions don't count!) at night or in the wee hours of the morning. And they usually deliver in the afternoon or early evening.

Q. What is labor anyway?

Labor means you have regular uterine contractions that make your cervix open (dilate) and thin out (efface). It is what allows the baby to descend from inside your uterus, through the birth canal to the outside. There are three stages of labor, defined by the changes that occur in your uterus and cervix.

First Stage

- ◆ Begins with the onset of labor and ends when your cervix is ten centimeters dilated and 100% effaced (completely thinned out).

- The average length of this stage for first-time moms is between ten and 14 hours.
- The length is shorter for women who've delivered babies before.

Second Stage (Pushing and Delivery)
- Begins when the cervix is completely dilated and ends with the birth of the baby (this is the pushing phase of labor).
- The average length for first time moms is between one and two hours.
- The length of this stage is shorter for women who've done this before, averaging less than an hour.

Third Stage (Afterbirth)
- Begins with the birth of the baby and ends with delivery of the placenta.
- The average length for this stage for all vaginal deliveries, whether this is your first or your fourth, is between five and 15 minutes.

Reality Check

Labor takes longer if you've never done it before.

For women who haven't had a child before, the average length of labor is anywhere from ten to 14 hours. This is broken down into eight to 12 hours for the first stage (see above) and one to two hours for the second stage.

For women who have had at least one baby, labor is usually much quicker. Typically, the more babies you have had, the quicker the labor. The average is four to six hours for the first stage and less than one hour for the second stage.

These ranges are slightly longer if you get regional anesthesia (epidural or spinal).

Q. How does it all work?

Delivering a baby is a fascinating, well-orchestrated process.

Labor involves a few key players: your cervix, your uterus, two hormones (oxytocin and prostaglandin) and, of course, your baby. The production and release of oxytocin from your brain tells your uterus (which is really just a big, specialized muscle) to contract.

The contractions are doing important work. They help to open the cervix, which has been tightly closed since the start of pregnancy. They also push the baby's head against the cervix—this helps to open the cervix further.

The cervix must be fully thinned out (effaced) and fully opened (dilated) to allow the baby's head to pass through the vagina. Contractions also help (along with your efforts) to push the baby through the vagina. They will become more intense, last longer, and come closer together until the birth of the baby.

During active labor, the fluid-filled amniotic sac where your baby has lived for the past nine-ish months may rupture (your "water" may "break") or your practitioner may rupture it for you. Once your water has broken, more prostaglandins are released and your contractions become more intense.

Q. What causes labor?

No one knows.

Yep, we've been able to map the human genome and invent vaccines to stop cancer . . . but we still don't know what actually causes a woman to go into labor.

One theory: baby triggers labor. At some late stage of pregnancy, your baby sends a signal (whether it is hormonal, from the baby's adrenal gland, or the release of a certain fetal protein) that enters into your bloodstream. This substance is thought to signal your body to start labor, probably through the release of maternal oxytocin. Oxytocin is the hormone that stimulates contractions. (Pitocin is a synthetic form of oxytocin that is routinely used to induce labor).

That's why all those tricks to induce labor (balsamic vinegar salad dressing, anyone?) don't work . . . until your baby tells your body to do its thing.

Q. Once my labor starts, how long does it usually take to deliver?

Everyone asks this question, but there is no easy answer.

Families often like to make bets and create large pools with spreadsheets that rival March Madness brackets. But even for someone like me who does this everyday, it's tough to predict. Here are the variables that are involved:

- How many babies you've had in the past.
- Duration of previous labors.
- Baby's estimated weight.
- The reason for the induction (if you are induced).
- Your Bishop score (see Chapter 12, Home Stretch) at the start of labor (or your induction).

Your practitioner can give you a ballpark estimate of how long you will be in labor. Just don't ask her to bet on it!

The Walk-Through: Hospital Experience

Q. Where am I supposed to go at the hospital?

Know where you are going *before* the big day. If you take a tour of the hospital/maternity floor, this is the perfect time to inquire. You can also just ask your practitioner.

Some hospitals want you to go through the emergency room and oth-

---

**DR H'S TRUE STORY:
DON'T PARK IN THE RED ZONE!**

It's also important to know where to park! One of my patient's husbands was so flustered by his wife's labor that he parked in a red zone outside the ER. When he went back down to get his wife's things, he found that his car had been towed!

labor day

ers prefer that you come straight to labor and delivery. Figure out which entrance is best (hospitals usually have several), and on which floor labor and delivery is located.

Q. Will I automatically get admitted to the hospital?

No. You only get to stay if you prove you are actually in labor. So, don't just show up at the hospital on the day you'd *like* to deliver and hope they will let you in.

Most labor and delivery units have a triage system to help decide who stays and who goes. Usually, a labor and delivery nurse will do your initial assessment and check your vital signs. You get to pee in a container (yeah, we know, again, and it's nearly impossible at this point) and change into a hospital gown. Heads up—it is open in the back, so if your whole family has come with you in hopes that today is the big day, turn with caution!

Then, you'll have to answer a million questions, some of which are irritating if you are actually in labor since you are trying to think and breathe at the same time. (You won't feel like discussing your dietary preferences or the last time you had a bowel movement!)

Next comes the monitor hookup. You will wear two small plastic devices that are fastened to your belly by Velcro straps. One is an external fetal monitor (a monitor used to pick up the baby's heart rate and pattern) and the other is a pressure-sensing device (TOCO; a monitor used to pick up uterine contractions).

If you are leaking, you will get a special examination to determine whether you've broken your water bag. Depending on the delivery hospital, it will be a nurse, midwife, resident (doctor in specialty training), or obstetrician who does the exam. That person inserts a sterile speculum into your vagina to collect a specimen of fluid and determine if it's really amniotic fluid (or just pee or vaginal discharge).

If you aren't complaining of leaking, the healthcare provider will examine your cervix with his or her fingers. This isn't very comfortable, but it's quick and necessary.

The hospital staff gives all of this information to your obstetrician. And if your water bag has broken or you are officially in labor, you will be admitted.

Q. What happens after I am admitted?

Once you get the green light for admission, one of the friendly hospital staff escorts you to the labor room. You'll either walk or catch a ride in a wheelchair.

All hospitals are different when it comes to labor rooms. You might spend some time in a smaller room in early labor, and then move to a larger room when you become more active and delivery is imminent. Or you'll labor in one room and deliver in an operating/delivery room. Or you may have one deluxe suite for the entire time.

After you get into bed and you're in that attractive hospital gown, the usual protocol is to hook you back up to the fetal monitors and give you an IV (that involves a needle going into a vein in your arm or hand, but your contractions are more painful than that so you really won't care).

IV stands for "intravenous" line—a small tube that allows access into one of your veins so that you can receive fluids and medications. The healthcare provider who starts the IV will collect some of your blood at the same time. That's used to check your blood type, a complete blood count (looking for signs of infection, anemia, or a low platelet count), and to obtain a specimen for a cord blood collection kit if you are doing one. It is standard to get IV fluid to keep you well hydrated, unless your doc specifies differently. Dehydration can be a risk factor for a labor that fails to progress (and leads to a C-section).

Note: You only get pain medication through that IV if you request it. Contrary to what you might hear in childbirth class, no one can give you ANYTHING without your consent.

Once you are settled in and the procedures are over with, you might as well get cozy (as much as possible). You'll be hanging out with your partner for the next ten to 14 hours as you go through the first stage of labor.

Q. I tested positive for Group B Strep during pregnancy. Is there anything special that needs to happen?

Yes.

If you tested positive for Group B Strep (GBS) during your pregnancy, you will get intravenous (IV) antibiotics during labor to protect your baby. We discuss why this is so important in Chapter 5, Tests.

Penicillin or ampicillin are the antibiotics specifically used for GBS. If you are allergic to penicillin or one of its relatives, there are other antibiotic options. Your prenatal records (which should be at the hospital) document medication allergies, but it's always a good idea to tell your nurse if you have any drug allergies.

Reality Check

If you go into labor before 37 weeks and haven't been tested for Group B Strep, you will be treated as if you are positive and you'll get IV antibiotics during labor. This is extremely important, since premature babies are at much higher risk of getting infected with GBS.

Q. Can I eat or drink anything while I am in labor?

Docs used to tell women that they could have nothing but ice chips once the labor process began. There are two reasons for that:

Labor makes some women queasy and that often leads to vomiting. It's easier to clean up water than a chicken burrito with extra hot sauce.

If you end up needing an emergency C-section, it's best to have an empty stomach during surgery. (If you need general anesthesia, that food could end up in your lungs and potentially cause pneumonia. More than you wanted to know, right?)

But those rules have changed a little bit. Ask your OB to find out the specific guidelines you should follow. Once you get to the hospital, you probably won't be allowed to eat, but most hospitals have relaxed their guidelines in recent years. At the very least, you can sip on liquids throughout labor. You might also be able to eat popsicles or suck on hard candy. Find out the answer to this question at your pre-labor hospital visit.

LABOR DAY

Partner Tip

If you decide to get a burger on the way in to the hospital, leave off the onions. Your laboring partner will smell your breath constantly for the next several hours . . . and we probably don't have to warn you about how moody she'll be during labor.

Vaginal Deliveries

New Parent 411: A Vaginal Delivery in 13 easy steps

Step 1: You go into labor and get admitted to your hospital or birthing center. Or you arrive for your induction.

Step 2: You move to your delivery or birthing suite.

Step 3: You get hooked up to monitors.

Step 4: You get an IV placed and blood drawn (it's only one needle stick!).

Step 5: You and your partner hang out while your contractions become more frequent and more uncomfortable during the first stage of labor.

Step 6: Your nurse checks on you often and your practitioner (or another healthcare provider) examines you to check your progress every couple of hours.

Step 7: You notify your medical team if/when you would like to receive any pain medication.

Step 8: If you desire pain medication by epidural, an anesthesiologist arrives to place it.

Step 9: You reach ten centimeters (cm) dilation and it's time to push.

Step 10: Find a position that works for you, and go for it. Your partner, support people, and medical team keep you focused and pushing.

Step 11: Your baby arrives! Piece-o-cake, right?

Step 12: Umbilical cord is cut.

Step 13: The placenta is delivered.

Q. Who will examine me?

This is going to depend on the hospital (see below) and where your practitioner is at the moment. If are going to a:

◆ *Public hospital:* a nurse or the obstetrician on call will examine you.

◆ *Community hospital:* a nurse, your practitioner, or the person on-call for your practitioner will examine you.

◆ *Teaching hospital:* a nurse, midwife, resident, or attending physician will examine you. However, even in a teaching hospital, it's possible that your own doctor is the one doing most or all of the internal exams.

While you are in the first stage of labor (remember, that's ten to 14 hours on average), your practitioner may need to check on other patients who are in labor, or she may need to run back to her office to see patients.

LABOR DAY

Vaginal Delivery, in nutshell

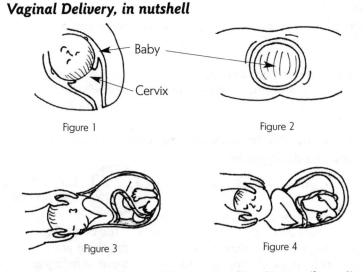

Figure 1

Figure 2

Figure 3

Figure 4

Baby remains in the uterus until the cervix is dilated ten cm (figure 1), then makes her way down the birth canal until the head emerges (figure 2). Your practitioner delivers your baby's head first, followed by the shoulders (figure 3). Then the rest of the baby is delivered (figure 4).

If there is a problem or your doc needs to know how far along you are after three or four hours (and she is at the office seeing patients), she may ask the nurse to examine you and relay the information to her.

If there is an absolute emergency requiring a procedure or intervention and she is not at the hospital, a resident or fellow (docs in specialty training) in a teaching hospital or a colleague in a community hospital might evaluate you.

Your job: trust that you will be in very capable hands.

Types of Hospitals

Public. These hospitals primarily (but not exclusively) care for indigent populations in cities. Some of them are also teaching hospitals.

Community. These are smaller hospitals that provide standard care. The doctors on the hospital staff usually have private practices near the facility.

Teaching. These hospitals are affiliated with medical institutions that train medical students, physicians in specialty training (interns, residents, fellows), and other healthcare professionals. Senior physicians (attending physicians) supervise those in training and see clinic patients or have their own private practices. Teaching hospitals are often regional referral centers for complex medical cases.

Q. How many internal exams will I have?

It depends. In general, you get one about every two to four hours during labor.

These exams help your practitioner figure out how your labor is progressing. If your labor is going slowly, expect more exams.

Here are a few rules:

You get *more* if you are being induced and you start with a low Bishop

labor day

Score (see Chapter 12, Home Stretch).

You get *less* if your water bag is broken right off the bat, particularly if you are known to be Group B Strep positive.*

Every internal exam introduces some bacteria into the cervix and uterus, even if your practitioner uses sterile gloves. That's why your doc will try to limit the number of internal exams once your amniotic sac is ruptured.

Q. Will I be able to walk around, take a shower, or use a bouncy ball during labor?

It depends on if you have an epidural or not.

If you *don't* have an epidural (or until you get one placed) and your baby's heart rate tracing looks good on the monitor, most practitioners will let you walk around, get into a bathtub, or use a birthing ball (see box below).

Most of the time, you just need to check in periodically. You get hooked up to the fetal heart rate monitor for 20 minutes to be sure all is well and then you get another 40 minutes of freedom.

If you really want to roam around during labor, see if your delivery hospital offers *"ambulatory monitoring."* That's a portable monitor that connects to a computer and allows staff to track your baby's heart rate while you pace the hallway and move into different positions.

If you *do* have a typical epidural, you won't be able to walk around because the nerves that are used to help your muscles move are being "blocked" by the pain medication. Some hospitals now offer *"walking epidurals"* that do allow for more movement. Talk to your practitioner about what is available to you.

> **DR H'S OPINION**
>
> *"You can bring anything you want to help you labor, but here's the bottom line: be flexible about how your labor will go. A successful delivery ends with a healthy mom and baby. It's doesn't matter how you accomplish that goal. And you don't get graded on style points!"*

Reality Check

Don't assume that your hospital's labor room will have a bathtub or shower. There may only be a few select rooms that offer those amenities. If you want one of those rooms, request it in advance or when you get admitted.

Q. How is the baby monitored while I am in labor?

In a hospital setting, an external fetal monitor (EFM) is used. It's a plastic monitor that is placed on your belly with a little bit of cold lubricant. Once a nurse finds the baby's heartbeat, it is secured with a large Velcro strap to hold it in place. It's the same monitor used for non-stress tests (NST's) in your OB's office.

This monitor gives a visual picture of your baby's heart rate and pattern, similar to an electrocardiogram (EKG). Unless you are up walking around

? ?

LABOR DAY

BIRTHING BALLS

Some women prefer to be sitting up and leaning forward during a contraction. A birthing ball may help you do this. Some updated birthing centers and maternity wards come complete with beds that have a trapeze bar above the bed, and side rails that moms can hold onto while laboring.

or going to the bathroom, you are hooked up to the monitor and there is a continuous reading of your baby's heartbeat.

The American Congress of Obstetricians and Gynecologists recommends that your healthcare provider check these monitor tracings every 30 minutes during your first stage of labor and every 15 minutes in your second stage of labor. For high-risk pregnancies, the provider should check the monitor tracings every 15 minutes during the first stage and every five minutes in the second stage.

If you deliver at home, your midwife will probably use a stethoscope to listen to the baby's heartbeat (fetoscope) or a hand-held Doppler device, like the one used to check the baby's heartbeat during your prenatal visits. Birthing centers also use Doppler devices to listen to the baby's heart rate.

Q. I've heard about a monitor that attaches to the baby's scalp. Is that necessary?

Occasionally, an *internal* monitor called a **FETAL SCALP ELECTRODE** (FSE) is necessary. This monitor does attach to the baby's head via a tiny little wire. Yes, the wire actually screws into the skin of the scalp. We know it sounds dreadful, but we only use them when we really need to get more information about your baby. These situations include:

◆ concern about the fetal heart rate or pattern.
◆ inability to use an external fetal monitor because mom is obese.
◆ position of the baby makes external monitoring difficult.

We know the thought of a tiny wire being put into your baby's scalp is the last thing that anyone would want (us included). But it's necessary sometimes. No, it can't do any permanent damage. And no, it can't go into your baby's brain. Most babies will have a little superficial mark on the scalp that ends up scabbing up and falling off, without any reminder that something was ever there.

Bottom line: monitors should only be used for good reason and your practitioner should explain to you why you need one.

Q. My friend's doctor put something inside of her to measure her contractions. What was that? Will I need that too?

This is a called an **INTRAUTERINE PRESSURE CATHETER** (IUPC).

The IUPC is a thin little sterile plastic catheter that slides up along the inner wall of your uterus (next to the baby) and measures the pressure of your contractions from inside your uterus. It is more accurate than the monitor placed on the outside of your belly.

An IUPC may be used in many situations such as when it is difficult to pick up contractions with an external monitor (often in obese patients), when it is unclear whether more or less Pitocin is needed, and to help predict uterine rupture in VBAC patients. Your practitioner will tell you if one is necessary.

Internal monitors are rarely needed in labor.

Q. I'm worried the umbilical cord will be wrapped around the baby's neck. Can we do an ultrasound when I go into labor to check for that?

Yes, it might happen. But, no, you shouldn't worry.

One quarter to 40% of babies are born with the cord around their neck (**NUCHAL CORD**). But doing an ultrasound to find out is not going to change the way your practitioner manages your labor or delivery.

The cord usually gets wrapped around some part of the baby (neck, shoulder, leg) during the first and second trimesters as he or she swims around in the amniotic fluid with a leash (the umbilical cord) attaching her to the placenta.

At delivery, your practitioner will sweep his or her fingers behind your baby's neck after the head comes out to feel for the umbilical cord. If it is present, it's usually loose enough for us to gently slip it over your baby's head.

Bottom Line

While you might think doing an ultrasound during labor to check for a cord wrapped around the baby's neck is a good idea, it won't really change what happens during delivery. Knowing that a cord is there would just freak out most women during labor—which is not a good thing!

Q. Will my practitioner know if the cord is wrapped around my baby's neck before delivery?

Sometimes yes, sometimes no.

If the cord is *loosely* wrapped around the baby's neck, shoulder, body or limbs, docs often have no idea until the baby is born.

Rarely, the cord is *tightly* wrapped around any one of the above-mentioned body parts—this can be "seen" by looking at the baby's heart monitor. If the umbilical cord is getting compressed when you are having contractions, it shows up on the fetal heart monitors as a very specific, recognizable pattern. If the pattern persists, it could mean the baby is not tolerating labor very well.

Sometimes changing your position helps the situation. If the baby's heart rate drops too low or too often, your practitioner may suggest doing an **AMNIOINFUSION**. Using a small catheter (called an intrauterine pressure catheter or IUPC), your practitioner puts sterile water into the uterus.

The increased water helps the umbilical cord "float" in hopes of lessening compression of the cord during each contraction. If that doesn't help and you are no where close to delivering and the fetal heart rate keeps dropping, your practitioner will probably recommend a C-section.

Q. Will my doctor hold my hand the entire time?

The answer is most likely no, but varies, depending on your doctor (or the doctor on call who manages your delivery). And it's a question you should ask at some point during your prenatal care so you feel comfortable with the plan.

Here are the different possible scenarios:

◆ *Scenario #1:* Your delivery doctor checks you at the beginning of labor, a nurse checks on you throughout labor and then your doc shows up as the baby's head is coming out.

◆ *Scenario #2:* Your delivery doctor checks on you a few times throughout the day or night, arrives when you are completely dilated or have started pushing, and stays with you until delivery.

◆ *Scenario #3:* Your delivery doctor checks on you frequently throughout your labor and stays with you the entire time you are pushing until you deliver.

Note: there is no right or wrong approach here—the key is you should be informed regarding what to expect.

How do docs know how your labor is going if they aren't in the room with you? Thanks to modern technology, many doctors can see their patients' heart rate tracing and contraction patterns on their home or office computers. Yes, there is even an iPhone/iPad/Blackberry app for that—AirStrip OB provides mobile monitoring for docs on the go.

As a result, your doctor can keep an eye on the whole process while a labor and delivery nurse is physically present at your side. Alternatively, your nurse can give periodic phone updates to your practitioner.

Q. Will my nurse hold my hand the entire time?

No. But you will see quite a bit of her and she'll be very helpful.

When you get admitted to the hospital, a labor and delivery nurse is assigned to you. She will help to get you settled in and comfortable. She'll check on you often, answer many of your questions, occasionally perform cervical exams, assess the baby's heart rate tracing, and support you during delivery.

However, your nurse will probably be assigned to more than one patient and she won't be in the room with you the entire time. It's also possible you will end up with one nurse during labor and another one for delivery if your labor goes beyond your first nurse's eight or 12 hour shift (but we'll be optimistic you won't be in labor that long!).

The positive here is that you and your partner will go through labor together without a third party constantly in the room with you. You can really let your hair down and swear like a sailor if you like.

Your nurse will be around if any problems arise during labor and with you (and only you) when it's time to push.

Reality Check

Occasionally, a laboring woman and the nurse assigned to her just don't see eye to eye. If this is the case, talk to your practitioner to see if you can have a new nurse assigned to your care.

LABOR DAY

? ?

You want to have a good birth experience so speak up for yourself if you feel uncomfortable (or make your partner do it!).

Q. If I have a doula, will she be there the entire time?

Yes. You hire her to be your personal labor coach/instructor/companion for the entire duration of labor and delivery.

Most doulas join you at your home when labor begins, and then transition with you to a birthing center or hospital.

Doulas are especially helpful if you choose to go through labor naturally without pain medication. This is a hard, but not impossible feat that's easier with a doula by your side.

Reality Check

Since a doula will be with you and your partner through the entire labor and delivery, make sure you both like her and agree with her philosophies.

Q. Can my partner hold my hand the entire time?

Yes! Gone are the days of making husbands or significant others cool their heels in the waiting room while their sons and daughters are being born down the hall.

Today, we encourage your partner to be with you the entire time. Your significant other's physical, mental and emotional support is critical and can help you have a smoother delivery.

Q. My doctor wants to use Pitocin to "augment" my labor? What does that mean?

Docs commonly use a medication called Pitocin (a synthetic form of oxytocin) to induce labor. Pitocin is also used to help move along (augment) your labor.

Sometimes, labor slows or contractions aren't strong enough or close enough together to dilate a woman's cervix and move the baby down the birth canal. Or, a woman's water bag may have broken and she isn't having any contractions at all. Helping your labor along may prevent the need for a C-section.

You'll get Pitocin through your IV. Usually the dose of Pitocin for augmenting labor is lower than what's needed for inducing labor. If you're at a birthing center and your practitioner decides that you need Pitocin, you need to be transferred to a hospital.

Before deciding to augment your labor, your practitioner will carefully assess your contraction pattern, how much your cervix is dilated, and how far your baby has descended into the birth canal. She'll also pay close attention to your baby's heart rate in response to your contractions, to make sure your baby will be able to tolerate the stronger contractions that will occur with Pitocin.

Whether to use Pitocin or not is a decision made by your doctor. Some doctors are more liberal about using it than others.

Insider Secret

Talk to your practitioner about any questions or concerns you may have. Keep the lines of communication open when any change in management occurs (a new nurse arrives, a decision to use Pitocin is made, etc.). You need to know what your practitioner is thinking and vice versa.

Q. Will my water break on its own? If it doesn't, what happens?

Your water usually breaks on its own, either at the beginning of labor (which is why you arrive at the hospital in the first place) or at some point before delivery.

If it doesn't happen spontaneously, your practitioner will probably break your water bag because it releases natural prostaglandins that move your labor along.

There are a few situations where your practitioner would want your bag to be left intact for as long as possible (or want it to happen naturally). Those include women with HIV, Hepatitis B and C, or those who are Group B Strep (GBS) positive who have *not* received antibiotics. It's best for GBS positive moms to get at least one dose of antibiotics before their water bag breaks.

It is rare for a baby to be born with a water bag intact.

Factoid: A baby who is born with its amniotic sac completely intact is called "en caul." This occurs in 0.1% of all deliveries. In medieval times, being born "en caul" was a sign of good luck. The family often kept the amniotic sac as an heirloom or sold it to others as a good luck charm to fend off witches and protect one from death by drowning. Since very few people today are familiar with this tradition, you won't get much for it on eBay. If this happens to you, just brag to your friends.

Q. My doctor says my labor is failing to progress. What does that mean?

As we discussed above, there is a typical pattern for labor. However, everyone is different and there is a range of what is considered normal.

Sometimes, the process of labor slows down too much or stops altogether. This is called **FAILURE TO PROGRESS** (FTP). There are very specific criteria that practitioners use to determine if your labor is officially failing to progress. And those criteria differ depending on if you have delivered a baby vaginally before and if you have an epidural.

Failure to progress can happen at any point during your labor—even if you're dilated at ten centimeters.

FTP can happen for the following reasons:

Problem with the uterus
 ◆ Cervix dilates very slowly.
 ◆ Cervix stops dilating.
Disproportion of baby's head size to mom's pelvic size or shape
 ◆ Baby's head is too large to fit through your pelvis.
 ◆ Your pelvis is too small or of a particular shape that doesn't allow the baby's head to fit through.

Abnormal presentation
◆   Baby's head is in a position that makes descent into the birth canal difficult or impossible.

If you have weak or infrequent contractions, your practitioner will probably start Pitocin to kick start contractions.

Reality Check:
Helping Mother Nature take its course

We realize there is a lot of pressure these days to have a natural child birth—no drugs, no interventions, etc. But there are situations where using a drug like Pitocin or breaking your water bag (or both) makes your labor progress more effectively. For a woman who has never gone through childbirth before, this may be just the ticket to avoid a C-section—the ultimate intervention. Here are the common scenarios where you might need help:

◆   Broken water bag without contractions.
◆   Contractions too far apart and thus the cervix stops dilating.
◆   Contractions are not strong enough to move baby's position.

Q. What are my delivery options if I have failure to progress?

The baby needs to come out eventually (as staying inside your uterus until kindergarten is not an option). Your practitioner keeps a close eye on your progress during labor and if he or she diagnoses you with failure to progress (and you are already on IV Pitocin and your water bag has broken), there are two options:

◆   *Option #1: **Operative vaginal delivery.*** This involves using forceps or a vacuum-extractor to help deliver the baby. This can only happen if you are already ten centimeters dilated (fully dilated) and your baby's head is low enough in your pelvis to safely help him out.

◆   *Option #2: **C-section.*** Talk to your practitioner before you go into labor about these alternatives so you will feel comfortable about Option #2, if Option #1 (an operative vaginal delivery) is not possible.

Q. Is it common to have an episiotomy?

Twenty years ago, it seemed like every woman delivering a baby vaginally had an episiotomy. That's because doctors thought that making a clean, surgical cut (**EPISIOTOMY**) to the area between the vagina and rectum (perineum) reduced the trauma to that area. And if that was the case, women after birth would have fewer bladder and bowel accidents (incontinence), problems having sex (sexual dysfunction), and body parts (bladder, uterus, rectum) sagging into the vagina (pelvic organ prolapse). It was also thought that a surgical incision was easier to sew up than the multiple tears that some women get during delivery.

However, here's what we know now, after many years of scientific research: doing routine episiotomies can lead to more third and fourth degree tears (see

DR H'S OPINION
EPISIOTOMIES

I don't commonly perform episiotomies. But I'll do one if a baby is large and mom will suffer more trauma if I don't. I might also do one if I need more room in the case of a vacuum-assisted vaginal delivery or a shoulder dystocia. It's a last minute judgment call after all the pros and cons have been weighed.

box below), ultimately leading to chronic vaginal pain, pain during intercourse and an anal sphincter muscle that doesn't function properly.

Episiotomies are also linked to an increase in bleeding (**POSTPARTUM HEMORRHAGE**) and infection at the surgical site. And the procedure does not protect a woman from incontinence or pelvic organ prolapse in the future, as previously thought.

So, episiotomies are no longer "routine."

However, there are still situations where you might need one. Your practitioner often has to make this difficult judgment call at the very end of delivery. For example, if your baby's shoulder gets stuck behind your pubic bone (**SHOULDER DYSTOCIA**), your practitioner will perform certain maneuvers to free the baby's shoulder. An episiotomy provides the extra room for the baby to deliver safely.

BOTTOM LINE: Episiotomies are no longer routine. You need a good reason to have one.

Factoid: There are about four million babies born every year. In 1992, 1.6 million episiotomies were performed in the United States. Today, only 10 to 17% of women with vaginal deliveries have an episiotomy.

Q. So how can I avoid tearing during delivery?

It's common to tear during delivery, especially if this is your first baby—

VAGINAL LACERATIONS

Here is how vaginal lacerations are graded. Warning: read this box only if you have a strong stomach and enjoy horror flicks. We're not kidding.

1st Degree: The cut/tear involves only the vaginal tissue.

2nd Degree: The cut/tear extends from the vagina into the tissue between the vagina and anus (the perineum).

3rd Degree: The cut/tear extends from the vagina, through the perineum and into part or all of the muscle of the anus (the anal sphincter).

4th Degree: The cut/tear extends from the vagina through the perineum and anal sphincter, into the lining of the rectum.

your vagina isn't the size of the Grand Canyon! And women who have shorter perineums, or more fragile tissue, may tear more. That's genetic and you can't control it. But here are two strategies that can help.

1. *Don't have an episiotomy unless it's medically necessary.* Talk to your practitioner about it.

2. *Have your practitioner massage mineral oil or another lubricant into your perineum while you are pushing.* That, and the pressure of the baby's head helps gently stretch the tissues out to minimize tearing. Having a trained practitioner help guide your baby's head and shoulders out also helps minimize tearing.

Q. I've heard about using different birthing positions. Must I be lying down to deliver?

Nope. There are a variety of positions you can use. There are only two rules:

Rule #1: You can't deliver standing up (because your practitioner cannot stoop beneath you to catch your baby)—although some women find squatting comfortable.

Rule #2: Birthing positions are limited if you have an epidural (but finding a comfortable position should be a non-issue if your epidural is effective). With an epidural, your options are lying down, lying on your side or lying in a reclined position.

Here are a few birthing positions if you don't have an epidural:

◆ Sitting   ◆ Squatting
◆ Lying on your side   ◆ Sitting on all fours
◆ Reclining on a bed or in a tub of water

There is no perfect position for labor and frequent changes of position can help you relax and get a little more comfortable with your contractions. As your labor progresses, try various positions until you find one that works for you.

Q. I've heard horror stories about "back labor" where all of the pain associated with contractions is in your back. Is there a way to prevent or avoid this pain?

Some laboring women feel most of the discomfort in their lower back during a contraction (back labor). Some women don't have any back pain with contractions, and a few feel pain both in the back and the lower abdomen.

Women who have back labor usually have a baby whose head is in the "sunny-side up" position (**OCCIPUT POSTERIOR** or "**OP**"). That means the baby is looking up instead of down (**OCCIPUT ANTERIOR** or "**OA**") 15 to 20% of babies are in the OP position during labor. But many of them rotate into a more favorable position during the later stages of labor . . . so only 5% to 10% are born OP or "sunny side up."

There is no way to prevent having your baby end up in the OP position. Some women have a certain shape to their pelvis that makes it hard for a fetus to be in a position other than OP. So, unfortunately, docs can't prevent back labor either.

But here are some tips to help relieve the discomfort of back labor:

- ◆ Massage.
- ◆ Warm compresses.
- ◆ Position yourself on all fours or on your side.
- ◆ Lie all the way on your side, almost on your stomach (which might help the baby turn), while hugging a pillow.

Q. What happens if I need to pee or poop during labor?

Yes, you will probably pee and poop when you are pushing. Now, take a deep breath and mentally prepare yourself and your partner for it.

During the early stages of labor, however, if you need to go to the bathroom there are a few options assuming you don't have an epidural (see question below). You can get up and walk to the bathroom and use the potty or you can have the nurse place a bedpan beneath you if you are too uncomfortable to move around.

Q. What if I have an epidural? Will I know if I need to pee or poop?

If you have epidural or spinal anesthesia, you won't be able to feel your bladder fill up with urine and you won't have the urge to urinate. So your nurse will insert a thin tube that goes through your urethra and into your bladder (a catheter) that will collect the urine. No worries—this procedure happens after the medication coming through the epidural has already kicked in. You will be numb and won't feel a thing. The catheter comes out right before you start pushing.

Pooping is another matter. Despite having an epidural, you will still be able to feel pressure, specifically rectal pressure. That pressure sensation is usually the baby's head as it descends into the birth canal, pushing down on the rectum below. It is the head pushing on the rectum that makes you feel like you have to have a bowel movement. So anytime a woman in labor says, "I feel like I have to poop," she gets a cervical exam first before she is allowed to try to poop. It's poor form to deliver a baby into a bedpan!

Partner Tip

You may witness your labor partner poop. That's only one of the visuals that partners can find disturbing. Try to erase those visions from your mind. Just remember how much you love this person, and how much of a sacrifice she is making to bring your baby into this world.

And try not to faint. The labor and delivery staff has more than enough to do without you becoming a patient, too. Stand with your knees partially bent and if you feel lightheaded, sit down and put your head between your knees. It's okay, it happens all the time.

Old Wives Tale

It's standard protocol to shave your pubic hair. *False.* Docs do not shave women for vaginal deliveries. Pubic hair only gets shaved if you are going to have a C-section.

Q. When will I know it is time to push?

This answer depends on whether you have an epidural or not.

*If you are laboring **without** an epidural*:

You'll probably feel the need to push when your cervix is dilated to eight or nine centimeters. While it's okay to bear down lightly, it's best to avoid pushing until the cervix has completely dilated to ten cm. Resist the temptation to push.

Why? You can cause tears in your cervix if you push at less than ten cm. These tears can be really difficult to repair and can make you bleed excessively (**POSTPARTUM HEMORRHAGE**). Not good. Your labor and delivery nurse or doula will help you breathe through your contractions and bear down lightly until you have reached ten cm and can really start pushing.

*If you are laboring **with** an epidural*: There are two scenarios.

◆ *Scenario #1:* You may start to feel rectal pressure (like you have to poop). At that point, your practitioner or an assistant will check your cervix to see how dilated you are and where the baby is situated in the birth canal. If you are ten cm and the baby's head has descended low enough in the birth canal, you get the green light to start pushing.

◆ *Scenario #2:* If the baby's head is still pretty high in the birth canal, your practitioner may decide to let you "labor down." That means your contractions can do a little more work on their own before you start pushing. Why? Pushing when the baby's head is still high in the birth canal (a "very high station") will tire you out. Once the head descends a little further, you can begin pushing.

Note: sometimes you won't feel anything and won't have a clue when it's time to push. Your practitioner will have to tell you that you are at ten centimeters, the baby's head is low enough, and you need to start pushing. If your epidural is that good, give your anesthesiologist a tip to pay for his next greens fees (or at least say thank you when he checks on you after delivery).

Factoid: With first-time deliveries, most women push 30 minutes to two hours.

Q. What's the best way to push?

Everyone finds her own best way to do it, and we trust that you will too. Push in the position that feels best to you. If you do not have an epidural, you will be more mobile and thus, have more options. Here are some of them (see pictures below):

◆ Lie on your back, slightly reclined. (This is the most effective way if you have an epidural.)
◆ Pull your legs back by reaching under your thighs, curl your chin to your chest, and push.
◆ Hold bedside rails or handles on each side and someone else holds your legs back.
◆ Sit more upright and hold onto a birthing bar above your head.
◆ If you feel like you aren't being effective in one position, try another until it feels right.

In any position, you'll be told to start pushing at the beginning of each contraction. And this is how pushing usually goes:

1. Take a deep breath in through your mouth and then let it out. (That's your cleansing breath to help open up your lungs and get your mind and body ready for what they need to do next.)
2. Your next breath is another deep breath in, which you HOLD in (do not exhale) as you bear down in your lower abdomen and vaginal/rectal area.
3. After pushing for approximately ten seconds (if you can only do it effectively for seven or eight, that's okay), you can exhale.
4. Take another deep breath in to do this all over again two more times.
5. Aim for three pushes in each contraction.
6. Some women want their "team" (partner, nurse, practitioner) to count for them and others do not. Tell your team what your preference is. Counting faster is not an option.

 ### Real World Tips on Pushing

If you begin to push while exhaling, all of your power leaves with the air you are exhaling. Just try doing a practice one right now. You'll see that things are more effective if you hold your air in and push, compared to if you let your air out while pushing.

Push like you are really constipated and you're trying to get the poop out (awful analogy, we know).

Yelling and screaming makes your pushing less effective and thus, makes your delivery even longer—the opposite of what you want. (But we do understand why you feel like doing this, as we've both been there.)

Q. Can I have a mirror to see the delivery?

Yes.

Of course, you are welcome to watch the baby being delivered. Some women are motivated by seeing that their pushing is effective. Other women, however, have no desire to see the show. It's your choice.

Q. What happens after the baby's head comes out?

At least 90% of the time, the head is the toughest thing to get out. So, the hardest part is usually over! Once the head comes out, your practitioner will likely ask you to rest for a second (that means don't push) so that he or she can quickly check to see if the umbilical cord is wrapped around the baby's head (don't panic, just read the question about that earlier in the chapter). Slowing down the delivery also reduces the trauma to you and your baby.

Once your doc knows the umbilical cord is safely away from your baby, she will tell you to push again to deliver the baby's shoulders and then the rest of the body.

LABOR DAY

? ?

Reality Check

You may say some pretty *#&%$! things while you are pushing. And there may also be some X-rated shots in there as well.

So, if you are recording the event, you may not want to share video footage of your child's birth with anyone else. It's always best to preview the video by yourself before sitting down in a home theater to view it with a 20-person audience.

Q. My sister has three children and they were all born "sunny-side up." What does that mean?

Let's first explain what all the positions are and what they mean. Your practitioner will know what position your baby is in by doing a cervical exam and feeling the bones that make up the baby's skull.

Docs locate the back part of the baby's head (the occiput) in relation to mom's body to figure out the position. So, envision that mom is lying down on her back. Here are the baby's possible delivery positions:

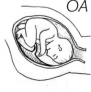

OA

♦ **OA (OCCIPUT ANTERIOR)**: Baby looks straight down as she comes through the birth canal (pictured at right).

♦ **LOA (LEFT OCCIPUT ANTERIOR)**: Baby looks down and the back of her head points towards mom's left side.

♦ **ROA (RIGHT OCCIPUT ANTERIOR)**: Baby looks down and the back of her head points towards mom's right side.

OP

♦ **OP (OCCIPUT POSTERIOR):** Baby looks straight up as she comes through the birth canal (a.k.a. "sunny side up"). Babies who look up and are pointing left or right (LOP or ROP) are also called sunny side up (pictured).

♦ **ROT** and **LOT (RIGHT OCCIPUT TRANSVERSE** or **LEFT OCCIPUT TRANSVERSE)**. See illustration below.

Factoid: How does the baby's skull manage to fit through the birth canal during delivery? A newborn's skull is not like an adult's—instead of a solid mass of bone, a newborn' skull is made up of several separate bones. These fuse together during the first year of life—but at birth, these bones are separated and that allows the skull to mold and squeeze through the pelvis.

Q. Can the baby be delivered vaginally if he is in an odd position?

Usually, the answer is yes.

Babies in the ROA, OA, or LOA positions (see above for discussion) are the easiest to deliver because it's easiest for the baby to maneuver through the pelvis when his head is looking down.

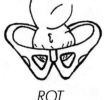

ROT

Babies can get where they need to go in other positions, but the delivery may take longer or require assistance (vacuum-extractor or forceps).

Occasionally, babies don't fit because of how they are presenting in the birth canal or because of the shape of the mom's pelvis. Babies whose heads are rotated sideways (**OCCIPUT TRANSVERSE POSI-TIONS**, referred to as ROT or LOT) are the ones most notorious for this problem. Moms with babies in these positions often require a C-section.

FYI: Refer back to Chapter 12, Home Stretch for more details on the position of baby (lie, station, presentation, etc).

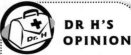

LOT

Q. Can my partner cut the umbilical cord? Is it okay if he doesn't want to cut the cord?

It is completely up to you and your partner.

Some partners are dying to do it and others don't even want to talk about it.

If your partner does want to cut the baby's cord, he will do it after the baby has come out and after your practitioner has placed two clamps (about one inch apart) on the cord. (Don't worry, your doc will tell him when it's his turn to go to work).

Your partner will cut the cord with a pair of scissors (provided by your practitioner) between the two clamps. The umbilical cord is a little rubbery so it often takes a few snips to complete the job. This never hurts mom or baby.

DR H'S OPINION

"I always ask my patients and their significant others in advance, and then I ask again on D-day. Sometimes people change their mind. If your partner doesn't want to cut the cord, that is perfectly okay."

Partner Tip

Sometimes there is quite a bit of blood still left in the vessels between the clamps. Cutting the cord can cause a little bit of a "spray effect" (which is why I always turn my head away when the cord is being cut). Be prepared to get a teensy bit messy!

Q. I've been told that we should wait to cut the umbilical cord until after it stops pulsating. Why?

This is an ongoing debate. Experts are at odds regarding the benefits of cutting the umbilical cord right after delivery or waiting for up to three minutes for the cord to stop pulsating (giving baby additional blood from the placenta).

In the U.S. and other developed nations, docs routinely cut a newborn's umbilical cord sooner rather than later. If your baby is in distress and there is a concern for his health, your doc wants to cut the cord right away and immediately hand the baby over to the pediatric team. *(Strauss RG, Chaparro CM)*. Your doc also needs cut the umbilical cord quickly if you want to store your baby's cord blood. Otherwise there is little, if any, cord blood to save.

Some studies, however, show a small benefit to waiting a few minutes and holding the baby below the level of the placenta (and mom's pelvis) when the cord is cut. Babies whose birth weights are five to six pounds or whose moms have low iron levels may get a boost from a mini-transfusion

labor day

of their own blood. Unfortunately, these are often preterm babies who are in distress and need a quick cord cutting and immediate care.

But do healthy, full-term babies benefit from delayed cord cutting? Some researchers say yes. Babies whose cords are cut sooner may have a greater risk of being anemic at four months compared to babies whose cords are cut after three minutes of life. (Of course, this doesn't happen that often as most babies are not at risk of anemia until after six months of age and this study did not look at long-term effects.) *(Andersson O.)*

So, should you cut the cord sooner or later? We think you have to weigh your options. If you have a family history of certain disorders that may benefit from cord blood banking, that may be a better option. If however, you don't, and are delivering a 35-week infant, delayed cord clamping may be a more reasonable choice.

Q. When will I be able to hold the baby for the first time?

If the delivery goes smoothly and the baby is doing well, you can hold your baby as soon as he comes out. The majority of moms request this to begin bonding with their baby.

However, if the baby has an immediate problem (such as trouble breathing), he may get whisked over to the warming table in your delivery suite or even off to the neonatal intensive care unit.

This is very unsettling to new parents who have a perfect vision planned of those first moments together with their newborn. If this should happen to you, remember that your baby's health is the utmost priority. Even if you don't get to bond in those precious minutes right after delivery, you still have time later—and we promise it won't impact your long-term relationship with your child.

Reality Check

Your newborn will be bloody, covered in cheesy white stuff (**VERNIX**) and sometimes poop (**MECONIUM**). If the thought of this happens to turn your stomach, you have the option of having the baby dried and warmed right next to you at the warming table, and then handed over to you. He won't have his first real bath for a couple of hours after delivery, so he won't be totally clean, however.

Q. When does the OB collect blood for cord blood banking?

Very shortly after delivery. Here is how the scenario usually goes:

The baby comes out and your practitioner (usually) puts her right up on your chest. If a couple wants to bank their baby's cord blood, your practitioner places two clamps on the cord right after delivery and the cord is cut (either by your partner or by your practitioner).

Once the cord is cut, your practitioner places a needle into the largest vessel in the umbilical cord to drain as much blood as possible into a bag or syringe. The goal is to get as much blood as possible before the vessels spasm and the placenta begins to separate from the wall of the uterus. Once that happens, no more blood flows through the umbilical cord.

Q. When do I get to feed the baby for the first time?

Assuming all is well after vaginal delivery and baby doesn't need to go to the nursery for any reason, you can start feeding him right away.

Some babies want to eat immediately. It is easy to tell because they start moving their lips and sticking out their tongues.

Other babies are rather sleepy—or coughing and sneezing to try to get all the fluid out of their lungs. Don't worry if your baby doesn't want to eat right away. Breathing is a higher priority than eating, so she will need to get the hang of it first (remember, she just learned how to do this the moment she came out).

Whether you are nursing or formula feeding, those first feeding moments can be awkward since you probably have no idea what you are doing. Don't be embarrassed to ask for help. Your baby is very forgiving.

Q. How/when does the placenta come out?

The placenta is typically delivered within five to 15 minutes after the birth of the baby. Trust us, it's a lot easier to deliver the placenta than the baby!

Most practitioners actively manage this stage of labor by gently pulling down on the umbilical cord, helping it separate from the wall of the uterus. You may also get a dose of Pitocin (through an IV) to help with delivery of the placenta and prevent excessive bleeding after delivery.

After you deliver your placenta, docs do a few things to help your uterus contract and reduce blood loss. Your uterus is massaged from the outside of your abdomen and you may get a dose of Pitocin (particularly if one was not given just prior to delivery of your placenta). The Pitocin helps your uterus contract even after you have delivered. The goal is to get your uterus to rapidly contract after delivery of the placenta—this helps slow bleeding. Your uterine contractions close off the arteries that previously supplied the placenta, which reduces blood loss.

Q. What if my placenta doesn't come out?

Occasionally, the placenta doesn't separate well and deliver.

Your practitioner can give a dose of Pitocin to help the uterus contract and expel the placenta. If that doesn't work, your doc may need to reach into your uterus with a gloved hand and separate the placenta from the wall of the uterus. This pleasant procedure is called a "manual extraction of the placenta." This is often very difficult, especially if the uterus has already started to shrink or if the placenta is really stuck to the uterine wall.

Very rarely, a woman has to go to the operating room to have the placenta removed with a surgical procedure.

BOTTOM LINE: The placenta needs to come out. In most cases (thank goodness!), it does so on its own.

Q. Does all the tissue from pregnancy come out by itself?

Your practitioner inspects the placenta once it is delivered to confirm that it is intact. A close inspection of the placenta, umbilical cord and associated membranes (amniotic sac) is made to make sure that there aren't any pieces missing. Every once in a while, part of the placenta or fetal membranes doesn't come out and remains in the uterus (**RETAINED PRODUCTS**

OF CONCEPTION).

Very rarely, a woman has to go to the operating room to have any remaining tissue removed with a surgical instrument (**POSTPARTUM D & C**).

FYI: Products of conception refers to all of the tissue that forms as a result of the sperm meeting the egg. That includes the fetus, placenta, umbilical cord and amniotic sac.

Q. Is someone gonna clean me up after all this?

Yes!

Either your practitioner or nurse will take care of that. It varies.

They'll use warm water with clean towels to clean up all the **VERNIX**, blood and sometimes **MECONIUM** that will be all over your thighs and genital area. You are cleaned up immediately afterwards because it is much easier to get everything off when it is wet.

C-sections

Q. Why would I need a C-section?

We can think of about 23 reasons. Check out Chapter 12, Home Stretch, in the box entitled 23 Reasons You Might Need a C-Section.

New Parent 411: A C-Section in 14 easy steps

Here's the basic rundown, whether you have an elective or an emergency C-section. Some things vary between individual doctors and hospitals. And unless it's a major emergency, you are awake for the whole experience.

Step 1: Your doctor explains why she feels it is necessary that you have a C-section. She explains the risks, benefits and alternatives and you ask all of your questions.

Step 2: You read and sign a consent form stating that you understand and accept the risks, benefits and alternatives.

Step 3: You drink a REALLY bad tasting antacid. (Part of you wants to drink it because you are beyond thirsty. The other part of you wants to puke just smelling it. Take it down like a tequila shot. You'll be sorry if you sip it.)

Step 4: You get wheeled or walked into an operating room (OR) and your partner waits outside while everything gets set up. Don't let the sterile environs of the OR scare you. The OR is a white room with big lights hanging from the ceiling. It looks just like a set from Grey's Anatomy. You'll see a big anesthesia cart, a bed where you will be lying, and a big table to the right with all of the surgical instruments, needles and towels on it (usually covered with a drape until just before surgery). There is also an incubator where the baby goes immediately after delivery.

Step 5: The anesthesiologist (your new best friend) inserts a small needle into your back and injects numbing medicine. You will probably have **SPINAL ANESTHESIA** (discussed later in this chapter) unless you have been in labor and already have an **EPIDURAL** in place. If your epidural is

? ?

LABOR DAY

already in place from being in labor, you will be given more medication through the catheter that is already in your back (no more needle sticks!).

Step 6: You lie down on the OR bed with your head on a pillow and your arms *out* to the side. I know you'd rather fold your arms on your chest or place them down at your side... but you might inadvertently move them into the surgical field where docs are operating (thus contaminating it), hit your doctor's hand while she has a sharp instrument in it (I don't need to explain why that might be bad), or accidentally grab your doctor's tush (which actually happened to me once!). You'll have an IV in one arm and a blood pressure cuff on the other, which both do better with outstretched arms. And your hands will stay out of trouble.

Step 7: A member of the OR team places monitors on your chest and one on your finger (see question below for details). FYI: all of this is really cold. The room, the air, the monitors. Ask for warm blankets if you are getting a chill.

Step 8: The anesthesiologist will test you (using a cold alcohol wipe or a sharp object) to make sure you are numb. Once that's certain, you have a catheter tube placed through your urethra into your bladder (I know it sounds bad but remember, you're numb!).

Step 9: You get "prepped" for surgery. Your pubic hair is shaved in the spot where the incision will be and you are painted with an antibacterial soap to sterilize the area.

Step 10: You get "draped" for surgery. The OR team arranges sterile towels all over your body to cover you up, leaving only a small area over your lower abdomen open for your doctor to work. The drapes (yes, like curtains) are hung from to two poles on either side so that your chest and head are visible but you can't see what is going on below.

Step 11: Now your partner arrives to be by your side, wearing disposable, sterile yet fashionable scrub attire. (If you've ever had fantasies of being with Dr. McDreamy, enjoy that visual now.)

Step 12: The OR team counts instruments and sponges—and then has a "Time Out." (No one's in trouble—this helps avoid medical errors.) Your surgeon states a few obvious things out loud (like your name and what surgery you are having) to make sure that everyone is in agreement.

Step 13: Your doctor tests once more that you are indeed numb, and begins the C-section.

Step 14: Your doctor begins surgery by making an incision (a cut) on the skin and works her way down to the uterus. Once she gets into the uterus, she will rupture the amniotic sac (if not already ruptured) and lift the baby out. (You will feel pressure on your chest just before delivery as the OB pushes the baby out—this is a weird tugging sensation.) Next, she removes the placenta. Then, all your body parts get sewn back together while you meet your baby. Voila!

FYI: The stitches (sutures) on the inside of your body are self-absorbable so they don't need to be taken out. Your doctor will close your skin with either stitches or staples. If she uses staples to close your skin, she'll take those out right before you go home from the hospital.

LABOR DAY

? ?

Q. Do I need an IV?

Yes, absolutely.

There must be immediate access to a vein for any type of surgery. Through the IV, you can get fluids, antibiotics, and medication.

Q. What if I need to pee?

You won't feel the sensation that your bladder is filling up if you have spinal or epidural anesthesia. That's dangerous because the bladder can stretch out and not correctly function later on—or may rupture. That's why docs put a tube (Foley catheter) into your bladder through your urethra to constantly collect your urine. The procedure is done after your numbing medicine has kicked in. And it is removed about 12 hours after surgery when you can again pee on your own.

Q. Why is my blood being drawn?

When your IV is placed, some blood is drawn at the same time to check your blood type, Rh type, and get a complete blood count (CBC). Yes, you had those same labs checked in your doctor's office, but the hospital needs it to match donor blood in the remote chance you need a blood transfusion.

The CBC reveals if you are anemic and if you have an adequate number of platelets to clot your blood.

Q. What are all the monitors for?

You are hooked up to several monitors when you have surgery (thankfully, none of them hurt). We'll go over them so you won't feel like an alien. They help your doctors make sure your body is tolerating surgery.

- ◆ *Blood pressure cuff.* The cuff wraps around the upper part of your arm and stays for the duration of the surgery. It periodically fills with air (and gets pretty darn tight), reads your blood pressure, and then deflates.
- ◆ *Heart monitor.* You'll have three sticky patches on your chest with wires that go to a heart monitor. (Warning: they are COLD when they go on.) The anesthesiologist uses this monitor to check your heart rate and pattern.
- ◆ *Pulse oximeter.* A small clip or sticker goes on your finger. This little thing, believe it or not, tells us how much oxygen is in your blood.

Q. What kind of anesthesia will be used?

Spinal anesthesia is the most popular choice for a C-section.

You'll feel a little poke and burn when the anesthesiologist injects local anesthesia to numb up your skin. Then, he uses another very thin needle to find the right space in your spinal canal and injects numbing medication.

The main difference between a spinal and an epidural is that with a spinal you get one shot and you're done. With an epidural, a tiny tube remains in your back to be able to periodically inject more medication.

Spinal anesthesia is used for C-sections because the operation is pretty quick. Epidural anesthesia is used for vaginal deliveries since a woman might be in labor for 18 hours and need more medication.

However, if your C-section is a non-elective one and you already have an epidural, this is kept going. Docs also use an epidural if you are having additional surgery at the same time as the C-section (like removing a large ovarian cyst) or your doctor projects that your surgery may go longer or be harder than usual (example: this is your third C-section).

It's rare to need general anesthesia (where you are asleep) except with some emergency C-sections. It's only used when there is an immediate concern about the well-being of a fetus, there is no time to put in regional anesthesia (a spinal or epidural), or there is a reason you cannot have regional anesthesia.

For details, see the medications section later in this chapter.

Reality Check

A C-section puts you at a higher risk of getting an infection than delivering vaginally. That's because making a cut in the skin can lead to a wound infection. To prevent this, doctors routinely give a dose of antibiotics through your IV before the start of surgery.

Q. Will I be cleaned up like I am having surgery?

Yes, because you are having surgery.

An antibacterial soap-like substance (usually dark brown and sticky, but there are many varieties) is used remove as much of the bacteria living on your skin as possible. We know you are clean, but no matter how clean you are, we all have bacteria living on the surface of our skin and these are the same bacteria that can cause wound infections after surgery.

Q. Is my partner allowed to be in the operating room?

Yes!

Your practitioner wants your partner or support person to be there with you. However, if he or she is the queasy type, tell him/her NOT to look over the sterile blue sheet! Even with a routine C-section, it looks like a war zone on the other side.

DR H'S TRUE STORY: FAINTING DAD

I once had a dad look over the curtain just as I was taking his wife's uterus out of her abdomen to start sewing it up. He politely asked what the purple thing was that I was holding in my hand. When I replied, "Oh, its just your wife's uterus," he turned bluish-white, started getting wobbly in the knees and almost passed out. A word to the wise: don't look if you have a weak stomach. We have two patients to take care of already (mom and baby); we don't need three!

Q. Can anyone else be in the OR?

Usually not.

But all hospitals have different policies. Some will allow two people to be with you. Just ask.

Q. Can we video the delivery?

This varies depending on the hospital and physician.

Here's a typical scenario: you can usually video the part of the delivery when the baby is actually coming out. Then, you can video the baby in the warmer and getting cleaned up. Often, you cannot video the surgery itself, leading up to delivery or afterwards. And really, unless you are a pre-med student, why would you want to?

Q. Can I view the delivery with a mirror?

It depends on your hospital's policies (and whether or not you have a strong stomach).

If this is important to you, ask in advance. It's common to be queasy during the surgery anyway, then consider whether you actually want to see someone cutting you open, touching your internal organs, covered in your blood.

It may be better to have someone videotape the delivery and then decide later whether or not you want to see it.

Q. How long will it take?

A routine C-section takes about 25 to 30 minutes.

But if you've had a previous C-section or prior abdominal surgery, scar tissue may increase the time needed to perform your surgery. Your anatomy is now different, so docs have to avoid damaging tissue that may not be in its usual place.

Emergency C-sections done for fetal distress are much quicker. If your baby is in severe distress, your practitioner can deliver him in a minute or two.

Q. Will my partner be able to cut the cord?

Yes, but it's not quite the same as in a vaginal delivery.

Because everything must be sterile in the operating room on the doctor's side of the blue curtain, your partner cannot come over to make the cut.

The delivery doctor initially cuts the cord. After the nurse or pediatrician takes the baby, a clamp is placed on the umbilical cord very close to the baby's skin. If desired, your partner can trim the remaining cord that is hanging above that clamp with a pair of scissors.

Q. Is it still possible to collect the cord blood for cord blood banking?

Yes.

It is just as easy to collect cord blood during a C-section as with a vaginal delivery. Just remember to bring your kit to the hospital and hand it to your nurse when you are admitted. Many hospitals carry cord blood collection kits in case you forget yours at home.

Q. Where will the scar be?

Usually, your doctor will make the cut horizontally (**PFANNENSTIEL INCI-SION**) across the lower part of your abdomen. These days, most docs try to make the cut as low as possible (in the upper part of your pubic hair) to avoid having a visible scar.

Some doctors make vertical skin incisions (from your belly button to your pubic bone)—but those are only usually done in emergencies.

Q. Will I have stitches or staples?

It depends on your doctor.

Most doctors use stitches on all the layers underneath the skin and staples to close the skin. Your doctor removes the staples right before you go home (three to four days after surgery). He will place Steristrips (little sterile pieces of surgical tape) over the incision after the staples are out.

Some doctors prefer to use stitches to close all the layers, including the skin.

Reality Check

There have been many studies on the method used to close a C-section incision. The conclusion: there is no cosmetic difference between using stitches and staples. *(Alderice F.)*

Q. When do I get to see the baby?

You will see the baby right after delivery. But where your baby goes next as you move from the operating room to a recovery room depends on the hospital.

Many delivery hospitals try to keep mother and baby together. If the baby does not have any medical issues requiring attention in the newborn nursery, mom and baby go to the recovery room together. A labor and delivery nurse looks after mom and a nursery nurse comes to evaluate the baby.

If the baby needs to be observed more closely, she goes to either the newborn nursery or the neonatal ICU (NICU). We know it's hard to be separated, but your baby's health is the first priority.

If you are in a hospital where it isn't possible to keep mom and baby together, you head to the recovery room and your baby goes to the newborn nursery for a while. You reunite about three to four hours later when you settle into your postpartum room. Truthfully, you will fall asleep so that time will pass quickly!

Q. When do I get to nurse the baby?

If you are delivering at a hospital where mom and baby stay together, you can nurse in the recovery room.

If you are delivering at a hospital where

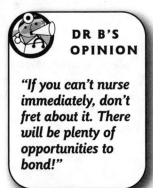

DR B'S OPINION

"If you can't nurse immediately, don't fret about it. There will be plenty of opportunities to bond!"

labor day

you need to recover first, you can nurse your baby when you are brought to your postpartum room a few hours later.

Reality Check

The operating room may feel chaotic to you—but it's really a highly organized place. Don't feel overwhelmed by it all. If you deliver twins or other multiples, expect two or more NICU teams and warmers in the delivery room.

Q. Who will be sure the baby is okay after delivery?

In the operating room, there is a team for you and a team for your baby. Every hospital has its own policies, but there is (at least) one specially trained pediatric nursery nurse at even the most routine, low-risk C-section. At the other end of the spectrum, there may be a neonatologist, NICU nurse, and a respiratory therapist in the OR—all awaiting the delivery of a newborn in a high-risk situation.

The pediatric team takes the baby from the sterile surgical field over to a warming table or "warmer" and dries off/warms up and stimulates your baby to take some nice big breaths. This clears out the fluid from her lungs.

Meanwhile, the team does an initial survey of your baby, including vital signs, **APGAR SCORES** and measurements (head, chest, length and weight). For details, see the "Once the Baby is Born" section at the end of this chapter.

If all is well, the nurse wraps your baby up like a little burrito and hands her to you and your partner.

Reality Check

Unless you live in a rural community, your own pediatrician will probably not be in attendance at your C-section. It will be a pediatrician or pediatric specialist on the hospital staff. Your personal pediatrician sees the baby within 24 hours of delivery.

Medications During Labor And Delivery

New Parent 411:
Anesthesia and Analgesia

There are special medications used to keep a person comfortable, relaxed, and pain-free during medical procedures. Docs categorize them based on how the medications work.

The two basic terms to remember are **ANALGESIA** (pain relief) and **ANESTHESIA** (the absence of pain AND immobilization, usually with sedation).

Medications are taken by mouth, inhaled, or given through an IV/shot. While some medications act locally at one site, others act regionally (over a larger area of the body). And general anesthesia acts on the whole body.

The list below covers the types of medication used in labor, delivery, and postpartum care:

LABOR DAY

◆ **Sedatives**: Drugs that calm you down, ease your agitation and let you sleep.

◆ **Narcotics**: Potent pain relievers derived from opium or an opium-like compound. They can also affect mood and behavior. People can become dependent on them if used long-term.

◆ **Epidural anesthesia:** Pain relief medication that numbs the nerves from the waist down. A small needle goes into the epidural "space" of the spine, and then a thin catheter tube remains to give continuous flow of pain medication for the duration of labor. It takes about ten to 20 minutes to kick in. The epidural provides excellent pain relief. You will have some leg weakness, but you should still be able to push effectively. Once the epidural is discontinued, you will regain full sensation and muscle strength.

Epidural

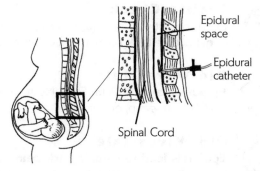

Epidural space

Epidural catheter

Spinal Cord

◆ **Spinal anesthesia:** Pain relief and numbing medication that affects nerves from the waist down. A small needle goes into the spinal canal for a single injection of medication. The medication begins to work immediately. You will be pain free and numb in the lower half of your body. It wears off after a couple of hours.

◆ **Pudendal block:** Local pain relief medication that is injected in the "pudendal nerve" (vaginal) area to quickly numb the vagina and vulva (perineum). It is used during the second stage of labor or after a delivery to do a repair.

◆ **Saddle block:** This is spinal analgesia that only numbs the buttocks, thighs, and genital area (perineum). It used to be popular, but it is rarely used today.

◆ **General anesthesia:** This is only used in true emergencies, when a baby needs to be delivered immediately, if you refuse regional anesthesia, or you are unable to receive regional anesthesia. You get a muscle relaxant, medication to fall asleep, and pain relief. If you are asleep and all your muscles are relaxed, you also need a ventilator to breathe for you while you are under anesthesia. Once you are asleep, a breathing tube is placed through your mouth into your windpipe (trachea) to attach to the ventilator. After the procedure is over, the medication is turned off, you begin to awaken, and the breathing tube is removed.

Q. I want pain medication! When can I get my epidural?

There are just two rules you need to remember here:

Rule #1: It's too early if you aren't in labor.
Rule #2: It's too late if the baby's head is coming out.

It takes about five minutes to set up and 15 minutes until pain relief is on board. Our advice: don't wait until pain is excruciating to request an epidural. Why? Because your friendly anesthesiologist may be busy helping another woman in labor and won't be able to get to you right away. So, if you know you want an epidural, speak up.

Here are the official guidelines on epidurals from ACOG: "Maternal request is sufficient medical indication for pain relief during labor." They also note that epidural anesthesia does not increase the risk of having a C-section. (ACOG.)

Reality Check
Once you get your epidural, you may want to read the paper or get out the backgammon board until it's time to push.

Old Wives Tale
Epidurals cause autism. *False*. Neither do cell phones, high fructose corn syrup, or vaccines!

Old Wives Tale
Epidurals lead to chronic back pain. *False*. You may be tender at the injection site for up to a week or two after delivery. If you have chronic back pain, it is more likely to be from the very awkward positions you are in while breast feeding, holding your newborn, and sleeping. (Russell R, MacArthur AJ.)

Q. I've heard that epidurals slow labor down. I don't want to be in labor any longer than I have to. What should I do?

Don't worry that the epidural will slow things down. In fact, some studies have shown that getting an epidural early may *decrease* the time to full dilation. This research is still up for debate, but the most recent data supports this theory. (Wong CA, Ohel G.)

However, your doctor should look at each patient individually. You'll have to ask your practitioner if she has any concerns.

Q. What is a spinal headache? How likely is it that I would get one?

A spinal headache (**POSTDURAL PUNCTURE HEADACHE**) occurs in one to three percent of women who receive epidural anesthesia.

The needle used in the procedure can puncture the membrane that surrounds the spinal cord. This causes a leakage of spinal fluid, leading to a severe headache and upper back/neck pain for a day or two.

The difference between a spinal headache and a regular headache is that a spinal headache goes away or improves when lying flat. Bright lights may also bother you.

Most anesthesiologists recommend simple treatment for the first 24 hours—bed rest, hydration, and pain medication. About one-third of patients have pain severe enough to need additional help.

If you fall into that group, you may need something called an *epidural blood patch*. This involves injecting a small amount of your own blood into the epidural space. The blood forms a clot and seals the hole like a patch on a tire. This will cure the headache almost instantly. Occasionally, the blood patch needs to be repeated, but this is not very common.

Q. What are the risks of having spinal or epidural anesthesia?

The risks are very low of having a problem if you have a well-trained anesthesiologist taking care of you. But you should be aware of potential side effects and complications before you sign off:

- Low blood pressure.
- Fever.
- Infection (abscess).
- Nerve damage.
- Itching.
- Large bruise (hematoma).
- Allergic reaction to medication.
- Inadequate pain relief.
- Spinal headache (Postdural puncture headache).
- Transient drops in fetal heart rate.
- Painful sensations in the buttocks and legs.
- "High spinal" where nerves to the neck and brainstem are numbed.
- Death. (Very rare, but possible.)

Q. The hospital that I am delivering at only provides laboring women with spinal anesthesia, not epidurals. Should I get one?

Spinal anesthesia only lasts for an hour or two. Once it wears off, you can't get any more. That's why it's better for C-sections than for vaginal deliveries. But it can be used for the second stage of labor (the pushing stage).

Remarkably, there are still some hospitals that don't offer epidurals to laboring women. If that is your only option, talk with your provider about when it might be right for you.

Q. Can everyone get an epidural?

Pretty much, yes. There are a few conditions that might make an anesthesiologist reluctant to place one. Doctors are very cautious about these things for safety reasons. Here are those situations:

- You are taking blood thinner medications.
- You have an extremely low platelet count.
- You have a bleeding disorder.
- You have a serious heart condition.
- Your blood pressure is unstable.
- You have had corrective spine surgery.

Anesthesiologist Dr. Steve Rutman has this advice: do a pre-labor visit with your anesthesiologist. "If you have a medical condition that you feel might complicate getting an epidural, have your OB call the anesthesia department at your delivery hospital and arrange a prenatal visit with an anesthesiologist. This allows the doctor to suggest additional tests before you go into labor to see if an epidural is safe. You can also make a plan for forms of pain relief so everyone knows what to expect when you arrive to have your baby."

Reality Check

Anesthesiologists do not like surprises!

Q. I've heard of women taking Demerol for pain relief before an epidural. What do you think?

Demerol is an IV narcotic medication used early in labor to dull the pain of contractions. It goes into your bloodstream, through the placenta, to your baby. If you have a long labor (that means you, first time moms), it can be taken early on because it usually wears off before delivery.

But if your labor is quick, your baby might be born with narcotics on board. In higher doses, it can make a baby's breathing rate dangerously slow and make him very lethargic. That's never a good way to start out life. Those babies need another drug after birth to reverse the narcotic's effects.

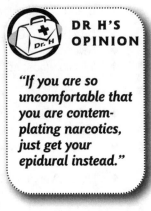

DR H'S OPINION

"If you are so uncomfortable that you are contemplating narcotics, just get your epidural instead."

Q. I don't want any pain medication. What are my options to reduce the discomfort of labor and delivery?

If you want to attempt labor and delivery without pain medication, we'd highly recommend having a doula. It is so important to have an experienced woman to coach, massage and encourage you through this very tough and painful process.

A doula will help you to relieve and cope with the pain by changing positions, breathing, sitting on a birthing ball, taking a bath, being massaged, and using different focusing techniques. Ask your friends, practitioner or local hospital for references.

Home Births

For this section, we recruited an experienced midwife to discuss the home birth experience. Heather Mancini, a Certified Professional Midwife (CPM) and certified pre-and postnatal massage therapist, has practiced in California and Hawaii. Heather is also Dr. H's sister, so the price was right.

Here's the take-home message: birthing at home with a skilled attendant can be a joyful and safe experience for low-risk women. Midwives provide both medical and emotional support during your prenatal care and labor.

When you go into labor, your midwife will likely come to your home during early labor and remain there through delivery. You may also have an assistant midwife, doula, or other healthcare practitioners present. Your partner and any other family members you desire to have with you can be your support team. The birth attendant will bring most of her own supplies, but will request you have some items on hand in advance.

The midwife monitors your progress by assessing your vital signs, doing periodic vaginal exams, and checking fetal heart tones using a fetoscope or Doppler. Home birth attendants try to avoid internal fetal monitoring, IV's, episiotomies, and artificial rupturing of the fetal membranes, unless it is absolutely necessary.

You can give birth on your bed, in a birthing tub, bathtub, or even on your living room floor if you like. You can decide where you feel the most comfortable.

Once you give birth, your baby is placed into your arms to begin bonding and breastfeeding. The midwife will examine your baby thoroughly, weigh and measure her, and administer Vitamin K and eye ointment.

After you deliver the placenta, the midwife will perform any necessary suturing and clean you and the birthing area. As Heather points out, "The only evidence that a birth just occurred is your new baby!"

The midwife stays for a couple of hours after your delivery to make sure both mother and baby are stable, to answer questions, provide care instructions, and ensure you have eaten a meal.

If a complication arises, midwives are trained in neonatal resuscitation and CPR. She will also have oxygen and medications to stop bleeding. But if you need advanced medical care, you are transferred to the nearest hospital or medical facility.

"When you choose to birth at home, you are free to wear what you want, labor and birth in any position, eat and drink freely, and have any friends and family present if you desire," Heather told us.

To help you cope with contractions, your midwife may suggest using herbal medicine, homeopathy, hydrotherapy, massage, acupuncture, and various breathing techniques. She'll also give continuous hands-on assistance.

If your birth is proceeding normally (which over 90% do), a midwife does little more than monitor the health and progress of you and your baby. She provides positive, loving support. Although every midwife brings her own style, there are standards of care that are universally followed.

 Insider Secret
Even though you deliver at home, your baby still needs close monitoring on a daily basis for weight loss and jaundice. Be sure your care attendants follow up at 24 and 48 hours of life in case your baby needs additional care. Your baby should also have a newborn follow-up appointment with your pediatrician at four to five days of life.

Birthing Centers

If you have a low-risk pregnancy and want a natural birth experience (but don't want to deliver at home), a birthing center might be right for you.

Most birthing centers *do not* do inductions, use pitocin or continuous external monitoring, offer epidurals or spinals, or perform operative deliveries (use a vacuum or forceps) or C-sections.

Birthing centers *do* provide a relaxed, comfortable setting with less intervention than hospitals and allow you to return home shortly after the birth if you so desire. Midwives or licensed nurses perform deliveries at birthing centers. Obstetricians typically do not.

The ideal birthing center experience closely follows the box earlier in the chapter on 13 easy steps for a vaginal delivery.

Reality Check

If there is a complication during your labor that requires immediate medical care, you will be transferred to the nearest delivery hospital. Even though this is not your ideal vision, remember the goal is a healthy baby and mom.

This WASN'T in the Birth Plan!

While one hopes for that picture perfect delivery, sometimes things don't go by the book. This section discusses items that weren't in the birth plan.

Freak-out warning: most of these complications are uncommon. This section is for those of you who want the complete picture. For everyone else who might find this material disturbing, you may want to skip to the next section called "Once the baby is born."

10 things that can go wrong during labor and delivery

Now for those who choose to read on, here are the top ten things that can go wrong with labor and delivery. If you end up in one of these scenarios, take a deep breath and let your healthcare team do what they are trained to do—get you and your baby through delivery safely.

1 **NONREASSURING FETAL HEART PATTERN.** If the monitors show that a baby is continually stressed during labor, your practitioner is going to move things along to get your baby out safely. That may mean doing an *"operative"* or *"assisted"* vaginal delivery (that is, using forceps or a vacuum extractor—more on this below) or a C-section.

2 **MALPRESENTATION:** Your baby may have his own idea of how he would like to make his entrance into the world. But sometimes his choice is unrealistic. If we know ahead of time that your baby is breech, you need a version or a C-section. But some malpresentations are discovered during labor. That makes for either a complicated vaginal delivery or an emergency C-section.

3 **FAILURE TO PROGRESS.** If you are exhausted AND your doc has already given you pitocin AND broken your water bag AND your baby is still high in the pelvis and not moving down the birth canal, yes, you will need a C-section.

4 **CHORIOAMNIONITIS.** About one to five percent of women get an infection in the placenta, amniotic sac and surrounding fluid. It's more common if your water has been broken for over 24 hours before delivery. Once your water breaks, the clock is ticking.

5 **MECONIUM.** Babies who are stressed prior to or at delivery may pass their first poop before they leave the womb. That poop can be seen in the amniotic fluid. If the meconium enters the baby's lungs, it can cause inflammation and problems breathing. So, it's important to clear the baby's airway. If your water breaks and your OB sees the meconium, a neonatal team is called to attend the delivery. Yes, even more people get to see you naked—you won't care at that point.

6 **SHOULDER DYSTOCIA.** After the baby's head comes out, the shoulder that is on top gets stuck behind mom's pubic bone. This is one of the few situations that will make your practitioner sweat (literally and figuratively). Your baby needs to be delivered pronto and she is going to do what it takes to make that happen. The forceful maneuvers can actually purposely break the baby's collar bone (**CLAVICULAR FRACTURE**) or cause a temporary (90 to 95% of the time) injury to the nerves of the baby's shoulder, arm, and hand (**BRACHIAL PLEXUS INJURY**).

7 **NEONATAL RESUSCITATION.** When your baby is born, the healthcare providers in the room make sure your baby is vigorous, breathing, moving, and turning nice and pink (see APGAR discussion below). If he is not doing what docs expect him to do, he may need to be warmed up, receive oxygen, have his nose and mouth suctioned, or even receive CPR. Your first reaction is, "Is my baby going to be okay?" The answer is almost always yes, but give your doc time to help baby make the big transition to the real world. And yes, some babies need more medical support in the intensive care nursery (NICU) until they prove they can manage life on their own.

8 **LABORED BREATHING.** Babies who are delivered by C-section don't get the amniotic fluid squeezed out of their lungs like those who get pushed through the birth canal. As a result, some babies may have temporary labored breathing for the first few hours after delivery (called **TRANSIENT TACHYPNEA OF THE NEWBORN,** or **TTN**). Occasionally, babies delivered vaginally will have this, too. If your baby has TTN, he is monitored for a little while in the nursery before getting his first snuggles with you.

9 **OPERATIVE VAGINAL DELIVERY.** An uncomplicated vaginal delivery is the goal, but sometimes that just isn't in the cards. If having a forceps or vacuum extraction will help get your baby out safely, it is the right answer.

10 **BIRTH TRAUMA.** If you have a vacuum extraction, your baby may have a very large goose egg on his head (a collection of blood called a **CEPHALHEMATOMA**). It's temporary, and you can cover it up with those cute little hats for his first baby pictures. Other babies may have bruised faces and little broken blood vessels from delivery. Medically, the only concern here is a slightly greater risk of your baby becoming jaundiced in the first few days of life.

labor day

LABOR DAY

? ?

Q. My doctor just broke my water bag and said that there was meconium (the fluid was greenish-brownish). That shouldn't happen before the baby is born right?

First of all, let's define **MECONIUM**. Meconium is a Latin word that means "poppy juice." It is a dark green sticky substance consisting of mucous and fecal material that forms in the fetal intestine (that is apparently the same color as poppy juice).

Meconium is released as the baby's first bowel movement at or near the time of birth. Typically, this does *not* occur prior to delivery.

Sometimes a fetus under stress will release meconium into the amniotic fluid prior to delivery. How do we know? There are two possible clues: once your amniotic sac is ruptured, the fluid is greenish/brownish. Or, in some cases, if there is no fluid leaking out at all after rupture of membranes, doctors may suspect meconium.

What causes this stress? Lack of sufficient blood supply and lack of oxygen. This may be caused by many things, including **PLACENTAL ABRUPTION**, **PREECLAMPSIA**, **FETAL GROWTH RESTRICTION**, **OLIGOHYDRAMNIOS** and fetal infection.

Q. Is there anything to do now that my baby has passed meconium and I am still in labor?

Yes and no.

If the amniotic fluid is only slightly tinged with what is called "light meconium" and your baby looks like she is doing well based on her heart rate pattern, there is nothing to do but observe.

If, on the other hand, the amniotic fluid is more like split pea soup in appearance or "thick meconium," it is likely that you will receive an **AMNIOINFUSION**.

This is a procedure where a very thin sterile catheter is placed through the vagina up into the uterus, next to the baby. This does not hurt nor bother your baby. Through this catheter, docs can infuse sterile water into the uterus to help "wash out" some of the thicker meconium. This is also done if a baby is showing signs of fetal distress based on a compressed umbilical cord.

Once your baby is delivered, he will have his nose and mouth suctioned (as well as the upper part of his throat) to remove any meconium prior to him taking his first breath. This prevents the meconium from getting beyond the baby's vocal cords and potentially into his lungs. As you might guess, this is a situation where your baby isn't immediately placed on your chest.

Q. My friend had a baby that got stuck after the head came out. Why does this happen and how do I know that won't happen to me?

This is called **SHOULDER DYSTOCIA**, when baby's shoulder gets stuck behind mom's pubic bone (after the head comes out).

Here's what you need to know: shoulder dystocia is rare, occurring in just 0.6% to 1.4% of all vaginal deliveries. It often happens without warning and is one of those unpredictable obstetric emergencies. So while there is no guarantee it won't happen during your delivery, you can rest somewhat easier by realizing it does NOT occur frequently.

There are some risk factors for shoulder dystocia (see below), but most cases just happen out of the blue.

And if it does happen, your practitioner will perform some special maneuvers to help free the little one's shoulder and deliver the rest of the baby.

Q. What are risk factors for having a shoulder dystocia?

A big baby (**MACROSOMIA**) is the number one risk factor. You are most likely to have a big baby if you have diabetes (either pre-existing or gestational, with poor sugar control), obesity, or a pregnancy that goes beyond its due date. Other risk factors include having a previous baby who was delivered with shoulder dystocia, who was large or needed a vacuum or forceps to help with delivery.

This is why practitioners recommend C-sections when the estimated fetal weight is 5,000 grams or more (11 lbs.) in non-diabetic patients and 4,500 grams or more (10 lbs.) in diabetic patients.

FYI: most cases of shoulder dystocia occur in patients with none of the above risk factors.

Q. Is it true that sometimes instruments are used to pull the baby out?

Yes.

This is called an *operative vaginal delivery*; it occurs in 10% to 15% of U.S.

POSSIBLE OPERATIVE VAGINAL DELIVERY COMPLICATIONS

Possible complications of vacuum extraction:
- ◆ Big bruise (collection of blood) under the baby's scalp and above the skull (**CEPHALOHEMATOMA**).
- ◆ Cut on the baby's scalp.
- ◆ **JAUNDICE.**
- ◆ Bleeding in the space between thin membrane that lines the bones of the skull and the thin membrane that covers the baby's brain (**SUBGALEAL HEMORRHAGE**).
- ◆ Bleeding in the back of the baby's eye (**RETINAL HEMORRHAGE**).
- ◆ Bleeding in the baby's brain (**INTRACRANIAL HEMORRHAGE**).
- ◆ **SHOULDER DYSTOCIA.**
- ◆ Soft tissue injury to the mother if vaginal or cervical tissue gets trapped under the suction cup.

Possible complications of forceps:
- ◆ Facial and head bruises on the baby.
- ◆ Facial nerve injury to the baby.
- ◆ Scratch on the outer part of the baby's eye (corneal abrasion).
- ◆ Skull fracture of the baby.
- ◆ Bleeding in the baby's brain (**INTRACRANIAL HEMORRHAGE**).
- ◆ **SHOULDER DYSTOCIA.**
- ◆ Soft tissue injury to the mother.
- ◆ Maternal bleeding.

labor day

deliveries. Operative deliveries use either forceps or a vacuum extractor.

The decision to do an operative vaginal delivery is often made in the heat of the moment—when it is clear there is either a risk to the mother or baby. Operative deliveries are also needed in cases of extreme maternal exhaustion where mom is just beat and can't push anymore. Additionally, they are used if mom suffers from a medical condition that requires her not to push during the second stage of labor. This might be severe maternal heart disease or certain rare conditions that increase the pressure in mom's brain, such as having too much spinal fluid and vascular aneurysms.

Talk to your practitioner about the hypothetical need for an operative vaginal delivery during one of your prenatal visits. You won't have time to have a relaxed discussion about it in the delivery room.

Here's an overview of each method:

Forceps: These puppies look like salad tongs on steroids. The practitioner places them on either side of the baby's head. Older physicians who are very experienced in this vanishing art occasionally choose this method of delivery.

Vacuum extractor: This is the instrument of choice for most OBs. The typical vacuum extractor is a flexible plastic suction cup (although a metal or inflexible cup is also occasionally used) placed over a specific area on the baby's head to help ease him out.

A practitioner can only perform an operative vaginal delivery in certain situations. To be successful, the cervix must be fully dilated and the baby's head must be low enough in the birth canal.

Here are three GOOD reasons to use forceps/vacuum extractor:

- *Lack of oxygen to the baby's brain:* if your doc sees the fetal heart rate dropping and not recovering, the baby must come out.
- *Mother's health at risk:* to shorten the pushing stage of labor if mom has severe heart disease or brain conditions that makes pushing risky.
- *Exhaustion:* if mom no longer has the energy to push.

And, by contrast, here are reasons NOT to use forceps/vacuum extractors:

- You should NOT have an operative vaginal delivery just because your OB is tired of watching you push and really wants to get home to catch the last few minutes of a basketball game.
- You should NOT have an operative vaginal delivery just because having an immediate C-section is not an option where you are laboring (such as a home birth or birthing center). You should be transported emergently to a hospital for a C-section.
- You should NEVER have an operative vaginal delivery without your consent.

WARNING: If you have a well-trained practitioner, it is relatively rare to have a complication from a vacuum extractor or forceps delivery (there is a 3% to 5% risk). But you need to be an informed patient, so that's why we list possible complications (see box earlier). If reading this will give you nightmares, just skip right over it!

Once the baby is born

Now let's pretend your baby was just born. Congratulations! What happens next? The order of things may vary a bit, but here's the general idea:

1 **DRYING AND STIMULATION**. Your baby will be covered in blood and vernix. In other words, he's all wet. And that means he is going to get cold pretty fast. So, the staff will vigorously dry him off with towels and either place him skin to skin on your chest or put him on a small exam table that has a heater (warming table). The vigorous rubdown stimulates your baby to breathe and gets his circulation going.

2 **SUCTIONING**. His mouth and nose get suctioned to remove thick secretions.

3 **APGAR SCORES**. Your baby gets graded on how he is adjusting to life outside the womb. He gets a score of zero to ten at one minute of life and again at five minutes (see more on APGAR below).

4 **MEASUREMENTS**. Your baby has his weight, length, and head circumference measured and recorded.

5 **ASSISTANCE AS NEEDED**. If your baby has a significant problem (limp, blue, not breathing, low heart rate), the staff provides any support necessary while he is on the warming table in the delivery room. If your baby needs ongoing support, he goes to the nursery or NICU. (If your delivery or birthing center does not have a NICU, and your baby is very ill, he may need to be transported to another facility.)

6 **FIRST MEAL**. If your baby is doing well, he should nurse or take a bottle of formula within the first hour of life. (He'll only be interested in sleep for the next few hours after that.) After baby and parents have time to bond, he has a few more things on his to-do list.

7 **EYE OINTMENT**. All newborns get antibiotic eye ointment to protect them from a serious eye infection.

labor day

WHAT APGAR SCORE DO YOU NEED TO GET INTO HARVARD?

This is actually a trick question—they only accept SAT or ACT scores. But the medical staff cares very much about your baby's APGAR scores because it tells them how your baby is transitioning to life outside the womb. Here's how we do the grading:

Appearance (color)
Pulse (heart rate)
Grimace (reaction to stimulation)
Activity (tone)
Respiratory rate

Each category is scored zero, one, or two, with a maximum of ten points (but it's rare to get a perfect score, even for babies born to moms who are doctors). Docs do an assessment at one minute of life, again at five minutes, and occasionally at ten minutes. Babies who go through difficult deliveries often have a low (less than five) Apgar at one minute, and then perk up (greater than seven) at five minutes. Babies that don't improve their scores may need observation and assistance by the medical staff.

LABOR DAY

WHAT HAPPENS TO THE PLACENTA?

The placenta is an amazing conduit of food and oxygen, a disposal system for fetal waste, and a manufacturer of hormones and amniotic fluid. But once the baby is born, the placenta's job is done. So, it gets delivered too.

The fate of your placenta depends on whether there were any problems during your pregnancy or labor. If so, your practitioner may ask a pathologist to take a look at it to help identify a placental abruption or infection.

Otherwise, your placenta ends up in a red biohazard bag and gets discarded with all other medical waste products.

If you want to keep your placenta for some reason (yes, a few people want to take it home with them), you should request it in advance to get clearance. If you deliver at home, you can do whatever you want.

You might decide to bury your placenta in the ground and plant a tree over it (like Matthew McConnaughy did). Let's hope Matthew's dog isn't a digger!

8 VITAMIN K SHOT. All newborns get one dose of Vitamin K as it's possible to be born with a Vitamin K deficiency (which can lead to significant bleeding into vital organs).

9 ID BAND AND SECURITY CLIP. Your baby is official now. He'll wear an ankle band bracelet that matches yours (so no one swaps babies in the nursery). Many facilities now attach security clips to newborns for additional peace of mind. We call them "Baby LoJacks."

10 OBSERVATION TIME. Your baby needs to be watched closely for the first couple of hours. The nursery nurses will do a complete head to toe exam, and monitor his heart rate, respiratory rate, body temperature, and oxygen level. That's the time your baby also gets any blood drawn for lab tests should any be necessary (blood sugar, blood count, blood culture). The nurses also notify your baby's doctor about the birth.

11 FIRST BATH, DOC EXAM. Your baby can get cleaned up after she proves she can maintain her body temperature. After all those hurdles, your baby is ready to join you in your postpartum room. Your baby's doc shows up within 24 hours of birth to check him out for the first time.

We could write a book on the details of your baby's first exam and what you're supposed to do next. Oh wait, we already did! Check out *Baby 411* for the sequel to this story.

Partner Tip

You will think of your beloved in a whole new light now after witnessing the miracle of birth together. Next time she yells at you for leaving the toilet seat up, remember this moment and how much you love her.

You now have a newborn in your arms. Whatever you went through to get here no longer matters. Enjoy!

Now that your baby is here, we'll walk you through your recovery and how to take care of yourself after delivery.

POSTPARTUM: WHAT'S NEXT?
Chapter 14

"Giving birth is like taking your lower lip and forcing it over your head!"
—Carol Burnett

This chapter will prepare you for the changes your body will go through after delivery, both immediately and a few weeks down the line. We are talking about physical, hormonal, and emotional changes—and there are plenty of them! Learn about them now so you'll know what is normal and what isn't. And you will be more prepared to deal with it all.

Reality Check: Postpartum Recommendations from 1949.

Let's pop into a time machine and read the recommendations for women who just gave birth back in 1949. Yes, this is from an actual hand-out given to women who just gave birth:

"If you smoke, try to limit your cigarettes to five a day, particularly if you are breastfeeding."

"If you drink, try to limit your drinking to one highball a day." (We love that term, highball!)

And our personal favorite: *"If you are having trouble breastfeeding, you may consider stopping and switching your baby to the bottle, as this will allow you to have more time to sew, cook, tend to your flowers and look well-maintained when your husband comes home from work."*

My, my . . we've come a *long* way ladies!

POSTPARTUM

? ?

Care after vaginal delivery

Q. Why is the nurse massaging my belly?

Your uterus needs to shrink down after delivery. A soft uterus whose muscles aren't contracting (**UTERINE ATONY**) can lead to excessive bleeding (**POSTPARTUM HEMORRHAGE**). This, as you might guess, is not good.

Your practitioner will massage your belly just after the placenta is delivered, then your nurses will do it periodically over the next 48 hours. In fact, you'll be sick of everyone touching your belly to see if your uterus is hard.

Q. How do I care for my episiotomy/tear?

Most women suffer some kind of trauma down there after a delivery. If you tore or had an episiotomy, healing can be pretty uncomfortable and may take a few weeks (particularly if this is your first). Here are some things that may help:

Put an icepack over your genital area (vulva/perineum) for the first 24 hours after delivery.

Use warm water (easiest if you put it in a squirt bottle) to cleanse the area after urinating or having a bowel movement. This helps ease discomfort and prevent infection.

Use a topical analgesic such as Dermaplast spray.

Use Ibuprofen around the clock (every six hours) for the first 48 hours after delivery.

Avoid lifting too much or being too active.

Avoid using soap directly on the outside of the vagina for a few days as it will sting like the dickens if you do.

Take a stool softener like docusate (Colace) to help with your first few bowel movements. Drink lots of water and eat prunes and fiber cereals.

If you are recovering from a third or fourth degree tear/episiotomy, use a donut (soft ring-shaped cushion) when you are sitting down.

Take sitz baths (your pelvic area sits in a few inches of warm water) two to four times a day to help with some of the discomfort.

Change your sanitary pads frequently.

---

5 AMAZING THINGS YOUR BODY DOES JUST AFTER DELIVERY

1. Your uterus shrinks from a size large enough to hold your baby to the size of a large grapefruit.
2. The lining of your uterus (the endometrium) begins to regenerate just 16 days later.
3. You lose more blood than would fill a pint-size container of ice cream . . . and live to tell about it.
4. Your body's hormonal changes (after the placenta is delivered) trigger your breast milk production.
5. You lose ten to 15 lbs. in a matter of minutes—eat your heart out, Jenny Craig!

Q. My vaginal area is bruised. How long will that last?

A bruise (or in medical lingo, a *hematoma*) can result from the veins in your genital area being torn during delivery. The blood gets trapped under your skin and your skin turns dark red, purple or black (sounds fun, right?).

Sometimes this can look dramatic and can extend up above your pubic hair line on your lower abdomen or down either thigh. Or this bruise can cause part of your vulva (the labia in particular) to swell.

Although it looks as if it will never go away, it will. But this takes time. A small vulvar hematoma may take only a week to disappear, just as a small bruise on your leg would. A large hematoma (particularly if your vulvar area is swollen) may take weeks or months to completely resolve. Using ice for the first 24 to 48 hours will help.

Q. I pushed for three hours and the outer part of my vagina is pretty swollen. What should I do?

Ice, ice, ice.

This is the best thing to do for the first 24 hours after delivery if you have a lot of swelling (**EDEMA**). If your swelling is pretty severe, keep the ice on for 48 hours. Most of the swelling is improved after 48 hours and your body will take care of the rest in the next week or so.

Q. I have a few tears on my vagina—how long will they take to heal?

It depends on how many and how deep.

Some women get tiny cuts and abrasions on either side of the urethra and into the vagina. Those usually heal up in three to four weeks.

But it may take six weeks or more to heal if you have deep tears along the sides of the vagina (**SULCAL TEARS**), lacerations of the cervix, or a third or fourth degree tear.

Partner Tip

Time heals all wounds. But tread lightly about lovemaking right now! Your partner won't get the green light for at least six weeks after delivery.

Care after a C-section

Q. When will I be allowed to drink something?

Usually, you can have a few sips of water four to six hours after surgery. But if you feel nauseated or you're puking, you don't get anything to drink until that subsides.

When they do hand you a drink, start with small sips even though you'd love to gulp it down (you'll feel like you just walked through the desert). Chugging it will only make you feel nauseated. Our advice: nurse your drink.

POSTPARTUM

Q. When can I eat something other than chicken broth?

You get a yummy liquid diet for the first 12 to 24 hours after a C-section. It's a very appetizing assortment of jello (you can select the color!), soup broth, juice, and teas. Yes, it feels like torture, but your doc wants to be sure your stomach and intestines are ready to handle liquids before moving up to solids.

If you are drinking like a champ and aren't nauseated or vomiting, you get to eat real food (if you call hospital food "real food") the next day.

If you have general anesthesia during a C-section, you may not even get liquids until 24 hours after surgery.

Reality Check

Although the tradition used to be that you needed to pass gas prior to eating after surgery, things have changed. Today, you can eat after showing that you can keep down liquids.

Passing gas usually happens within a day or two after surgery. Be prepared to answer the question "Have you passed any gas?" about 12 times a day as everyone coming into your room (the nurse's aid, the nurse, your doctor and maybe even your mother-in-law) will certainly ask.

Partner Tip

As long as you get approval from the doctor, bring in a nice meal from the real world for your recovering partner. Whether it's her favorite pasta dish or the sushi she's been craving for nine months, it will be very much appreciated. No matter where you deliver in this country, we guarantee that hospital food isn't like home cooking!

Q. My practitioner wants me to take a few laps up and down the hall. Why?

There are a few reasons.

First of all, you are still at risk for blood clots even though you aren't pregnant. Up to 30% of all blood clots (**DVTs**) associated with pregnancy occur AFTER delivery.

Moving around makes your veins work to move blood around and prevents stagnation, which is a risk factor in developing a blood clot.

Second, many women experience gas pain and constipation after a C-section. Walking helps to pass gas (bet you didn't know that!). So put your little darling in her mobile bassinet and hit the hallways. You don't have to go very far, but walking two to three times a day is the goal.

Factoid: After World War II, doctors started recommending that women walk the day after having a baby. Prior to this, women stayed in bed for about a week.

Q. How do I care for my healing body? How do I care for the wound until it heals? Can I take a shower or a bath?

Every doctor has his own recommendations, so find out from yours what he suggests.

Most doctors remove your bandages before you leave the hospital. If

HOW TO PREVENT A BLOOD CLOT

The last thing you want after surgery is a blood clot in your leg (**DEEP VEIN THROMBOSIS** or **DVT**). There are two things you need to do to prevent this:

1. *Get out of bed.* Start pacing the halls (feel free to count all the different colors of jello you see in food trays).
2. *Wear your TED hose.* These are attractive stockings that help prevent blood clots.

If you have additional factors putting you at risk for developing a blood clot, your doctor may prescribe a blood thinning medication for additional prevention. Who is at risk? Here are the factors:

◆ Obesity.
◆ Advanced maternal age (over 35).
◆ Family history of blood clots.
◆ Anti-Phospholipid antibody syndrome.
◆ Other inherited blood clotting disorders.
◆ C-section.
◆ Immobilized.
◆ Twins or other multiples.

Remember, every postpartum woman is at increased risk for blood clots. So, your doctors and nurses are watching you closely!

you had staples closing a skin incision, they will be removed as well. These are replaced with small little pieces of surgical tape. Ask your doctor when you can put ointment, salves, or scar treatments on your incision.

Your doctor will probably tell you that it is okay to take a shower, but make sure to dry your wound area with a clean towel (bacteria grows when things are moist). Some doctors say taking a bath is okay; others disagree.

Taking good care of your body is the best way to help your incision heal. Avoid heavy lifting, avoid being on your feet for too long, and avoid constipation. Drink lots of liquids, eat well, and sleep when you can.

We know this is tough because between the two of us, we have four children—so we know that the advice "sleep when you can" may seem like a cruel joke!

Q. My wound seems to be opening up and draining. This is bad, right?

Right!
You need to call your doctor right away—it doesn't matter how minor this seems.

Q. Do my stitches/staples need to be removed?

The stitches that are on the inside of your body dissolve on their own. And if you've got stitches on your skin, those usually dissolve as well.

If your doctor used staples on your skin, they will be removed three to five days after your surgery if you had a low horizontal incision in or just

? ?

POSTPARTUM

above your pubic hair (**PFANNENSTIEL INCISION**). This is done at the hospital before you go home. It sounds painful, but most people feel nothing more than a little pinch and it takes only a few minutes. Then, the incision is covered with pieces of sterile paper.

If you had a vertical skin incision (from your pubic bone to your belly button), your doctor will take the staples out after seven to ten days at his or her office.

Insider Secret

Some doctors prefer stitches, others prefer staples. It's merely personal preference. There is no advantage of one over the other.

Postpartum care for both vaginal and Cesarean deliveries

Q. I've got the shakes. Is something wrong with me?

Nothing is wrong with you—and you are NOT cold (although that won't stop well intended family members from covering you with blankets).

No surprise here, but you've got some major hormonal shifts happening. That's what makes you shake.

You may shake as you transition in labor from the first stage to the second stage, after you get a spinal or epidural block, and after delivery. Some women shake so severely that their teeth chatter and it's difficult for them to hold their baby.

Yes, it's annoying, but it's normal and it goes away within 30 to 120 minutes after delivery.

Q. I'm having lots of bleeding. Is this normal?

Yes.

Don't be concerned if you have some gushing in the first day or two after delivery. It will be worse when you nurse your baby and when you stand up. Occasionally, you'll even pass small clots. You'll wear the equivalent of Depends for the first few days. (How nice, you and your baby can both wear diapers!)

Expect to bleed for about four to six weeks after delivery. It should slow down in volume and become darker until it is brownish-yellowish. So what is and isn't normal?

Here are a few red flags:

- ◆ Bleeding that is continuously dripping or pouring out of you (like an open faucet).
- ◆ Continuously passing large clots (the size of a golf ball or larger).
- ◆ Bleeding that starts getting heavy again a week or two after delivery.
- ◆ Feeling lightheaded or dizzy.
- ◆ Loss of consciousness.
- ◆ Feeling your heart beating rapidly.

If you have any of the above symptoms and are still in the hospital, call your nurse immediately. If you are at home, call your practitioner immediately.

POSTPARTUM

Q. What happens if I have too much bleeding?

It's normal to lose a lot of blood during delivery. So what's *abnormal*?

A **POSTPARTUM HEMORRHAGE** is defined as losing more than 500ml (half a liter) of blood following a vaginal delivery, or 1,000ml of blood after a C-section.

Your body does just fine losing up to 1,000ml of blood because your blood volume increased during the last nine months that you were pregnant. Losing *more* than that can be dangerous.

Here's what happens if you lose too much blood:

◆ You will get more fluid running in through your IV.
◆ Your practitioner will do pretty aggressive uterine massage to help the uterus firm up and stop bleeding. She'll also order some medication (usually methergine or Hemabate) while she investigates the reason behind the bleeding.
◆ You may have blood drawn to check your blood count and to determine the levels of certain proteins and blood clotting factors.

The next step depends on why you are bleeding. If you have an undiagnosed laceration on the cervix or vagina, your doctor will repair it. If there are some pieces of placenta or membranes still stuck in the uterus (**RETAINED PRODUCTS OF CONCEPTION**), your doc will check your uterus to remove any remaining tissue. If you had a previous C-section or other uterine surgery, your practitioner needs to check to see if your old scar has opened up.

If your bleeding does not slow down despite intervention, you may need to have surgery. Depending on the reason, surgery can range from a D&C (cleaning the inside of the uterus with a surgical instrument) to major abdominal surgery to stitch the uterus in order to help it contract or tie off certain arteries supplying blood to the uterus.

A blood transfusion is necessary if your heart rate, blood pressure, or oxygen saturation is unstable and your practitioner is concerned you have lost too much blood. You may also get some blood clotting medication.

Very rarely, if nothing else works, a hysterectomy needs to be performed in order to save your life. Don't panic. Did we mention this is extremely rare?

Factoid: If you had a postpartum hemorrhage with your first pregnancy, you have a ten to 15% chance of having it again with your second delivery. If you have had it in two previous deliveries, the risk rises to 20% with your third.

FYI: In some emergencies, women may need blood products other than red blood cells. Some people get platelet transfusions and blood clotting substances. This is more often necessary for women having a postpartum hemorrhage compared to almost any other kind of hemorrhage occurring in non-pregnant patients.

Q. Why do the nurses have to keep checking me all night long? I just want to get a little sleep!

POSTPARTUM

? ?

BLOOD TRANSFUSIONS

No one gets a blood transfusion unless it is absolutely medically necessary. It is recommended only when your health is seriously at risk. Your doctor may decide that you need a blood transfusion because you have lost at least 30% of your total blood volume . . . or your heart rate, blood pressure, or oxygen saturation is unstable.

But you still have to sign the consent form to authorize it. Our advice: sign off if your doctor recommends it. But do so only after all of your questions have been answered and you understand her reasoning for recommending it.

If you end up in this situation, you won't have time to use donor blood from a friend or family member (designated donor). Even if your spouse or mother has the same blood type, there isn't time to have their blood checked and matched to yours (that can take days, and you need that blood within a matter of minutes to hours).

You will receive a blood transfusion from the blood bank. Blood donations are thoroughly screened to minimize any spread of infection, including HIV.

What are the risks? Although donor blood is extensively screened, the risk of contracting Hepatitis B from a transfusion is one in 200,000 if you haven't already been vaccinated. The risk of getting Hepatitis C is one in almost 2,000,000 and the HIV risk is one in 2,100,000.

It's also possible to have a mild immune reaction with fever, chills or hives. That's why patients sometimes get a dose of acetaminophen (Tylenol) and diphenhydramine (Benadryl) prior to getting a blood transfusion to prevent these symptoms. Rarely, a person has a more severe immune reaction where antibodies are made against the blood being transfused. *(Dodd RY)*

We know and agree with you.

You were up all night in labor, pushed for an hour, finally got the hang of breastfeeding, kicked out all the visitors, and dozed off for a few minutes.

Next thing you know, a nurse or nurse's assistant waltzes into your room to chat (and they are all so dang perky at 2 am!), pushes on your belly, listens to your chest, checks your pad (your diaper equivalent) and takes your vital signs.

It's true—the hospital is the worst place to get some rest.

However, the first 24 hours after delivery are important. There are rare, but serious, complications that can occur after having a baby. So the hospital needs to keep a close eye on you. A change in your vital signs can be an early sign of infection, bleeding, or a blood clot.

So how's a girl supposed to get some sleep? Here are two tips:

1. Ask your nurse to put a note on your door to request that all hospital personnel visit you during a certain window of time. That way you won't have someone waking you up every time you've just fallen asleep. It works great at night, but you can also request this during the day. (Murphy's Law says that the birth records per-

? ?

POSTPARTUM

son, the food tray delivery, cleaning person and staff photographer will all pop by when its nap time).
2. See if your doctor can write an order to let your nurse skip one set of vital signs at night. Assuming all is well, this is usually possible.

Q. I'm having some trouble peeing. Is this common?

Many women have trouble urinating after delivery (especially the first few times).

If you had an epidural or spinal, you also probably had a catheter draining urine from your bladder during labor. Occasionally, those catheters cause some temporary bladder irritation. And very rarely, a woman actually gets a bladder infection.

Catheter or not, you may have some trouble. You might not have the same sensation of your bladder filling up, or have trouble stopping your urine stream, or have a few accidents (leak a little) for several weeks after delivery. Fun, we know.

Rarely, women sustain a temporary nerve injury that leads to difficulty urinating. If you can't pee within six hours after delivery, you'll probably need to have a catheter placed to drain the urine from your bladder. (You don't want a stretched out bladder that doesn't function well later on.) Once that catheter goes in, your practitioner might decide to leave it in overnight and let your bladder rest.

Q. I'm feeling a bit short of breath. Is this okay?

No.

This can be one of the first signs of a problem. Tell your nurse or practitioner, especially if you are also having chest pain.

Here's a scary list of possible reasons for shortness of breath after delivery. We realize that this may give you an anxiety attack . . . which also causes shortness of breath! The possible causes for shortness if breath:

◆ Anxiety attack.
◆ Asthma flare-up.
◆ A temporary condition where a portion of the lungs does not expand completely (**ATELECTASIS**)—more common with C-sections and prolonged Pitocin use.
◆ Congestive heart failure (an overworked heart).
◆ Infection in the lungs (**PNEUMONIA**).
◆ Fluid build-up in the lungs, seen occasionally after C-sections and with preeclampsia (pulmonary edema).
◆ Blood clot that gets stuck in the lung's blood vessel (**PULMONARY EMBOLISM**).
◆ Amniotic contents enter a woman's bloodstream (**AMNIOTIC FLUID EMBOLISM**).

The take-home message: hit that nurse call button if you have shortness of breath.

Q. I'm having some pretty bad smelling vaginal discharge. Is this normal?

No, usually not.

The concern here is an infection in the lining of the uterus (**ENDOMETRITIS**). Besides foul smelling discharge, you can have fever, chills, lower abdominal pain, abnormal vaginal bleeding and exquisite uterine tenderness (severe pain when the top portion of your uterus is pushed upon).

So, who's most likely to get endometritis? Moms who have had a:

- ◆ C-section—especially if it is done before 28 weeks or you had a prolonged labor before having an emergency C-section.
- ◆ Prolonged rupture of membranes (your water bag was broken for 12 to 24 hours prior to delivering).
- ◆ Long labor with multiple vaginal exams.

Postpartum endometritis is pretty rare in vaginal deliveries (less than 3%) and scheduled C-sections (5% to 15%). It's most common in emergency C-sections done after labor starts (up to 20% of the time).

Reality Check

Your vaginal discharge may have an unpleasant odor as your bleeding decreases in the days and weeks after having a baby. Old blood is kind of stinky.

Q. My legs and feet are swelling. Is this a bad sign?

Not necessarily.

Many women get more swollen *after* having a baby than beforehand. Your body has a lot of extra fluid circulating around (remember your blood volume is double that of a non-pregnant woman). Until your kidneys can filter out all that extra fluid, you may be a little puffy, particularly in your legs and feet. Waking up on postpartum day number two and having cankles is usually nothing to panic about.

So, when does swelling need immediate attention? A **DEEP VENOUS THROMBOSIS** (DVT) is a blood clot that usually forms in the lower legs. Watch for pain and swelling in one leg more than the other. A clot can dislodge and travel though the heart to the lungs, where it gets lodged in an artery. This is called a **PULMONARY EMBOLISM** (PE).

The other potentially serious issue is called **PREECLAMPSIA**. Only pregnant and postpartum women get this disorder—high blood pressure and leaky kidneys, which allows protein to seep from your bloodstream into the urine. It usually occurs in the later stages of pregnancy (after 32 weeks), during labor and delivery, or up to six weeks after delivery.

Surprisingly, one-fourth of all cases of preeclampsia happen *after delivery*. Not every woman with preeclampsia has swelling. But tell your doctor if you notice severe swelling of the legs, hands or face.

Q. I am not going to breastfeed. Do I need to take something to make my milk dry up?

In the past, doctors used to prescribe a medication to stop milk production. But the FDA no longer approves this drug because of safety concerns.

If you do not desire to breastfeed or have decided to stop breastfeeding, here are a few helpful steps in making it as easy as possible:

◆ Talk with your practitioner and/or pediatrician first.
◆ If you started nursing, drop one session every two to three days.
◆ Wean your feedings to once or twice a day before stopping altogether.
◆ After you nurse or pump for the last time, bind your breasts tightly with an Ace bandage followed by a tight sports bra.
◆ If you are full of milk (**ENGORGEMENT**), use ice packs to help with the swelling. Avoid taking a hot shower (turn your back so that the hot water doesn't hit your breasts directly, just your back) or stimulating your breasts since this will cause more milk production. Then you have to start the process all over again!
◆ Use ibuprofen every six hours as directed to help with pain.

It can take up to two weeks for breast milk to dry up. It does not happen overnight.

Q. How long will I stay at the hospital/birthing center?

If you have a vaginal delivery at a hospital, you will usually stay there for 24 to 48 hours. If there are complications, you may have to stay longer.

If you deliver at a birthing center (all deliveries there are vaginal deliveries), you will usually go home after six hours. Most women do not stay past 24 hours.

If you had a Cesarean delivery, the typical stay is three to four days.

Reality Check

If you deliver at a birthing center or at home with a midwife, most practitioners will do a home visit the day after you deliver to check on you and your baby.

Q. Can my partner sleep with me at the hospital?

Usually, yes.

We won't guarantee that your partner's foldaway cot will feel like your Tempur-pedic mattress at home, but it sure is nice to have a support person there day and night. Even if it's not your partner, it's nice to have a will-

**DR B'S OPINION
HOSPITAL STAY LENGTH**

If this is your first baby, stay at the hospital as long as you can. Most insurance companies cover the cost (48 hours for a vaginal delivery and 96 hours for a C-section) and the clock begins the moment you deliver (not when you are admitted in labor). Your real labor begins once you take your newborn home—take advantage of all the "free" help.

Heck, even if its your fifth baby, you may want to stay as long as someone is lined up to care for your other children!

? ?

POSTPARTUM

ing relative or close friend there with you.

Ask your practitioner, hospital or birthing center to get specifics.

Q. Can my baby stay in the same room with me at the hospital?

Yes, it's called "rooming-in."

This is encouraged because rooming in promotes breastfeeding and bonding with your newborn. The only time this is not possible is if your baby needs to be observed or treated in the nursery or the NICU for a medical problem. If that situation arises, you can visit, cuddle, and feed your baby in a comfy recliner in the nursery. Not ideal, we know, but it's all about your baby's health.

FYI: you are also allowed to ask the nursery to babysit for an hour or two if you really need to get some shut-eye. Yes, the nurses will bring your baby back if she needs to eat. No one tries to sneak formula into a breast-fed baby while she is camping out in the nursery!

Q. What are my pain medication options? Are they safe for breastfeeding?

You have a few options, and all of them are safe to take while you are breastfeeding.

Vaginal delivery. Women vary in how they deal with pain, and some women have more pain than others due to circumstances surrounding delivery. Some women have extraordinary pain with breastfeeding. Others have pain as their uterus starts to shrink back down to its normal size.

Most women need some type of pain medication, at least for the first few days. Overall, the number-one pain medication of choice for postpar-tum women is ibuprofen (Motrin, Advil). It is both a pain reliever and an anti-inflammatory agent (that is, it reduces swelling). That makes it superior to acetaminophen (Tylenol), which is only a pain reliever. As an OB, I rec-ommend taking ibuprofen every six hours around the clock for the first two to four days and then as needed. Just be sure to take it with a little bit of food in your stomach since it can cause some stomach irritation.

Cesarean delivery. Virtually all women need pain medication after hav-ing a C-section. Remember, it *is* major surgery. You will have pain at the incision (wound) site, as well as from all the layers of stitches that were put in underneath the skin and on the uterus. You may also have discomfort as your uterus contracts to shrink back down.

Sometimes in the early stages of recovery when you aren't yet eating (or you've just puked for the fourth time), you are given something called Toradol, which is an intravenous form of ibuprofen. You may also need to take narcotic medication by mouth in addition to ibuprofen for the first week or two. Most women who have had an uncomplicated C-section do not need to take pain medication regularly after two and a half weeks.

How do you know you need more than ibuprofen? If you cry every time you think about nursing or pooping or you can't walk around due to pain, you need more than ibuprofen.

Your options include acetaminophen with codeine (Tylenol #3), Vicodin and Percocet. These are narcotic pain medications that are safe when used in prescribed dosages for short periods of time. They are a problem for breastfeeding moms only if you take them in large doses (above and beyond what is prescribed) or you take them for a long period of time. Using them for a short time after delivery is okay.

Note: Narcotic/opioid medications can make you constipated. Our advice: take a stool softener if you are on these medications.

FYI: Often, the anesthesiologist will administer a pain medication called Duramorph (a longer acting opioid medication) when they are doing spinal anesthesia for a C-section or an epidural. This provides very good pain relief for the first 24 hours after you deliver.

Q. I'm worried about how my three year old will react when she comes to visit me for the first time after having the baby. Is there anything I can do to help make things easier?

Yes.

Most siblings do just fine. Usually they are very nice to their new brother or sister (and *not* so nice to their parents who have the gall to shake up their little self-centered world).

What can you do to make that first meet and greet a good one?

- ◆ Greet your older child *without* the new baby in your arms.

- ◆ Let your older child jump in your arms, give you a big hug, and chat.

- ◆ Ask your child if she wants to hold her new sibling while sitting on your lap. If she doesn't, that is ok.

- ◆ Have a large picture of your older child prominently displayed in your hospital room. (Thanks to Bess, my child's pediatrician, for this recommendation as well as many others!)

- ◆ Have the new baby give a gift to the older sibling. And yes, your older child can also select a gift to bring to the new baby. (You may have to remind your child that newborns have no use for Thomas trains or Barbie dolls just yet!)

- ◆ Have a "birthday party" for the new baby. What toddler can resist cupcakes?

DR B'S OPINION
HELPING OLDER SIBLINGS ADJUST

Older siblings take about six to eight weeks to adjust to the "new normal." They are going through a grieving process of sorts. Expect some acting out. To a toddler or preschooler, any attention—good or bad—is attention. Give your child attention so he doesn't have to resort to acting out.

> ### DR H'S OPINION:
> ### ALONE TIME AND OLDER CHILDREN
>
> It's nice to set aside some "alone time" with your older child or children. Let them pick somewhere they want to go or something fun they want to do and have a little "date" with them. Even if you sneak away from the baby for an hour, it's a very special thing for your older child.

Q. What if I want to have my tubes tied? When is this done?

If you are having a C-section, you can have your tubes tied just after the baby is delivered and the uterus is sewn up.

If you are having a vaginal delivery, you have one of two options.

Option #1: Postpartum tubal ligation, done right after delivery. If you have an epidural, we'll just continue using it so that you won't need general anesthesia for the surgery. Your doctor makes a small incision just below the belly button and then brings each tube up to the incision, so they can be tied and cut.

Option #2: Tubal ligation, done at least six weeks after delivery. Most doctors nowadays perform tubal ligations *laparoscopically*. That means your doctor makes two or three tiny incisions in your belly and operates through long instruments placed in those incisions. This is day surgery (outpatient surgery) and requires general anesthesia.

Once You Go Home: General Questions

Q. When do I follow up with my OB in the office?

Vaginal delivery. Your OB will probably want to see you in two weeks unless there is a specific concern, although sometimes your practitioner will ask to see you in six weeks.

Your doctor will tell you the plan when you are discharged home from the hospital. You will also get a list of symptoms that deserve an earlier appointment. Those include: fever, breast pain/redness, worsening pain, or more bleeding instead of less.

Cesarean delivery. Most OBs see C-section patients back in the office in one to two weeks. Check prior to discharge for a recommendation.

No matter when you see your practitioner for the first time in the office, you will most likely be asked to come back a few weeks later for a "final six week postpartum visit." This visit almost always includes a Pap test (most women haven't had one for about a year), a discussion of birth control methods or IUD placement, and advice on returning to pre-pregnancy activities. Then with a touch of separation anxiety (we feel it too!), you say good-bye to a familiar face for six to 12 months!

Q. I have a fever. My doc says I need to see her. Why?

Having a fever (temperature greater than 100.4° F) between one to ten days after delivering a baby ALWAYS warrants a call to your practitioner. These are the top seven reasons for fever:

◆ *Endometritis.* Look for foul smelling discharge, abdominal tenderness, chills.
◆ *Surgical site infection.* Look for pus or discharge from your abdominal incision or episiotomy site and redness of the skin surrounding it.
◆ *Mastitis.* Look for flu-like symptoms (fever, chills, muscle aches), redness/pain in one breast.
◆ *Bladder infection (UTI).* Look for pain with urination, lower abdominal pain, urinary frequency.
◆ *Atelectasis.* Look for shortness of breath, difficulty breathing.
◆ *Pneumonia.* Look for difficulty breathing, coughing.
◆ *Pelvic abscess.* Look for abdominal tenderness, bloating, fatigue.
◆ *Deep Venous Thrombosis.* Look for leg swelling/pain and possible redness, typically in just one leg.

7 good reasons to call your doc once you're home

1. Fever, defined as greater than 100.4° F and/or chills.
2. Excessive bleeding.
3. New or increasing pain in your genital or rectal area.
4. Pain with urination or inability to urinate.
5. Leg pain or swelling, particularly on one side.
6. Breast pain or redness.
7. Severe abdominal pain not responding to or requiring more pain medication.

Q. When can I drive a car?

Whether you had a vaginal delivery or C-section, OB's have one simple rule: do not operate heavy machinery (car, truck or large farm equipment, if you are so inclined) while under the influence of narcotics! That includes Tylenol #3, Vicodin, Percocet or any other narcotic.

Here are some general guidelines; be sure to check with your practitioner before hopping into the driver's seat.

Vaginal delivery. If you are just taking ibuprofen and you had an uncomplicated vaginal delivery, you should be able to drive again within a week. If you had a third or fourth degree tear or episiotomy, you may want to check with your doctor first.

Cesarean delivery. Your doctor will probably tell you not to drive for two weeks after surgery. This is frustrating, but there are good reasons.

1. You'll be taking narcotic pain medication longer than your friends who delivered vaginally (probably at least a week or two).

2. You use your abdominal muscles when you drive, especially when you move your foot quickly from the gas pedal to the brake. It may be difficult, if not impossible to slam on the brakes in the days following major abdominal surgery. So, bite the bullet for a mere 14 days and ask a friend or your mother-in-law to pick you up to take you to your next appointment.

Reality Check

You will be very tired during your first few months as a new mom, so be extra careful on the road. Sleep deprivation can take a real toll on your driving ability.

Q. When can I walk upstairs?

Vaginal delivery. You can walk upstairs right away if you didn't tear or have an episiotomy, or your tear was very small. Just do it very carefully.

If you had a more substantial vaginal tear or episiotomy, it takes more time to heal. Going up and down stairs will hurt. You may want to use one level of your home or apartment for most of your daily activities and limit stair walking during the first week or two.

Cesarean delivery. You should also camp out on the first floor of your house if you have lots of stairs. It's okay if you need to go up or down once or twice a day. Just be careful and take it slow. Plan to have your baby sleeping nearby at night so you aren't going up and down the stairs after sundown. The chance of slipping is greater at night because it's dark and you are tired.

Two to three weeks after delivery, you should be able to go up and down stairs without any difficulty.

Q. When can I lift my toddler again?

Yes, your maternal instincts (and guilt) will make you want to pick up your toddler and show her the love. But listen to your practitioner before you act on that instinct.

Vaginal delivery. You can lift your child as long as you had an easy delivery. If you had major complications at delivery or you are healing from a large vaginal tear or episiotomy, you are in the "I have more healing to do" category. For you, wait a week or so before lifting or carrying your toddler. But ask your practitioner for a specific plan. Your toddler can still jump up on you and sit in your lap, just without you assisting her.

Cesarean delivery. Avoid lifting your toddler for four to six weeks. Your toddler can crawl up or be placed on your lap by someone else, but it's not a good idea to carry her around after major surgery. Why? Your wound (incision) is weaker than the surrounding tissue while it is healing. It is much easier to have an incision open up during the first few weeks after surgery than at any other time. You won't want to deal with the consequences of that! This includes cleaning the wound and packing it with sterile gauze everyday. If it doesn't heal on its own, you will have to go back to the operating room to have it closed surgically, weeks or months down the line. This is not a fun experience, trust us!

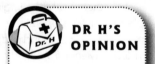

DR H'S OPINION

"I hate to see the look on my patients' faces when I advise them not to lift their older kiddos for at least four to six weeks after a C-section. I know you are dying to pick your toddler up (I was too) but it's just not worth the risk."

Q. When can I start exercising again?

Check with your provider before you start doing any kind of exercise after delivery. OB's usually give the green light after six weeks (occasionally longer with C-sections), but your personal history determines when it is safe for you. Ask first.

ACOG says that women can gradually resume exercising when they feel ready. Some women who have had uneventful vaginal deliveries with little genital (perineal) trauma feel well enough to take a light, brief walk a week or so after delivery. But if you had a third or fourth degree laceration, you may need to hold off exercising for up to eight weeks.

Once your practitioner gives her official blessing, you can resume all pre-pregnancy activities and exercise regimens. But remember to START SLOW. Begin with walking, yoga, mild hiking and swimming. You can't expect to jump back into the 60 minute weight and cardio routine that you were doing prior to getting pregnant. Remember that all of your joints and ligaments can be loose for up to five months after delivery.

And let's talk about those abdominal muscles. Most women develop some degree of a gap between their abdominal muscles as their pregnancy progresses. That gap (called the **DIASTASIS RECTI**) takes about two months to close. In some women, it never closes and there's always a gap. It's important to let your body heal and close the muscle separation prior to beginning any intense abdominal workouts. Start easy and save the heavy-duty crunches for eight to ten weeks after delivery.

Exercise tips:

◆ Stretch for five to ten minutes before *and* after exercising.
◆ Wear comfortable clothing.
◆ Keep well hydrated with water or a sports drink.
◆ Wear a comfortable and supportive bra.
◆ Clear your mind of all the other things going on.
◆ This is your time to relax, think, meditate, and get back into shape.

Q. Umm, I still look pregnant. When will this baby bump go away?

Yep, none of your friends told you that either did they?

Why? Remember there are two things that grow during pregnancy: your uterus and the skin over it.

After delivery, your uterus shrinks down to the level of your belly button immediately and stays there for a day or two. By two weeks after delivery, the uterus has gone down to half way between your belly button and your pubic bone.

In most women, the uterus returns to normal size (about the size of your fist) by six to eight weeks after delivery. As your uterus shrinks down in size, your tummy will too.

The skin covering your belly is another story. It has been stretched out over the last nine months by your expanding uterus (rivaling Santa Claus' physique). This takes time and then some hard work to put it back the way it was.

Reality Check

In some women, the skin over the abdomen is so stretched during a pregnancy it never really goes back. In these cases, no amount of diet or exercise will return the elasticity of the skin to its pre-pregnancy form. If this bothers you, options include wearing support garments (like Spanx) or having a plastic surgeon surgically remove the excess skin (**ABDOMINOPLASTY**).

Q. I feel like I am having contractions again. Is this okay?

Just when you thought it was over, right? Actually, you continue to have contractions after delivery because this helps your uterus shrink. That, in turn, decreases postpartum bleeding and gets your uterus back to its normal size (about the size of a fist).

You'll probably feel contraction pain while nursing—and don't be shocked to see a gush of blood that follows. Contractions decrease in frequency and intensity and you won't even notice them five to seven days after delivery.

FYI: Postpartum contractions are more intense (but go away more quickly) with each subsequent delivery.

Q. I am having bloody discharge. How long does that last? Can I use tampons?

The bloody discharge is called **LOCHIA**. What you see is blood and sloughed-off tissue from the lining of the uterus. That lining was held in check by hormones during your pregnancy and now it's time to clean house.

It's normal to have lochia for 30 to 45 days after you've given birth. Here's the 411 on lochia after birth:

- ◆ *Days 1-7:* Lochia contains quite a bit of blood so it will be bright red.
- ◆ *Days 7-10:* Lochia is less bloody and more watery and pinkish in color.
- ◆ *Day 10 until four to six weeks:* Lochia turns brown, then yellowish in color.

Lochia should progressively decrease in volume and get less bloody in appearance.

Bottom line: most women have lochia for four to six weeks.

There may be some days during this time that you think, "Oh, wow, I've stopped bleeding!" only to be met with more lochia the next day. This is normal and the flow may wax and wane over a few weeks.

And, no, tampons are not recommended. Sorry, but you've got to stick with pads until six weeks have passed from the time of your delivery.

Red Flag

If your bleeding/lochia is becoming heavier and is bright red, contact your practitioner.

? ?

POSTPARTUM

KEGEL (KAY-GULL) EXERCISES

So, you've probably already figured out that you don't quite feel the same below your waistline. Don't be too dismayed. You need to give your body time to heal—and that takes six to eight weeks. Just look at your baby's noggin and you'll understand why your muscles are so stretched out right now!

Good news: you can actively help your pelvic floor muscles get back in shape. Kegel (KAY-gull) exercises help tighten up all of the muscles in the vaginal area, including the muscle that keeps you from having pee pee accidents (urethral muscle). These exercises not only help reduce incontinence, but they get you back in shape for the day you are ready for sexual intercourse. We promise that desire will return at some point.

Here is a step-by-step guide to all things Kegel:

◆ Start this process while you are urinating.
◆ After you begin to urinate, try to stop the stream of urine.
◆ Hold this position for a few seconds.
◆ Release and resume urinating.
◆ Do this a few times each time you go to the bathroom.

When you first start, you probably won't be able to stop the entire flow of urine (or any of it if you are like we were!). Don't panic. Keep trying. As your muscles get stronger, you might win the gold medal when Kegels become an Olympic sport. Just kidding on that one, but you will be surprised at what you will be able to do.

Besides Kegels, your regular exercise regimen will help tone your pelvic floor muscles too.

postpartum

Q. When do I get my period again?

It really varies from woman to woman. It also depends on whether or not you are breastfeeding.

Many women who are breastfeeding do not have periods at all. Some have irregular spotting and even fewer have regular menstrual cycles.

If you are not breastfeeding, you will probably see your period (menstrual cycle) return within six to ten weeks after delivery. Sorry, the party's over. It's back to the "Feminine Hygiene Products" aisle because by 12 weeks, up to 80% of non-breastfeeding women have resumed their menstrual cycle.

And here's a little fact you need to know: about 75% of women do *not* ovulate prior to their first period. But that means a quarter of all moms CAN get pregnant right after having a baby. And yes, this includes those of you who needed assisted reproductive technology like IVF to get pregnant the first time!

Q. How long after delivery should I wait to have intercourse?

Docs usually advise waiting six weeks after having either a vaginal delivery or a C-section to resume intercourse.

This will probably be an easy sell for you. Most women do not feel like being intimate right after having a baby. Do not be discouraged! You will eventually get your groove back.

You are going through a lot right now. Here is just a small sampling of reasons why you feel like you do after delivery:

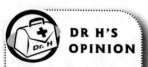

DR H'S OPINION

"Most of the time, we docs don't have to twist your arm when it comes to refraining from sex. In fact, most of my patients are begging me to tell their partners that they can't have intercourse for even longer!"

- ◆ You are exhausted beyond belief.
- ◆ Your hormones are all over the place, making you an emotional wreck.
- ◆ You have a few extra pounds to lose and don't feel very sexy.
- ◆ Your boobs leak all the time (also not very sexy).
- ◆ Your baby is attached to your body 24/7 and you just want a few moments in the day where no one is touching you.
- ◆ Your baby needs you all the time. You think your spouse also "needs" you. There is not enough of you to go around.
- ◆ You had a big vaginal tear with delivery and the thought of sex makes you cry.

The best advice we can give you is to talk to your partner about your feelings. The sexual part of your relationship is as important as any other aspect of your relationship.

Make sure your doc gives you the green light before proceeding. For instance, if you had a big vaginal tear (4th degree laceration) or a wound infection, you may need to wait longer than six weeks.

Always, always use lubrication jelly for the first several times you get back in the saddle and if you are breastfeeding.

Reality Check

As doctors, both authors have endured sleep-depriving residency training programs. Back in our day, there was a rite of passage in medicine that required us to work 80+ hours a week (for about $4 an hour) to somehow prepare for a medical career. After finishing this experience, we both thought having a newborn in the house would be a piece of cake.

WRONG!

By far, new parenthood is the most exhausting job we have ever had. When you are a resident, you get to go home and sleep after being up all night on-call. When you are a new parent, you are up every two or three hours for two to four months straight!

Who'd be interested in sex with that kind of sleep schedule?

Partner Tip: Tread lightly

Don't feel rejected if your partner doesn't share your desire to be intimate. Just be patient—REALLY patient.

Q. I've heard having sex for the first few times is really painful. Is that true?

We're sorry to say that usually the answer is yes, especially if you are breastfeeding.

The walls of the vagina are thinner than usual after having a baby and continue to be that way while you breastfeed, due to the lower levels of estrogen. So, even if you didn't have a tear or episiotomy, sex may be uncomfortable or even painful.

Sometimes, women who had episiotomies or natural tears/lacerations have more discomfort with intercourse initially. It depends on the degree or severity of the cut or tear, whether or not there was a subsequent infection, how quickly your body heals, and a few other factors. Check with your practitioner before having intercourse. If you had a fourth-degree laceration or episiotomy, you may need to wait longer than the typical six weeks.

FYI: Always use a lot of lubrication since your body won't lubricate normally for a while. Buy the industrial-size drum of Astroglide—does Costco sell this yet?

Q. I'm breastfeeding and I have absolutely no interest in being touched at the end of the day. Is this normal?

Yes, this is normal.

Your estrogen levels are extremely low and you are exhausted from having a new baby around.

Many breastfeeding women feel like they get plenty of touching by having a baby at their breast all day long. While breastfeeding is not sexually arousing, it's common to feel like you don't have anything left at the end of the day for another person that wants to touch you.

Some breastfeeding moms may also feel their breasts are for baby now, not for playing around. Your partner may feel frustrated, so talk about your concerns and fears. Your desire will return after your baby gets a little older and you stop breastfeeding.

We hope you will successfully breastfeed for your baby's entire first year of life (this is the official recommendation from the American Academy of Pediatrics). But we don't want you to wait an entire year to have intercourse again. So here are a few ways to breastfeed and make love:

After the first few weeks, you can begin pumping or "expressing" breast milk. Let your partner do a bottle feeding or two of expressed milk in the

DR H'S OPINION: BACK IN THE SADDLE

Many of my patients are so uncomfortable that they swear they will only have one child because there is no way they would ever be able to get pregnant again! The good news is that a) once you are done breastfeeding, the symptoms typically go away, and b) there are a plethora of water-soluble lubrication options (including Astroglide, which I think is one of the best). Use it every time you have intercourse to help prevent chafing and tearing.

evening. This gives you a mental and physical break. Hopefully, you'll be more interested in sex if you get a respite from breastfeeding. Added bonus: some women find it arousing for their partners to have spit up on their shoulder. (Really! Once you see it, you'll understand.)

Lubricate, lubricate, lubricate.

Q. When do I need to use birth control again?

Easy—once you start having intercourse again.

Assuming you are healing well, you can resume sexual relations at six weeks. Even though you are breastfeeding, you can still get pregnant. Let's put that in bold caps: **YOU CAN STILL GET PREGNANT.**

And even if you needed assisted reproductive technology to become pregnant last time, YOU CAN STILL GET PREGNANT!

Your practitioner will go over your birth control options at the six-week postpartum visit. If you are breastfeeding, you still have a variety of options. Those include a progesterone-only pill, the Depo-provera injection, an IUD, or condoms.

If you aren't breastfeeding, in addition to the items just mentioned, you have the option of using combination oral contraceptive pills ("the pill"), a contraceptive patch or ring.

If you are finished having babies, you might consider permanent sterilization in the form of Essure, a tubal ligation, or a vasectomy for your other half. See Expecting411.com/extra for full details on birth control options.

Q. Does breastfeeding work as contraception?

The short answer is NO.

Do not use breastfeeding as a form of birth control unless you want to have a toddler and a newborn in your house. I've seen countless, utterly shocked, moms get a positive pregnancy test . . . before their baby's first birthday.

It's true that most women who are breastfeeding on a regular basis do not menstruate regularly or at all. But this DOES NOT MEAN that you can't get pregnant. You can ovulate at any time and this is especially true as you begin to wean your baby and breastfeed less. And all it takes is one little sperm making his way down the right tube at the right time.

If you don't want to use other forms of birth control, at least use a condom.

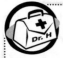

DR H'S TRUE STORY: MURPHY'S LAW AND PREGNANCY

I can't tell you how many patients I have who didn't use contraception after having a baby because . . . "We got pregnant using IVF so there is no way I can get pregnant again," "We got pregnant using medication and IUI so there is no way I can get pregnant again," "It took us ten months to get pregnant the first time so there is no way I can get pregnant right away." These are the same patients who are frantic on the phone (while holding a four month old in their arms) because they took a pregnancy test after feeling weird symptoms and it was positive.

Having another child

At some point, you will actually have sexual intercourse again. I remember a patient who, after my six-week pep talk, had a horrified look on her face. She literally begged me to tell her husband that the "no sex" rule ends at six MONTHS and not six weeks. However, her second child was born when her first was 15 months old.

Even if you don't think you will feel like having sex again in this lifetime (and most of us don't), at some point you will! That said, you have to consider if/when you want to have another child.

Q. How long should I wait between one pregnancy and the next?

For your own health and your next baby's, a recent study by the U.S. Centers for Disease Control and Prevention concluded that the optimal gap between births is at least 18 to 23 months.

It is especially important to wait to conceive again if you had a C-section so that the uterine muscle can fully heal before carrying another pregnancy.

We asked Dr. Kaylen Silverberg, Medical Director of Texas Fertility Center in Austin, TX, for his advice. He recommends having children at least two years apart. Why? It provides quality time with the first baby and time for a woman's body to recover from pregnancy, delivery, and breastfeeding. And he says, "most importantly—it gives couples time to reconnect!"

Q. How will I know if I am ready to have another baby?

There are many things to think about before getting pregnant again. Everyone is different.

Some women are ready to have another baby with one still in diapers and others don't even want to start trying until second grade is over. But if you are planning another one, you may want to ask yourself a few tough questions first:

Do you work? If so, do you have time for another baby right now?

If you have a baby or toddler at home, are you getting enough rest or still waking up repeatedly in the middle of the night?

Will you be financially ready to have another baby?

How does your partner feel about having another baby?

Do you have enough time and energy right now to give attention to a newborn and still continue to care for your other child/ren?

Do you have help (parents, siblings, other relatives, friends, a nanny)?

BOTTOM LINE: There is no perfect time to have another baby. And it often happens without much planning.

Partner Tip
Your vote is equally as important when it comes to your family planning. It takes two to tango. Speak up!

General appearance

Q. I have an outie belly button right now. Will it go back to being an inny?

Most of the time your belly button goes back to what it was, albeit a little bigger. If you had an inny, you'll have an inny again, and the same goes if you started with an outie. This process may take some time, though.

Q. I feel like I have a "bowl full of jelly" in front of me. My stomach is so stretched out and it jiggles every time I walk around. Will I be like this forever?

I know it's strange. Before you deliver, your belly is hard and tight. Now there's a crazy amount of skin that seems to move with your every move!

Your growing baby and uterus stretched out your skin and the underlying tissue and muscle over the past nine months. Now that your uterus is empty and the baby is out, that same skin has nothing big to cover.

You will notice a big decrease in size over the first 14 to 21 days after having your baby. Then, just as it took nine months to stretch out, it often takes a long time for everything to go back down.

Q. My aunt told me that she wore her pre-pregnancy jeans home from the hospital after she had her baby. Is that possible?

No, she is lying. Really. We know she swears she did, but believe us, she didn't. Either that or her doctor kept her in the hospital for three to six months after having her baby.

Your uterus will be at about the level of your belly button and your hips are wider from the normal expansion that occurs prior to delivery. Don't even attempt to try on pre-pregnancy jeans until it's been at least six months. Otherwise, you will find yourself sweating and cursing on the floor as you try to inch them up your thighs (yes, I was dumb enough to try that!).

Hormones, diabetes

Q. I'm sweating all the time. Has my body thermostat changed or is this just hormonal?

It is very normal to find yourself waking up in a puddle in the middle of the night, to the point where you need to change your shirt. These "hot flashes" can also happen in the middle of the day.

Experts believe this is due to the drastic change in hormones that has just occurred in your body. You delivered a baby and with that event, a huge cascade of hormonal changes happened in your body. Your estrogen levels have plummeted and you are in a temporary state of "menopause."

Don't panic, we said *temporary*. The constant feeling of being hot and bothered usually doesn't last more than a month or two.

Q. I had gestational diabetes. What happens now that I'm not pregnant anymore?

The beauty of gestational diabetes is that it goes away after delivery. Human placental lactogen (a hormone made by the placenta) is what usually causes gestational diabetes. Since the placenta is gone now, so is the culprit, uh, we mean, the hormone.

You are no longer classified as a diabetic and can eat normally. Yay!

But you still have a few things to be aware of.

1. You are at risk for having gestational diabetes with your next pregnancy.
3. You are at risk for developing Type II (adult onset) diabetes later in life.
3. You need to do another glucose challenge test (very similar to the one you took during pregnancy when you drank that really sweet, flat syrupy drink) at your six-week postpartum visit (if not then, within 12 weeks of delivery).
4. If you pass the test, tell your general practice/family practice/internist that you were diabetic during your pregnancy. They need to follow you more closely to watch for diabetes in the future.
5. If you fail the test, you get referred to your general practice doctor for an evaluation.

Cardiovascular System

Q. I had preeclampsia. What happens after I deliver?

Preeclampsia is a disease that is specific to pregnancy (we discuss this in detail in Chapter 16, Complications, #20). Most cases occur after 32 weeks gestation or during delivery. Occasionally, it develops after pregnancy in the postpartum period.

If you had preeclampsia during your pregnancy or delivery, your doctor will monitor your blood pressure closely in the postpartum period. If you were placed on magnesium sulfate to prevent seizures, your doctor checks your lungs regularly to make sure there isn't any fluid buildup (pulmonary edema).

The good news: your blood pressure should return to normal shortly after birth.

The bad news: you have a greater risk of preeclampsia with future pregnancies.

Skin/ Hair

Q. My hair texture is changing again and I am starting to lose my hair. Do I need Rogaine?

Wasn't it fantastic to have massive hair growth and shiny, radiant hair during your pregnancy? You can thank your high estrogen levels for that.

But now that your pregnancy is over (yet those pesky little hormonal shifts continue to happen), many women begin to notice something new—hair loss.

We aren't just talking about a little more hair on the brush. Nope, we are referring to chunks of hair falling out in the shower, while brushing or styling, and even while just resting your head on a pillow or your loved one's shoulder.

You'll only appreciate this hair loss if you were one of the unlucky ones who suffered from facial and body hair during your pregnancy. That will start to fall out too!

It's a long time to wait, but most women get their pre-pregnancy hair back six to 18 months after delivery.

Q. Ugh, those stretch marks—will they ever go away?

Unfortunately, once stretch marks appear, they are there to stay. If you want to feel a little better, their initial reddish, purplish color does fade over time to a silver-gray color.

If you don't want to wait or are done having kids and can't take the lines anymore, consult a dermatologist or plastic surgeon about using laser therapy. Just make sure to lose all of your baby weight first.

Q. I have splotches on my skin now (melasma/chloasma). Will they go away?

The splotches may fade, but they typically do not go away completely on their own. Stay out of the sun, because that will only make it worse.

If it doesn't fade and still bothers you, consult with a dermatologist. She may offer certain prescription creams or laser treatment. Neither treatment may work completely, but it might help severe cases.

Q. When can I start using all of my retinal-based creams that I had to stop during pregnancy?

When you are done breastfeeding.

Q. When can I get Botox again?

When you are done breastfeeding. Hang in there, mama, you've made it this far.

DR H'S TRUE STORY: ALARMING HAIR LOSS!

I used to wonder why my office got so many frantic phone calls from women who were one, two, three . . . or six months postpartum, stating that a lot of hair was falling out. I would tell my nurse to reassure them; I didn't really know why they were so upset. After having my first child and seeing the equivalent of a full wig plastered across the shower floor, I finally understand how this process could be so alarming!

POSTPARTUM

Blood

Q. I am Rh negative. I got Rhogam during my pregnancy. Is there anything else I need to do?

It depends on whether your baby is Rh negative or Rh positive.

All babies that are born to Rh negative women get their blood type checked in the first 24 to 48 hours of life. If your baby is Rh *positive*, you should receive another dose of Rhogam. You need to receive your dose of Rhogam within the first 72 hours after delivery to be fully protected.

Q. My practitioner said I lost a lot of blood during my delivery and that I was anemic (based on a blood test done after delivery). What should I do?

Most of the time, taking an iron supplement and eating foods that are rich in iron will correct the anemia.

The typical advice is to take the iron supplement once, twice or three times a day (your practitioner will get more specific). Yes, iron supplements are constipating. Ask for one that is less constipating or take it with a stool softener. (See Expecting411.com/extra for details).

Iron-rich foods include chickpeas, lentils, chicken, turkey, red meat, liver, spinach, dried apricots, prunes, raisins, egg yolks, iron-enriched cereals and grains (read the label), artichokes and mollusks (oysters, clams and scallops).

Immune System

Q. I wasn't immune to rubella when I had my prenatal blood work done. What do I do now?

You should receive a rubella vaccine. This is routinely given before you leave the hospital—it is safe to receive while breastfeeding.

Q. I wasn't sure if I had chickenpox when I was little and when my practitioner checked at the beginning of pregnancy, it showed that I hadn't. What should I do now?

You should receive a varicella vaccine. It is a two-part vaccine, with the

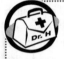

**DR H'S OPINION:
VITAMIN C**

Vitamin C helps your body absorb iron better. So have a Vitamin C-rich food or drink along with your iron supplement. Foods containing higher amounts of Vitamin C include guavas, strawberries, citrus fruit (lemons, oranges, grapefruit), kiwi fruit, rose hip extracts, raspberries, nectarines, mangoes, peaches, peppers, broccoli, curly kale, tomatoes, cauliflower, and brussel sprouts.

postpartum

? ?

POSTPARTUM

second dose given four to eight weeks after the first dose. This vaccine is also safe to receive while breastfeeding.

Q. Do I need any other vaccinations?

Yes!

If you received your last tetanus shot prior to 2005 (or the last one you remember getting was at your own pediatrician's office), you need to get the Tdap—T stands for Tetanus, D stands for Diphtheria, and "ap" stands for acellular pertussis (you might know it better as whooping cough).

Before 2005, adults used to get Td for their tetanus booster shots (recommended every ten years)—there was no "P".

We know that our immunity to whooping cough wanes over time, but there was never a booster vaccination available for pertussis before now. Because of that, adults would be the ones to get whooping cough and go undiagnosed (thinking it was a cough they just couldn't shake or bronchitis). Sick adults would then spread it to those who were the most vulnerable—infants too young to be vaccinated. Yes, that includes your newborn.

Today, all moms, dads, grandparents, and adult caretakers should get the Tdap vaccine if they spend time around a newborn baby. Mom can get her Tdap shot during pregnancy or shortly after delivery. It's also safe to get while breastfeeding. Dads—you can get your shot today. Don't procrastinate!

Reality Check

Tell your newborn's adoring fans (grandparents, aunts, uncles, etc) to get their Tdap shots if they want to hold your new baby.

Partner Tip

If you don't have a personal doctor, now is the time to get one. You should get your Tdap shot as well as the seasonal flu vaccine to protect your precious cargo at home.

Tummy Issues & Nutrition

Q. Are there any special vitamins or nutrients I need more of?

You should continue taking your prenatal vitamins (preferably with DHA) for as long as you breastfeed.

Breastfeeding women also need 1300mg calcium and 800IU of Vitamin D. Your prenatal vitamin probably won't have enough calcium in it, so take a calcium supplement to make up the difference. It's also important to get calcium from your diet. Your body absorbs the calcium from food better than the calcium found in a supplement.

One eight-ounce glass of milk contains about 300mg of calcium. Other ways to get about 300mg of calcium include one cup (eight ounces) of yogurt, two cups of cottage cheese, one cup of orange juice fortified with calcium, one cup of soy milk fortified with calcium, six oranges or two slices of calcium-fortified bread.

Insider Secret

Take your prenatal vitamin and your calcium supplement at different times of the day. All that calcium cannot be absorbed into your system at the same time.

Q. I managed to escape pregnancy without developing hemorrhoids, but boy do I have them now after pushing. What can I do?

Hemorrhoids are just varicose veins that develop around the anus due to the pressure of the baby during pregnancy and the pushing forces that occur during a delivery.

They can get pretty big (like the size of a large grape or even bigger) and sometimes they actually hurt more than your genital area after delivery!

You can use ice packs, Witch Hazel pads, and a topical steroid cream or suppository (like 1% hydrocortisone) to help shrink them back down to normal. Being constipated doesn't help matters. So, take a stool softener and eat anything that is high in fiber (fruits, vegetables, whole grains, prunes, bran).

Red Flag

If you are having excruciating pain from hemorrhoids, contact your provider right way. That's because a clot can form in the vein—although this is rare.

Q. I had my baby three days ago and still haven't had a bowel movement. Is that normal?

Yes.

Many women will not poop for a few days after delivery. The good news is that it gives some time for your girl parts to heal before having to bear down while pooping and stretch out some tender, healing tissue.

However, you will do yourself a big favor if you go when you feel the urge to go. We know you are scared to go, but holding it in will only make things worse a few days down the line. And load up on fiber, water, and a stool softener shortly after delivery so you aren't in misery when nature calls. If you had a third or fourth degree tear, ask your practitioner about taking something more than a run-of-the-mill stool softener. You may benefit from something a little stronger, at least until you have a few BMs.

Reality Check

As we discussed, narcotic pain medication can cause constipation as a side effect. So, either take a stool softener and increase your fiber to combat the effects of the medication . . . or you can try switching over to ibuprofen for pain relief instead.

Q. How much weight will I lose now that I have delivered?

The good news: You will lose quite a bit of weight right after delivery. Specifically, you lose seven to eight pounds of baby, one to two pounds of placenta, and at least two pounds of amniotic fluid and blood.

That's a ten to 12 lb. weight loss at the time of birth!

Then, you get rid of your extra fluid in the week or so after delivery just by peeing and sweating it out. That's another two to four pounds without even heading to the gym.

The bad news: it takes some time to get back to your pre-pregnancy weight. So be realistic . . . and optimistic!

Q. Can I go on a diet if I am breastfeeding?

For a full discussion of this answer, see Expecting411.com/extra on breastfeeding. Here's the Cliffs Notes version:

We know you don't want to hear this, but the answer is no.

You actually need about 300 to 500 calories more than what you normally eat while breastfeeding. If you aren't getting enough to eat or drink, you and your breast milk will suffer.

Your baby is still somewhat of a parasite—taking what he needs at your body's expense. For instance, if you don't get enough calcium in your diet to provide an adequate amount in your breast milk, your body conveniently takes it out of your own bones. And if you are truly starving yourself to lose weight, your milk quality and quantity will suffer. As a result, you aren't doing your baby any favors.

The goal: be healthy, make wise food choices and exercise—but save the dieting until after you are done breastfeeding.

Urinary Tract

Q. I pee a bit every time I laugh—and that's not very funny. What do I do?

It is very normal to leak a little urine after having a baby. This may last for a few days or up to a few months.

Many women also report not having great bladder control until after they are done breastfeeding, their estrogen levels rise again and the vaginal/vulvar/urethral tissue gets "plumped" up. The very first step is doing Kegel exercises. (See the box earlier in this chapter for Kegel How-To's).

If you feel Kegel's haven't cured the problem, there are some other options:

◆ **Topical estrogen cream.** If you apply this cream religiously once or twice a day, it may help revitalize the tissues down there. It's available by prescription only, so you will need to ask your doc for it.

◆ **Timed voiding.** This means that you go into the bathroom, sit down and try to urinate every two hours whether you feel like you have to go or not. Many of us tend to "hold" our urine thinking, "Oh I will just do one more thing before I go." Try to train yourself to empty your bladder regularly.

◆ **Surgery.** Bladder reconstructive surgery is a last resort and reserved for severe cases. A woman must have completed childbearing and be unsuccessful with all other treatments.

Most of the time, your symptoms will resolve by six months after delivery.

Nervous System

Q. How long am I going to feel exhausted?

Let's see here. You just worked really hard to deliver a baby. Regardless of whether you had a vaginal delivery or a C-section, you body has been through a lot and is expending a lot of energy toward healing.

You also lost quite a bit of blood during delivery and you are likely a little bit (or a lot) anemic.

And now for the biggie, you have a newborn and are likely not sleeping well through the night. Newborns sleep a lot, but not all at the same time. You'll probably be awakened every two to three hours at night for the next eight weeks.

No one can really prepare you for the sheer exhaustion you will experience. But it is a rite of passage for all new parents. You will survive, even though some days you might wonder!

It's critical to take care of yourself, for your baby's sake. Eat well. Nap when your baby naps. Do not be tempted to clean up or do laundry during naptime. And believe it or not, regular exercise actually helps lessen fatigue.

While some parents report that they are exhausted until their kids go off to college, expect to start feeling better after three months (assuming your baby starts sleeping longer at night).

Emotional/Mental Health

Q. I just had my baby a week ago and I find myself crying for no apparent reason. I'm also really irritated with my husband. Is this normal?

Yes.

In fact, it's so normal that up to 80% of women feel this way. It's called **POSTPARTUM** or **"BABY" BLUES**. This is different than postpartum *depression*.

Postpartum blues typically occur in the first four to five days after delivery and can last for up to two weeks. You might feel moody, anxious, impatient, irritable, or weepy. It's kind of like PMS.

The blues occur for a number of reasons: major hormonal shifts, lack of sleep, and anxiety over caring for a new baby. You may not always feel sad when you are crying. In fact, you may sob as you say out loud, "I have no

DR H'S TRUE STORY: POSTPARTUM BLUES

No one really tells you about postpartum blues. I sure didn't learn about it in medical school, residency or from any of my girlfriends. It wasn't until I went through it myself that I learned about it.

I now make it a point to tell my patients before sending them home so that they know what to expect and know that they aren't the only one in the world experiencing these feelings.

idea why I am crying!"

When you have the baby blues:

1. You are eating normally.
2. You have no difficulty sleeping (when you get a chance to!)

Remember these key points when we compare the blues to postpartum *depression*.

Q. I just had my baby ten weeks ago and I am still crying everyday. I'm having a hard time getting out of bed to take care of my baby. Is this normal?

While it's *not* normal, there is an explanation. It's called **POSTPARTUM DEPRESSION (PPD)** and it happens to as many as 10% of all new mothers.

Symptoms may occur a few days after delivery or not until months afterwards. Symptoms may be mild or severe, and often alternate . . . so that some days seem okay but other days are really tough to get through.

The difference between postpartum blues and postpartum depression is that PPD does not go away.

Symptoms include severe fatigue, overwhelming feelings of sadness and guilt, and trouble sleeping and eating.

It is vitally important that you speak to your practitioner about your feelings and if possible, include your partner or other loved ones in the visit. The more help you can get, the quicker you can begin to feel better.

Reality Check

Psychiatrist and author Dr. Lucy Puryear shares her insider tip on deciphering postpartum depression: "In my experience, the single best question to ask a new mother who I suspect is suffering postpartum depression is, 'Are you able to sleep when the baby is sleeping?'" If the answer is no, seek professional help.

Puryear is the Director of Baylor Psychiatry Clinic and specializes in women's reproductive mental health. She is the author of *Understanding Your Moods When You're Expecting* (Houghton Mifflin, 2007). We recommend this book for further reading.

POSTPARTUM DEPRESSION: WHO'S AT RISK?

According to Dr. Lucy Puryear, certain women are at greater risk of developing postpartum depression. These are women who are more vulnerable to hormonal changes than others. For them, those major hormone shifts cause depression. Here are the top six risk factors:

- History of depression at any point in life.
- Symptoms of depression during the third trimester of pregnancy.
- Previous history of postpartum depression.
- Family member with bipolar disorder.
- Severe premenstrual syndrome (PMS).
- Poor marital support.

Partner Tip

As you may know, partners sometimes gain sympathy weight. Well, partners are also at risk for having postpartum depression. Seek help if you have some of the warning symptoms we've discussed.

Q. I know this sounds strange but I'm having thoughts of harming my baby. Is this normal?

No, this is not normal.

This may be a symptom of severe postpartum depression or postpartum psychosis. Postpartum psychosis occurs in one out of every 1,000 pregnancies. The onset is sudden and usually occurs two to three weeks after giving birth (but it can happen as quickly as a few days after delivery).

Symptoms include bizarre behavior, hallucinations (hearing or seeing things that are not really there and can't be heard or seen by others), delusions, suicidal thoughts and thoughts of harming others, including your newborn.

Postpartum psychosis is a medical emergency because it is extremely dangerous for you and your baby. You should contact your practitioner immediately and have another adult with you and your baby at all times.

Partner Tip

Often times, the support person is the one to identify a problem. Keep your eyes open and get help for your partner if you have concerns. Trust your instincts—you know your partner best and if she seems depressed or you are concerned about other behavior, call her practitioner. Check out the Red Flags for postpartum depression below.

Q. I keep having these horrible thoughts that something terrible will happen to my baby and it will be my fault. Is it normal to feel this way?

Every once in a while, a mom might come up with a worst case scenario in her mind—such as, "If I fall asleep while I am nursing in this rocking chair, I might drop my baby." That's normal (and probably wise to consider!).

But occasionally moms find themselves having these thoughts all the time. They have no desire to intentionally harm their babies and they are very scared of these crazy thoughts. This is called *postpartum obsessive-compulsive disorder*.

If you feel this way, do not be afraid to ask for help!

Red flags for Postpartum Depression *(Puryear L.)*

◆ Lots of crying.
◆ Sad mood.
◆ Short temper.
◆ Feeling hopeless or worthless.
◆ Lack of desire to be around family and friends.
◆ Lack of caring for self.

postpartum

◆ Change in appetite or eating pattern.
◆ Difficulty sleeping, even when the baby is sleeping.
◆ No desire to get out of bed.
◆ Not wanting to hold or touch the baby (not enjoying the baby).
◆ Difficulty thinking clearly.
◆ Thoughts about your own death, or death of the baby.

Q. Where do I turn if I need help?

The first place to start is with your practitioner. She can help you immediately, and then refer you to local professionals and support groups in your community. There is nothing to be embarrassed about. And believe us, you are definitely not alone!

The next section of this book covers special concerns and problems. We hope you don't have to read the next few chapters—but they are there just in case!

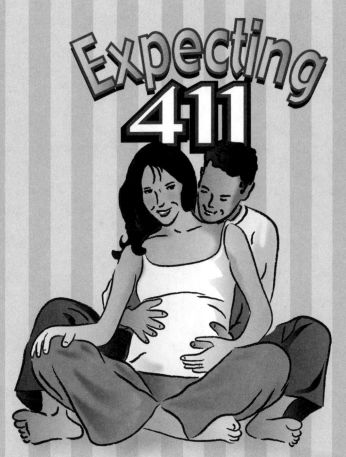

section five

Special Concerns
& Problems

PREGNANCY 911

Chapter 15

"'Don't worry, I've never lost a patient. I never lose anything. Have you seen my stethoscope?"
—Hawkeye, M*A*S*H*

Let's face it. We all pause for a moment before calling our doctor about a concern. We don't want to sound like complete idiots, obsessing over something that is probably nothing. We don't want to wake our overworked practitioners up at 3am over something that could wait until the morning.

This chapter should help you troubleshoot the most common and the most urgent medical problems during your pregnancy. It will help you determine when you really do need to call your practitioner (even at 3am) and when it's probably okay to wait until the office opens. It also prepares you for what your doc will ask you when you call.

A key point: this chapter does not, in any way, replace the need to check in with your practitioner. If you are worried, pick up the phone! Your practitioner will not get upset with you. But having this information on your nightstand may help you worry less and trust your instincts more.

The goal of this chapter is to help you troubleshoot, and do it quickly. If you want to read up on the topics we refer to here, head over to Chapter 16, Complications for all the ugly details.

 On-Call Etiquette
Before we get into specifics on emergencies, let's go over a few tips on how to best communicate with your practitioner:

1. **Who you gonna call?** *Before the need arises,* find out how your practitioner handles phone calls during the day and after hours. Who answers the phone? And what number do you call?

2. **Volunteer information.** If your practitioner shares on-call responsibilities with other doctors (which is likely), don't expect the on-call doc to know your medical history or have it accessible. Tell the on-call doctor how far along you are and if you've had any complications, as well as the problem you are calling about.

3. **Skip the snack.** If you have to head to the hospital, do *not* eat before you go. It's better to do certain tests and procedures on an empty stomach. Since you don't know what lies ahead, hold off on the food. Do grab a toothbrush and some reading material.

4. **Call before running anywhere.** If you think there is a problem, you should always call your doctor before rushing to the emergency room (unless you are calling 911). Your doctor may be able to manage things over the phone, and if not, your doc can notify the hospital that you are coming in (and be ready to meet you there).

5. **Take your temp.** If you think you have a fever, take your temperature with a thermometer *before* calling. The practitioner will ask, so you might as well be ready to tell her exactly what your temperature is instead of saying "I think I feel warm."

6. **You make the call.** While it's nice for your husband or partner to speak with your practitioner, it's best if you call yourself. Your practitioner will ask a number of questions that will be tough for your partner to answer, such as "How many days ago did your green vaginal discharge begin?" or "When was the last time you had a bowel movement?"

7. **Make sure your phone accepts anonymous calls.** Most docs call from blocked phone lines—make sure your cell phone is not blocking such calls.

Insider secret

Just a head's up—if you encounter one of the problems in this chapter during office hours, your practitioner may manage it differently than in the middle of the night or on a weekend. During normal business hours, your doctor will be able to see you in his or her office and have full access to a lab or imaging facility. If you need urgent attention at other times, the only way to accomplish an evaluation is through an urgent care facility, emergency room or admission to the hospital.

Q. How do I decide what is a medical emergency?

Much of this is just common sense.

Unless your life or the life of your fetus is in imminent danger, it's best not to call 911. But there are situations when you need paramedics and a rapid trip to the Emergency Room.

Let's go over a little doctor lingo before we discuss specific emergencies. If you've ever watched Grey's Anatomy or ER, you know that doctors will "triage" or prioritize patients to be treated based on the severity of their problem.

For the purposes of this chapter, this is how we will triage (that is, categorize) pregnancy emergencies:

? ?

911

- **911:** call 911.
- **Priority 1:** Needs medical attention NOW!
- **Priority 2:** Needs appointment in the next day or two.
- **Priority 3:** Watch and wait. Needs appointment if there is no improvement or worsening of symptoms.

Red Flags: When do I call 911?

Here are the top pregnancy emergencies that require immediate attention by a trained medical provider and immediate transport to the nearest hospital. Call 911 if you experience:

- **Severe vaginal bleeding**—extremely heavy vaginal bleeding that does not stop, or gets worse. Bleeding along with abdominal pain or dizziness/faintness is also a red flag.
- **Severe chest pain**—especially if you are also short of breath.
- **Labor and rectal pressure**—if your labor has progressed at home, your contractions are coming every two to three minutes, and you feel rectal pressure. You don't have to poop—it's the baby's head!
- **Blood when water bag breaks**—if you break your water bag and there is a large amount of blood.
- **Water bag breaks and you feel something in your vagina**—it could be the umbilical cord or a fetal part (head, hand or foot).
- **Severe abdominal pain**—a sudden onset of severe, constant abdominal pain . . . especially if you also have vaginal bleeding.
- **Sharp abdominal trauma**—yes, this can happen. If it does, have someone call 911 immediately if you are stabbed or take a gunshot wound to the belly.
- **Severe blunt abdominal trauma**—if you have a bad fall or motor vehicle accident that results in direct abdominal contact.

Red Flags: When to head to the ER

There are times you need urgent care even if you don't need an ambulance. For example, if your emergency happens after office hours (at night, early in the morning or on a weekend), it's often best to go straight to the ER. Presuming you have a cell phone, you can call your doctor while you are en route. The ER doctor who sees you will likely give your practitioner a call to discuss your case and make a follow-up plan.

Here are a few of the top reasons to head to the nearest ER without waiting for the on-call doctor to call you back:

- Abrupt onset of a severe headache that is not responding to pain medication (Tylenol).
- Extreme, unrelenting vomiting.
- Excruciating abdominal pain, especially when associated with nausea, vomiting, diarrhea, and/or fever.
- Moderate or heavy vaginal bleeding.

If you have an emergency when your doctor's office is open, it's best to call there first. Your doctor will either want you to come to the office for an immediate evaluation or go to the ER.

911: emergencies

Q. How do I take my vital signs?

For certain problems, it's helpful to report your vital signs to the doctor on call. If it's not an extreme emergency, take your temperature, pulse (heart rate), and breaths per minute (respiratory rate) before picking up the phone.

How to check your pulse: The easiest places to find your pulse are your neck (just under your jaw bone on either side) or the inner part of your wrist. Count how many times you feel a beat in 15 seconds and then multiply that by four. That equals your pulse (how many times your heart beats in a minute). The average heart rate for an adult is 60 to 100 beats per minute.

How to check your breaths per minute: Watch your chest as it moves in and out. Count one breath for each time you breathe in for 15 seconds and then multiply that by four. This is your respiratory rate. The average respiratory rate for an adult is 12 to 20 breaths per minute.

We assume you know how to use a thermometer, so we won't go through an explanation of checking your temperature. We just have one bit of advice, however: report the actual reading on the thermometer (by mouth or ear or temporal artery scanner) to your practitioner. Do not add a degree, subtract a decimal point, or do a calculus equation on the number!

Partner Tip

If you are there during an emergency, one helpful role is to get your partner's vitals. Stay calm and follow the above procedures to get accurate readings.

Top 12 Obstetrical Emergencies

We will triage symptoms that require medical attention and discuss how quickly you need to act in each scenario. While this is not an exhaustive list, it covers the most common and the most serious issues you may encounter.

We are keeping our fingers crossed that you won't ever need this chapter! Remember, this is how docs handle emergencies *when the office is closed.*

1. Headache

Being pregnant can give anyone a headache! So, don't be surprised if you have one here or there. They are typical in the first and early second trimesters, even in women who don't have a history of frequent headaches. Headaches are rarely a sign of something serious. But on occasion, your body is telling you that something is very wrong.

Common diagnoses:
- Tension headache from stress or work.
- Dehydration.
- Lack of sleep.
- Discontinuing caffeine from your diet (caffeine withdrawal).
- Elevated hormone levels.
- Migraine sufferers sometimes have more migraines during pregnancy.

Uncommon diagnoses:
- High blood pressure (severe **PREECLAMPSIA**).
- Stroke.
- Bleeding between the brain and surrounding tissues (subarachnoid hemorrhage).
- Bleeding in the brain (**SUBDURAL HEMATOMA**).
- Infection in the tissue around the brain (**MENINGITIS**).
- Trauma.

What to do:
- Drink water.
- Rest in a cool, quiet room.
- Take acetaminophen (Tylenol) as directed on the bottle. Do NOT take ibuprofen (Advil, Aleve, Motrin) or aspirin.
- Have a caffeinated drink (coffee or cola . . . no it won't hurt the baby).
- Ask for a shoulder/neck/head massage if your partner is around.

Take home tips:
Most pregnancy headaches resolve with drinking fluids, rest, acetaminophen (Tylenol) and caffeine. If yours does not, or this is the worst headache you have ever had in your life, call your practitioner.

What the practitioner will ask you about your HEADACHE:
- Do you have a previous history of frequent headaches or migraine headaches?
- When did it start?
- Did it wake you from sleep?
- How long has it been going on?
- Have you had a recent head injury?
- Have you tried taking acetaminophen (Tylenol), resting, drinking fluids or having some caffeine?
- Are you having any other symptoms: Fever? Nausea or vomiting? Stiff neck? Blurred vision? Sensitivity to light? Pain in the upper right side of your belly? Abdominal pain or vaginal bleeding? Dizziness? Loss of consciousness? Seizures? Confusion? Slurred speech?

911: Call an ambulance.
- Severe headache and loss of consciousness/confusion.
- Severe headache and seizure.
- Severe headache and uncontrollable vomiting.
- Severe headache after head injury (car accident, fall, violence).
- The worst headache you have ever had, particularly if it wakes you from sleep.

Priority 1: Needs medical attention now.
- Severe headache and onset of blurred vision.
- Severe headache and dizziness.
- Severe headache and sudden onset of hand/feet swelling.
- Severe headache with fever and/or neck stiffness and light sensitivity.

911: emergencies

Priority 2: Needs appointment in the next day or two.

◆ Constant headache without other symptoms that comes and goes, despite trying the above mentioned measures.

Priority 3: Watch and wait.

◆ Frequent headaches that resolve with the above mentioned measures.
◆ A dull, intermittent headache with no other symptoms.

Red Flag
If this is the worst headache of your life, call 911.

FYI: Acetaminophen (Tylenol) is okay to take during pregnancy. Ibuprofen (Motrin, Advil) is not. Ibuprofen is fine to take *after* delivery.

2. Vomiting

Almost every pregnant woman tosses her cookies at some point, particularly in the first trimester. But vomiting can also be a sign of something more serious, especially when it occurs without "morning sickness" or when morning sickness has already come and gone.

Common diagnoses:
◆ Morning sickness.
◆ Food poisoning.
◆ Eating too much, especially in the later stages of pregnancy.
◆ Labor.

Uncommon diagnoses:
◆ Gallstones/gallbladder inflammation (**CHOLECYSTITIS**).
◆ Inflammation or infection of the liver (hepatitis).
◆ Inflammation of the pancreas (**PANCREATITIS**).
◆ Inflammation or infection of the appendix (appendicitis).
◆ Kidney infection (**PYELONEPHRITIS**).
◆ Twisted ovary (ovarian torsion).
◆ High blood pressure (**PREECLAMPSIA**).
◆ Acute fatty liver.

What to do:
◆ Rest.
◆ After vomiting, wait five to ten minutes and try to take a small sip of liquid. The best liquids to try are those with a little bit of sugar (instead of straight water), like ginger ale, 7-UP, Sprite, or Gatorade. You can also try clear chicken broth.
◆ Hold off on milk or dairy products while your stomach is unsettled.
◆ If you can keep the sips down after ten minutes, try a few more sips every five minutes.
◆ If you are actively vomiting or extremely nauseated, wait one hour before you test the waters with those sips of fluid.

- ◆ If you cannot stop vomiting and/or you are NOT able to keep down those sips of liquids, call your practitioner.
- ◆ Remember to take your temperature first and take note of any other symptoms you may have (see below).

Take home tips:
The priority is to keep liquids down to prevent dehydration. It's less important whether or not you can tolerate solid food right now. Call your practitioner if you are vomiting so often that you cannot keep liquids down for three to four hours.

What the practitioner will ask you about your VOMITING:
- ◆ How many times have you vomited?
- ◆ What color is it? Green? Yellow? Bloody? Coffee grounds?
- ◆ What have you eaten in the last 12 hours?
- ◆ Have you been able to keep any liquids down in the last few hours?
- ◆ Have you been around anyone who has been sick?
- ◆ Do you have a fever?
- ◆ Do you have any of these other symptoms: diarrhea? Abdominal pain? Low back pain? Headache? Pain with urination?

911: Call an ambulance.

- ◆ Vomiting a significant amount of blood (red or brownish fluid).
- ◆ Vomiting associated with severe, constant abdominal pain.

Priority 1: Needs medical attention now.

- ◆ Vomiting a small amount of blood.
- ◆ Vomiting so much you haven't been able to keep fluids down in four hours.
- ◆ Vomiting and dizziness.
- ◆ Vomiting and chills, low back pain and painful urination.
- ◆ Vomiting and a fever greater than or equal to 102° F.
- ◆ Vomiting bile (yellow/bright green fluid).
- ◆ Vomiting and head injury.
- ◆ Unrelenting vomiting that has continued for more than six hours.

Priority 2: Needs appointment the next day.

- ◆ Vomiting throughout the day, but you're able to keep some liquids down.
- ◆ Persistent vomiting and diarrhea.
- ◆ Vomiting associated with a fever greater than 100.4° F but less than 102° F.

Priority 3: Watch and wait.

- ◆ Sporadic vomiting associated with morning sickness in the first trimester.
- ◆ One or two episodes of vomiting with no other symptoms.

911: emergencies

911

Red Flag

Keeping liquids down is key. If you have not been able to keep any liquid down in the past four hours, call your doc.

3. Fever

Fever is an elevation of the body's regular temperature. Contrary to what you probably learned in school, our body temperature is not 98.6° F, 24 hours a day. It varies on a daily cycle based on hormone levels. Our body is coolest at 4am (as low as 97.6° F) and hottest at 7pm (as high at 100° F). So, the true definition of a "fever" is a body temperature of 100.4° F or higher.

Fever is your body's way of responding to an infection or inflammation. You should contact your practitioner any time you have a temperature of 100.4° F or greater.

Common diagnoses:
- ◆ Common cold or flu virus.
- ◆ Stomach virus.
- ◆ Food poisoning.
- ◆ You just received a vaccine (seasonal flu shot, etc.)

Uncommon diagnoses:
- ◆ Lung infection (**PNEUMONIA**).
- ◆ Inflammation of the pancreas (**PANCREATITIS**).
- ◆ Inflammation and infection of the appendix (appendicitis).
- ◆ Blood clot.
- ◆ Inflammation or infection of the liver (hepatitis).
- ◆ Gallstones/inflammation of the gallbladder (**CHOLECYSTITIS**).
- ◆ Infection of the placenta and amniotic sac (**CHORIOAMNIONITIS**).
- ◆ Parvovirus infection.
- ◆ Listeria infection.
- ◆ Kidney infection (**PYELONEPHRITIS**).

What to do:
- ◆ Rule #1: before you panic, take your temperature. . . just because you feel hot doesn't mean your core body temperature is actually over 100.4° F (what we consider to be a fever).
- ◆ Take acetaminophen (Tylenol) 650mg by mouth every four to six hours.
- ◆ Drink more fluids.
- ◆ Take note of other symptoms (see below).

Take home tips: Have a thermometer at home!

What the practitioner will ask you about your FEVER:
- ◆ What is your temperature?
- ◆ How long have you had it?
- ◆ Have you taken any medication? Acetaminophen (Tylenol)? How much? When was your last dose?
- ◆ Do you have any other symptoms: headache? Cough? Runny

nose? Sore throat? Nausea? Vomiting? Diarrhea? Abdominal pain? Vaginal bleeding or leaking? Painful urination? Back pain? Chills? Body aches?

◆ Is anyone at home sick or have you had any sick contacts in the past week?

◆ Do you have a rash?

Priority 1: Needs medical attention now.

◆ Fever at or over 102° F.
◆ Fever and back/flank pain with or without chills.
◆ Fever with body aches and chills.
◆ Fever and intractable vomiting or diarrhea.
◆ Fever and foul-smelling vaginal discharge.
◆ Fever and severe abdominal pain.
◆ Fever and difficulty breathing.

Priority 2: Needs appointment in the next day or two.

◆ Fever and severe sinus pain.
◆ Fever and upper respiratory symptoms (cough, runny nose, ear pain, sore throat).

Priority 3: Watch and wait.

◆ Fever less than 102° F that responds to acetaminophen (Tylenol) and resolves.
◆ Fever less than 102° F with no other symptoms.

Red Flag
If you have a persistent fever and you cannot figure out why, call your practitioner.

4. Abdominal pain

Everyone gets some belly discomfort during pregnancy. It happens in the first trimester as your uterus begins to grow . . . and in the second trimester as your round ligaments get pulled. Inevitably, it also happens in your third trimester, either due to the extreme discomfort from having a big baby in your belly or secondary to uterine contractions and labor. The key is to be able to figure out when abdominal pain is normal, and when it is not.

Common diagnoses:

◆ A growing uterus (menstrual-like cramps without vaginal bleeding).
◆ Round ligament pain.
◆ Muscle strain.
◆ Constipation.
◆ Bladder infection.
◆ Uterine contractions/labor.
◆ Stomach virus (**GASTROENTERITIS**).
◆ Food poisoning.

Uncommon diagnoses:

◆ Appendicitis.

◆ Benign tumor in uterus outgrows its blood supply (**DEGENERATING UTERINE FIBROID**).

◆ Rupture of an ovarian cyst.

◆ Gallstones/inflammation of the gallbladder (**CHOLECYSTITIS**).

◆ Liver inflammation or infection (hepatitis).

◆ Inflammation of the pancreas (**PANCREATITIS**).

◆ Kidney infection (**PYELONEPHRITIS**).

◆ Hernia.

◆ **ECTOPIC PREGNANCY** (first trimester).

◆ **PLACENTAL ABRUPTION.**

What to do:

◆ Rest. Sit down or lie down on your left side.

◆ If your pain persists, gets worse, or you have additional symptoms, call your practitioner.

◆ Take note of whether you have any additional symptoms (see below).

Take home tips:

◆ It's common to have random, short-lived episodes of abdominal pain during any trimester.

◆ Docs worry MORE about dull, crampy abdominal pain than sharp, knife-like pain.

What the practitioner will ask you about your ABDOMINAL PAIN:

◆ Where is your pain located? Upper abdomen? Lower abdomen? In the middle? More to one side?

◆ Does the pain radiate or travel anywhere? Your back? Your leg? Your chest?

◆ How long have you had the pain?

◆ Is it constant or does it come and go?

◆ Does anything you do make it better? Worse?

◆ Do you have any underlying medical problems (such as high blood pressure or lupus)?

◆ Are you having any vaginal bleeding or leaking of fluid from the vagina?

◆ Is your baby moving (if past 26 weeks)?

◆ Are you having any other symptoms: Fever? Chills? Nausea? Vomiting? Diarrhea? Pain with urination? Low back pain?

911: Call an ambulance.

◆ Severe pain that comes on suddenly and there is no relief for an hour or more.

◆ Severe abdominal pain and heavy vaginal bleeding.

◆ Severe abdominal pain and constant vomiting.

◆ Severe one-sided abdominal pain in the first trimester with vaginal bleeding and/or dizziness before you have had an ultrasound showing that your baby has correctly implanted in your uterus.

Priority 1: Needs medical attention now.

◆ Abdominal pain and fever, chills, low back pain or painful urination.
◆ Abdominal pain with nausea and intermittent vomiting.
◆ Abdominal pain and small amounts of vaginal bleeding.
◆ Abdominal pain and watery vaginal discharge.
◆ Severe abdominal pain with known uterine fibroids or an ovarian cyst.

Priority 2: Needs appointment in the next day or two.

◆ Intermittent abdominal pain and no other symptoms.
◆ Mild abdominal pain and a visible bulge in your groin area.

Priority 3: Watch and wait.

◆ Abdominal pain that gets better and resolves with no other symptoms.
◆ Abdominal pain that improves with rest or use of a maternity belt.

5. Contractions

Unless you have a scheduled C-section, you will encounter contractions when you go into labor. It's also natural to have **BRAXTON HICKS CONTRACTIONS** sporadically towards the end of pregnancy. If this is your second, third or (wow, we salute you) fourth pregnancy, Braxton Hicks contractions may be felt as early as 24 to 28 weeks.

If you have real contractions in the second or early third trimester, you definitely need to chat with your practitioner!

Common diagnoses:
◆ Braxton Hicks contractions.
◆ Dehydration (leading to contractions).
◆ A bladder infection (leading to contractions).
◆ Labor (real contractions in a pregnancy beyond 37 weeks gestation).

Uncommon diagnoses:
◆ Preterm contractions (uterine contractions occurring after 22 weeks and before 37 weeks that, although uncomfortable, do not cause dilation of the cervix).
◆ Preterm labor (uterine contractions occurring after 22 weeks but before 37 weeks, that *do* lead to dilation of the cervix).

What to do (these are all things that my mother-in-law, married to an obstetrician for over 30 years, would tell my father-in-law's patients on the phone when he was away delivering another baby):
◆ Rest. Sit down or lie down on your left side.
◆ Hydrate. Drink a lot of water/fluids.
◆ Time your contractions over the course of an hour. How? Time them from the start of one to the start of the next.
◆ Take note of other symptoms such as vaginal bleeding or leaking of water from the vagina, pain with urination, or constant pain.

911: emergencies

Take home tips:

◆ **If you are less than 35 weeks:** call your practitioner if you are having more than four to six contractions in an hour.

◆ **If you are more than 35 weeks:** call your practitioner if you are having regular uterine contractions every five to seven minutes for an hour.

◆ If you are carrying more than one fetus, have a **CERCLAGE** or any other type of high-risk pregnancy, discuss *all* contractions with your practitioner.

What your practitioner will ask you about your CONTRACTIONS:

◆ What is your due date?

◆ How often are your contractions occurring?

◆ How long have you been having contractions?

◆ Does your pain come and go or is it constant?

◆ Are you carrying one fetus or do you have twins? Triplets? More?

◆ On a scale of one to ten with ten being the most pain you have ever felt, how painful are your contractions?

◆ Do you have a history of preterm labor in this pregnancy or any previous pregnancies?

◆ Are you having any vaginal bleeding or leaking of fluid from the vagina?

◆ What were you doing when your contractions began? Exercising? On your feet all day? Having intercourse?

◆ Have you been getting enough to drink? Are you well hydrated?

◆ Do you have any pain with urination? Fever? Frequent urination?

911: Call an ambulance.

◆ Severe, constant abdominal pain, especially with vaginal bleeding.

◆ Regular, painful contractions occurring every two to three minutes with rectal pressure (particularly in a woman who has already had one or two children).

Priority 1: Needs medical attention now.

◆ Painful uterine contractions occurring more frequently than four to six times an hour if you are less than 35 weeks gestation.

◆ Painful regular contractions occurring every three to five minutes, for at least an hour or two if you are over 35 weeks gestation.

◆ Painful uterine contractions with leaking of fluid/blood from vagina.

◆ Painful, regular uterine contractions with a high-risk pregnancy (breech baby, **PLACENTA PREVIA**, **VASA PREVIA**, previous C-section, multiples).

Priority 2: Needs appointment the next day.

◆ Intermittent contractions that are becoming more regular but are still 15 to 30 minutes apart.

◆ Uterine contractions and frequent urination.

Priority 3: Watch and wait.

◆ Intermittent contractions occurring at 35 weeks or beyond.

- ◆ Uterine contractions with dehydration that resolve when you increase your fluid intake.
- ◆ Uterine contractions occurring with over-exertion that resolve when you rest.

6. Vaginal bleeding

About 10% of all pregnant women have some vaginal bleeding, with most of these episodes occurring in the first trimester. Typically, a small amount of vaginal bleeding is nothing serious. But, it's always a good idea to run it by your practitioner.

Docs are most concerned when the bleeding persists or when it is extremely heavy and accompanied by large clots. Practitioners get clues from what color the blood is, how much is coming out, whether or not clots are present, and when in a pregnancy the bleeding occurs.

Common diagnoses:
- ◆ **IMPLANTATION BLEEDING** (first trimester).
- ◆ Vaginal irritation or injury (from intercourse).
- ◆ Vaginal or cervical infection.
- ◆ Partial placental separation.
- ◆ Labor (**BLOODY SHOW**).

Uncommon diagnoses:
- ◆ Ectopic pregnancy (1st trimester).
- ◆ Threatened miscarriage (1st trimester).
- ◆ Cervical cancer.
- ◆ Death of one fetus in a multiples pregnancy (**VANISHING TWIN**).
- ◆ **CERVICAL INSUFFICIENCY** (2nd/3rd trimester).
- ◆ Premature labor (2nd/3rd trimester).
- ◆ **PLACENTA PREVIA** (2nd/3rd trimester).
- ◆ **VASA PREVIA** (2nd/3rd trimester).
- ◆ **PLACENTA ABRUPTION** (2nd/3rd trimester).

What to do:
- ◆ Rest. Lie down if possible.
- ◆ Use a feminine pad so that you can quantify how much blood you are losing.
- ◆ Note any other symptoms: abdominal pain, decreased fetal movement (if you are more than 26 weeks), dizziness, lightheadedness.
- ◆ Bring any blood clots/tissue you pass with you to the medical facility.
- ◆ Call your practitioner with any amount of bleeding.

Take home tips:
At least half the time, your practitioner will not know exactly why you have vaginal bleeding. If there is no obvious diagnosis, docs assume that it is due to a small degree of placental separation that isn't visible on ultrasound.

What the practitioner will ask you about your VAGINAL BLEEDING:

◆ How much blood are you passing? Is it spotting or are you bleeding as much as a period?

◆ How far along are you? What is your due date?

◆ Are you passing any blood clots or any tissue?

◆ Are you having any abdominal pain or cramping?

◆ Do you feel faint, dizzy, or lightheaded?

◆ Is this the first episode of vaginal bleeding you have had during this pregnancy?

◆ Have you ever lost a pregnancy/had a miscarriage in the past?

◆ Have you had intercourse recently?

◆ Have you had any recent abdominal trauma?

◆ If you are past 26 weeks, do you feel your baby moving around?

911: Call an ambulance.

◆ Severe abdominal pain with moderate to heavy vaginal bleeding.

◆ Moderate to severe bleeding with a known **PLACENTA PREVIA.**

◆ Moderate to severe bleeding with a known chronic **PLACENTAL ABRUPTION.**

◆ Moderate to severe bleeding and dizziness or lightheadedness.

◆ Moderate to severe bleeding after having direct abdominal trauma.

Priority 1: Needs medical attention now.

◆ Continuous vaginal bleeding.

◆ Spotting with a known **PLACENTA PREVIA, VASA PREVIA OR CHRONIC PLACENTAL ABRUPTION.**

Priority 2: Needs appointment in the next day or two.

◆ Minimal red spotting without pain.

Priority 3: Watch and wait.

◆ Intermittent brownish spotting once you have already confirmed that the fetus is implanted in your uterus (i.e., you've had an ultrasound).

MISCARRIAGE

If you miscarry before six to seven weeks, you can usually manage things at home. You will have bleeding like a heavy period and you may pass a few blood clots. You can treat the pain with ibuprofen (Advil, Motrin).

Signs of a potentially more serious condition include severe, unrelenting pain, particularly on one side versus the other, excessive vaginal bleeding (as if a faucet has been opened up), continuous passage of large blood clots, dizziness or faintness.

See Chapter 21, When It Doesn't Work, and Expecting411.com/extra for details.

911

7. Decreased fetal movement

A happy, healthy fetus is one that moves around. Most women cannot feel their baby moving around until 18 to 22 weeks. And even at this point, the movement is sporadic. You may feel movement one day and then not again for two more days. But after about 26 weeks, you should begin to notice the baby moving around every day and this is when we recommend that you start doing **FETAL KICK COUNTS**. Be sure your baby is moving during each 12 to 24 hour period.

Common diagnoses:
◆ Your baby is sleeping (fetal sleep cycle).
◆ Your baby is hiding behind the placenta (an *anterior placenta* cushions the fetus' movement making it more difficult to feel).
◆ You have been moving around all day and although baby has been moving, you have not been aware of it.

Uncommon diagnoses:
◆ Low level of amniotic fluid (**OLIGOHYDRAMNIOS**).
◆ Fetal distress.
◆ Stillbirth.

What to do:
◆ Many times a mother suspects that she is not feeling her baby move because she has been moving around all day at home or at work. Stop your activity and see what happens.
◆ Sit down or lie on your left side.
◆ Drink something sweet like orange juice or lemonade.
◆ Eat a snack or your meal if it is mealtime.
◆ Take your hands and lightly move your belly around.
◆ Count how many times the baby moves over the next hour.
◆ If you still cannot feel movement over the next hour, call your practitioner.

Take home tips:
Most women who have had stillbirths report a decrease or absence of fetal movement for the two to five days prior to diagnosis. If you are uncertain about how much your baby is moving around, and you have tried all the tips above, call your practitioner.

What the practitioner will ask you about DECREASED FETAL MOVEMENT:
◆ How far along are you? What is your due date?
◆ When was the last time you felt the baby move?
◆ When was the last time you ate or drank anything?
◆ Are you having contractions?
◆ Are you leaking any fluid?
◆ Are you having any vaginal bleeding?

911: emergencies

? ?

911

Priority 1: Needs medical attention now.

◆ Lack of fetal movement for 24 hours, after 26 weeks, despite attempting all the efforts listed above.

Priority 2: Needs appointment the next day.

◆ Baby is still moving around, but there's been less movement in the past day or two.

Priority 3: Watch and wait.

◆ Your baby's movements change from quick punches and jabs to larger, rolling body movements, but she is still moving. This typically happens after 34 to 35 weeks.

8. Leaking fluid from the vagina

It's normal to have quite a bit of vaginal discharge during pregnancy (**LEUKORRHEA OF PREGNANCY**). Discharge typically is whitish-clear, odorless, and the consistency of mucous. Tell your practitioner if you have leakage of a watery substance from your vagina.

Common diagnoses:
◆ Increased vaginal discharge.
◆ Vaginal infection.
◆ Semen leaking out after intercourse.
◆ Leaking urine.

Uncommon diagnoses:
◆ Water bag breaks (rupture of your amniotic sac).

What to do:
Now, don't get grossed out when we tell you what to do here, but:

◆ Take a look at the fluid—check the color, texture (watery or mucousy) and odor.
◆ Try to figure out when the fluid came out. Did you have a full bladder on the way to the toilet? Was it just after urinating? A few hours after having intercourse?
◆ If the fluid is a mystery to you, always call your practitioner. It is better to play it safe and check things out, even if your doc tells you that you peed on yourself. You don't want to have a broken water bag undiagnosed for days.

Take home tips:
Most of the time when you break your water bag, you will leak continuously and start having uterine contractions within 24 to 72 hours. It's pretty rare to be leaking once every few days from a broken water bag.

What your practitioner will ask you about LEAKING FLUID from the vagina:
◆ How far along are you? What is your due date?

- What color is it?
- How much came out?
- Is the fluid thick, thin, watery, or mucousy?
- Is there an odor?
- Are you having any vaginal symptoms? Itching? Burning?
- Was it one time or is it still happening?
- Was there any bleeding associated with it?
- Are you having contractions?
- Did you just have intercourse? Take a bath? Go swimming?
- Do you have to go to the bathroom? Is your bladder full?

911: Call an ambulance.

- Massive bleeding from the vagina.
- Fluid leaking from the vagina with the feeling or sight of something in the vagina—particularly when the baby is in the breech position.

Priority 1: Needs medical attention now.

- Watery fluid continuously leaking from the vagina.
- Discolored fluid (dark green, brown, black) leaking from the vagina.
- Fluid leaking from the vagina with uterine contractions.
- You have leaked once or twice without other symptoms or contractions and you are less than 37 weeks.

Priority 2: Needs appointment in 1 to 2 days.

- You have leaked once or twice without other symptoms or contractions, you are more than 37 weeks pregnant and it has stopped.

Priority 3: Watch and wait.

- "Leaking" that occurs only with a full bladder, on the way to the bathroom or just after you think you are done urinating.

Reality Check

Most women will leak urine at some point during their pregnancy. For some it happens only with coughing, laughing or sneezing. For others, it's a daily occurrence. It's not pretty, but it's normal.

9. Trauma

Trauma simply means injury to the body. This includes car accidents (minor or major), falls, domestic violence, and assault (burns, gunshot wounds, stabbings, kicks and punches).

Believe it or not, pregnant women suffer trauma more frequently than the average person. Your center of gravity is off and you are more likely to suffer a fall by tripping on uneven ground, falling down stairs or even walking your dog. Your belly sticks out and it is something you aren't used to. You are more likely to bump into things (the corners of countertops for example) and get burned at the stove.

And unfortunately, pregnancy is a time when domestic violence occurs more frequently. As hard as it is to imagine, women do get beaten by husbands and boyfriends during pregnancy, including being punched or kicked in the abdomen.

It's possible for the fetus to be harmed any time there is direct trauma to the abdomen. The placenta can be injured and pull off the wall of the uterus (**PLACENTAL ABRUPTION**), interfering with the fetus' blood and oxygen supply. Trauma can also cause first trimester miscarriage, premature rupture of membranes, uterine rupture, and stillbirth.

You need to contact your practitioner if you have *any* abdominal trauma, blunt or sharp—no matter how minor it seems.

Common diagnoses:
- ◆ Falls.
- ◆ Burns.
- ◆ Minor car accidents.

Uncommon diagnoses:
- ◆ Major car accidents.
- ◆ Domestic violence.
- ◆ Assault.
- ◆ Gunshot wounds.
- ◆ Stabbings.

What to do:
Call your practitioner ANYTIME you have had an injury to your belly. Seek medical care as soon as possible if you were in a car accident and had direct abdominal trauma (contact between your belly and the steering wheel, dashboard, airbag or even tightening of your seatbelt). The same goes for any assault injury or fall where you had a direct injury to your abdomen.

Take home tips:
- ◆ The bottom portion of the seatbelt (the belt) should be placed BELOW your belly across your lap (see illustration, right). Avoid placing it across your belly near your belly button.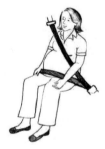
- ◆ Be careful: your center of gravity has shifted and you are more likely to trip and fall when pregnant.
- ◆ Avoid things that will increase your risk of falling: walking dogs, riding horses, wearing high-healed shoes (As you already know—I'm a shoe-lover so this one was tough for me to put in here ladies, but it's the truth). Or say, playing in a co-ed rugby tournament.
- ◆ If you are in an abusive relationship, seek out help and formulate a plan to leave. National Domestic Abuse Hotline info: ndvh.org or 1-800-799-SAFE (7233) or 1-800-787-3224.

What your practitioner will ask you about the TRAUMA you sustained:

◆ How far along are you? When is your due date?

◆ What kind of accident was it?

◆ Was there any direct abdominal trauma?

◆ If so, how hard was the impact?

◆ Do you have any bruising or abrasions on your skin where the trauma occurred?

◆ Are you having any abdominal pain right now?

◆ Are you having any vaginal bleeding?

◆ Are you leaking any fluid from the vagina?

◆ Is the baby moving (if greater than 26 weeks)?

◆ Do you have any other associated injuries? Sprains? Open wounds? Abrasions? Head injury?

◆ Was this injury the result of an assault or domestic violence? Are you currently still in danger?

◆ If you sustained a burn, where is it? How much of your abdomen is involved? Is the skin coming off or is it just red? What did you get burned with—hot water? Coffee? Something on the stove?

911: Call an ambulance.

◆ You were in a major car accident.

◆ You sustained major blunt trauma to your abdomen.

◆ You were stabbed.

◆ You were shot.

◆ You were in a minor car accident but have severe abdominal pain and/or vaginal bleeding.

◆ You fell and have severe abdominal pain and/or vaginal bleeding.

Priority 1: Needs medical attention now.

◆ Direct abdominal trauma (by any method) not fitting into the categories above.

◆ Decreased fetal movement hours or days after direct abdominal trauma.

◆ Severe abdominal pain hours or days after direct abdominal trauma.

◆ Vaginal bleeding hours or days after direct abdominal trauma.

Priority 3: Watch and wait.

◆ A minor fall. You did not directly hit your belly. You have no vaginal bleeding, abdominal pain, or obvious injury. It's still a good idea to talk to your practitioner, but you probably won't need an office visit.

Factoid: Major trauma complicates three to eight percent of all U.S. pregnancies.

Reality Check

Up to 40% of severe blunt trauma injuries in pregnancy lead to a placental abruption.

But here's a surprise. About three to five percent of *minor* abdominal trauma also leads to placental abruption.

911

? ?

So even if you think that you are absolutely fine after your little fender bender, it's best to talk with your practitioner and get checked out. *(Brown HL.)*

10. Swelling of your lower extremities (legs/feet)

Cankles happen.

Nine out of ten pregnant women lose sight of their ankle bones as their pregnancy nears the end. It's frightening, shocking, and often sad when this day happens. And it happens earlier for some women than others.

Although most of the time swelling is a normal phenomenon, sometimes it is a sign that something more serious is happening.

Common diagnoses:
◆ Normal swelling (**EDEMA**) that occurs at the end of pregnancy.
◆ Increased salt intake (as a Texan and a Californian, we know how hard it is to say "no" to chips and salsa).
◆ Blood vessel changes with pregnancy (venous insufficiency).
◆ Just got off the plane.
◆ Forgot to wear your support stockings!

Uncommon diagnoses:
◆ High blood pressure (**PREECLAMPSIA**).
◆ Blood clot (**DEEP VENOUS THROMBOSIS**), particularly if only affecting one leg.
◆ Inadequate heart (congestive heart failure) or kidney function.

What to do:
◆ Rest.
◆ Elevate your legs with a stool or a few pillows.
◆ Drink more water.
◆ If one leg is more swollen than the other, call your practitioner.

Take home tips:
◆ Prevention of swelling is the best medicine. Here are a few tips:
◆ Put your feet up whenever possible. Use a stool or low table with pillows stacked on top.
◆ Decrease your salt intake.
◆ Exercise.
◆ Wear comfortable shoes and socks . . . you may have to get a size bigger than you normally wear to accommodate the swelling that happens as the day progresses.

> **DR H'S OPINION**
>
> *"TED hose were a lifesaver for me! They are not sexy, but neither are the cankles you are trying to prevent."*

◆ Don't cross your legs while sitting down.
◆ Drink tons of water because this actually helps your body retain less water (we know this is counter-intuitive since you are swollen, but it's true).
◆ Eat a well-balanced diet.

◆ Ask your practitioner about using support stockings.

What your practitioner will ask you about your SWELLING:
- ◆ How far along are you? What is your due date?
- ◆ Did it come on suddenly or has it been going on for a while?
- ◆ Is it symmetrical in both legs or is there more swelling in one leg/foot?
- ◆ Are you having any pain with your swelling?
- ◆ Is there any discoloration to the skin of your lower extremities?
- ◆ Do you have any chest pain? Shortness of breath? Dizziness? Feelings of anxiety?
- ◆ Do you have any medical problems?
- ◆ Have you had a lot of salt intake over the last few days?
- ◆ Have you been diagnosed with high blood pressure or **PREECLAMPSIA**?
- ◆ Are your hands and face swollen too?
- ◆ Are you having headaches, blurry vision, changes in your vision or right upper abdominal pain?
- ◆ Did you just get off an airplane?

911: Call an ambulance.

- ◆ One leg dramatically more swollen than the other and chest pain, shortness of breath, dizziness or a feeling of impending doom.

Priority 1: Needs medical attention now.

- ◆ One leg more swollen than the other.
- ◆ Experiencing pain in one leg in the presence of swelling.
- ◆ Rapid onset of swelling in legs, feet, hands and face.

Priority 2: Needs an appointment in 1 or 2 days.

- ◆ Gradual increase in swelling in the lower extremities prior to 28 weeks.
- ◆ Gradual increase in swelling in the lower extremities and discomfort in both legs.

Priority 3: Watch and wait.

- ◆ Gradual onset of swelling in the third trimester, in just the lower legs, ankles and feet.

11. Seizures

A seizure occurs when something (lack of oxygen, lack of nutrients, toxins, drugs, blood, trauma) interrupts the normal electrical circuitry in the cells of the brain (neurons). Seizures are RARE during pregnancy and it is a true medical emergency for both mom and baby.

The key is being able to determine what is really a seizure and what is not. Many people report that they saw a loved one have a "seizure" when in fact that person fainted, lost consciousness, passed out or had some involuntary body shaking (tremors or chills). While there are a few different

911: emergencies

types of seizures, here are the key points:

The person having the seizure:

- ◆ Loses consciousness or cannot remember a certain period of time.
- ◆ Feels a sensation in their skin, muscles, vision, or sensation of taste.

The person witnessing a seizure may see the person:

- ◆ Lose consciousness, faint, or appear spaced out.
- ◆ Have rigid muscle tone.
- ◆ Clench jaws and teeth.
- ◆ Have involuntary muscle movements that are jerky and repetitive.
- ◆ Pee or poop involuntarily (incontinence).

Common diagnoses:

- ◆ Not enough blood gets up to the head while standing or sitting up too fast (**VASOVAGAL EVENT**).
- ◆ Dehydration.
- ◆ Fainting.
- ◆ Seizure when someone has a known seizure disorder (epilepsy) prior to pregnancy.

Uncommon diagnoses:

- ◆ Seizure from severe, uncontrolled **PREECLAMPSIA** (called **ECLAMPSIA**).
- ◆ Seizure from another rare cause such as drugs or recent head trauma.

What to do:

- ◆ If you have a seizure, someone should call 911 first and then notify your practitioner immediately!

Take home tips:

- ◆ Although it is rare to have a seizure caused by **PREECLAMPSIA**, any pregnant woman who has a seizure needs immediate medical attention to rule that out.

911: Call an ambulance.

- ◆ A true seizure during pregnancy is ALWAYS considered a medical emergency.

Reality Check

I had a patient, who, bless her heart, called me at 9am on a Saturday morning. She said, "Sorry to bother you Dr. H, but my husband told me that while we were having breakfast at 6:30 this morning, my eyes rolled back and I started shaking uncontrollably. I don't really remember what happened after that. I knew I should call you but I didn't want to wake you up".

Moral of the story: for something like this, WAKE UP YOUR DOCTOR!

12. Shortness of breath and/or chest pain

It's normal for a pregnant gal to get short of breath occasionally. Especially near the end of your pregnancy, you may have a brief sensation where you can't take in a big breath of air. This feeling should resolve with rest.

Why do you feel this way? Your growing uterus puts pressure on the diaphragm muscle above your belly and below your lungs. Your lungs have less room to expand. And you weigh more and need more oxygen.

Chest pain is *never* a "normal" symptom of pregnancy and always needs medical evaluation.

Common diagnoses:
◆ End of pregnancy.
◆ Overexertion.
◆ Asthma flare-up.

Uncommon diagnoses:
◆ Blood clot in the blood vessel supplying the lungs (**PULMONARY EMBOLISM**).
◆ Severe allergic reaction where your throat begins to swell (anaphylaxis).
◆ Worsening of a previously known heart condition.
◆ Initial symptoms of a previously undiagnosed heart condition.
◆ Fluid build-up in the lungs from congestive heart failure or severe preeclampsia.

What to do:
◆ Rest. Sit down and put your feet up.
◆ If you are still short of breath after resting, call your practitioner.
◆ If you have asthma, try using your inhaler (that your doc has previously approved).
◆ If you have a lung or heart condition, call your practitioner.

What your practitioner will ask you about your CHEST PAIN AND/OR SHORTNESS OF BREATH:
◆ How long have you been having chest pain?
◆ How long have you been having shortness of breath?
◆ Do you have any medical problems? Heart conditions? Asthma?
◆ Do you have any allergies?
◆ What were you doing when your symptoms began?
◆ Does it improve with rest?
◆ Do you have any abdominal pain? Dizziness? A rash or hives? A severe headache? Blurry vision?
◆ Does your chest pain travel anywhere? Your back? Your abdomen? Your arm? Your neck?
◆ Are you having any swelling in your legs and feet? If so, is one leg/foot more swollen than the other?

911: Call an ambulance.

- Severe, unrelenting chest pain.
- Unable to catch your breath/severe difficulty breathing.
- Total body swelling with or without hives/rash and difficulty swallowing or breathing.

Priority 1: Needs medical attention now.

- Difficulty breathing and you have asthma.
- Difficulty breathing, with or without a cough, with known preeclampsia (some women with mild preeclampsia are managed at home and the development of shortness of breath could signal pulmonary edema, or "water in your lungs").
- Any type of chest pain other than the 911 emergency kind.

Priority 2: Needs an appointment within a day or two.

- Asthma flare-up that is not improving with your rescue inhaler medication.

Priority 3: Watch and wait.

- Intermittent shortness of breath that resolves with rest (particularly in the third trimester).

If you have already delivered your baby and think you have a medical emergency, check out Chapter 14, Postpartum for guidance.

Now that you know when to call an ambulance and when to stay home, we'll tackle the details of these pregnancy complications.

THE COMPLICATED PREGNANCY

Chapter 16

"Love is all fun and games until some-one loses an eye or gets pregnant."
—Jim Cole

WARNING: This chapter may induce restless nights full of anxious worrying (as if you already didn't have insomnia). Yes, there are many things that CAN happen during pregnancy. But most of them DON'T happen. View this chapter as a reference if you have concerns about a condition or if you have been given a specific diagnosis. We haven't listed every possible complication in pregnancy, just the most common ones.

Bottom line: this is a scary chapter. It is full of medical scenarios without any sugar-coating. And some of the discussion here can get rather technical—but we figure if you are dealing with one of these complications, you want a detailed picture of what's happening.

Here's our advice: ***do NOT read this chapter unless a concern arises.*** You have enough to worry about.

This chapter is divided into two major sections:
- ◆ Medical complications: Health issues that complicate pregnancy.
- ◆ Obstetrical complications: Issues specific to pregnancy itself (either a problem with the mother or the baby).

To make it easier to find what you are looking for, we've grouped these by body system (urinary tract, blood, etc).

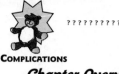

??

Chapter Overview

Medical Complications

A. The Gut (Stomach, Intestines, Liver, Gallbladder & Pancreas)
1. Excessive Vomiting (Hyperemesis Gravidarum)
2. Liver Problem (Cholestasis)
3. Liver Problem (Acute Fatty Liver)
4. Liver Problem Plus Other Problems (HELLP Syndrome)
5. Gallbladder Problem (Cholecystitis)
6. Pancreas Problem (Pancreatitis)
7. Appendicitis

B. Girl Parts (Uterus, Ovaries, Fallopian Tubes)
8. Ovary Problem (Ruptured Ovarian Cyst)
9. Ovary/Tubes Problem (Adnexal Torsion)
10. Fibroids (Degenerating Uterine Fibroid)

C. Urinary Tract (Bladder & Kidneys)
11. Kidney Stones
12. Acute Urinary Retention
*Bladder And Kidney Infections Are Covered In Chapter 17, Infections.

D. Blood
13. Anemia
14. Rh Incompatibility
15. Sickle Cell Anemia
16. Thalassemias
17. Low Platelet Count (Thrombocytopenia)
18. Blood Clot In Your Leg Or Lung (Deep Venous Thrombosis, Pulmonary Embolus)
19. Blood Clotting Disorders (Thrombophilias, Factor V Leiden, Prothrombin Gene Mutation, Protein C Or S Deficiency, Antithrombin III Deficiency, Antiphospholipid Syndrome)

E. Heart And Blood Vessels
20. High Blood Pressure And Protein In Urine (Preeclampsia, Eclampsia)
21. Preexisting Hypertension, Gestational Hypertension

F. Lungs
22. Asthma

G. Hormonal Issues (Endocrine)
23. Underfunctioning Thyroid Gland (Hypothyroidism)
24. Overfunctioning Thyroid Gland (Hyperthyroidism)
25. Diabetes, Pre-Existing
26. Diabetes, With Pregnancy (Gestational Diabetes)

H. Collagen Vascular Diseases
27. Lupus (Systemic Lupus Erythematosus)

I. Brain And Nervous System
28. Seizure Disorder
29. Migraine Headaches

J. Mental Health
30. Depression
31. Anxiety Disorder
32. Bipolar Disorder
33. Schizophrenia

Obstetrical Complications (Mother)

K. Uterus
34. Cervical Problem (Cervical Insufficiency)
35. Abnormal Uterus (Uterine Didelphys, Bicornuate Uterus)
36. Preterm Labor

L. Placenta
37. Problem With Placental Position (Placenta Previa)
38. Problem With The Umbilical Cord Position (Vasa Previa)
39. Problem With Placenta Attachment (Placenta Accreta, Increta, Percreta)
40. Placenta Separates Too Early (Placental Abruption)

M. Amniotic Fluid
41. Too Much (Polyhydramnios)
42. Too Little (Oligohydramnios)

Obstetrical Complications (Fetus)

N. Position
43. Breech
44. Transverse Lie

O. Size
45. Too Big (Macrosomia/Large For Gestational Age)
46. Too Little (Intrauterine Growth Restriction)

P. Other
47. Genetic/Chromosomal Defects
48. Past Your Due Date (Post Term Pregnancy)

Insider Secret
There's a "Rule of Three's" in pregnancy when it comes to many pre-existing health conditions. That means, one-third of people's symptoms get better, one-third of people's symptoms get worse, and one-third stay the same during pregnancy.

Medical Complications of Pregnancy

A. The Gut (Stomach, Intestines, Liver, Gallbladder & Pancreas)

Q. I'm throwing up all day, every day. I can't keep anything down. What now?

COMPLICATION:
HYPEREMESIS GRAVIDARUM

What is it? Supersized morning sickness. Constant nausea and vomiting causes dehydration and weight loss. It occurs in up to 2% of all pregnancies.

Usual time of onset: First trimester.

Symptoms: Severe vomiting, weight loss of more than 5% of your pre-pregnancy weight, scant/dark urine, headaches, confusion, fainting, occasionally jaundice.

Cause: Unknown. It's thought to be due to elevated hormone levels (especially hCG) during pregnancy.

Treatment:

◆ Hospitalization.

◆ Fluid and electrolyte replacement through a vein (IV).

◆ Anti-nausea medication.

◆ Vitamin B supplements.

◆ Once the vomiting is under control and you are rehydrated, start with small, frequent bland meals and take oral anti-nausea medication.

◆ If you cannot tolerate food over a long period of time, you may need to get your nutrition through an IV.

◆ Complementary therapies: acupuncture, acupressure and hypnosis.

Issues for Mom: If not treated, hyperemesis can have seriously bad results—malnutrition, jaundice, kidney failure, blood clotting disorders, tears in the esophagus.

Issues for Baby: None immediately. A fetus who endures prolonged stress (which occasionally happens with hyperemesis) may be at risk for medical issues later in life such as high blood pressure, heart disease and diabetes. *(Kajantie E.)*

Reality Check
Your doc will make sure it's not something else causing all your vomiting before chalking it up to hyperemesis. Thyroid disease, gallbladder disease, hepatitis, or even the stomach flu can make you puke excessively.

Q. My palms and soles are extremely itchy and my husband says I look a little yellow. Is this a problem?

2 COMPLICATION: CHOLESTASIS OF PREGNANCY

What is it? The normal flow of bile in the gallbladder and liver is decreased or stops altogether. Eventually, the excess bile can enter the bloodstream (which makes your skin yellow or jaundiced and itchy).

Usual time of onset: Almost always third trimester, but occasionally earlier.

Symptoms: Intense itching, particularly on the palms and soles, particularly at night, dark-colored urine, light-colored bowel movements, yellowing of the eyes or skin, abdominal pain. These symptoms make it easy to diagnose. But often intense itching is the only symptom.

Cause: Elevated hormone levels in pregnancy cause a dilation and slowing of the bile ducts, slowing the passage of bile through the liver and gallbladder.

Treatment:

◆ Anti-itch creams and lotions (calamine, aloe, steroid cream) to relieve itching.

◆ Soak in cold water or take an oatmeal bath to relieve itching.

◆ Prescription medication (such as ursodeoxycholic acid) to treat the problem.

◆ Immediate delivery, if cholestasis is severe.

◆ Even with mild cholestasis, you will still likely deliver early to help prevent possible fetal complications.

◆ Your doctor will check your liver and bile acid levels with regular blood tests, and perform non-stress tests to assess your baby's well being. Your job is to do daily fetal kick counts and report any abnormality to your practitioner.

Issues for Mom: Using creams and oatmeal baths may do nothing to help relieve the misery. And if cholestasis goes on for a while, you will not absorb fat-soluble vitamins (A, D, E and K) very well.

Issues for Baby: This complication is more dangerous for the fetus than for the mom. There is a risk of preterm birth (since early delivery is often recommended), passing meconium early (in the womb), and fetal death.

complications

Your abdomen

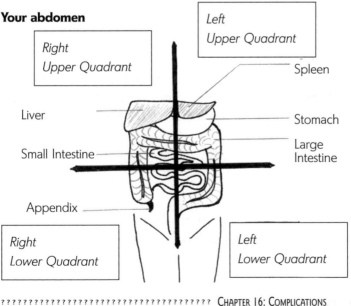

Reality Check

If you have cholestasis with this pregnancy, you have a 70% chance of having it again with a future pregnancy. Ugh.

Q. I'm 35 weeks but it seems that the nausea and vomiting from my first trimester have returned and I don't have any appetite. I also have pretty severe pain in my upper abdomen. It's been going on for a few days. Should I tell my doctor?

3 COMPLICATION: ACUTE FATTY LIVER

What is it? Rare, life-threatening condition where a pregnant woman's liver stops working as it normally does.

Usual Time of Onset: Third trimester, but occasionally in the second trimester or immediately postpartum.

Symptoms: Nausea, vomiting, lack of appetite, upper abdominal pain, particularly on the right side, fever and **JAUNDICE** (yellowing of the skin and eyes).

Cause: The theory—an enzyme deficiency leads to abnormal metabolism of fatty acids during pregnancy.

Treatment:
◆ Admission to hospital with an OB, a high-risk obstetrical specialists, liver doc and liver transplant surgeon all taking care of you in an intensive care unit (ICU).
◆ Sugar and fluid replacement through a vein (IV).
◆ Blood transfusion and transfusion of blood clotting factors if needed.
◆ Liver transplant (rare).
◆ Immediate delivery after you are medically stabile (usually vaginal but occasionally C-section is necessary).

Issues for Mom: Liver dysfunction/hepatitis, inability to clot blood, pancreatitis, brain swelling and coma, liver rupture.

Issues for Baby: Prematurity.

Q. My doctor has discovered through a blood test that my platelets are low and my liver tests are elevated. She says I need to be induced right away. What does this mean?

4 COMPLICATION: HELLP SYNDROME

What is it? A severe form of **PREECLAMPSIA** (see Complication #20). HELLP stands for "H" hemolysis, "EL" elevated liver enzymes and "LP" low platelets. Very rarely, it develops without any high-blood pressure or other symptoms of preeclampsia.

Usual Time of Onset: Third trimester.

Symptoms: See Complication #20 later in this chapter. Bleeding from gums, nose, urethra, rectum. Pain in the upper right side of the belly, yellowing of the skin (**JAUNDICE**).

Cause: Unknown. Theories include a disruption in the balance of hormones that control blood vessels, a decreased amount of blood flow to the uterus, injury to uterine blood vessels and calcium deficiency.

Treatment:
- ◆ Immediate delivery.
- ◆ Steroids, platelet transfusion, and plasma exchange if necessary.

Issues for Mom: Very low platelet count, liver dysfunction, severe anemia. It's possible (but rare) to have a whole body reaction called **DIC** where your body is unable to clot blood.

Issues for Baby: Prematurity (if you have HELLP before 37 weeks). And since HELLP is essentially a severe variation of preeclampsia (and therefore causes subsequent placenta problems), there is also a risk of growth restriction and fetal death.

Q. I'm having a lot of nausea and vomiting and the right side of my upper abdomen is really hurting. I can't even eat. What could this mean?

5 COMPLICATION: CHOLECYSTITIS

What is it? An inflammation and/or infection of the gallbladder.

Usual Time of Onset: Late second or third trimesters.

Symptoms: Pain in the middle of or right upper side of the belly that sometimes spreads to the flank area or shoulder blade. Pain is often worse after eating. Sometimes there is also nausea, vomiting, fever, and yellowing of the skin and eyes (**JAUNDICE**).

Cause: Most often, it's because a gallstone forms in the gallbladder. This blocks the passageway that bile uses to travel from the gallbladder to the small intestine. The bile thickens and then becomes infected with bacteria. Women with sickle cell disease or similar conditions are at increased risk for **CHOLECYSTITIS**.

Treatment:
- ◆ Temporary fasting with fluid and electrolyte replacement through an IV.
- ◆ Pain medication.
- ◆ Antibiotics.
- ◆ A tube is temporarily placed from nose to stomach (nasogastric tube) to help drain the stomach, if necessary.
- ◆ Surgery to remove gallbladder, if all else fails. Optimal timing of surgery is the second trimester. Minimally-invasive (laparoscopic) surgery is safe during pregnancy.

Issues for Mom: Anyone, including pregnant women can have complications from gallbladder disease including infection, perforation, or slowing of the intestine. But for a pregnant woman, these complications can lead to preterm labor. Pregnant moms with cholecystitis are also at risk for pneumonia, adult respiratory distress syndrome (**ARDS**), and inflammation of

complications

the pancreas (pancreatitis).

Issues for Baby: Preterm labor and delivery.

Reality Check

Any abdominal problem (from appendicitis to gallstones) can lead to preterm labor.

Q. I am having nausea, vomiting, and severe pain in the upper part of my belly. The pain is spreading to my back—like I'm being stabbed with a knife. What could this be?

6 COMPLICATION: PANCREATITIS

What is it? An inflammation and/or infection of the pancreas.

Usual Time of Onset: Late second or third trimesters.

Symptoms: Sudden and severe abdominal pain in the middle to upper abdomen that often spreads to the back, nausea, vomiting, fever, jaundice.

Cause: Many causes, but in pregnancy it is almost always due to a gallstone blocking the connection from the gallbladder and pancreas to the small intestine. Pancreatic enzymes back up and cause inflammation of the pancreas.

Treatment:

- ◆ Temporary fasting with fluid and electrolyte replacement through a vein (IV).
- ◆ Treat any electrolyte or blood sugar abnormalities.
- ◆ Pain medication.
- ◆ Fetal monitoring, if needed.
- ◆ A tube is temporarily placed through the nose to the stomach to help drain the stomach, if necessary.
- ◆ Total nutrition through IV, if needed.
- ◆ If all else fails, surgery to remove the gallbladder (if this is the cause).

Issues for Mom: Pain control—it really hurts. Acute symptoms last for five to eight days. Ninety-five percent of women recover.

Issues for Baby: Preterm labor and delivery. Fetal death is rare (<10%) but the chance goes up with the severity of the illness.

Q. I started off with some pain around my belly button. The pain is worse and has moved to the right of my belly button. And now I am vomiting. What is it?

7 COMPLICATION: APPENDICITIS (assuming you still have yours)

What is it? An inflammation of the appendix.

Usual Time of Onset: Second trimester.

Symptoms: Pain first, then nausea, vomiting, fever and sometimes decreased appetite. Although appendicitis pain classically starts around the belly button then moves to the lower right side of the belly, it may not happen that way during pregnancy. The position of your appendix moves as your pregnancy progresses.

- ◆ First trimester: pain is in the lower right side ("right lower quadrant" see illustration on page 417).
- ◆ Second trimester: pain is to the right at the level of the belly button.
- ◆ Third trimester: pain is in the middle or on the upper right side ("right upper quadrant" see page 417).

Cause: The appendix gets blocked (often by poop), then swells up and can get infected.

Treatment: Immediate surgery.

Issues for Mom: Pregnancy prolongs recovery from surgery and increases the risk of complications. Worst outcome (which is rare): leads to widespread infection into the belly and bloodstream.

Issues for Baby: Preterm labor and delivery from the disease or the surgery. Timely diagnosis and treatment significantly reduces risk of death to mother or baby.

B. Girl Parts (Uterus, Ovaries & Tubes)

Q. My doctor told me I had a cyst on my ovary at my first ultrasound. Now I am having a lot of pain on one side. Should I call my doc?

8 COMPLICATION: RUPTURED OVARIAN CYST

What is it? It's very common to have a cyst on your ovary during pregnancy. That cyst can go on to rupture and leak fluid into your abdominal cavity—which causes inflammation and pain. Call your doc.

Usual Time of Onset: Often late first and second trimesters.

Symptoms: Chronic, mild pain in lower belly that suddenly changes in intensity after a minor fall or intercourse. Or it can just happen out of the blue.

Cause: Most of the time it is the corpus luteum—a cyst on the ovary that initially produces the progesterone needed to sustain a pregnancy until the placenta takes over this job at about ten weeks. Most corpus luteum cysts start leaking and slowly go away on their own. Occasionally, the hormones produced during pregnancy can stimulate these cysts to get very large.

Treatment:
- ◆ Take it easy at home.
- ◆ Drink lots of fluids.
- ◆ Pain medication.
- ◆ As long as you do not have a lot of bleeding and the cyst goes away, you can recuperate at home. It's rare to have complications that require hospitalization or surgery.

Issues for Mom: Pain management, bleeding/hemorrhage into the abdomen if the ruptured cyst bleeds. Surgery, if necessary.

Issues for Baby: Possible preterm labor and delivery.

Q. **I'm in my second trimester and my doctor has been watching a big cyst on my ovary. I'm now doubled-over in pain and I've been vomiting. What could this mean? I'm really scared. Do I need surgery?**

9 COMPLICATION: OVARIAN/ADNEXAL TORSION

What is it? The ovary and tube twist upon one another, compromising the blood supply to both. The tissues will die if this condition is not resolved.

Usual Time of Onset: 12 to 20 weeks.

Symptoms: Acute, severe, one-sided lower pelvic pain, nausea, vomiting and fever. You may have had similar episodes in the past.

Cause: Often, a mass in the pelvis (such as a dermoid tumor or other cyst of the ovary). The mass makes the tube and ovary heavier than usual and they are more likely to twist upon themselves.

Treatment:

- ◆ Surgery.
- ◆ Progesterone supplements if a "corpus luteum" cyst needs removal before ten weeks gestation.
- ◆ If it is caught early enough, your OB will untwist the tube and ovary and blood flow resumes without tissue damage. And she'll remove the mass. If your OB sees that there is tissue death, she will remove the tube/ovary and mass.

Issues for Mom: Pain control, recovery from surgery.

Issues for Baby: Possible preterm labor and delivery.

Q. **I have a history of fibroids, even before I got pregnant. They have gotten a lot bigger during my pregnancy and the dull ache in my lower pelvis that I've been having is now excruciating. Why is this happening?**

10 COMPLICATION: DEGENERATING UTERINE FIBROID

What is it? Fibroids are benign tumors in the muscle of the uterus. If the blood supply to the fibroid is altered, the fibroid tissue dies. It occurs in 5% to 10% of pregnant women with fibroids.

Usual Time of Onset: 12 to 20 weeks.

Symptoms: You may or may not have had bouts of pain earlier in the pregnancy. But now you have severe abdominal pain in one area (where the fibroid is located on the uterus). Most women can pinpoint the pain with one or two fingers. Nausea, vomiting, and tenderness over the area.

Cause: Rapid growth of uterus during pregnancy decreases the blood flow to the fibroids, which leads to tissue death. When the fibroid breaks down, prostaglandins are produced which can cause pain and uterine contractions. This condition resolves on its own.

Treatment:
- Supportive care with pain medication (narcotics and anti-inflammatory medication such as indomethacin or ibuprofen if used before 32 weeks).
- Prevention of preterm labor.
- Surgery is not an option for this condition during pregnancy.

Issues for Mom: Pain control.

Issues for Baby: Potential adverse effects of indomethacin. Occasionally preterm labor and delivery. See Expecting.411.com/extra for details on this medication.

C. Urinary Tract (Bladder & Kidneys)

Q. I have excruciating pain on my left side. I can't tell if it's coming from my belly or my back. And now there is blood in my urine. What could this be?

11 COMPLICATION: KIDNEY STONES

What is it? A kidney stone is made of minerals that have crystallized in the urine. This small mass (which looks like a rock and can sometimes be sharp as hell) gets stuck as it makes its way down from the kidney into the bladder. Kidney stones occur in one of every 1500 pregnancies.

Usual Time of Onset: Second and third trimesters.

Symptoms: Flank pain (usually one-sided), pain spreads to the groin or labia, painful urination, blood in the urine. Less common: nausea, vomiting, lower abdominal pain, fever, chills.

Cause: Family history or personal history of kidney stones, recurrent bladder infections, increased age, low water intake, hot/dry climate, diet high in calcium/sodium, obesity and pregnancy. Pregnancy puts women at risk because the tubes (ureters) from the kidney to the bladder function poorly during pregnancy. You also excrete more calcium in your urine when you're pregnant, which is a set up for stones.

Treatment:
- Hospitalization/bedrest.
- Fluid replacement through IV.
- Pain medication.
- Anti-nausea medication.
- Antibiotics, if necessary.
- 60-80% of stones pass by themselves, 20% need surgical intervention.
- Afterwards, drink plenty of water and keep your calcium intake at a normal level (1200mg/day). Too much or too little calcium puts you at risk for stones. And it's possible to get these more than once!

Issues for Mom: Severe pain, preterm labor, possible need for surgery, bloodstream infection, pneumonia, **ARDS.**

Issues for Baby: Possible preterm labor and delivery.

COMPLICATIONS

? ?

Reality Check

Passing a kidney stone may be as painful as childbirth—at least that's what men think!

Q. It's been harder and harder for me to urinate but today I haven't been able to go at all. I'm starting to have a lot of lower abdominal pain. What's going on?

12 COMPLICATION: ACUTE URINARY RETENTION.

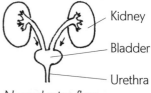

Normal urine flow.

What is it? You can't pee even though you want to.

Usual Time of Onset: First and early second trimesters.

Symptoms: Inability to urinate, lower abdominal pain, occasionally fever.

Cause: Your enlarging uterus blocks the passage of urine from the bladder to the urethra (see graphic above). Good news—it's usually no longer a problem when the uterus grows and gets even bigger.

Treatment:

◆ A tube (catheter) is placed into your urethra to release the urine.
◆ A tube (Foley catheter) remains in place until the issue resolves.
◆ Move the position of the uterus by manually repositioning the uterus or inserting a device called a pessary.

Issues for Mom: Failure to get emergency care can lead to bladder tears and rupture, and occasionally a build-up of waste products in the bloodstream.

Issues for Baby: None.

D. Blood

Q. I'm in my second trimester now and I am still so tired all the time. Shouldn't I have my energy back by now?

13 COMPLICATION: ANEMIA.

What is it? Less than the normal number of healthy red blood cells or hemoglobin that carries oxygen to the body.

Usual time of onset: Second or third trimester.

Symptoms: Fatigue (beyond your usual pregnancy fatigue), a whiter, paler color to the skin, a whiter color on the insides of the eyes (instead of the usual pinkish or reddish color)

Cause: Numerous! The top reason is your body needs more iron during pregnancy. And your blood volume doubles during pregnancy but the number of red blood cells does not. The increased liquid (blood volume) "dilutes" out the red blood cells (hence, it's called a **DILUTIONAL ANEMIA**). Double whammy. That's why you need an iron-rich diet and a prenatal vitamin with iron. Other causes: chronic bleeding (such as

? ?

COMPLICATIONS

from hemorrhoids or vaginal bleeding from a chronic placental abruption), inherited anemia (such as thalassemia or sickle cell anemia).

Treatment:
- ◆ If you have an inherited anemia, see details later in this chapter.
- ◆ Eat iron-rich foods (raisins, dried apricots, clams, shrimp, chicken, liver, red meat, breakfast cereals, dark green vegetables like spinach and kale, as well as lentils).
- ◆ Take an iron supplement, which unfortunately, can cause constipation (try Slow Fe if you are already having problems with that).
- ◆ Iron replacement through an IV for severe cases.
- ◆ Blood transfusion for really severe cases.

Issues for Mom: Common problem: fatigue. Uncommon problem (with persistent, severe anemia): heart failure. Your practitioner checks your hemoglobin level at your first prenatal visit and usually again at 24 to 28 weeks. Anemia at the end of pregnancy is risky because you are about to lose 300 to 1000 ml of blood during your delivery, and potentially become severely anemic afterwards. The goal is to prevent the need for a blood transfusion.

Issues for Baby: A few studies show a link between maternal iron deficiency anemia, preterm birth, and subsequent low birth weight. *(Robinson JN.)* Severe anemia (defined as a hemoglobin level less than six) reduces oxygen delivery to the fetus and that can be serious, as you might imagine.

Q. I have a "negative" blood type. My doctor says I need to have some shots to protect the baby. Why?

14 COMPLICATION:
RH ISOIMMUNIZATION (INCOMPATIBILITY) OR RH DISEASE.

What is it? An Rh-negative mom is carrying an Rh-positive fetus. See box, Hemoglobin Diseases, later in this section.

Usual time of onset: Second trimester, in pregnancies other than a woman's first.

Symptoms: None.

Cause: An Rh-negative mom and an Rh-positive dad conceive a baby. There is at least a 50/50 chance of the fetus being Rh-positive. If there is any crossover of blood from the fetus to the mom (which can occur with minor trauma, vaginal bleeding, CVS, amniocentesis, external cephalic version procedures, placental abruption, miscarriage, abortion procedures, or at the time of delivery), mom's immune system makes antibodies against the foreign Rh-positive proteins. In any subsequent pregnancies, mom's antibodies can cross the placenta and "attack" and destroy fetal red blood cells (if the fetus is Rh-positive) causing severe anemia in the baby or even fetal death. This usually occurs in pregnancies other than the first.

Treatment:
- ◆ Rh immune-globulin (Rhogam) shot at 28 weeks of pregnancy.
- ◆ A second Rhogam shot is given within 72 hours after delivery only if the baby is Rh positive.
- ◆ You also need a Rhogam shot if you have a miscarriage, abortion, ectopic pregnancy, CVS, amniocentesis, percutaneous umbilical

complications

cord blood sampling (PUBS), external cephalic version or any bleeding during your pregnancy.

◆ Rhogam prevents mom's body from producing any potentially harmful antibodies and complicating any future pregnancies. Rhogam is mercury-free and there is no risk of contracting Hepatitis or HIV.

Issues for Mom: No problems.

Issues for Baby: If you have already developed Rh antibodies, your practitioner will closely monitor the fetus for anemia (*hemolytic anemia*). This anemia is rare (less than one percent of the time), but a severely anemic baby needs a special blood transfusion (exchange transfusion) that replaces the damaged red blood cells with healthy ones. A baby with severe Rh disease often needs to be delivered prematurely. Undiagnosed and untreated Rh Disease can lead to severe anemia, jaundice, brain damage, heart failure and death in extreme cases.

Reality Check

The only way to avoid a Rhogam shot is to test the baby's father. If you can prove he is Rh-negative (and that he's the father), your baby is Rh-negative and Rhogam isn't needed. You'll need his blood, though, and that requires a needle. This, of course, could lead to an ugly picture of you, your practitioner and the tow truck guy outside having to tie your beloved down for the blood test! So, you can see why it's easier just to get the Rhogam for you!

Q. I have sickle cell anemia. Am I at risk for complications during my pregnancy?

15 COMPLICATION: SICKLE CELL ANEMIA.

What is it? An inherited blood disorder that affects red blood cells. The red blood cells carry an abnormal type of hemoglobin (the part of the red blood cell that helps carry oxygen). The abnormal hemoglobin causes the red cells to have a crescent shape as opposed to a spherical shape and they don't live as long as normal red blood cells. These "crescents" can get stuck in the smaller blood vessels in the body, causing less blood and therefore less oxygen to reach the tissues and organs. Tissue damage eventually occurs.

Usual Time of Onset: You are born with it. Sickle cell crises, however, are more common during pregnancy, specifically in the second and third trimesters.

Cause:

◆ An inherited disease that's more common in people of African, South and Central American, Saudi Arabian, Indian and Mediterranean (Turkey, Greece, Italy) descent.

◆ Sickle cell disease occurs when someone inherits two abnormal hemoglobin genes, one from their mom and one from their dad. Sickle cell "trait" occurs when someone inherits a normal gene from one parent and an abnormal gene from another parent.

? ?

COMPLICATIONS

People with sickle cell trait are generally healthy, although they can have crises in these situations: dehydration, high altitude, activities that have increased pressure (scuba diving) or lower oxygen (excessive exercising or mountain climbing).

Treatment:
- ◆ Avoid potential triggers (see above).
- ◆ Get a flu shot.
- ◆ Take 4mg of folic acid a day.
- ◆ Hospitalization for a sickle cell crisis.
- ◆ Fluid replacement through IV for a crisis.
- ◆ Pain medication for a crisis.
- ◆ Blood transfusion for severe anemia.

Issues for Mom: Pain (when the abnormal red blood cells get stuck in the blood vessels causing lack of oxygen to the tissues), increased risk for infection (because the disease causes you to have a non-functioning spleen), severe anemia that may require a blood transfusion, increased risk of gallstones and gallbladder inflammation (see cholecystitis in gastrointestinal section earlier in this chapter).

Issues for Baby: If mom has sickle cell disease, it is important to know if the father of the baby has sickle cell disease or trait. See the box on hemoglobin diseases below. Preterm labor and delivery are also a risk.

BOTTOM LINE: Women with sickle cell disease have a higher risk of preterm labor and delivery. And sickle cell crises are more common during pregnancy. Good prenatal care is essential.

Reality Check

All states screen newborns for sickle cell disease with a simple blood test done after 24 hours of life. Early detection allows for early treatment. See Chapter 10, Parenthood Prep, for details on newborn metabolic screening.

Q. **I was anemic at my first visit so my doctor ordered another specialized test. She said I have thalassemia. What does this mean for me and my baby?**

16 COMPLICATION: BETA-THALASSEMIA (MINOR)

What is it? An inherited form of anemia more common in people of Middle-Eastern or Mediterranean descent.

Usual Time of Onset: Congenital (you are born with it).

Symptoms: Many patients don't have any symptoms. Some have symptoms of anemia (fatigue, lack of energy).

Cause: Abnormal gene causes abnormal hemoglobin, so red blood cells are less able to carry oxygen to other organs/tissues.

Treatment:
- ◆ None, unless you also have iron-deficiency anemia.
- ◆ Genetic counseling for parents, particularly if both parents are carriers.
- ◆ Take 4mg of folic acid a day.

complications

COMPLICATIONS

? ?

Issues for Mom: None.

Issues for Baby: It's only an issue if the father of the baby also has a hemo-globin abnormality. For details, see box on hemoglobin disease below.

Q. **I've been bleeding from my gums and nose daily, but now I have been bruising like crazy from the smallest injury. My doctor told me to come in to get a blood test. What is he looking for?**

17 COMPLICATION: THROMBOCYTOPENIA.

What is it? A low platelet count. Platelets are cells that clot blood. Normal ranges are between 150,000 and 400,000 per microliter. It occurs in 7% of all pregnancies and can be part of HELLP syndrome.

Usual Time of Onset: Third trimester.

Symptoms: Bleeding from the nose and gums, easy bruising, and *petechi-ae* (pronounced pe-teek-E-eye), which are flat, purplish, pinpoint dots that almost look like freckles. Some women have no symptoms. Good news: it's very rare to just bleed excessively.

Cause: Several. The most common reason is benign gestational thrombo-cytopenia. Others are lupus, idiopathic thrombocytopenia (ITP), throm-botic thrombocytopenic purpura (TTP), **HELLP SYNDROME** (Complication #4 in this chapter), medications (such as heparin), certain viral infections, and having an enlarged spleen.

Treatment: Treatment depends on the cause.

◆ For gestational thrombocytopenia: observe and check platelet counts periodically.

◆ For HELLP syndrome: delivery, magnesium sulfate (See Expecting411.com/extra for details on this medication).

◆ For ITP: possible platelet transfusion, steroids, IVIG (See Expecting411.com/extra for details on this medication).

◆ Rarely, surgical removal of spleen when there is no improvement in first/second trimesters. This is only necessary in extremely rare cases of ITP but never for HELLP Syndrome.

Issues for Mom: Platelet transfusions, like blood transfusions, carry a small risk of acquiring HIV, Hepatitis B and C. HELLP syndrome is often asso-ciated with **PREECLAMPSIA** (Complication #20).

Issues for Baby: It depends on the cause. For gestational thrombocytope-nia, there are no major concerns for baby. In maternal ITP, there is a small risk (12%) that the newborn will also have a low platelet count and could be at risk (1%) of having bleeding inside the brain. In HELLP syndrome, docs worry about prematurity, growth restriction, and rarely, fetal death (from placental abruption, lack of oxygen, or extreme prematurity).

Reality Check

If your platelet count is too low, you may not be able to have an epidural or spinal anesthesia. Why? Because you risk suf-fering from excessive bleeding in the area where the needle is placed.

HEMOGLOBIN DISEASES

The formal name for a bunch of different diseases that affect hemoglobin (the oxygen-carrying component of our red blood cells) is hemoglobinopathies. They are genetic defects, passed on through your family. You can blame your parents, but it's just your fate . . . not your fault.

While there are quite a few hemoglobin diseases, the most common are sickle cell anemia, alpha-thalassemia and beta-thalassemia. State mandated newborn screening tests can detect these diseases in babies. Since they all cause anemia, they also can be picked up on a routine blood test called a complete blood count (CBC). If the CBC is abnormal, additional testing can determine exactly which hemoglobin disease you have.

Why is this important? If you have a hemoglobinopathy, your partner should be tested to see if he has one too. This helps identify couples at risk for having a baby with hemoglobin disease. It's just a blood test (**HEMOGLOBIN ELECTROPHORESIS**). Considering all the testing you've been through, it's the least your partner can do! Here are a few scenarios:

◆ If both parents have sickle cell disease, the baby will have sickle cell disease.
◆ If the mother has sickle cell disease and the father has sickle cell *trait*, the baby has a 50% chance of having the disease.
◆ If both parents have only the sickle cell *trait*, there is a 25% chance that baby will have the disease.
◆ If mom has beta-thalassemia, the baby only has a potential issue if his dad is also a beta-thalassemia carrier or a carrier of another hemoglobin abnormality (such as sickle cell trait)—then there is a 25% chance of baby being severely affected.

A CVS or amniocentesis can determine if the baby will be affected, be a carrier or remain unaffected.

In all hemoglobin diseases, your body breaks down more of your red blood cells than normal. You'll need more folic acid to help make new red blood cells. You should have 4mg (milligrams) a day of folic acid, instead of the 400mcg (micrograms) a day recommended for other pregnant women.

Q. One of my legs is much more swollen than the other one and it really hurts. What should I be concerned about?

18 COMPLICATION: DEEP VENOUS THROMBOSIS (DVT)/PULMONARY EMBOLUS (PE).

What is it? A blood clot in the deep veins of the legs or pelvis.
Usual Time of Onset: Second or third trimester and immediately postpartum.
Symptoms: **DVT**: Swelling in one leg that is more pronounced than the

other one, pain in the same leg, typically in the calf, difficulty walking and sometimes redness at the site of the clot. **PE**: shortness of breath or difficulty breathing, chest pain, severe anxiety, lightheadedness, dizziness and loss of consciousness.

Cause: You are at risk for blood clots during pregnancy because blood pools in your veins due to your increased weight and big uterus. The uterus is a roadblock which puts pressure on the blood vessels and restricts blood flow from the legs and pelvis back to the heart. Plus, all that progesterone you're making causes the walls of the veins to relax and encourages clotting.

Treatment:
- ◆ Blood thinners—heparin, Lovenox (see Expecting411.com/extra).
- ◆ Sometimes a small piece of mesh needs to be placed in the major vein (vena cava) to catch any potential clots that break free before they make their way to the lungs.

Issues for Mom: DVTs are a concern because they have the potential for a piece of the clot to break off and enter the lung blood vessels, causing a **PULMONARY EMBOLISM** (PE). This is a life-threatening condition, as oxygen flow to other parts of the body can be severely compromised.

Issues for Baby: A DVT itself poses no major risk for the baby. An untreated PE, on the other hand, can lead to very low blood pressure and impaired oxygen delivery, which can compromise the fetus. And since a PE is life-threatening for mom, it is obviously life-threatening for baby, too.

Q. I have been diagnosed with a clotting disorder after having multiple miscarriages. What do I need to be concerned about during my pregnancy?

19 **COMPLICATION:**
THROMBOPHILIA/CLOTTING DISORDER (Factor V Leiden mutation, Prothrombin gene mutation, Protein C or S deficiency, Antithrombin III deficiency, antiphospholipid syndrome).

What is it? They are genetic (hereditary) or acquired defects that affect the blood clotting system, making it easier to form clots in the blood vessels. Five to 7% of the population have the more common disorders (Factor V Leiden and prothrombin gene mutation). The others are much more rare. Most people who are born with these mutations will never have a blood clot, though their lifetime risk is higher than for other people. So you may not know you even have this disorder, despite being born with it. Among these, only antiphospholipid and other autoimmune antibodies that predispose to blood clots are acquired (meaning you are not born with them).

Usual Time of Onset: High-estrogen states (like pregnancy or taking birth control pills), extended periods of bedrest or immobilization, and major surgery increase the risk in people already predisposed to clotting.

Symptoms: Usually there are no symptoms until someone develops a blood clot (in the leg or lungs). Only the autoimmune/antiphospholipid antibodies are associated with recurrent first trimester pregnancy losses and women who have this history can be tested.

Cause: You inherit abnormal genes from one or both parents (depending on the particular disorder you have). Autoimmune antibodies, however, are acquired later in life, and can be recurrent in some families (but they do not occur in a predictable pattern).

Treatment: It depends on the particular disorder and whether or not you have had affected pregnancies or blood clots in the past.

◆ Low-dose aspirin and/or heparin or Lovenox (see Expecting411. com/extra).

◆ Stay well hydrated.

Issues for Mom: For people with antiphospholipid antibodies, there are risks for the mother (blood clots) and the pregnancy (miscarriage, growth restriction, preeclampsia). For the other clotting disorders, the risk is only for the mother.

Issues for Baby: See issues for mom.

BOTTOM LINE: Not everyone with a clotting disorder needs to be treated during pregnancy. A high-risk pregnancy doctor (perinatologist), along with your doctor, will discuss management options with you.

E. Heart And Blood Vessels

Q. My blood pressure was elevated at my doctor's visit today. He told me I have preeclampsia and wants to induce my labor. What does this mean?

20 COMPLICATION:
PREECLAMPSIA (OLD TERM: TOXEMIA).

What is it? Preeclampsia only happens during pregnancy (lucky you!). There are two things required for the diagnosis: 1) you have high blood pressure (higher than 140/90) beginning after 20 weeks of pregnancy (when you previously had normal blood pressure) and 2) you have protein in your urine. Preeclampsia can be mild or severe. It occurs in 5% to 8% of all pregnancies.

Usual Time of Onset: Almost always in the third trimester, rarely in the second trimester (usually only in women with pre-existing medical conditions like lupus or kidney disease), or after recently delivering (postpartum period).

Symptoms: Feeling blah/fatigued, severe headaches that start showing up out of the blue and don't go away with traditional measures, blurred vision, nausea/vomiting, sharp pain under your ribs, on the right side or upper belly area that spreads around the sides or goes deep to the back, and sometimes swelling in the legs/feet/hands/face.

Cause: We don't know. The result, however, is poor placental function. It is more common in first time pregnancies, women under 18, over 40, having multiples, and those with a pre-pregnancy BMI over 30.

Treatment: Very mild preeclampsia, very early in pregnancy may be observed. Otherwise, delivery is the optimal treatment. If you have severe preeclampsia, you need to deliver regardless of the gestational age of the baby because of the health risk to you and baby.

Observation:
- Nonstress tests (NSTs) twice weekly.
- Periodic ultrasounds.
- Bed rest.
- Check daily fetal kick counts.
- Lab work to look for HELLP Syndrome (see box below).
- Regular blood pressure checks and OB visits.
- Possible blood pressure lowering medication.

Delivery:
- Deliver at hospital that handles high-risk deliveries and newborns, with obstetrician, perinatologist, and neonatologist.
- IV of magnesium sulfate to prevent seizures (**ECLAMPSIA**) through labor, delivery and even for a bit afterwards (postpartum period).
- Possible blood pressure lowering medication.

Issues for Mom: Without treatment, preeclampsia can progress to full-blown eclampsia (seizures). In rare cases of severe preeclampsia, HELLP Syndrome can occur (see box below) as well as fluid in the lungs (pulmonary edema), serious problem with blood clotting (**DIC**), eye problems (retinal detachment), liver rupture, stroke and kidney damage.

Issues for Baby: Poor placental function can lead to growth restriction, too little amniotic fluid (**OLIGOHYDRAMNIOS**), **PLACENTAL ABRUPTION** and prematurity. *(ACOG, Wu CS.)*

Q. Before becoming pregnant, I was taking medication for high blood pressure. Now that I'm pregnant, should I be concerned?

21 COMPLICATION:
HIGH BLOOD PRESSURE, either pre-existing or occurring first in pregnancy (**GESTATIONAL HYPERTENSION**).

What is it? Your blood pressure is higher than it should be, typically higher than 140/90. It occurs in 5% of all pregnant women.

Usual Time of Onset: Either this is a pre-existing condition before pregnancy, or it is diagnosed after 20 weeks gestation.

Symptoms: Usually no symptoms. A person with long-standing, untreated high blood pressure might have headaches, visual changes, or dizziness.

Cause: Several. It can be genetically inherited, or due to other diseases (such as lupus, diabetes, or obesity).

Treatment:
- Close observation by an OB who is comfortable with high-risk pregnancies, along with a perinatologist.
- Frequent lab tests (tests for kidney/liver function, **HELLP SYNDROME**).
- Urine samples (looking for protein in the urine, found in **PREECLAMPSIA**).
- Increased fetal surveillance (growth scans every three to four weeks), amniotic fluid level checks weekly or every other week, daily fetal kick counts, sometimes non-stress tests (NSTs) or biophysical profiles beginning at 28 to 32 weeks.
- Blood pressure medication, if needed (see Expecting411. com/extra).

HELP, I HAVE HELLP!

H stands for Hemolysis
EL stands for Elevated Liver enzymes
LP stands for Low Platelet count

HELLP syndrome is a serious pregnancy complication that usually occurs with preeclampsia, but occasionally happens on its own. About 0.4% of all pregnancies and up to 15% of all women with preeclampsia suffer from HELLP. Why does it happen? We don't know. It usually shows up in the third trimester, but 8% of cases occur after delivery.

This is the basic chain of events:

1. Your red blood cells get destroyed, leading to anemia.
2. Your liver malfunctions, leading to poor blood clotting and a build up of toxins normally processed by the liver.
3. Your platelet count drops, making it harder for your blood to clot.

If you also have preeclampsia, you will have the symptoms discussed in complication #20 (see earlier). Without preeclampsia, the symptoms can be pretty vague. You may feel crummy, with nausea, vomiting, headaches, all-over itching, and pain or tenderness in the upper right side of the abdomen. Rarely, women who have HELLP syndrome after delivery are only diagnosed when they go into shock. This is really serious. All obstetricians respect the fact that women with preeclampsia can get very sick, very quickly. Don't ignore symptoms and don't be afraid to ask questions.

 About one in four women with HELLP has complications if they are not diagnosed and treated quickly. And even with treatment, there is still a small chance of death (one in 100). Complications include placental abruption, severe blood clotting problems (**DIC**), acute kidney failure, bruising on the liver, and eye problems (retinal detachment).

Women at the greatest risk of having HELLP syndrome have baseline high blood pressure, high blood pressure with pregnancy (**GESTATIONAL HYPERTENSION**), preeclampsia or HELLP in a previous pregnancy, are carrying multiples, have other medical conditions, or are of advanced maternal age (over 35).

If you have HELLP Syndrome, your baby needs to be delivered immediately. You may also need blood, platelet and clotting factor transfusions, as well as steroids, if the condition becomes severe.

Issues for Mom: There is an increased risk of **PREECLAMPSIA, PLACENTAL ABRUPTION**, preterm delivery, delivery by C-section, and stillbirth. Rarely, pregnancy can worsen high blood pressure and lead to having a stroke, kidney or heart failure.

Issues for Baby: **INTRAUTERINE GROWTH RESTRICTION**, prematurity, increased risk of death as a newborn. *(ACOG)*

F. Lungs

Q. I had asthma before I became pregnant. Can pregnancy make it worse? And what can I do if I have a flare up?

22 COMPLICATION: ASTHMA.

What is it? Asthma is fairly common and it's the most common chronic medical condition seen during pregnancy. The tiny airways of the lungs swell up, making it harder to breathe and get enough oxygen into the lungs. People have certain triggers (exercise, allergies to indoor or outdoor pollens, respiratory infections, emotions).

Usual Time of Onset: Before pregnancy. It can worsen (30%), stay the same (47%) or improve during pregnancy (23%).

Symptoms: Shortness of breath, difficulty taking a deep breath, chest tightness/pain/pressure, wheezing and coughing, particularly at night.

Cause: Unknown. Asthma is to the lungs as hay fever is to the nose. It is an allergic response in the lungs. It is unclear why certain triggers cause an attack.

Treatment:
- ◆ Avoid potential triggers (if you know what they are).
- ◆ Keep your home clean.
- ◆ Stay inside on ozone action days (high pollution days).
- ◆ Have a home nebulizer.
- ◆ Treat any heartburn or acid reflux since it can trigger asthma flare-ups.
- ◆ Review your asthma medications with your doctor ((See Expecting411.com/extra for details about albuterol and steroids).
- ◆ Increased fetal surveillance (ultrasounds, non-stress tests).

Issues for Mom: Discomfort, possible worsening of symptoms during pregnancy, possible hospitalization, risk of serious labored breathing. Severe or poorly controlled asthma can lead to **PREECLAMPSIA,** and significant bleeding after delivery.

Issues for Baby: Moms with mild to moderate asthma have healthy babies. Moms with severe, uncontrolled asthma chronically deprive their fetuses of oxygen. That increases the baby's risk of preterm birth and low birth weight. *(ACOG)*

Reality Check
It's safer for you to take your asthma medication than to have asthma symptoms and flare-ups. Not getting enough oxygen is bad for both you and your baby. Get your asthma under control.

G. Hormonal Issues (Endocrine)

Q. My doctor just told me that my thyroid gland is not working. I'm worried because I'm eight weeks pregnant. What does this mean?

23 COMPLICATION: HYPOTHYROIDISM

What is it? Underactive thyroid makes too little thyroid hormone.

Usual Time of Onset: Before or during pregnancy.

Symptoms: All body systems slow down. Severe fatigue, constipation, hair loss, very dry skin, muscle aches and cramps, cold intolerance, weight gain, intellectual slowness, insomnia (sounds like all pregnant women, right?).

Cause: Hashimoto's disease, subacute thyroiditis, a prior history of complete or partial removal of the thyroid for tumors or cancer, history of Graves' disease that has been treated.

Treatment:
- ◆ Thyroid replacement hormone (levothyroxine).
- ◆ Increased fetal surveillance (nonstress tests, ultrasounds).
- ◆ Consult perinatologist and endocrinologist.

Issues for Mom: Untreated hypothyroidism increases the risk of severe preeclampsia.

Issues for Baby: Low-birth weight. Moms who are hypothyroid because of iodine deficiency risk having a baby with an intellectual disability (cretinism). This is luckily a rare complication in the U.S. today. *(ACOG)*

Factoid: Your thyroid gland sits at the base of your neck and controls many of your body's functions, including metabolism.

Reality Check

Women who have one autoimmune disease (such as lupus or diabetes) are at greater risk for developing autoimmune thyroid disease.

Q. My doctor just told me that my thyroid is overactive. I'm worried because I'm eight weeks pregnant. What does this mean?

24 COMPLICATION: HYPERTHYROIDISM

What is it? Overactive thyroid makes too much thyroid hormone.

Usual Time of Onset: Before or during pregnancy.

Symptoms: All body systems speed up. Nervousness, tremors, weight loss, excessive vomiting (**HYPEREMESIS**), intolerance to heat, excessive sweating, rapid heartbeat, palpitations, weight loss, a bulge in the lower portion of your neck (enlarged thyroid gland), frequent, loose stools, insomnia.

Cause: 95% of cases are caused by Graves' disease, an autoimmune condition where your body makes antibodies against your own thyroid gland. Other causes: benign tumors of the thyroid, **MOLAR PREGNANCIES**, ingestion of thyroid hormone (yes, some people take thyroid hormone when they don't need it for a medical reason), toxic multinodular goiter.

Treatment:
- ◆ Medications to decrease thyroid hormone production (propylthiouracil or PTU, methimazole).

- ◆ Medications to control tremors/palpitations (beta-blockers like propranolol).
- ◆ Increased fetal surveillance (nonstress tests, ultrasounds).
- ◆ Consult perinatologist and endocrinologist.

Issues for Mom: Inadequately treated thyroid disease can lead to preterm labor, increased risk of developing severe **PREECLAMPSIA**, and increased risk of heart failure. Pregnant women with untreated hyperthyroidism may have a medical emergency when excessive amounts of thyroid hormone are released quickly, causing acute heart failure (thyroid storm). Before you go into heart failure reading this book, the risk is quite low—about one percent. Just take good care of yourself!

Issues for Baby: If mom is untreated or inadequately treated, there is a greater risk of preterm delivery, low birth weight, and possible stillbirth. There's also a two percent chance your newborn will have thyroid dysfunction if you have Graves' disease (because those thyroid antibodies can also affect the baby's thyroid gland). Your baby's pediatrician can check the baby for this at birth and two weeks of age. *(ACOG)*

Q. I have insulin-dependent diabetes. I'm now 12 weeks pregnant and worried about all of the potential complications. What do I need to know?

25 **COMPLICATION:**
PRE-EXISTING TYPE 1 DIABETES MELLITUS (not to be confused with gestational diabetes, which starts during pregnancy)

What is it? The pancreas stops making insulin in normal amounts. Insulin is needed to help glucose (sugar) move into the cells of the body. Lack of insulin makes glucose levels rise, causing complications.

Usual Time of Onset: Before pregnancy.

Symptoms: Excessive thirst, excessive urination, fatigue, dizziness spells, sweating.

Cause: Diabetes mellitus can be inherited (genetic). It can also be caused by certain viral infections and exposures. They trigger an abnormal immune response, making antibodies that attack and destroy the cells in the pancreas that make insulin.

Treatment:
- ◆ Consult a diabetic nutritionist/nurse, perinatologist, obstetrician who cares for high-risk pregnancies.
- ◆ Eat a diabetic diet.
- ◆ Check your sugars regularly.
- ◆ Keep your blood sugar under excellent control to prevent numerous complications.

Issues for Mom: Be diligent about controlling blood sugar or deal with these ugly possibilities: vision problems, kidney disease, high blood pressure, diabetic ketoacidosis, preterm labor, **POLYHYDRAMNIOS**, **PREECLAMPSIA**, and increased risk of C-section.

Issues for Baby: In poorly controlled mothers: increased risk of intrauterine growth restriction, preterm delivery, stillbirth, **SHOULDER DYSTOCIA.** Up to 12% of infants born to diabetic moms have a risk of birth defects.

These include: major heart defects and defects of the brain, spine, and skeleton (**SPINA BIFIDA**, **ANENCEPHALY**). There are also potential risks for a newborn after delivery: low blood sugar, seizures, respiratory distress syndrome, jaundice. *(ACOG)*

FYI: Type 2 Diabetes Mellitus is yet another form of diabetes where someone may make enough insulin but the body becomes relatively resistant to its effects. Type 2 diabetes is due to lack of activity, elevated body mass index, and poor dietary habits.

BOTTOM LINE: Up to 10% of pregnant women with pre-existing Type 1 Diabetes end up in diabetic ketoacidosis (DKA), a life-threatening emergency. Please control your sugars!

Q. I failed my three-hour glucose tolerance test. What does this mean? What do I do now?

26 COMPLICATION:
GESTATIONAL DIABETES (**GDM**).

What is it? Problem controlling blood sugars during pregnancy.
Usual Time of Onset: Typically, late second trimester.
Symptoms: None.
Cause: A hormone made by the placenta (human placental lactogen, hPL) makes it harder for your body to use insulin. Sugar levels rise and your pancreas begins to secrete more insulin. But for some women, the demands on the pancreas are too much and it can't keep up with the amount of insulin needed by your body. This causes *temporary* diabetes during pregnancy. About 4% of women get it, but it's more common in women over the age of 35.
Treatment:
- ◆ Check blood sugar levels daily using a home glucose meter and maintain a diary of all your readings. Do your homework because your diabetic counselor and practitioner will ask to see it. They need to be sure you are on track to having normal blood sugars.
- ◆ Consult a diabetic nurse, dietician or counselor to help plan meals/snacks and discuss sugar levels.
- ◆ Don't skip meals. Although it seems counterintuitive, skipping meals will only make things worse. In fact, you'll probably be told to eat a bedtime snack to keep glucose levels constant overnight.
- ◆ Moderate exercise (30 minutes a day) improves glucose control— so do it! But check first with your practitioner before you begin an exercise plan.
- ◆ If diet and moderate exercise are not controlling your blood sugars, you will need an oral hypoglycemic (sugar-lowering) pill or insulin.
Issues for Mom: With gestational diabetes, there is an increased risk of **PREECLAMPSIA** (Complication #20), recurrent urinary tract infections, yeast infections, gestational diabetes in future pregnancies, and diabetes as you get older.

Issues for Baby:

◆ If mom has excellent blood sugar control: slim to no health risks for baby.

◆ There are several health concerns if mom has poorly controlled sugars throughout pregnancy. See below.

BOTTOM LINE: Only 15% of all women with gestational diabetes require medication to control blood sugars. Don't worry—the medication is safe. The danger to baby of this disease going untreated is much more serious.

Reality Check

Women with gestational diabetes have a greater risk of developing diabetes later in life. Make healthy lifestyle choices after delivery (diet and exercise) and reach your ideal body weight. Your chance of getting diabetes later drops to less than 25% if you take these steps. If not, the risk is 50%. Docs are really aggressive about treating even mild gestational diabetes since this lowers complications at birth. *(NIH)*

Why you need to keep your blood sugar under control

Here are the major health concerns for your baby from untreated diabetes. We'd suggest skipping reading this section unless it applies to you. Otherwise, you may not sleep at night. *(Tam H)*

1. *Big baby* (**MACROSOMIA**). These babies weigh over the 90th percentile at birth (which means at least 8 1/2 lbs.). Infants of diabetic mothers (IDM) are bigger because of the extra sugar and altered metabolism during development. The bigger the baby, the harder it is for him/her to pass through the birth canal. So there's a greater risk of having a baby's shoulder get stuck behind mom's pubic bone (**SHOULDER DYSTOCIA**). This can lead to use of forceps or a vacuum during delivery, birth trauma for you (large tears in your genital area or need for an **EPISIOTOMY**) and the baby (nerve injury, broken collar bone or other fractures, insufficient oxygen at birth). And there's a greater risk of needing a C-section.

2. *Delayed lung maturation.* High insulin levels affect the fetus' lung maturation (his ability to utilize the air in his lungs once born). An IDM baby's lungs may be immature prior to 39 weeks.

3. *Low blood sugar (hypoglycemia).* This one may be hard to follow but stick with us. While an IDM fetus is in the womb, he has very high blood sugar levels if mom's blood sugar is too high. So his body (pancreas, specifically) makes extra insulin to deal with the excess sugar. Once the baby is born and the umbilical cord is cut, he no longer has excess sugar (since he doesn't see mom's blood anymore). But the baby still has excess insulin for the first 48 hours until his body's metabolism adjusts. The high insulin levels can lead to a plummeting of baby's blood sugar. Typically, very low blood sugar causes jitteriness, lethargy, and lack of interest in eating (which would fix the problem).

4. *Jaundice (hyperbilirubinemia).* Any newborn can have tempo-
    rary jaundice (yellowing of the skin). But IDM newborns have a
    greater risk of having jaundice due to higher levels of bilirubin
    (body garbage). IDM babies make more bilirubin than other
    newborns, so they have more to break down and eliminate. It can
    be a potential health problem until the body eliminates it prop-
    erly around five days of age.

5. *Stillbirth* (fetal death inside the uterus occurring after 20 weeks).
    The more uncontrolled your sugars are, the higher the likelihood
    of having a stillborn. If you require medication to control blood
    sugar, your risk of stillbirth is the same as women who have dia-
    betes prior to pregnancy.

H. Collagen Vascular Diseases

Q. I was diagnosed with lupus four years ago. I had a hard time getting pregnant and now that I am, I'm worried about the baby. What do I need to know?

27 COMPLICATION:
SYSTEMIC LUPUS ERYTHEMATOSUS—LUPUS, FOR SHORT.

What is it? Your own immune system attacks you, causing a chronic inflammatory disease.

Usual Time of Onset: It usually occurs before pregnancy, but a few cases
start during pregnancy or right after delivery.

Symptoms: No two cases of lupus are exactly the same. Flares (symptoms)
may be mild or severe, and may come on slowly or suddenly. It
depends which part of your body is currently inflamed. Common symptoms include: fever, fatigue, joint pain, stiffness and/or swelling, skin
rashes, mouth sores, hair loss, chest pain, dry eyes, shortness of breath,
weight gain or weight loss, easy bruising.

Cause: Autoimmune disease. Instead of your immune system making antibodies that attack foreign threats (like bacteria and viruses), it makes antibodies that fight against your own healthy tissue. Many different body
systems can become inflamed (joints, skin, kidneys, blood vessels, heart,
lungs, brain), and ultimately, damaged.

Treatment:

◆   Anti-inflammatory medications (aspirin, ibuprofen, plaquenil,
    steroids; see Expecting411.com/extra for details on these meds).

◆   Possible blood thinners (heparin, Lovenox—see Expecting411.
    com/extra for details on these meds).

◆   If you have *antiphospholipid antibodies (lupus anticoagulant* or
    anticardiolipin antibodies) or *Antiphospholipid Syndrome,* you'll
    get daily heparin or Lovenox injections.

◆   Consult with team of specialists regarding management and med-
    ication options: high-risk obstetrician, perinatologist, rheumatologist.

complications

◆ Fetal monitoring (nonstress tests, biophysical profiles, periodic ultrasounds—see Chapter 5, Tests) starting at 26 to 28 weeks.

◆ Special ultrasound of the baby's heart (fetal echocardiogram) to check for heart defects.

◆ Closely monitor platelet counts, kidney and liver function.

Issues for Mom: Miscarriage, stillbirth, **PREECLAMPSIA**, **GESTATIONAL DIA-BETES**, urinary tract infections, and lupus flares during and shortly after pregnancy (first or second trimester or up to four months after delivery). Most flares are mild and can be treated with steroids. But women taking steroids during pregnancy are at higher risk of developing diabetes and high blood pressure. One key point: women with lupus may have antiphospholipid antibodies, which can lead to a miscarriage late in pregnancy. You need to be checked for this prior to or just after you find out you are pregnant.

Issues for Baby: Most babies do fine. Small risk of: miscarriage, stillborn, preterm birth, **INTRAUTERINE GROWTH RESTRICTION**, and in three percent of babies, *neonatal lupus*. Neonatal lupus causes a rash that resolves within six months of life . . . but more importantly, half of these babies have a heart defect that requires a permanent pacemaker. Consult your rheumatologist and pediatrician about which medications are safe for you to take while breastfeeding.

FYI: Yes, you can get pregnant if you have lupus and take medications to control your symptoms. It's a good idea, though, to visit with your obstetrician BEFORE getting pregnant. And be sure to get checked for antiphospholipid antibodies.

FYI: Women with lupus have a higher risk of chronic kidney disease. This should be checked before trying to get pregnant (this can be done with a few simple blood tests), since pregnancy risks are extremely high with both lupus and kidney disease.

Reality Check
Flares may occur in some pregnancies and not in others.

I. Brain And Nervous System

Q. I have epilepsy and I take medication every day. Are my baby and I at risk?

28 COMPLICATION:
EPILEPSY, ALSO CALLED SEIZURE DISORDER.

What is it? Abnormal pattern of electrical impulses in the neurons (specialized cells) of the brain. Epilepsy is when you have at least two seizures at least 24 hours apart that are not caused by fever or substance abuse. There are several types of epilepsy (see below).

Usual Time of Onset: Before pregnancy.

Symptoms: Depends on the type of seizure. Generalized seizures: total body stiffening with rhythmic movements of arms and legs, open eyes, involuntary urination, temporary lapse of breathing, frothing at the mouth, confusion afterwards. Partial or focal seizures: may be only one area of body affected (such as rhythmic jerking of one hand).

Cause: Unknown most of the time.

Treatment:

◆ Consult with obstetrician and neurologist, preferably before pregnancy to get seizures under control. This is a condition where pre-pregnancy counseling is critical. Some medications can cause neural tube defects and other deformities in the fetus. Use lowest possible dose of anti-seizure medication and take only one anti-seizure medication if possible (instead of two or three). You may be able to switch to a newer medication that is less risky for the fetus. If you haven't had a seizure in two to five years, you may be able to discontinue all medication.

◆ If you didn't know you were pregnant and you take valproate (valproic acid), you need to talk with your doctor prior to stopping your medication. Although valproate is not something docs want pregnant women taking, it should NEVER be stopped cold turkey. Talk to your neurologist.

◆ Take higher dose folic acid (4mg per day) preferably before pregnancy or starting right now as it may lower the risk of neural tube defects and other birth defects.

◆ Get early genetic counseling.

◆ Get a special ultrasound to look for malformations of the face, brain, spine, heart.

◆ Consider doing an AFP test at 15 to 20 weeks or an amniocentesis to screen for neural tube defects.

◆ If you take medication, see your OB and neurologist regularly to check medication levels.

◆ Vaginal delivery is preferable unless you have repeated seizures in labor.

◆ Monitor medication levels closely after delivery since they can change quickly.

Issues for Mom: Seizures. Up to one third of pregnant women with seizure disorders have more seizures during pregnancy. Here are a few reasons: lack of sleep, the liver metabolizes anti-seizure medication differently during pregnancy, and women often stop taking their medications because they worry about adverse effects to the baby. Slightly higher risk of **PREECLAMPSIA**.

Issues for Baby: Most babies do fine. Risk of miscarriage, stillborn, growth restriction. Greater risk (two to five times greater) of birth defects—heart defects, **CLEFT LIP/PALATE**. Older children may have abnormal brain wave activity (found on EEG), developmental delays, and lower IQ's. The biggest problems are the anti-seizure medications. Carbamazepine and valproic acid increase the risk of neural tube defects. Valproic acid is also associated with an increased risk of autism. Phenytoin can cause a constellation of birth defects in about one third of fetuses. It's called *Fetal Hydantoin Syndrome* (facial defects, abnormal finger development, and developmental delay).

Q. I have had migraines since I was a teenager. They seem to be getting worse. What should I do?

29 COMPLICATION: MIGRAINE HEADACHES.

What is it? Headaches brought on by certain triggers.

Usual Time of Onset: Usually before pregnancy, sometimes new onset in first trimester.

Symptoms: Some people know a migraine is coming on about 30 minutes before the pain starts, but many don't. That sixth sense is called an aura (seeing spots, flashing lights or wavy lines, or numbness/"pins and needles" sensation in the hands, arms or face). Headache: throbbing pain usually on one side of the head, worsening with routine activity, nausea and/or vomiting, sensitivity to light/noise/smell.

Cause: Genetics (other family members have them, too), environmental. Certain triggers: caffeine, lack of sleep, alcohol, MSG, stress, change in environment (changing elevation or climate), bright lights, loud sounds and intense smells (such as cigarette smoke and perfume), certain medications, extreme physical exertion, and fluctuations in estrogen levels—during the menstrual cycle, menopause and pregnancy.

Treatment:

Lifestyle measures
 ◆ Relaxation exercises (meditation or yoga).
 ◆ Get enough sleep.
 ◆ Keep a headache diary.
 ◆ Avoid known triggers (alcohol, chocolate, caffeine, MSG).
 ◆ Exercise.

Alternative Medicine therapies
 ◆ Acupuncture.
 ◆ Massage.
 ◆ Biofeedback.
 ◆ A few helpful supplements include riboflavin (vitamin B2), coenzyme Q10, magnesium sulfate supplements. Although there is some evidence that the herbal meds feverfew and butterbur can help prevent or reduce the severity of migraines, DO NOT USE these while pregnant.

Medication options
 ◆ Acetaminophen.
 ◆ Consider taking medication to prevent migraines (stopping them before they start) with calcium channel blockers or beta-blockers.
 ◆ Sumatriptan (Imitrex), rizatriptan (Maxalt), zolmitriptan (Zomig). These medications (called triptans) are possible if absolutely necessary but are not usually recommended due to their ability to increase blood pressure and cause heavy bleeding after delivery.
 ◆ Anti-nausea medication.
 ◆ Opiates (as a last resort—they are addictive).

Issues for Mom: Many women have fewer migraines during pregnancy. Great! Others have more frequent and more intense migraines. Not so great. You're also more likely to have nausea, vomiting and **HYPEREMESIS GRAVIDARUM** (Complication #1).

Issues for Baby: None.

Reality Check

You should NOT take Migerot, Cafergot, or Migranal (collectively called "ergot" medications) during pregnancy since they can cause uterine bleeding and miscarriage.

J. Mental Health

For a complete list of medications typically used for mental health, see Expecting411.com/extra for details.

Reality Check

Mental illness is not anything to be embarrassed about. There are about four million pregnancies in the U.S. annually, and over 500,000 of these women have a psychiatric illness. That may occur before pregnancy, or happen for the first time during pregnancy. It is estimated that up to 33% of all fetuses are exposed to some type of psychotropic medication at some point during pregnancy.

Q. **I have a history of depression. I'm 12 weeks pregnant and feeling OK now, but I'm worried that as my pregnancy progresses, all my symptoms will come back again. What do I need to know?**

30 COMPLICATION: DEPRESSION.

What is it? This disorder interferes with your ability to carry out activities of daily living. It occurs in 10% to 16% of all pregnancies.

Usual Time of Onset: It usually begins before pregnancy, but some cases arise during pregnancy or in the first four to six weeks after delivery.

Symptoms: Not enjoying life/pleasurable activities, weight loss or weight gain, loss of energy, sleep disturbance, excessive feelings of guilt or worthlessness, depressed mood, and in severe cases, thoughts of committing suicide.

Cause: A chemical imbalance in the brain that may be genetic, environmental (recent loss of a friend, spouse, child or other family member, loss of a job, loss of finances, divorce), or secondary to substance abuse. The massive hormonal surges that occur during pregnancy and in the postpartum period can trigger an initial episode of depression or can worsen symptoms in someone who was previously doing well.

Treatment: Get treatment, especially during pregnancy, because there are consequences for both mom and baby if you don't get help. Report any of the above symptoms to your practitioner.

◆ Confirm the diagnosis and receive care from mental health providers (psychologist, psychiatrist, support groups, substance abuse treatment if needed).
◆ Consult a perinatologist.
◆ Eat well, exercise, get enough sleep.
◆ Anti-depressant medication, if needed.

Issues for Mom: If you aren't treated, you probably won't take good care of yourself. Poor prenatal care, nutrition, and lifestyles can lead to health risks for you and baby and poor maternal-fetal bonding. Depressed pregnant moms are also more likely to be substance abusers.

Issues for Baby: Vicious cycle. Poor prenatal care means pregnancy complications may be missed—which could mean preterm delivery. Growth restriction from poor nutrition. Issues related to substance abuse. Poor maternal-fetal bonding. Possible side effects/withdrawal from psychiatric medications if mom uses them during pregnancy. Newborns of women with untreated depression often cry more and are much more difficult to console.

Q. **I have an anxiety disorder that has been well-controlled. I'm in my first trimester and I'm feeling all my symptoms again. What should I do?**

31 COMPLICATION: ANXIETY DISORDER.

What is it? Excessive or irrational response to stress, which, if severe, can affect performing activities of daily living. There are five types: panic disorder, obsessive-compulsive disorder (OCD), generalized anxiety disorder (GAD), posttraumatic stress disorder (PTSD), social anxiety disorder/phobias.

Usual Time of Onset: Usually before pregnancy, but some cases first arise during pregnancy or four to six weeks after delivery. PTSD and OCD may worsen after delivery.

Symptoms: It depends on the disorder, but include: anxiety, stress, sleep disturbances, feeling of dread, feeling out of control, heart pounding, tingling fingers, avoidance of certain places or activities, ritualistic behavior, irrational fears.

Cause: Genetics, brain chemistry, certain life experiences. Massive hormonal surges during pregnancy and in the postpartum period can trigger an initial episode of anxiety or can trigger symptoms in a person whose anxiety was under good control.

Treatment:
◆ Consult psychologist, psychiatrist, and support groups.
◆ Anti-anxiety medication, if necessary (see Expecting411.com/extra).

Issues for Mom: Excessive worrying, lack of good prenatal care, worsening of symptoms (particularly in women with panic disorder, PTSD and OCD), postpartum depression. Moms with severe stress and anxiety have a higher risk of miscarriage, preterm labor, and delivery complications (prolonged labor, precipitous labor, fetal distress, use of forceps or vacuum during delivery).

Issues for Baby: Anti-anxiety medications can cause problems for a newborn including: **"FLOPPY BABY" SYNDROME**, low body temperature, lethargy, trouble breathing, and feeding. Babies can also go through drug withdrawal syndrome and have restlessness, increased tone, diarrhea, vomiting and tremors. These symptoms may persist up to three months after delivery. These symptoms are most common in pregnancies where benzodiazepine medications were used shortly before delivery.

Factoid: Anxiety disorders are the most common psychiatric disorders in the U.S. About 18% of American adults have one these disorders.

Reality Check

Some anti-anxiety medications taken during pregnancy can affect your newborn. Talk to your doctor about it.

Q. I've had manic depression since I was in my teens. I am happily, but unexpectedly pregnant. What do I need to worry about?

32 COMPLICATION:
BIPOLAR DISORDER (used to be called "manic-depression").

What is it? Distinct episodes of highs and lows (abnormal elation and/or irritable mood and separate episodes of depressed mood).

Usual Time of Onset: Before pregnancy, sometimes new onset during pregnancy, or within six weeks of delivery.

Symptoms: Depression symptoms: lack of pleasure in anything, weight loss or weight gain, loss of energy, sleep disturbance, excessive feelings of guilt or worthlessness, depressed mood and in severe cases, thoughts of committing suicide. *Mania symptoms*: sleeplessness, extremely elevated mood, spending sprees, travel, and often substance abuse.

Cause: Genetic, chemical imbalance in the brain. Those hormone surges in pregnancy and after delivery can set off bipolar disorder or trigger symptoms in someone who already carries the diagnosis.

Treatment:
- ◆ Care team: obstetrician, perinatologist, psychiatrist.
- ◆ Support groups.
- ◆ Medication, which is usually necessary (mood stabilizing medication, antidepressants, antipsychotics, antiepileptics). See Expecting411.com/extra for details on these meds.

Issues for Mom: If you are not appropriately treated, you may not follow-up with your prenatal care, eat poorly, abuse substances, and have poor maternal-fetal bonding. Warning: many women will have relapses after delivery (30% to 70%). And up to 45% of women develop postpartum psychosis.

Issues for Baby: If you don't take care of yourself, you probably won't follow up with your prenatal care (that detects complications early). So your baby has a higher risk of growth restriction, preterm delivery, substance abuse withdrawal, and psychiatric medication withdrawal. Newborns whose moms had untreated depression often cry more and are more difficult to console.

Partner Tip

If your pregnancy partner has these symptoms, speak up and get her help.

Q. I have schizophrenia. It is under control with medication. Will my pregnancy be affected?

33 COMPLICATION:
SCHIZOPHRENIA AND SCHIZOPHRENIA-LIKE DISORDERS.

What is it? Losing touch with reality. People have false ideas or see or hear things that are not there.

Usual Time of Onset: Before pregnancy (late teens to mid-thirties).

Symptoms: Out of touch with reality, hearing voices that are not there, seeing things that do not exist, completely unemotional, dysfunctional in social situations.

Cause: Combination of genetics, brain chemistry and life experiences/situations. It runs in families.

Treatment:

◆ Care team: High-risk obstetrician, perinatologist, psychiatrist.

◆ Medication, if necessary. Use one medication instead of several, if possible. Older "typical" antipsychotic medications are safe for pregnancy. Newer "atypical" ones lack safety data on use in pregnancy or breastfeeding right now. See Expecting411.com/extra.

Issues for Mom: If you don't take care of yourself, you're likely to have poor nutrition, substance abuse, preterm delivery, increased chance of vaginal delivery with forceps/C-sections, and poor bonding with your baby. If you aren't treated, you may harm yourself or your baby because you are out of touch with reality or hear voices that tell you to do so. Get treated! Beware: You are at risk of severe postpartum depression and psychosis.

Issues for Baby: Preterm delivery, low-birth weight, higher risk of birth defects (especially the heart). If you aren't treated, you may harm your baby. Get treated!

Obstetrical Complications (Mom)

K. Uterus/Cervix

Q. I had a miscarriage at 18 weeks and my doctor says I have an "incompetent cervix." She wants to do a procedure to try to prevent this with my current pregnancy. What is usually done?

34 COMPLICATION:
CERVICAL INSUFFICIENCY (previously called "Cervical Incompetence")

What is it? Cervix begins to open (dilate) very early in pregnancy, often leading to loss of a pregnancy, sometimes as early as 13 to 15 weeks.

Usual Time of Onset: Anytime between 13 to 24 weeks.

Symptoms: You usually don't know your cervix is dilating because it doesn't hurt. One scenario: you have some light spotting and then your membranes rupture abruptly and you deliver.

Cause: Previous surgery on the cervix (LEEP, cold knife conization), overdilation during pregnancy termination, cervical lacerations from previous deliveries, congenital abnormalities of the female genital system, a deficiency of collagen and elastin in the cervical tissue, and women who were exposed to DES (diethylstilbesterol) while they were fetuses.

Treatment:
- ◆ Placement of a *cerclage* at 13 to 16 weeks if you have true cervical insufficiency. (What is a cerclage? Your OB sews a large piece of string (suture) around the cervix like a purse-string and ties it.) The cerclage is removed around 36 weeks, just before you would normally break your water or go into labor.
- ◆ Bedrest until you deliver.
- ◆ Periodic transvaginal ultrasounds measure the actual length of the cervix to determine whether or not you have cervical insufficiency. This is helpful for women who've had cone biopsies or multiple cervical procedures, as it reduces the need for "preventative" cerclages and gives time to place one if the cervix starts to shorten too early.

Issues for Mom: Recurrent miscarriage, possible surgical procedure (if you need a cerclage), prolonged bed rest, preterm delivery, risk of cervical insufficiency in subsequent pregnancies.
Issues for Baby: Risk of preterm delivery. *(ACOG)*

Factoid: A cerclage is 75% to 90% effective in preventing preterm delivery.

Q. **My doctor just did an ultrasound. She said I'm nine weeks but that my uterus had two cavities and that I am considered a high-risk pregnancy. What does this mean?**

35 **COMPLICATION:**
UTERINE DIDELPHYS OR BICORNUATE UTERUS.

What is it? You have an abnormally formed uterus.
Usual Time of Onset: You're born with it. Many women don't know they have this malformation until they have an ultrasound with a first pregnancy.
Symptoms: Symptoms depend on the actual defect. Some women have no symptoms at all. Possible symptoms: no periods, infertility, recurrent miscarriage, pain.
Cause: It happened as your female organs developed when you were a fetus. The two Mullerian ducts in the embryo develop into the "female organs," the vagina, cervix, uterus and fallopian tubes. In this complication, your Mullerian ducts formed abnormally.
Treatment: It depends on the abnormality.
- ◆ Didelphic uterus: none.
- ◆ Uterine septum: removing the abnormality with a surgical procedure decreases miscarriage rates.

Issues for Mom: It's possible to have a normal pregnancy even if you have a double uterus. But it can increase the risk of miscarriage, premature birth, unusual baby positions (breech, transverse), and delivery by C-section.
Issues for Baby: Possible growth restriction, premature birth.

Reality Check
No surprise, women with a double uterus can have difficulty getting pregnant.

COMPLICATIONS

Q. I'm 24 weeks and I'm starting to have contractions. My doctor has put me on bed rest but I'm worried about the baby. Why is this happening?

36 COMPLICATION: PRETERM CONTRACTIONS/PRETERM LABOR.

What is it? Uterine contractions before 37 weeks gestation.
Usual Time of Onset: Between 22 to 37 weeks.
Symptoms: Painful cramping or tightening in your lower abdomen or back that occur at regular intervals.
Cause: Unknown about half the time. The other half are caused by:

- Stress to mom or baby (severe emotional stress, exhaustion, medical condition, malnutrition in mom and a poor blood supply or birth defect in baby).
- Infections (**BLADDER INFECTIONS**, some vaginal infections and sexually transmitted infections).
- Bleeding (**PLACENTAL ABRUPTION**, subchorionic clot).
- Over-stretching of the uterus (multiple fetuses, too much amniotic fluid, uterus that is abnormally shaped).
- Cervical insufficiency (Complication #34; where the cervix opens too early often without warning).

Treatment: It depends on the cause of the preterm labor, severity of your contractions, whether your water bag has broken and whether or not your cervix has dilated.

- Call practitioner if you have more than four to six contractions in an hour and you're less than 35 weeks pregnant.
- Possible bed rest.
- Hydration.
- Possible hospitalization (definitely if your water bag has broken).
- Medication to help stop contractions (**TOCOLYTIC** medication). See Expecting411.com/extra.
- Antibiotics if an infection is suspected or diagnosed.
- Steroids to mature the baby's lungs if delivery is thought to be imminent.

Issues for Mom: Depends on the cause of the preterm labor.
Issues for Baby: Preterm birth.
See Chapter 19, Preterm Labor for more details.

 Reality Check
Going on bed rest is not only boring as all heck, it also puts you at risk for having blood clots in your legs (**DEEP VENOUS THROMBOSIS** or DVT). Your muscles can get a little weaker as well. Ask your practitioner about getting massages, physical therapy and doing light weights in bed to help keep your muscle tone and prevent a DVT. Support stockings are also a good idea.

L. Placenta

Q. I just had a 20-week ultrasound and was told I have a placenta previa. What does this mean?

37 COMPLICATION: PLACENTA PREVIA.

What is it? The placenta implants over part of or all of the cervix. Bleeding when contractions begin and/or the cervix starts to dilate. There are three types:

◆ *Complete previa*: placenta completely covers the cervical opening.
◆ *Partial previa*: placenta covers a portion of the cervix.
◆ *Marginal previa:* placenta extends to the edge of the cervix.

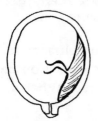
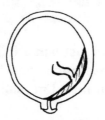
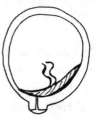

Marginal placenta   *Partial Placenta Previa*   *Complete Previa*

Usual Time of Onset: The placenta implants at the beginning of pregnancy, so that's when the problem starts. The good news: many placenta previas that are diagnosed early in pregnancy move to a safer spot higher up on the uterine wall as the uterus grows.

Symptoms: Painless bleeding, usually in the third trimester. This ranges from a little bit of spotting to a significant hemorrhage. But you may also be symptom-free during your entire pregnancy.

Cause: Unknown. Several risk factors: mom over 35 years old, previous uterine surgery (C-section, myomectomy), carrying multiple fetuses (twins, triplets, etc.), history of more than four pregnancies.

complications

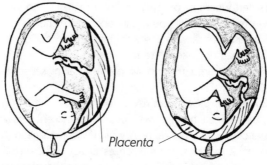

Placenta

Normal Placenta   *Placenta Previa*

Treatment: Depends on the severity of symptoms.
◆ Bed rest.
◆ Pelvic rest (no intercourse or pelvic exams).

◆ Hospitalization, if there is constant or chronic bleeding.

◆ Steroid injections to mature your baby's body organs, in case of preterm delivery.

◆ C-section for complete or partial previas. Some marginal previas can deliver vaginally.

Issues for Mom: Prolonged bed rest, hospitalization, anemia from chronic or severe blood loss (occasionally requires a blood transfusion). See Reality Check below for more info.

Issues for Baby: Premature birth. Fetus is also at risk for not getting enough blood or oxygen from the placenta. Occasionally, it can be fatal.

Factoid: Placenta previa occurs in one out of every 200 pregnancies.

Reality Check

PLACENTA PREVIA is sometimes associated with **PLACENTA ACC-RETA** (see Complication #39), which can cause excessive bleeding after delivery and possibly require a hysterectomy.

Q. I'm 20 weeks and just had a follow-up ultrasound. I was told I have a vasa previa and I was placed on bed rest. I Googled it and now I'm really scared. What do I need to know?

38 COMPLICATION: VASA PREVIA.

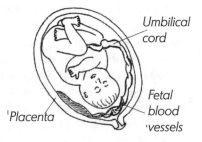

Umbilical cord

Fetal blood vessels

Placenta

What is it? The umbilical blood vessels either insert on the amniotic sac that is overlying the cervix instead of the placenta...or there are two lobes to the placenta and the vessels running between the two lobes cross over the cervix. If your water bag breaks, those blood vessels tear and there is excessive bleeding. This can be very serious.

Usual Time of Onset: The situation occurs when the placenta develops in the first ten weeks of pregnancy. But if there are no symptoms, it may not be diagnosed until you are in labor. It's sometimes possible to discover a vasa previa with a special ultrasound that uses color Doppler (like the Weather Channel) to map blood flow.

Symptoms: There are either no symptoms at all or severe vaginal hemorrhage.

Cause: Cause is unknown, but risk factors include: carrying multiple fetuses (twins, triplets, etc), having two lobes to the placenta, having a low-lying placenta or placenta previa, history of in vitro fertilization (IVF), prior uterine surgery (C-sections, myomectomies, D&C), or the umbilical cord inserts into the amniotic sac rather than directly into the placenta (velementous cord). It is also sure to happen if you are a labor and delivery nurse, doctor or ER doctor's wife (a little hospital humor, as there is an unwritten rule that really bad things only happen to health care personnel).

? ?

COMPLICATIONS

Treatment:

Plan A: If the diagnosis is *known* prior to delivery:
- ◆ Bed rest.
- ◆ Hospitalization in the third trimester.
- ◆ Early delivery (often at 35 weeks) by C-section.

Plan B: If the diagnosis is *unknown* prior to delivery:
- ◆ Emergency C-section is immediately performed. The mother usually has severe vaginal bleeding and the fetus is in distress. (A pathologist confirms the diagnosis after delivery when the placenta and fetal membranes are examined.)

Issues for Mom: Bed rest if diagnosed prior to delivery. Planned C-section at 35 weeks.

Issues for Baby: Fetal distress and unfortunately, often fetal death. Since the blood vessels running over the cervix are those that take blood to and from the fetus, rupture of the amniotic sac leads to rupture of the blood vessels and significant fetal hemorrhage. If hemorrhage occurs, treatment after delivery includes aggressive fetal resuscitation and blood transfusion.

Q. I was told on a recent ultrasound that it looks like my placenta has attached to my uterus in an abnormal way. My doctor called it a placenta accreta. What is this?

39 COMPLICATION: PLACENTA ACCRETA, INCRETA, PERCRETA.

What is it? Placenta attaches too deeply to the wall of the uterus. Typically as the placenta develops, there is a thin layer that forms separating the placenta from the uterine wall. There is no layer with placenta accreta, increta and percreta. See box below for details.

Usual Time of Onset: It occurs during development of the embryo and placenta. Sometimes it is identified during pregnancy by using ultrasound and Doppler flow technology. But more often it is diagnosed after delivery of the baby and/or the placenta.

Symptoms: None, unless an accreta is present with a placenta previa.

Cause: Unknown. More common with placenta previa (present in five to ten percent), women who have had previous uterine surgery (previous C-sections fibroid removal), and those who have had multiple previous C-sections (60% of women with placenta accreta).

Treatment: There is nothing that can be done to prevent a placenta accreta from happening and there is very little that can be done once diagnosed. If you are diagnosed prior to delivery:
- ◆ Periodic ultrasounds assess the severity/degree of the accreta.
- ◆ Scheduled C-section, usually.
- ◆ Discuss the game plan with your practitioner regarding possible hysterectomy and blood transfusions (the worst case scenario).

Issues for Mom: Risk of significant bleeding when an attempt is made to separate the placenta from the uterine wall. If severe, blood loss can be life-threatening and could require further uterine surgery, a hysterectomy and/or blood transfusions. It's important to diagnose and treat it quickly.

Issues for Baby: Premature delivery if bleeding occurs.

FYI: Placenta accreta occurs in one in every 2500 pregnancies.

ABNORMAL PLACENTAL ATTACHMENTS

There are three different types of abnormal placental attachments:

◆ *Placenta accreta*: Placenta attaches in an abnormal way to the uterine wall. It does not, however, invade the uterine muscle. This is the most common of the three abnormalities and accounts for 75% of all cases.

◆ *Placenta increta*: Placenta invades the uterine muscle, but does not extend through the wall of the uterus. It occurs in 15% of all cases.

◆ *Placenta percreta*: Placenta penetrates through the entire uterine wall and attaches to another organ such as the bladder or intestine. This is the least common of the three and accounts for three to five percent of all cases.

Q. I'm 35 weeks and I am having heavy vaginal bleeding and some really painful belly cramps. What is wrong?

40 **COMPLICATION: PLACENTAL ABRUPTION.**

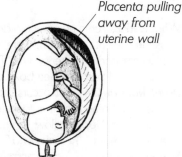

Placenta pulling away from uterine wall

What is it? Placenta separates (partially or completely) from the wall of the uterus PRIOR to delivery of the fetus. It can be serious (depending on the severity of the separation) and occurs in about one in 150 deliveries.

Usual Time of Onset: Mostly third trimester, but any time after 20 weeks.

Symptoms: Usually vaginal bleeding (either slight or heavy) AND abdominal pain (with or without contractions), back pain, uterus sometimes tender to touch. If contractions are present, they are usually back-to-back, coming one after another. The amount of blood that is coming from the vagina does not necessarily correlate with how much of the placenta has separated from the wall of the uterus. In one out of five cases, the bleeding is hidden and a woman can be very ill from losing a large amount of blood before she is diagnosed (dizziness, low blood pressure, rapid heart rate, shock).

Cause: Often, there is no specific reason. Direct abdominal injury (such as a car accident or a fall) can cause it. Other risk factors are:

◆ High blood pressure (chronic or **PREECLAMPSIA**).
◆ You've had a previous **PLACENTAL ABRUPTION** (your risk is about 15% in subsequent pregnancies).
◆ You've been pregnant before.

- Excessive amount of amniotic fluid (**POLYHYDRAMNIOS**).
- Premature rupture of membranes.
- Age (this is more common in women over the age of 35).
- Substance abuse, particularly cigarettes, alcohol, cocaine or methamphetamines during pregnancy.
- Carrying multiples (twins, triplets or more).

Treatment: Treatment depends on severity of abruption, how far along the pregnancy is, and if the fetus is in any danger. Unfortunately, docs can't reattach the placenta once it has separated from the uterine wall. If you are Rh negative, you will need Rhogam.

Scenario #1: Mild abruption, and you are beyond 36 to 37 weeks:

- Delivery likely. You will either be induced if it is safe to do so, or have a C-section.

Scenario #2: Mild abruption, and you are less than 36 weeks:

- Check for reassuring fetal heart rate tracing.

BLOOD TRANSFUSIONS: WHAT YOU NEED TO KNOW

We know that getting a blood transfusion sounds scary. Rest assured that it is NOT common to receive blood, either during your pregnancy or afterwards. But some women with chronic medical conditions (such as sickle cell anemia) need a blood transfusion during pregnancy.

However, the most common reason for needing a transfusion is excessive bleeding after delivery (**POSTPARTUM HEMORRHAGE**). Everyone loses a lot of blood during the delivery of a baby, whether it's a vaginal delivery or a C-section. The average amount of blood lost in a vaginal delivery is about ten to 13 oz. (300 to 400ml). In a C-section, the average is about 20 to 27 oz. (600 to 800ml). Anything greater than a 16 oz. (500ml) blood loss in a vaginal delivery and 34 oz. (1,000ml) blood loss in a C-section is considered to be a postpartum hemorrhage.

Around the world, a postpartum hemorrhage happens every four minutes. And 140,000 women die each year from this pregnancy complication. Most of those deaths do NOT occur in the U.S. because of good medical care and the availability of resources, particularly blood and blood products. If you have so much blood loss that your blood pressure is dropping, a blood transfusion will save your life. Period. About 0.4 to 0.6% of American women need a postpartum blood transfusion.

Obviously, this is not a decision that is taken lightly. If ordered, your practitioner feels the benefits outweigh the potential risks. The risks of transfusion include: a transfusion reaction (an allergic reaction to the blood you receive, even if it is the same blood type), a reaction due to receiving the wrong blood type (pretty rare), or a risk of contracting an infection. Donor blood is screened very thoroughly to prevent infectious disease transmission, so the general risks are about one in a million to get HIV or Hepatitis C from a blood transfusion and one in 500,000 for Hepatitis B.

complications

- ◆ Hospitalization for observation.
- ◆ Bed rest at home if bleeding stops and you and baby are stable.
- ◆ Frequent follow-up office visits.

Scenario #3: Severe abruption:
- ◆ Immediate delivery (usually emergency C-section) no matter how far along you are if you have massive, uncontrollable vaginal bleeding or if you or your baby is unstable.
- ◆ Possible blood transfusion, if bleeding is excessive.

Issues for Mom: Bleeding, sometimes excessive. Yes, it's rare, but possible to go into shock or bleed to death without quick medical intervention. Possible C-section, possible hysterectomy after delivery if bleeding cannot be controlled.

Issues for Baby: Premature birth. If too much of the placenta separates from the uterus, the baby can be deprived of oxygen and nutrients. That has the potential to cause neurologic problems or rarely, stillbirth. The babies at highest risk are those who are unstable before delivery and those delivered by emergency C-section. These babies also have a slightly higher risk of Sudden Infant Death Syndrome (SIDS). *(Gabbe SG)*

Factoid: 85% of placental abruptions are mild to moderate ones. That's the good news. The bad news: almost half the women with placental abruptions deliver before 37 weeks. *(Gabbe SG)*

M. Amniotic Fluid

Q. An ultrasound showed I have too much amniotic fluid. What's the matter?

41 COMPLICATION:
POLYHYDRAMNIOS.

What is it? Too much amniotic fluid. This occurs in one to two percent of all pregnancies. Most cases are mild and rarely result in any complications. As the level of fluid increases, so does the risk of problems.
Usual Time of Onset: Usually third trimester, sometimes second trimester.
Symptoms: None, except for a big belly.
Cause: Over half of the time, the cause is unknown. In other cases, the causes could be:
- ◆ Birth defects. If a fetus has a malformation (gastrointestinal tract, nervous system) that affects his ability to swallow/digest amniotic fluid, it builds up.
- ◆ **RH INCOMPATIBILITY.**
- ◆ Maternal Diabetes, poorly controlled.
- ◆ **TWIN-TO-TWIN TRANSFUSION SYNDROME (TTTS)** –One twin gets too much blood flow and the other too little due to connections between blood vessels in their shared placenta. This leads to too much amniotic fluid for the twin with too much blood flow and too little amniotic fluid for the twin without enough blood flow.

Treatment: Usually none. Increased monitoring by frequent ultrasounds and tests of fetal well-being (nonstress tests, biophysical profiles). Depending on each individual situation, treatments may include:

♦ Medication: reduces fluid production. It is effective up to 90% of the time, but is not generally used after about 28 to 32 weeks gestation.

♦ Amnioreduction procedure: a needle drains excess fluid from within the uterine cavity (exactly like an amniocentesis). Risks are premature rupture of membranes, infection, and fluid can build back up again. This procedure is usually only done if the size of the uterus is impairing the ability of mom to breathe.

♦ Delivery, if baby is at risk (poor growth, lacks signs of well-being).

Issues for Mom: As more fluid accumulates, there is greater risk of premature rupture of the membranes (PROM), increased risk of the umbilical cord protruding through the cervix (**CORD PROLAPSE**) with rupture of membranes, preterm labor and delivery, placental abruption, increased risk of needing a C-section, and postpartum hemorrhage.

Issues for Baby: Increased risk of stillborn (although rare, it is twice the risk of a normal pregnancy), possible complications of maternal diabetes (hypoglycemia, seizures, jaundice) if present, possible fetal growth restriction, preterm birth.

Q. My doctor discovered that I did not have enough amniotic fluid and I'm only 34 weeks. Now what needs to happen?

WHY IS AMNIOTIC FLUID SO IMPORTANT ANYWAY?

Your baby develops in a fluid-filled bubble. This is why her fingers and toes at birth will look like yours do after a leisurely bath.

Your baby's bubble (the amniotic sac) starts to form just 12 days after conception. Mom makes the initial amniotic fluid (which is mostly water) in the early stages of pregnancy. After about 12 weeks, the placenta and your baby make amniotic fluid. Yes, amniotic fluid is actually your baby's urine—but don't worry, it's all sterile!

The amniotic fluid has several important jobs. Babies not only make the amniotic fluid, they also breathe it into their lungs and swallow it to go through the digestive tract. This helps the lungs and digestive tracts develop properly. The fluid cushions and protects your baby, provides her with fluids, allows for fetal movement, allows growth, and helps strengthen the baby's muscles and bones. It also allows the umbilical cord to float around freely. You can see why it's so essential.

Having too much amniotic fluid can be a sign that your baby is not ingesting it as he should or too much is being made. Having too little may mean your baby or the placenta is not producing enough of it, or your membranes have ruptured.

The level of amniotic fluid increases until about 28 to 32 weeks of pregnancy, at which time it plateaus and then begins to decrease when your baby reaches 37 to 40 weeks.

complications

42 COMPLICATION: OLIGOHYDRAMNIOS.

What is it? Too little amniotic fluid. If you are past your due date by at least two weeks, you may be at risk. Oligohydramnios complicates 12% of pregnancies that go beyond 41 weeks.

Usual Time of Onset: Usually third trimester, but it also happens in the second trimester.

Symptoms: Sometimes, none. Or, you might feel a decrease in the size of your belly or decreased fetal movement.

Cause: Often unknown. Possible causes include:

◆ You ruptured your membranes and you are leaking fluid (preterm or at term).

◆ You go past your due date, so your placental function declines (see FYI below).

◆ Birth defects: your baby's kidneys make urine (amniotic fluid). A problem with the kidneys or urinary tract development can lead to too little amniotic fluid.

◆ Problems with placenta.

◆ Maternal complications: dehydration, high blood pressure (either chronic/pre-existing or **PREECLAMPSIA**), diabetes, lupus, or chronic lack of oxygen that can sometimes occur at higher altitudes or with some diseases.

Treatment: It depends on how far along you are in your pregnancy and the presumed cause. In any scenario, it's possible you will need to get hydrated with either liquids by mouth or an IV.

Scenario #1: You are not full term and not in labor.

◆ Close monitoring with periodic ultrasounds, nonstress tests, biophysical profiles (see Chapter 5, Tests).

◆ Possible hospitalization for observation.

◆ Possible bed rest.

◆ Possible infusion of fluid by amniocentesis, if necessary.

Scenario #2: You are full term (or close to it) but not in labor.

◆ Probable delivery, especially if your membranes are ruptured.

◆ Antibiotics, if it is suspected or confirmed that your membranes are ruptured.

◆ Close monitoring if your membranes are intact and you and baby are stable.

◆ Delivery if you are at term or there are any signs of fetal distress.

Scenario #3: You are in labor.

◆ Delivery.

◆ Amnioinfusion: obstetrician infuses sterile saline (salt water) through the cervix into the amniotic cavity to help increase buoyancy and prevent compression of the umbilical cord and subsequent fetal distress.

Issues for Mom: Increased risk of C-section if the baby is in distress (**CORD COMPRESSION, MECONIUM STAINED FLUID**).

Issues for Baby: It depends on when in the pregnancy it occurs. Amniotic fluid is essential for your baby to develop appropriately (see box above). The baby begins to breathe and swallow the fluid in the second trimester to help her lungs grow and mature. If oligohydramnios occurs earlier in pregnancy (the second trimester), the complications are often more serious: increased risk of miscarriage or stillbirth, birth defects because developing fetal organs are compressed (lung and limb defects). Too little fluid later in pregnancy can lead to growth restriction, preterm birth, passing the first poop (**MECONIUM**) while in the womb (see details below), or cord compression which stresses the baby. *(March of Dimes)*

FYI: Certain diseases will make the placenta "age" prematurely, and as a result, it doesn't function as well (called *placental insufficiency*). There is less amniotic fluid when there is placental insufficiency since the placenta helps make amniotic fluid. Example: High blood pressure leads to placental insufficiency, which can lead to oligohydramnios.

Red Flags

Healthy amniotic fluid is clear to straw-colored. If your baby is stressed before delivery, he may poop (pass **MECONIUM**) for the first time while in the womb (instead of afterwards like he is supposed to), making the amniotic fluid stained green/yellow/brown. If you have **CHORIOAMNIONITIS** (an infection), the amniotic fluid can be cloudy and foul smelling.

BOTTOM LINE: Your baby may be in distress if he doesn't have enough amniotic fluid. There are two ways your doc will know:

1. *Cord compression:* Umbilical cord (and its blood vessels) is compressed because it can't float around freely. Less oxygen goes to the baby and a non-reassuring fetal heart pattern is seen on the monitor or picked up while listening with a Doppler.
2. *Meconium stained fluid:* Fetuses do not ordinarily poop while they are in the womb. They poop for the first time once they are born. But they will poop in the womb if they are stressed. So when your water breaks, the fluid looks yellow/green/brown because it is meconium-stained. Unfortunately, this is not only a sign of distress but it can also become a problem since the baby can swallow this meconium into his lungs and have temporary breathing problems after birth.

Obstetrical Complications (fetus)

N. Position

See Chapter 12 and 13, Home Stretch and Labor Day for details on different fetal positions

Q. I'm 35 weeks and my baby is breech. What does that mean exactly, and how will that complicate the pregnancy?

43 COMPLICATION: BREECH POSITION.

What is it? It's normal for a baby to come out of the birth canal with his head first. In a breech position (3% of full term pregnancies), your baby's head is up, not down near your cervix. So he plans to exit the womb bottom first. There are three types of breech presentations:

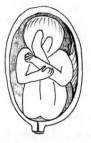

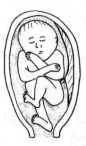

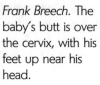

Frank Breech. The baby's butt is over the cervix, with his feet up near his head.

Complete Breech. The baby's butt is over the cervix, but his knees are bent and tucked up against his chest.

Footling Breech. One or both feet are over the cervix.

Usual Time of Onset: A baby can be breech at any point during the pregnancy. Many babies start out in the breech position. However, if a baby has not turned by the end of 36 weeks, it is unlikely that she will do so in the remaining few weeks of the pregnancy.

Symptoms: Usually none, but some women can feel their baby's head in their upper abdomen. More kicking may occur lower in the belly, near the cervix and bladder (ouch!).

Cause: Unknown, most of the time. Remember that!

♦ Most breech babies are completely healthy and have no medical issues whatsoever. Some situations make a baby feel "more comfortable" with her head up, instead of down. These include maternal uterine abnormalities (see Complication #35), large uterine fibroids or other pelvic tumors, **POLYHYDRAMNIOS** (baby has a lot of fluid to move around in), **OLIGOHYDRAMNIOS** (not enough fluid for a baby to move into head down position) **PLACENTA PREVIA**, birth defects (**HYDROCEPHALUS, HIP DYSPLASIA** for example), multiples.

Treatment: It is much safer to deliver them by C-section. There is substantially less risk of injury to the baby. ACOG recommends delivering all breech babies by C-section (except in the case of twins, when the second twin is breech). But there are some treatments that have been tried to move the fetus from a breech position to a head down position before delivery. These include:

♦ Acupuncture.

♦ Prenatal chiropractor (ALWAYS check with your practitioner first!).

♦ **EXTERNAL CEPHALIC VERSION** (see box nearby).

Issues for Mom: Increased chance of more procedures (external cephalic version, possible amniocentesis to assess lung maturity), increased risk of C-section.

Issues for Baby: Growth restriction, possible birth defects, **CORD PROLAPSE** if rupture of membranes occurs, premature birth (breech position does-n't cause preterm labor...many preterm babies just haven't had time to flip around or they are multiples). Check for hip dislocation at four to six weeks of life (see below).

Insider Secret

Breech babies have a slightly higher risk of having a hip defor-mity called **DEVELOPMENTAL DYSPLASIA OF THE HIPS**. English translation: it's a hip dislocation similar to what you might see in pure-bred dogs. The abnormal formation of the hip(s) is what triggers the baby to move into a breech position. Pediatricians screen all breech babies at four to six weeks of life with a simple hip ultrasound to rule it out. NOTE: hip dislocations are uncommon, even for breech babies. They are just more common for them and something docs don't want to miss.

WHAT IS EXTERNAL CEPHALIC VERSION ANYWAY?

This is a procedure that obstetricians use to try to turn a baby who is currently NOT poised to come out head first (vertex presentation). Docs usually attempt this procedure at about 37 weeks of pregnan-cy in a hospital that is equipped to offer an immediate C-section, should the need arise. Don't worry: the need rarely arises!

Here's how it goes:

◆ At the hospital, you get hooked up to a fetal heart monitor.
◆ You have an ultrasound done to be sure there is plenty of amniotic fluid and to reconfirm the position of the baby (because its really embarrassing to try to turn a baby who is already in the head down position).
◆ You will have an IV put in and your blood type should be known (because if you are Rh negative you will need to be given a shot of Rhogam).
◆ Someone slathers a bunch of mineral oil or ultrasound gel (hopefully warm) over your belly.
◆ This is when the fun begins.
◆ Have you ever watched Wrestle Mania? One (or sometimes two) OBs put their hands on your belly and by applying lots of pressure, attempt to turn the baby via a forward or back-ward somersault, into the head down position.
◆ It hurts.
◆ After this attempt, you get another ultrasound to see if your baby moved.

Why bother with all of this? If it turns your baby around, you have the chance to have a vaginal delivery.

Are there risks? Yes, but they are quite rare. It's possible to cause a placental abruption, premature rupture of membranes, labor and need for emergency C-section. So if your baby is breech, you should talk with your practitioner to see if an external cephalic version is an option for you.

complications

COMPLICATIONS

? ?

 DR H'S OPINION

External cephalic version is a procedure that is being done less and less in this country. Most breech babies are born via Cesarean section.

 Reality Check
Don't worry if your newborn looks frog-legged or his head is flat instead of round. It comes from lying in your womb right-side up instead of down. His head will round out and his legs will straighten out over the next several weeks!

Q. I'm 24 weeks and the fetus is lying sideways. What are the odds he will turn the right way?

44 COMPLICATION:
TRANSVERSE LIE.

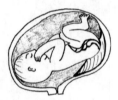

What is it? The baby lies horizontally (sideways) across your belly instead of head down (**CEPHALIC/VERTEX**) or bottom/feet down (**BREECH**). In 99.5% of all term pregnancies, babies are either head down or breech. In 0.5%, they are lying in another plane, such as transverse. There are two types of transverse lie:

◆ *Back up.* The spine of the fetus is oriented upward. His arms, hands, legs and feet are the parts intending to exit the birth canal first (the "presenting part" at the cervix).

◆ *Back down.* The spine of the fetus is oriented downward. His shoulder intends to exit the birth canal first (the presenting part at the cervix).

Most fetuses that are in the transverse position in early pregnancy, turn themselves into a head down (**CEPHALIC/VERTEX**) or feet/butt down (**BREECH**) position by the time labor occurs.

Usual Time of Onset: A baby can be transverse at any point during the pregnancy. It is often seen on ultrasound early in pregnancy. If your baby has a transverse lie between 20 to 25 weeks, there is only a 2.5% chance she will be transverse at delivery. After 36 weeks, she has an 11.5% chance of being transverse at the time of labor.

Symptoms: Usually none. A woman might notice a different shape to her belly and feel the fetus' head on one side of her belly.

Cause:

◆ *Preterm delivery before 32 weeks*: Fetuses often don't turn into their final delivery position until after 32 weeks.

◆ *A uterus and abdomen with poor muscle tone*: You've had multiple previous pregnancies.

◆ *Twins:* The second baby to deliver is more likely to be transverse.

◆ *Polyhydramnios*: Too much amniotic fluid.

◆ *Pelvis issue*: Mom's pelvis is too small or abnormally shaped.

- *Extremely large pelvic tumors*: Fibroids or ovarian cysts limit the baby's ability to get into the desired delivery position.
- *Uterus issue:* Mom's abnormal uterus (see Complication #35) also limits the baby's delivery position options.

Treatment: Don't panic. Most babies will turn themselves before labor begins.

- Attempt external cephalic version (see box on previous page)—there is a 50% to 60% success rate.
- Consider acupuncture (unknown success rate).
- C-section, if baby remains in a transverse lie position.

Issues for Mom: Easily treated and unlikely to cause any problems in the good ol' USA. You might have to endure an external cephalic version or C-section. Very rare problem: your rupture of membranes might allow the umbilical cord to come through the cervix into the vagina because there is no head or bottom "blocking" the cervical opening (**CORD PROLAPSE**). Even with a cord prolapse, in developed countries, you would probably have enough time to get to the hospital and undergo a Cesarean delivery.

Issues for Baby: Risks associated with C-section, lack of oxygen or nutrients if cord prolapse occurs (very rare).

FYI: In underdeveloped countries with inadequate prenatal care, trying to deliver a baby in a transverse lie can be fatal for both mom and baby. That's because these countries may lack adequate medical facilities to perform a C-section. That is NOT the case where you live. You can take that sigh of relief now.

O. Size

Q. The fetus is measuring bigger than he is supposed to for his age. How will this affect my pregnancy (and, gulp, delivery)!

45 COMPLICATION: MACROSOMIA OR "LARGE FOR GESTATIONAL AGE" (LGA).

What is it? Big baby. An LGA baby's birth weight is equal to or greater than the 90th percentile for a specific gestational age. Macrosomia means the baby weighs over four to 4.5 kilograms (8 lbs, 13oz–10 lbs), regardless of gestational age. Ten percent of all babies born in the U.S. weigh more than eight lbs, 13 oz, but only 1.5% weigh more than ten pounds, thank goodness!

Usual Time of Onset: Usually diagnosed in the third trimester. Difficult to diagnose. Ultrasounds can be imprecise.

Symptoms: None, other than a really big belly. Your practitioner suspects it when your **FUNDAL HEIGHT** measurements exceed what she expects for your due date. Periodic ultrasound measurements also show a larger weight than expected.

Cause: Here are your risk factors:

COMPLICATIONS

? ?

◆ You've already had one or more big babies.
◆ You were overweight before pregnancy.
◆ You gain excessive weight during pregnancy.
◆ You go beyond 40 weeks.
◆ You were a big baby. (You can't control that one!)
◆ You had diabetes before pregnancy or have gestational diabetes.
◆ You are younger than 17 years.
◆ You are Latina. Unfortunately, you have a better chance of having a big baby than your white, black or Asian friends.

Treatment:
◆ Diabetes—control your blood sugars.
◆ Excessive weight gain—meet with nutritionist to control further growth.
◆ Discuss delivery risks with your practitioner, especially if your doc suspects your baby will weigh over 4 kg (8 lb. 13 oz.) and you are diabetic. Or your baby is over 4.5 kg (10 lbs.) and you're not diabetic.
◆ Planned C-section for fetuses suspected to be over 4.5 kg (10 lbs.), or if you are anyone else who would appreciate not delivering a baby vaginally who is the size of a two month old.

Issues for Mom: Increased risk of a C-section (due to labor abnormalities), genital trauma during delivery (vaginal and perineal lacerations/episiotomies), **SHOULDER DYSTOCIA**, and excessive bleeding after delivery (**POSTPARTUM HEMORRHAGE**).

Issues for Baby: Shoulder dystocia can rarely cause nerve injury and occasionally collar bone fractures. Most babies recover without long-lasting problems. Big fetuses also have more trouble with the initial transition to life outside the womb, resulting in lower APGAR scores at five minutes and a chance of spending some quality time in the newborn intensive care unit. Overweight babies may also remain overweight as they grow up. *(ACOG)*

Q. The fetus is measuring much smaller than she should be for her age. Is this a problem for the baby?

46 COMPLICATION: INTRAUTERINE GROWTH RESTRICTION (**IUGR**) OR "SMALL FOR GESTATIONAL AGE" (**SGA**)

What is it? The short answer: small baby.

The long answer is complicated, so stick with us. IUGR refers to the growth restricted *fetus* who is still inside you and SGA refers to the small *newborn*. A fetus with IUGR is estimated to weigh below the 10th percentile for his gestational age. A newborn with SGA has a birth weight below the 10th percentile for gestational age.

SGA babies are either *symmetrically* growth restricted (the entire body is affected) or *asymmetrically* growth restricted (body weight is low, but head and length grow normally). This distinction is important because it helps determine the cause of the problem.

Usual Time of Onset: IUGR is typically diagnosed in the late second or third trimester, sometimes earlier in the second trimester. Diagnosis is difficult and ultrasound can be imprecise.

Symptoms: None. Sometimes a woman notices that her belly has not grown or seems small. Your practitioner discovers that your **FUNDAL HEIGHT** measurements are below what is expected for how far along you are. And periodic ultrasound measurements of your baby will also show a smaller weight than expected.

Cause: IUGR risk factors are listed below. It's also possible to have small parents and just be a small baby.

- ◆ *Certain maternal medical conditions*: high blood pressure (pre-existing and **PREECLAMPSIA**), kidney disease, lupus, blood clotting disorders (**THROMBOPHILIAS**) like antiphospholipid antibody syndrome, chronic anemia, preexisting diabetes.
- ◆ *Abnormal placenta*: placenta previa, partial placental abruption, placental mosaicism, subchorionic hematoma, placental tumors (very rare).
- ◆ *Maternal substance abuse*: alcohol abuse, smoking, cocaine abuse, heroin abuse, methadone abuse.
- ◆ *Multiples*: with twins, the placenta is less able to handle nutrition for both (especially when there is only one placenta in monozygotic twins).
- ◆ *Certain infections*: CMV, rubella, chicken pox (varicella), syphilis, toxoplasmosis, trypanosoma (Chagas disease).
- ◆ *Genetic disorders*: chromosome defects cause symmetric growth restriction.
- ◆ *Structural defects*: **ANENCEPHALY**, pyloric stenosis.
- ◆ *Teratogen exposure*: amount and timing of exposure impact the severity of the growth restriction. Examples: phenytoin (Dilantin), warfarin (Coumadin), methotrexate.

Treatment:
- ◆ If possible, figure out the cause. There's usually not much you can do, though, to improve a fetus' growth.
- ◆ Get tested for medical disorders, medication use, substance abuse.
- ◆ Deliver, if you are at term.
- ◆ Measure your baby by ultrasound every three to four weeks, if you are not at term.
- ◆ Periodically assess fetal well-being (nonstress tests, biophysical profiles, Doppler studies on the umbilical arteries).
- ◆ Deliver anytime after the baby is viable, if the fetus is not growing at all after three to four weeks or if there is immediate concern for fetal well-being.
- ◆ Stop smoking, if you are doing so.
- ◆ Bed rest (even though no studies show that it helps improve a baby's weight).
- ◆ Consider: zinc supplementation, low dose aspirin use, calcium supplementation, heparin and maternal oxygen therapy. None of these have been proven to work, however.

Issues for Mom: Possible C-section, and lots of worrying.

Issues for Baby: Although IUGR is defined by being less than the 10th percentile, the babies most at risk are less than the third to fifth percentile. One-fourth of all stillbirths are SGA (some of whom also may have too little amniotic fluid).

So when does your doc decide to proceed with delivery? It depends on your situation and involves your team of specialists. It's time if the fetus has not grown at all between ultrasounds three to four weeks apart or when tests don't confirm fetal well-being.

Your docs weigh the risks of premature birth against the risk of potential fetal death. C-sections are more common because half of IUGR fetuses have abnormal heart rate patterns in labor. Then these babies can have lower APGAR scores initially, and newborn problems that land them in the newborn intensive care unit. *(ACOG)*

Reality Check
If you smoke, your baby has a three times greater risk of being small for gestational age.

Old Wives Tale
A pregnant woman who eats poorly will have a small baby. *False.*

Studies of women living during famines at the time of World War II showed it takes a diet of less than 1500 calories per day to affect fetal growth. It is highly unlikely that any poor diet in the U.S. would be less than that amount.

P. Other

Go to Expecting411.com/extra for a comprehensive list of fetal malformations detected on ultrasound.

Q. My CVS/Amnio was abnormal. Now what?

47 COMPLICATION: GENETIC/CHROMOSOMAL DEFECTS

Several abnormalities may be detected by CVS or amniocentesis. If your baby is diagnosed with one of these disorders, you should have a consultation with a perinatologist or genetic counselor so that you and your partner will have a better idea of what this all means.

Q. Okay, I have watched my due date come and go, and I'm still pregnant. I don't want to be induced. Are there any potential problems for me or the baby?

48 COMPLICATION: POST TERM PREGNANCY.

What is it? You have gone past 42 weeks. We don't wish this on anyone, but it happens in seven to ten percent of all pregnancies.

Symptoms: You feel as big as a house and have irrational thoughts on how to induce labor.

Cause: Usually unknown. First pregnancies, boys more than girls, or your dates may be off. Rarely, things like a placental problem or fetal malformation can prolong a pregnancy.

Treatment:

◆ Tests of fetal well being (nonstress test, amniotic fluid index) after 40 to 41 weeks.

◆ Labor induction if your cervix is favorable (see "Bishop score" in Chapter 12, Home Stretch).

◆ Deliver by 41 completed weeks (42 weeks) due to risks to baby and mother.

◆ *Issues for Mom:* Longer and more difficult delivery, genital trauma due to the increased size of the baby, double the chances of needing a C-section, greater risk of stillbirth. Anxiety!

◆ *Issues for Baby:* big baby, **SHOULDER DYSTOCIA**, low blood sugars, seizures, temporary respiratory problems (**MECONIUM ASPIRATION**), infection, too little amniotic fluid, malnourished, increased risk of stillbirth. *(ACOG)*

OVERRIPE

Although we say pregnancy lasts nine months, it's really more like 9 1/2 or 9 3/5 months. A post-term pregnancy (overripe) is one that has gone beyond 42 weeks. About seven to ten percent of all pregnancies go post-term.

We know that it is every pregnant woman's nightmare to go a DAY over your predicted due date. You feel tired and heavy, and you are suffering from leg cramps and heartburn. Every night before you go to bed you pray to the Labor gods to please, please, please, at some point before sunrise, make you wake up in a puddle of water or with painful contractions.

From a medical standpoint, docs also prefer that women don't go too far past their due dates. Why? Why not just let everyone continue until that magical day comes and labor occurs? Well, there are a few risks, both to mom and to baby.

Your baby has an increased risk of stillbirth (the odds are four to seven per 1,000 versus three per 1,000 in babies less than 42 weeks), very large size (**MACROSOMIA**), breathing problems (**MECONIUM ASPIRATION SYNDROME**) as well as problems related to outgrowing the womb (fetal dysmaturity).

Some recent studies suggest that there is an increased risk of all of the above even after 41 weeks. *(Norwitz ER)* Big babies (we are talking about ten-pounders) may have trouble getting through the birth canal, which occasionally leads to broken collar bones and nerve injury. Big babies also have trouble keeping their blood sugars up, which requires close monitoring.

Moms face risks, too. You're more likely to have complications during labor and delivery due to the baby's larger size. These include longer, more difficult labors, increased risk of injury to your vagina, bladder, and rectum, and an increased risk of C-section.

So for all these reasons, your practitioner will probably suggest an induction if you are post-term.

complications

??

BOTTOM LINE: For pregnancies that go past 42 weeks, the risk of still-birth is doubled compared to deliveries at term (37 to 40 weeks). Get the bun out of the oven!

DR H'S OPINION:
DESPERATE FOR LABOR?

I know you are desperate enough to do just about anything to go into labor. If you are considering eating hot sauce straight from the bottle . . . drinking gallons of red raspberry leaf tea . . . or walking for hours in the hot sun at an amusement park, without drinking water, while purposefully forgetting the stroller in the car and then having to carry a three year old around ... we have a word of advice: don't. I tried all these things with my second pregnancy and none of them worked!

Well . . . that was enough doom and gloom for anyone! But wait! There's more! Infections are coming up next.

??

INFECTIONS
Chapter 17

"I don't think nuclear war will ever get us, but germs will."
—Raymond Martin

G erms don't really care if you are pregnant or not. They follow their mission statement: infect whoever comes along.

Of course, *you* care about getting sick. First, you will worry that your infection might harm your unborn baby (see—you are already a parent!). Then, you will worry about yourself. It is true that you might become more ill because pregnancy lowers your defenses against infection (on the plus side: this is only temporary).

The good news is that most of the usual players that cause infection—the common cold or stomach virus, are unlikely to have a major impact on your unborn baby.

But there are some infections that can be real problems for both of you, and we'll let you know which ones those are. We'll also cover the routine prenatal infectious disease screening tests and what they mean if they are positive. And since vaccines protect against infections, they are covered here as well.

Let's take a look at some of the common bugs (and vaccination issues) during pregnancy:

◆ *Infections found on routine pregnancy tests.* These include Chlamydia and Hepatitis B.
◆ *Other serious infections.* Chickenpox and toxoplasmosis are included in this group.

THE LOWDOWN ON ANTIBODIES

If infections are the offense, antibodies are your body's defense—after your body sees a threat (virus, bacteria, parasite or even a different type of blood), it goes into high gear and cranks out antibodies. These proteins are made by special white blood cells and are sent by your immune system to attack and kill the invaders.

Here's the important part to remember: tests for infections actually look for antibodies. These antibodies come in several types: two of the most common are IgM and IgG.

Let's use chickenpox as an example. If you are infected by this bug, your body makes IgM antibodies right away. Hence, a test that is positive for IgM means you've had a recent infection.

After the initial antibodies (IgM) do their magic, the body makes a clean up crew: the IgG antibodies. These protect you in the future should the chickenpox make a return visit.

Bottom line: testing your blood for antibodies tells whether you have:

◆ Ever come in contact with the germ in question.
◆ Been exposed recently.
◆ Been exposed in the past.
◆ Been vaccinated against a certain bug, in some cases.

◆ *Common infections.* From the common cold to sinus infections, this section also includes the flu and bladder infections.
◆ *Girl problems.* These include yeast infections, bacterial vaginosis and genital warts (HPV).
◆ *Vaccines.* We'll cover all the recommended vaccines in this section.

Infection 411: TORCH

TORCH is shorthand for a list of infections that can cause birth defects during pregnancy. If you test positive for one of these infections, you'll be followed more closely for the rest of your pregnancy. We'll discuss these throughout this chapter, but here are the offenders: Toxoplasmosis, Other (Syphilis, Varicella, Parvovirus B19 or "Fifth Disease", HIV), Rubella, CMV, Herpes. (*Children's Hospital, Boston.*)

Infections found on routine screening

CHLAMYDIA/GONORRHEA

Q. I tested positive for Chlamydia/gonorrhea. What does that mean?

Chlamydia and gonorrhea are sexually transmitted infections. During pregnancy, you are screened for both in the first trimester so that if you test positive for one or both, you can be treated early in your pregnancy. Women at higher risk may also be screened again in the third trimester.

It's easy to treat both infections with antibiotics. All sexual partners must

? ?

INFECTIONS

be treated as well.

After finishing the antibiotics, return to your doctor for re-testing to confirm the infection is completely gone.

Note: it is very important that you NOT resume sexual relations with anyone who has not been treated. Talk with your provider for exact details.

Gonorrhea 411

Disease A bacterial infection spread by sexual contact with the penis, vagina, mouth, or anus of an infected partner. It can also spread from mother to baby during delivery. The bacteria grows and multiplies easily in the tissues of the female genital tract (cervix, uterus, fallopian tubes). Hence, an untreated infection can lead to premature rupture of membranes, preterm labor and delivery.

Symptoms Often, none. Even when women do have symptoms, they are nonspecific and can mimic other infections. Symptoms may include burning with urination, increased vaginal discharge that has a different color or odor than usual, and lower abdominal pain.

Risk to the baby? Premature birth, if you go into preterm labor. It can also lead to blindness, bloodstream infection and joint infection in the newborn.

Treatment: Antibiotics.

Chlamydia 411

Disease A bacterial infection spread by sexual contact with an infected partner. It initially infects the cervix and the tube leading from the bladder to the outside (urethra). It can also spread into the fallopian tubes. If untreated, Chlamydia can lead to premature rupture of membranes and preterm labor and delivery.

Symptoms Often, none. Half to 75% of infected women have no symptoms (and up to 45% of men don't have symptoms either). When symptoms are present, they can include abnormal vaginal discharge, a burning sensation when urinating, lower abdominal pain, low back pain, nausea, fever, or pain during intercourse.

Risk to the baby? Chlamydia is a leading cause of early infant pneumonia and conjunctivitis (pink eye) in newborns. Your baby could also be premature if you go into preterm labor.

Treatment: Antibiotics.

2 RUBELLA

Q. My doctor told me that I am not immune to Rubella. What is Rubella and what does this mean during my pregnancy?

Rubella (also called German measles or three-day measles) is an infection caused by a virus. Most adults of childbearing age today are immune to rubella because they were vaccinated during childhood (MMR vaccine).

Ideally, it would be nice to know *before* you got pregnant if you were immune to rubella. If not, you could then be vaccinated before conceiving.

Women are routinely tested at the beginning of pregnancy to see if they are immune to rubella. If your blood work shows that you are not immune, either you were never vaccinated for rubella, your body never

infections

mounted an appropriate response to the vaccine (your body didn't make enough antibodies to protect you) or your immune response has worn off over time (your antibody levels have declined).

Rubella is not an infection you want to get when pregnant. Why? If infected with rubella in the first trimester, there is an 85% chance your baby will develop congenital rubella syndrome, which can lead to miscarriage, growth restriction, intellectual disability, blindness, deafness, heart defects and other problems. Exposure to rubella later in pregnancy is also dangerous, but the risk is greatest in the first trimester.

The good news: most folks are immune. In the U.S. today, *fewer than ten babies* are born every year with congenital rubella syndrome. Compare that to the 1964 epidemic (prior to the development of rubella vaccine), where 20,000 American babies were born with congenital rubella syndrome.

See information at the end of this chapter regarding the rubella vaccine.

Q. I got vaccinated for rubella and then found out I was pregnant! I'm really worried that I've done some kind of damage to my baby. Have I?

First of all, don't panic.

It is true that the rubella vaccine is not routinely given to pregnant women because it contains a live-attenuated virus. However, there has NEVER been a single documented case of a fetus developing congenital rubella syndrome (severe birth defects) when a mom has been accidentally vaccinated during pregnancy.

Bottom line: it is extremely unlikely your baby has suffered any damage as a result of this vaccine. Of course, docs err on the side of caution, so you'll probably be monitored more closely and have a few extra ultrasounds.

3 HIV

Q. Why am I being tested for HIV?

HIV (human immunodeficiency virus) is the virus that causes AIDS. It is spread through sexual contact with an infected person or when infected body fluids (like blood and breast milk) come in contact with mucous membranes (inside the eyes, nose, throat, mouth, urethra, rectum, or vagina) or broken skin.

Babies can potentially get infected while developing in the uterus, at the time of delivery, and during breastfeeding. All women should be routinely screened for HIV at the beginning of their pregnancies. There are two key reasons:

- If you are HIV positive, you can get treated with antiviral medication. This is important because babies who are born to UNTREATED women with HIV have a 25% to 35% risk of being infected. If you *do* get treated and don't breastfeed, your baby's risk of getting HIV is less than 2%.
- If HIV screening was only offered to women who were thought to be at high-risk, practitioners would miss many women who didn't know they were HIV positive. And those women would unwittingly pass along HIV to their babies. Remember, HIV is just a virus—its job is to find another person to infect.

Q. I have had HIV for over five years. What do I need to know now that I am pregnant?

As you probably know, you can have the HIV virus without actually having developed AIDS (Acquired Immune Deficiency Syndrome).

Over time, the virus can replicate and may eventually decrease the strength of your immune system. This leaves you susceptible to infections and tumors. Symptoms may include the development of certain cancers (such as cervical cancer, skin cancer or lymphoma), recurrent infections (such as pneumonia or chronic diarrhea), as well as symptoms of fever, night sweats, chills, weakness, weight loss and swollen glands.

If you are HIV positive, your healthcare team will include an OB, perinatologist, and an infectious disease specialist. To prevent spreading the infection to your baby, you should take an antiviral medication (such as AZT) during pregnancy.

While a detailed discussion of HIV and pregnancy is beyond the scope of this book, the goal for any HIV positive woman is to keep her viral load less than 1000. This reduces the risk of transmission to your baby and fewer complications for mom-to-be. *(ACOG)*

4&5 HEPATITIS B AND C

Q. I don't have any risk factors but my doctor wants to test me for Hepatitis B and C. Why?

Hepatitis B and C are two of at least six hepatitis viruses that infect the liver. Both viruses spread through sexual contact or contact with infected body fluids (like blood).

As you might know, those at high risk for Hepatitis B and C are people who are sexually promiscuous, IV drug abusers/needle sharers or who have received multiple blood transfusions throughout their lives (hemophiliacs).

However, up to one-third of adults who get a Hepatitis B infection are NOT in those high-risk categories and have no idea where they contracted the illness.

Hepatitis B became part of the routine childhood vaccination series in 1991. So many adults of childbearing age have been vaccinated. Docs routinely screen all pregnant women to test for immunity or evidence of active or previous infection with Hepatitis B. Women with certain risk factors are selectively screened for Hepatitis C (for instance, if you have Hepatitis B, you also might have Hepatitis C).

Pregnant women who are carriers of the hepatitis virus require more specialized prenatal care. Your practitioner can discuss medication options as well as questions about delivery and breastfeeding.

Bottom line: knowing whether you have Hepatitis B or C is best for you and your baby. The result is better care for mom and lower risk of spreading the infection to baby.

Factoid: 90% of babies that are born to women with Hepatitis B will become lifelong carriers of the disease *unless* they get readily available preventive treatment in the first 12 hours of life.

Factoid: If you contract Hepatitis B in your first trimester, the fetus has a 10% chance of getting infected. If infected during third trimester, there is an 80-90% risk of fetal infection.

Q. I tested positive for Hepatitis B. What comes next?

The test for Hepatitis B gives one of three results:

◆ You have been vaccinated against Hepatitis B.
◆ You were infected with Hepatitis B in the past but no longer have the virus.
◆ You are a chronic carrier of the infection.

If you are a chronic carrier, your healthcare team should include an OB, a perinatologist, and an infectious disease specialist. You should avoid procedures like a CVS or amniocentesis (discussed in Chapter 5, Tests), if possible, because they risk introducing the infection to the fetus.

You will be able to breastfeed, as long as your baby receives immune globulin and a Hepatitis B vaccine after birth. *(ACOG)*

6 SYPHILIS

Q. Why am I being screened for syphilis? Does that disease really still exist?

Yes. In fact, syphilis is more popular than ever, unfortunately.

Syphilis is more apparent in men than women—an ugly lesion on the penis is a dead giveaway (yuck, we know). But women with syphilis may not know it, since a lesion may not hurt or be visible.

A test for syphilis is routine at the first prenatal visit (and again in the third trimester for some high-risk populations).

What is the risk for babies? Syphilis infects babies through the placenta or during delivery. If mom is infected and does not receive treatment, there is an increased risk of miscarriage and stillbirth. If the baby survives, he may have congenital syphilis—which can cause blindness, deafness, and bone deformities among other problems. These are preventable with treatment.

FYI: Looking for more info on sexually transmitted infections? Check out the Centers for Disease Control website at cdc.gov/std or at 1-800-CDC-INFO.

7 GROUP B STREP

See Chapter 5, Tests, for information about this infection, screening tests, and treatment.

Other problem infections

8 CHICKENPOX (VARICELLA)

? ?

INFECTIONS

Q. I've never had chickenpox so my doctor tested me for it. She told me that I was not immune. What does this mean? Can this hurt the baby?

It's easy to do a blood test to see if your immune system has made antibodies to fight off the chickenpox virus (**VARICELLA-ZOSTER VIRUS**). If your test comes back negative, it means one of three things:

◆ You have never had chickenpox.

◆ You have never been vaccinated against chickenpox.

◆ Your body did not mount an appropriate response to the disease or the vaccine.

Why is this important? Because contracting chickenpox for the first time during pregnancy can have a devastating impact on baby (see discussion below).

If you are not immune to chickenpox, it's best to stay away from young children. We know that is pretty tough if you are, say, a mom already . . . or your job puts you in contact with kids (school teacher, etc).

If avoiding little people is impossible, here is the next best advice: stay home from work if there is a chickenpox outbreak. If your kids were vaccinated against chickenpox (at the 12 to 15 month well check), they probably won't bring it home.

Insider Secret

The best time to discuss chickenpox is (ideally) at the pre-conception visit you have with your practitioner. Then you can do the test to see if you have immunity. If you are immune, you won't have to worry if you actually get exposed to someone with chickenpox (varicella) or shingles (zoster). If you are not immune, you can get vaccinated prior to getting pregnant.

Q. How is chickenpox spread?

Chickenpox is spread by coming into contact with an infected person's respiratory droplets (secretions from the nose and mouth in the air) or skin lesions (clear, fluid filled mini-blisters).

Chickenpox is caused by **VARICELLA-ZOSTER VIRUS** or "VZV," which is a member of the Herpes virus family (not the kind that is sexually transmitted, however). Like all herpes viruses, VZV lies dormant forever in previously infected people. So it's possible for the infection to reactivate later in life and cause something called shingles.

Unlike chickenpox, shingles infects only one group of nerves and causes painful blisters. These blisters contain the virus and are also contagious. Therefore, someone who isn't immune can get chickenpox by direct contact with the lesions of a person with active shingles.

Here is the biggest issue for exposure: a person is contagious for 24 hours (via those respiratory droplets) *before* the classic chickenpox rash appears. So a non-immune person might be exposed to someone who doesn't know he has chickenpox until the next day. That's how these germs used to spread like wildfire through childcare centers and schools before the vaccine came out in 1995. And it's how a non-immune person might get exposed today.

infections

? ?

INFECTIONS

People with chickenpox and shingles are contagious until all the lesions are crusted over.

Factoid: It takes about ten to 21 days to come down with chickenpox after you have been exposed. So, breathe a sigh of relief if you are chickenpox free after three weeks.

Q. I have a one-year old and I am pregnant again. Is it safe for my one-year old to get her chickenpox vaccine and be around me afterwards?

Yes! In fact, you WANT your child to get this shot and be protected as soon as possible.

The varicella vaccine is a live-attenuated vaccine, which means that your child will mount an immune response to it within one to four weeks of getting the shot.

Occasionally, children will develop a rash that looks like chickenpox when their immune system responds to the vaccine. That rash does *not* mean she has the disease. So you do not have to worry about getting chickenpox from your child.

After 30 million doses of the vaccine, there have been a grand total of *three* people who got chickenpox after exposure to a recently-vaccinated person with a rash.

Q. I found out I was not immune to chickenpox at my preconception visit so I got the vaccine. I was already pregnant though, and didn't know it. Will my baby be ok?

Chickenpox is not routinely given to pregnant women since the vaccine contains live viral particles. However, here's the bottom line: there has NEVER been a documented case of birth defects or congenital varicella syndrome (see question below) in a fetus born to a pregnant woman who mistakenly received the chickenpox vaccine.

If this happens to you by mistake, yes, your practitioner will watch you more closely. No, you don't need to worry.

Q. I'm in my late 2nd trimester and just got diagnosed with chickenpox. I'm freaking out. What do I need to know?

First of all, don't freak out.

Congenital varicella syndrome (fancy words for a baby getting infected with the chickenpox virus while still in the uterus) most often occurs from exposure during the first 20 weeks of pregnancy. It is quite rare, occurring in just one to two percent of fetuses whose mothers have been infected.

Let's be clear, however: the syndrome is devastating. Babies have skin lesions that scar, abnormal limb formation, eye inflammation, small heads, and varying degrees of intellectual disability.

The other inopportune time for a pregnant woman to get chickenpox is five days before or up to 48 hours after delivery. The concern here is the newborn getting chickenpox (neonatal VZV infection). Because newborns have little defense to fend off the infection, death is often the result.

Perhaps the only time your baby would be unaffected by your chickenpox would be during the later part of second trimester. Your doctor will, however, keep a closer eye on the pregnancy. *(ACOG)*

9 CMV

Q. I am pregnant with my first child and work as a kindergarten teacher. My doctor said she wants to check to see if I have ever been exposed to something called CMV. What is that? Do I have to be worried?

CMV (cytomegalovirus) is another type of herpes virus that spreads through infected blood, saliva, urine, or sexual contact.

Most of the time, people don't even know when they have the infection (which is why it's difficult to diagnose during pregnancy—or any other time for that matter). Occasionally adults have a mono-like illness with severe fatigue, chills, muscle aches, fever and abnormal liver function.

So docs usually diagnose a CMV infection after discovering something unusual at the second-trimester ultrasound. The diagnosis is confirmed with an amniocentesis.

If a woman gets CMV during pregnancy, her fetus has a 30% to 40% chance of becoming infected. Fetal CMV infection can lead to hearing loss, a small head, varying degrees of intellectual disability, blindness, and death.

Although CMV is not part of the routine pregnancy screen at the first OB visit, many doctors do check patients who are at higher risk. Those patients include women who have other children at home, those who work with young children (school teachers, daycare workers, pediatricians or pediatric nurses) or work with immuno-compromised individuals (the elderly or AIDS patients).

If blood work shows that you have already been exposed to CMV, you cannot be infected again and your baby is not at risk. If you are not immune to CMV, you don't have to quit your job and live in a bubble. But you should take preventative measures to help decrease the risk of getting a CMV infection. These include:

- ◆ Wear gloves when handling dirty diapers, cleaning small children or coming in contact with immune-compromised individuals.
- ◆ Wash hands vigorously after diaper handling.
- ◆ Wash hands vigorously after coming in contact with nasal and respiratory secretions.

Factoid: CMV is the most common of all congenital infections and affects up to 2% of all newborns. It is the leading cause of congenital hearing loss.

10 PARVOVIRUS B19 (A.K.A. FIFTH DISEASE, "SLAPPED CHEEK")

Q. I work with kids and was exposed to a child with Fifth

Disease (parvovirus) and I am totally freaked out. Will my baby be okay if I get the infection?

Parvovirus is a very common viral illness that most people get in childhood. It's also called Fifth Disease because it was the fifth viral illness identified to have a classic rash (called "slapped cheek").

And true to the name, kids will get rosy red cheeks about a week or two *after* they were contagious with this minor illness. The most annoying part of this infectious disease is that kids have absolutely no symptoms when they are contagious. We only find out two weeks later that the kid had it and exposed his pregnant kindergarten teacher.

Most adults are immune to parvovirus because they had it in childhood. For the rare pregnant woman who actually isn't immune, parvovirus has the potential to cause anemia in the fetus and **very rarely**, fetal death.

Relax. This is extremely rare. Most fetuses born to women who got parvovirus during pregnancy do just fine. Even if a fetus gets this infection, they tend to "clear" it all by themselves with no long-term impact. And it doesn't produce birth defects.

The greatest risk to your fetus is if you get parvovirus infection *before* 20 weeks gestation. However, you should talk with your practitioner if you feel you have been exposed at ANY point during your pregnancy.

If you have been exposed, first get a blood test, no matter how far along in your pregnancy. Odds are, you are immune already and your blood work will confirm that. Case closed.

If you are one of the few adults who isn't immune, you should get retested three to four weeks later to see if you were, in fact, infected.

If you do contract parvovirus, your practitioner will check your fetus regularly by ultrasound to make sure she isn't becoming anemic, a very rare result of this infection. Docs can also detect fetal infection by testing the amniotic fluid via an amniocentesis.

TOXOPLASMOSIS

Q. I have three cats at home and my doctor wants to do a special blood test on me. What is he looking for? Should I be worried?

Your doctor wants to test you for toxoplasmosis.

Toxoplasmosis is a parasite that many animals, including cats, can carry. Humans can get the infection by being in direct contact with cat poop (changing the litter box), being scratched or bitten by an infected cat, eating infected meat (particularly pork, lamb or venison), coming in contact with soil contaminated with infected cat poop or with unwashed, raw vegetables that were in contact with contaminated soil.

Just a few more drops of blood from you (but really, who's counting at this point) and the lab can see if you have two different toxoplasmosis antibodies, IgM and IgG (see discussion earlier). Here's what the results mean: if you are negative for both, you have never been exposed to toxoplasmosis. You are *not* immune. Be very careful around your cats or any other cats, particularly strays, outdoor cats and kittens. Do not change your litter

? ?

INFECTIONS

box. Call your practitioner if you are scratched, bitten or come in direct contact with cat feces, so you can schedule a blood test.

If you are negative for IgM, but positive for IgG, you have been exposed to toxoplasmosis in the past. You *are* immune, so neither you nor your baby can become infected even if you are exposed to it again. Whew.

If you are positive for IgM and negative for IgG, it's possible you had a recent infection. But no test is perfect, and neither is this one. Sometimes, a patient's IgM antibody remains high for years after the initial infection.

Q. My test came back positive for toxoplasmosis. What are the risks to my baby?

It depends. The key issue: when where you infected? That impacts your baby's risk of getting the disease.

In the first trimester, there is a 10% to 15% chance that your baby will be infected. The chance is 25% in the second trimester. In the third trimester, it is more than 60%.

The earlier in pregnancy the fetus is infected, the more severe the consequences. Most infants do not show signs of infection at birth, but between 50% and 80% of infected infants later develop problems such as eye damage/blindness, hearing loss, or intellectual disability. Other features of congenital toxoplasmosis infection include a rash, enlargement of the liver and spleen, fever, brain abnormalities, and seizures.

Q. Is there any treatment for toxoplasmosis?

Yes.

There is an antibiotic called spiramycin that may reduce fetal transmission by 60%.

Unfortunately, even if mom is treated, this doesn't *eliminate* the risk of baby contracting the disease.

Doctors can tell if the fetus is infected by ultrasound, amniocentesis, and fetal blood sampling. If so, mom takes three more medications in addition to the spiramycin to attempt to lower the severity of the infection. Unfortunately, these meds rarely cure the infection. A perinatologist will do periodic follow-up ultrasounds to make sure the baby is growing appropriately.

FYI: If your practitioner suspects you have a new infection with toxoplasmosis, you will probably need to get your antibody levels retested every three weeks.

12 GENITAL HERPES (HSV)

Q. I am 22 weeks pregnant and have a red bump on the outside of my vagina that is really painful. My doctor told me to come in for a culture. What is she going to do? Can this hurt my baby?

infections

INFECTIONS

Your practitioner probably wants to do a herpes culture or a more specific test (polymerase chain reaction or PCR) on your lesion.

She will examine you first and decide if this painful red bump (or cluster of fluid-filled bumps) looks enough like herpes to warrant further testing. She needs to take a bit of fluid from the lesion for the culture and PCR tests. It can be a little painful, especially if you have a fluid-filled blister (vesicle) because your doctor needs to open it up to swab some of the fluid.

Your doctor may also do a blood test to see if this is your first episode of herpes. Antibody tests help determine if you have been exposed to herpes in the past or if the exposure is recent. Unfortunately, herpes tests aren't as helpful or specific as other infectious disease tests. Talk with your practitioner about the pros and cons of herpes testing, given your personal medical history.

People can harbor the virus for years before they have a first outbreak. And a first outbreak during pregnancy doesn't mean you were just infected (so resist making that phone call to the divorce attorney!).

A quick definition: *primary herpes infection* is the first time you have a herpes infection (painful bumps or vesicles in the genital or rectal area) *and* have evidence that this is a new exposure (through a combination of blood work and a herpes culture).

It is rare to have a primary herpes infection during pregnancy. More common is a first outbreak with a known prior exposure—that is, you knew you had been exposed to herpes in the past.

It's more dangerous to have a primary herpes infection in pregnancy because it poses a greater risk to the fetus than if you have a recurrent herpes outbreak.

If you get a primary infection in the first trimester, the fetus is at risk for eye inflammation, a small head, and rarely, skin lesions.

If you have a primary outbreak at delivery, the baby has a 30% to 60% risk of becoming infected. And once you have herpes, you have it for life. Newborns, in particular, can get very sick with a primary herpes infection. That's why a C-section is recommended if your practitioner detects an active outbreak at the time of delivery.

But don't get too alarmed. You can take prescription antiviral medication (acyclovir) once you recognize you have an outbreak or your practitioner diagnoses it. This helps decrease the duration of the infection and the risk of transmission to baby. Acyclovir is very safe during pregnancy.

 Reality Check

Women who have a known history of genital herpes get acyclovir every day, three times a day, starting at 36 weeks. The reasons:

◆ To decrease the amount of virus that is being shed from the cervix and vagina, therefore decreasing the risk to your baby as she makes her way down your birth canal.

◆ To decrease the chance of having an outbreak in labor and needing a C-section.

Q. **I have had genital herpes for many years, long before getting pregnant. What precautions do I need to take? Can I still have a vaginal delivery?**

? ?

INFECTIONS

You are in good company: over 45 million adults in the United States have been infected with genital herpes.

Although it's possible recurrent herpes outbreaks can spread the infection to the fetus, the risk is very low (thought to be less than 1%). Scientists theorize this is because mom's anti-herpes antibodies pass through the placenta and protect the baby. Even if there is an active herpes lesion at the time of delivery, the risk of transmission to the baby is only about 3%.

Despite the low risk, be sure to report all outbreaks to your practitioner so that you can be treated with antiviral medication.

Starting at 36 weeks, you should take daily antiviral medication until you deliver your baby (see previous Reality Check for details).

Q. I've heard there are three medications that can treat herpes. Why is acyclovir preferred?

There are three prescription antiviral medications that are used to prevent and treat herpes: acyclovir, famcyclovir, and valacyclovir (Valtrex).

We have the most safety information on acyclovir because the Centers for Disease Control and Prevention (CDC) asked drug makers to keep a registry of all pregnant women being treated with this drug since 1999.

In this study, over 700 women took acyclovir and their babies were all healthy. Unfortunately, there isn't as much data on women taking famcyclovir and valacyclovir during pregnancy, which is why they are prescribed less frequently.

All three medications have been proven safe in animal studies, though. (See explanation of categories of drug safety in Expecting411.com/extra).

However, valacyclovir is converted to acyclovir in the body, so most docs are fine with its use. This drug is only taken twice daily—but is A LOT more expensive than acyclovir, not available as a generic medication, and not covered on all insurance prescription plans.

BOTTOM LINE: It is much safer to take acyclovir than not to take it. The alternative (developing an active herpes infection that in turn infects your baby) is much worse.

Q. Do I need to have a C-section if I have an outbreak at the time I go into labor?

Yes.

A C-section is recommended for all women who either have an active lesion or feel an outbreak is imminent (burning, pain or itching in the vaginal/vulva area) at the time of delivery. In one study, only 1.2% of babies born by C-section to moms with active HSV outbreaks contracted the infection versus 7.7% of infants who were born vaginally.

You can still have a vaginal delivery if you don't have an active outbreak or early symptoms that a herpes outbreak is about to happen (itching, tingling or burning).

Q. Can I still breastfeed my baby if I have active genital herpes?

Yes.

Unless you have a lesion on your breast, you can absolutely breastfeed your baby. You can prevent spreading your infection by washing your hands obsessively. If you have an outbreak, make sure you wash your hands very well before coming in contact with baby. FYI: Acyclovir is safe to take while breastfeeding.

Q. I always get my outbreaks on the back of my thigh and butt. Can I still have a vaginal delivery?

Yes.

Your practitioner can simply cover the lesion with a bandage. But it is very important for your practitioner to closely examine your cervix, vagina, vulva and rectum to ensure that there are no active lesions elsewhere. The good news: the odds are pretty low of you passing HSV to your baby when you have a recurrent outbreak—in fact, it's less than 1%.

13 ORAL HERPES

Q. I get cold sores. Are these dangerous during pregnancy?

No.

Cold sores are those painful blisters on the lip that are fluid-filled and then scab over. They are caused by a different form of herpes simplex virus (HSV-1). They are not a problem for your fetus, but they can pop up more often during pregnancy while your immune system is suppressed. You can be treated with a topical medication or with antiviral medication taken by mouth, if necessary.

The biggest issue for the baby is *after* he is born. A person with active cold sores can spread the herpes virus to a newborn, who can in turn get pretty sick. Don't kiss your baby if you have an active cold sore.

Factoid: Herpes Simplex Virus-2 (HSV-2) is the most common cause of genital herpes. It's cousin, Herpes Simplex Virus-1 (HSV-1) is the most common cause of cold sores. But yes, you can get HSV-1 in your genital area (and vice versa) if your partner has an active cold sore and you receive oral sex.

NEONATAL HERPES

So what's the big deal about passing herpes on to your newborn? A herpes infection can go anywhere—including the brain, spinal cord, or eyes. While death rates from neonatal herpes are declining, 20% of babies that survive neonatal herpes have long-term neurological issues. There are about 1500 cases each year in the U.S., and one-third of them are due to HSV-1 (oral herpes). About 80% of babies who have neonatal herpes are born to moms who have no history of herpes infections.

? ?

INFECTIONS

Insider Secret

If you suffer from cold sores or genital herpes, you may have more flare-ups during pregnancy.

14 LISTERIA

Q. I accidentally ate some unpasteurized cheese last night and this morning I have a high fever with nausea and vomiting. Could this be Listeria?

Yes.

Listeria is a bacterial infection most often caused by eating uncooked or undercooked meat (hot dogs, deli meat, lunch meats unless cooked until steaming), refrigerated pate or meat spreads, uncooked vegetables, smoked seafood (lox, kippered, jerky), unpasteurized dairy products (soft cheeses like brie) and random events like contaminated cantaloupes in 2011.

Symptoms include fever, body aches, chills, stomach pain, nausea and diarrhea. It can feel like the flu or food poisoning. Occasionally, pregnant women infected with Listeria can become very ill as the bacteria infects the bloodstream, lungs (pneumonia) or the lining of the spinal cord and brain (meningitis). Some infected pregnant women may only experience mild flu-like symptoms.

Your doc can prescribe antibiotics that can often prevent infection in the fetus . . . but only if symptoms are reported early. It can take several weeks before you feel ill so report any symptoms to your doctor immediately.

If you have Listeria, you will be followed more closely with ultrasounds to ensure the health of your baby. Rarely, the bacteria crosses the placenta and can lead to miscarriage, stillbirth, preterm delivery or neonatal infection.

Q. How can I protect myself from getting this infection?

The best defense against Listeria infection is a good offense. Here's how to avoid it:

- ◆ Thoroughly cook all meat such as beef, pork and poultry.
- ◆ Thoroughly wash all raw vegetables before eating them.
- ◆ Keep uncooked meat in separate packaging and be sure to keep any liquid from the meat away from other foods.
- ◆ Avoid all unpasteurized dairy products.
- ◆ Avoid deli meats, cheeses and hot dogs unless cooked until steaming.
- ◆ Wash your hands, and all utensils (knives, cutting boards) thoroughly after coming in contact with uncooked meat.

FYI: Pregnant women are twenty times more likely to get Listeria infections than other healthy adults.

INFECTIONS

? ?

Common infections

15 COMMON COLD

Q. I have a cold. Will this harm my baby?

No. Your baby will be fine.

While the common cold is a minor illness, you are more susceptible if you are pregnant. And you'll probably feel more miserable with a cold when pregnant because your immune system isn't firing on all cylinders.

Check in with your doctor if you:

◆ Run a fever over 100.4° F for more than two days straight
◆ Run any fever over 102° F or . . .
◆ Continue to have a runny nose or cough for more than a couple of weeks.

Check out the Appendix A, Medications, for approved over-the-counter medications to take for a cold while pregnant.

16 SINUS INFECTION

Q. I have had a cold for the last two weeks and it is only getting worse. Do I have a sinus infection? Do I need to be treated?

Yes, and you may need an antibiotic to clear it up.

Pregnant or not, a cold that lingers for an extended time or seasonal allergies can be a perfect nesting ground for bacteria to invade your sinuses.

Even during pregnancy, you can use many of the same treatments that you would sans pregnancy. Try taking a hot shower or breathing in warm steam a few times a day. Saline nasal spray, acetaminophen (Tylenol), an expectorant (like Robitussin DM), or decongestant (like Sudafed) are all safe to use.

If you are not getting better after a few days or you have a fever (over 100.4° F), it's time to call your doc. There are many prescription antibiotics

DR B'S OPINION
IT'S OK TO HAVE A COLD

I was a senior pediatric resident when I was pregnant with my first child. Needless to say, I suffered my fair share of viral illnesses, thanks to my patients. But like you, I worried when I sniffled for the first time during my pregnancy. My OB's comment was, "This is the first of many colds. Relax."

She went on to remind me that it was a good thing because I was giving the antibodies I made to my unborn baby. Not that I felt a whole lot better coughing and sneezing while being pregnant, but at least I was reassured!

and nasal steroid sprays that are safe during pregnancy. (See Expecting411. com/extra for details).

17 THE FLU

Q. I have a fever, bodyaches, and chills. Do I have the flu? What do I need to do?

Yes, it sounds like you have the flu (technically, an influenza infection).

Although many people refer to the common stomach virus as "stomach flu," this *isn't* the flu. Influenza is a respiratory infection. You start off with fever, chills, bodyaches, and fatigue. The runny nose, sore throat, and cough come later. Every once in a while, you're unlucky enough to have some vomiting or diarrhea too.

As a pregnant and thus temporarily immune-compromised person, you are more likely to suffer the complications from the flu—dehydration, pneumonia, meningitis, or bloodstream infection. This infection can also set off preterm labor.

So what should you do? See your practitioner pronto. You can take antiviral medication (like Tamiflu) to lessen the severity and length of your illness if you start it within 48 hours of the first symptoms. You can also take acetaminophen (Tylenol) and cough medication to relieve your symptoms. (See Expecting411 com/extra for details on medications.)

And drink lots of fluids to stay hydrated.

Reality Check
Pregnant women are five times more likely to be hospitalized for the flu than non-pregnant women. That's why it is so important for you to get your flu shot!

Bottom Line
Influenza virus spreads by contact with an infected person's cough or sneeze droplets. You can catch it by touching contaminated surfaces like a door handle or ATM keypad.

Avoid catching the flu by frequently washing your hands and avoiding contact with people who are sick (folks are contagious for one day before symptoms start and until they are fever free for 24 hours). Also limit touching your nose, mouth and eyes. Lastly, get a flu shot.

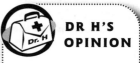

DR H'S OPINION

"When it comes to flu prevention, I no longer think the people who reach for the public bathroom door with a paper towel are nuts!"

18 STOMACH VIRUS

Q. My toddler came home from daycare with a stomach virus and now I have it too. How can I tell if I am getting dehydrated?

People like to call it the "stomach flu," but this illness is not caused by an influenza virus.

If you get a stomach virus (rotavirus, adenovirus, norovirus), you may have one or more of these symptoms: nausea, vomiting, diarrhea (usually watery), abdominal pain/cramps, tired, achy, and maybe a fever.

Less commonly, "the runs" can be caused by bacterial food poisoning (E. coli, Shigella or Salmonella), or a parasitic infection (Giardia, for example). Any of these can cause wicked diarrhea. Red flags for these illnesses are blood or mucus in your diarrhea or more than a few days of symptoms.

The goal is to stay hydrated since you will lose tons of water in your poop. Dehydration can be pretty serious for pregnant gals, sometimes leading to preterm labor.

After your vomiting stops, try to take small sips of a fluid other than water or milk (Gatorade, Vitamin water, 7-Up, Gingerale) at five to ten minute intervals. If a little sip stays down, wait five to ten minutes and take another little sip.

If you take a big gulp, you will regret it—it will come right back up again.

Take acetaminophen (Tylenol) if you have a fever of 100.4° F or greater.

When to call the doc: if you are unable to keep liquids down for over four to six hours. You might need to be admitted to the hospital for intravenous fluids if you and the toilet bowl are spending too much time together. You can also call your practitioner from the get-go to help determine whether you have a run-of-the-mill stomach bug or something more serious.

19 BLADDER INFECTION

Q. I'm peeing all the time and not that much comes out. It doesn't hurt like it normally does when I've had bladder infections in the past. Should I tell my practitioner?

Yes, you probably have a bladder infection or urinary tract infection (UTI).

UTI's are more common during pregnancy and women often have no symptoms. That's one reason docs check your pee at every visit. Typical symptoms include:

- ◆ frequent urination.
- ◆ urgency (the need to urinate immediately).
- ◆ blood in the urine.
- ◆ painful urination.

Your doc will prescribe antibiotics to treat it. Drink more cranberry juice and water, and try to urinate often (don't hold it). Untreated UTI's can progress to kidney infections, which are far more serious.

BOTTOM LINE: Bladder infections during pregnancy may not hurt.

Reality Check
Up to 10% of pregnant women get bladder infections.

20 KIDNEY INFECTION

Q. My doctor is treating me for a bladder infection. I just started taking antibiotics but now I have back pain, chills and a fever. Is this a kidney infection?

Yes. Unlike urinary tract infections (which may not have symptoms), this time you'll know you're sick.

Symptoms include back pain on one or both sides, high fever, chills, nausea, vomiting, the need to pee immediately, painful urination, or blood in the urine.

Kidney infections require hospitalization for IV fluids and antibiotics. Your doc will probably order an ultrasound to look for kidney stones or any obstruction. Once you improve, you can go home and take oral antibiotics for seven to ten days.

Practitioners are aggressive about treating kidney infections because they can lead to:

◆ an infection in the bloodstream that can quickly spread to other organs.

◆ pneumonia.

◆ preterm labor and rarely (gulp!) death.

Since women who are susceptible to kidney infections can be repeat offenders, docs usually recommend a daily low-dose antibiotic after the first infection.

Factoid: One to two percent of women get a kidney infection during pregnancy.

Girl Problems (genital infections)

21 YEAST INFECTION

Q. I am battling a yeast infection that just won't clear up. Is this a problem for delivery or for the baby?

It's not a problem for your baby, but it's a real pain for you. And it certainly interferes with any desire to have intercourse.

Yeast infections occur more often during pregnancy because of your temporarily depressed immune system. We all have a little yeast growing down there, but pregnancy allows overgrowth and thus, you end up with white cottage cheesy vaginal discharge (sometimes it's yellow or green), vaginal irritation, burning, and itching. You'll look like a rap singer because you are reaching for your crotch every few minutes.

The over-the-counter anti-fungal creams (clotrimazole, miconazole) are safe to use during pregnancy. But if you need a prescription anti-fungal, you and your practitioner will have to weigh the risks and benefits. See Expecting411.com/extra for details.

If you are prone to yeast infections, it's wise to take a probiotic (the stuff found in yogurt and kefir) every day for prevention. The more good germs you have living in and on you, the less the yeast is able to grow.

22 Bacterial Vaginosis

Q. I have vaginal discharge, but it doesn't seem like a yeast infection. Is this a problem?

This may be a bacterial infection that causes irritation of the external genital area. Symptoms can mimic a yeast infection because external vaginal itching and burning are common. The increased vaginal discharge is often gray or yellow-white and has a "fishy" odor, particularly after intercourse. As opposed to a yeast infection that often has "cottage cheesy" discharge, this discharge is often thin and sometimes frothy. Now that we have forever ruined your appetite for cottage cheese, seafood and beer, be sure to keep reading!

The bacterial culprit here is *Gardnerella vaginalis*, which all women carry around (it's not a sexually transmitted infection). Gardnerella overgrowth is the problem.

In pregnancy, this can be more than just an issue of your bedroom smelling like Eau-de-Salmon after lovemaking. It has been linked to miscarriage, preterm labor and delivery, breaking your water bag prematurely, and low-birth weight babies. Obviously, it's very important to tell your practitioner if there is a change in the color, smell, or volume of vaginal discharge!

It is easily treated with oral antibiotics or those inserted directly into the vagina.

Factoid: Ten to 30% of pregnant women will develop bacterial vaginosis (BV) during their pregnancy.

23 Trichomonas

Q. I had a lot of vaginal discharge so I went in to see my doctor. She just called and told me that I have something called Trichomonas. Will this hurt my baby?

This is a sexually transmitted bacterial infection caused by *Trichomonas vaginalis*. It infects the vagina and the cervix. In men, it infects the penis.

It causes yellow-green vaginal discharge, vaginal irritation, and lower abdominal pain. But about 40% of women don't have any symptoms at all. It's a problem during pregnancy because it can lead to premature rupture of membranes, preterm labor and delivery, low birth weight babies, and possible stillbirth. Very rarely, a baby can get infected while going through the birth canal.

If you test positive for Trichomonas, your doc will prescribe an antibiotic. The cure rate is between 90% and 95%, assuming that both you *and* your partner are treated. If you are in a relationship where one or both of you are sexually active with more than one person, you should always use a condom during intercourse. Refrain from having intercourse with your partner or with anyone new until you and your partner have been fully treated with antibiotics.

24 GENITAL WARTS (HPV)

Q. I have genital warts. Do these need to be treated while I am pregnant?

Yes, genital warts should be treated.

Genital warts are a sexually transmitted infection caused by Human Papilloma Virus (HPV). The warts show up on your external genital area, around your anus, or on your cervix. They look like flesh-colored growths that often occur in clusters. Some are little bumps and others resemble cauliflower. They do not hurt, but often cause itching.

Pregnancy can trigger an outbreak or allow existing lesions to grow more rapidly because of your depressed immune system and hormones gone wild.

Warts should be treated because their increasing size can obstruct the urethra (making it next to impossible to pee), the cervix and vagina (making it difficult to have a vaginal delivery).

Warts are also a possible health risk for baby. It's rare, but newborns can

acquire HPV infection from their moms and get warts on the eyelids or in their throats (laryngeal papillomatosis).

Here are the safe treatment options during pregnancy: trichloroacetic acid (TCA), freezing (cryosurgery), burning (electrocautery), laser treatment or rarely, surgical removal.

FYI: HPV is one of the most common sexually transmitted infections in the

DR H'S OPINION: MORE THAN YOU WANTED TO KNOW

Aaahh, vaginal discharge, the topic of many dinner conversations. . . at least the dinner conversations in my household as there are four OB/GYNs and a midwife in my immediate family!

The big question in pregnancy is what is normal and what is not? There is something called **LEUKORRHEA OF PREGNANCY** that usually starts to happen in the early first trimester. It's a set of big words that basically mean you will begin to suffer from a lot of vaginal discharge, and I mean A LOT.

This is a normal phenomenon that occurs in most pregnant women as a result of the increased blood flow to your cervix and vagina. You will notice large amounts of thin to moderately thick, whitish-yellowish vaginal discharge. It is not clumpy. It is not brown or green. There is no strong odor. You will not have vaginal or external genital pain, burning or itching. But I can tell you one thing—it is annoying. Any questions? Talk to your practitioner about it. She can decide if this is normal and rule out any infection.

INFECTIONS

? ?

world. There are approximately 5.5 million new cases of sexually transmitted HPV infections annually. At least 20 million Americans are already infected.

Vaccines for you

The Flu Shot and Pregnancy

This has been a hot topic for the past decade and recommendations have changed several times.

Here's the latest advice from both ACOG and the Centers for Disease Control: ALL pregnant women should get a flu shot—no matter what stage of pregnancy you are in during flu season.

The advice changed when a 17-year study showed that pregnant women who received the flu shot had a significantly lower risk of complications from the flu—particularly heart and lung problems. *(ACOG, CDC)*

Remember, you are a temporarily immune-compromised sitting duck. You're more likely to get extremely ill or even die (it is rare, but possible) from the flu. Studies also show that the flu shot does not harm the fetus at any point during pregnancy. In fact, the flu shot you get during pregnancy may give your baby some short-term immunity to the flu virus as well.

Flu shot do's and don'ts:

- ◆ Check with your allergist if you are allergic to eggs or egg products. Some egg-allergic people can get the flu shot with appropriate testing and careful supervision.
- ◆ You cannot get the flu vaccine in the nasal spray form while you are pregnant.
- ◆ You CAN and should get either the flu shot or the nose spray *while you are breastfeeding*.
- ◆ The flu vaccine immunizes against the most likely influenza strains expected each season. There are two A strains and one B strain.
- ◆ If you are going to be pregnant during flu season (October through March), talk with your practitioner about getting the flu shot.

Old Wives Tale
You can catch the flu from the flu shot. *False.*

Reality Check
What about that mercury-containing preservative in flu vaccines? Yes, thimerosal is in some flu vaccines. However, you can request a vaccine that doesn't contain this preservative.

What if the only flu vaccine in stock at your doc's office contains thimerosal? We recommend getting the shot anyway, even if it has thimerosal. The amount of mercury present in this vaccine is tiny—probably less than the piece of sushi you stole off your husband's plate last week. By contrast, the downside to *not* getting the vaccine (and catching the flu) far exceeds any risk from thimerosal. And, just so you know, ACOG advises all pregnant women get vaccinated, thimerosal or no thimerosal.

Rubella

The rubella vaccine cannot be given during pregnancy. But if you discover you are not immune, you should absolutely be vaccinated after delivery. Then there are no worries about rubella if you get pregnant again.

Currently, the rubella vaccine is not available in the U.S. as a single shot. Therefore, you will be vaccinated after delivery with the MMR (measles, mumps, rubella) vaccine. It is safe to get this vaccine even if you are nursing.

Tdap

This is a combination vaccine that protects against tetanus, diphtheria, and pertussis (whooping cough). If you can't remember the last time you

DR B TRUE STORY

A few years back, a mother that I knew well brought her four-week-old son into my office. After having three kids, her mommy instinct told her something was wrong.

The baby was having difficulty breathing. Yes, some newborns have "periodic breathing," where they pant for several breaths, pause, and then breath again. But this was different. The baby would stop breathing and seemed like he couldn't catch his breath. He was having these episodes a few times a day, and it scared even this seasoned mom.

When I examined him, he appeared perfectly normal until he started choking. I turned to her and asked, "Are you afraid to sleep at night?" Her response: "YES!" That was enough for me: this baby needed to be in the hospital.

The diagnosis: whooping cough. The baby had horrible coughing spells where he would turn red, choke, and gasp for breath.

It turns out that his mom had a hacking cough towards the end of her pregnancy that she just couldn't shake. It continued in the weeks after she delivered, but she was too busy taking care of her newborn to worry about herself. Mom had whooping cough and gave it to her son.

Fortunately, there was a happy ending. After several scary days in the hospital receiving oxygen and constant monitoring, the boy went home and made a full recovery. Today, he is a healthy, thriving kid.

But not all babies who get whooping cough are so lucky.

That's why it is so important to get vaccinated against this disease. Whooping cough often spreads from adults to those who are the most vulnerable—our babies, who, like my patient, are too young to be vaccinated.

Bottom line: anyone who is going to take care of your baby should be vaccinated—dads, grandparents and so on. Teens and adults can receive a whooping cough booster vaccine that's given in combination with their tetanus shot (called the Tdap vaccine). Moms-to-be should get a Tdap shot after 20 weeks of pregnancy or at least after delivery if they have never had it.

Remember, your baby can only be protected if everyone around him is vaccinated.

If you can't remember the last time you got your tetanus shot, or you got your last one when you were still seeing *your* pediatrician, it's time to do it!

got your tetanus shot (or had one prior to 2005), you need a booster dose *now* preferably or at least *after* delivery.

As of 2011, the Centers for Disease Control have new recommendations for pregnant women and whooping cough protection. The advice: all pregnant women who have not gotten the Tdap vaccine should get it after 20 weeks of pregnancy. Most newborns and infants contract whooping cough from their moms, but they can't get the vaccine until two months of age (because the vaccine isn't very effective prior to that). The vaccine is safe during pregnancy and if mom gets the shot during the second or third trimester, temporary immunity can be passed from mother to baby. *(Centers for Disease Control)*

Even with vaccination, immunity to whooping cough wanes with time. The best way to protect your newborn is to protect yourself and others who spend time with him (including all family members and caregivers).

Hepatitis A

The Hepatitis A vaccine can be given to pregnant women if they are planning to travel to areas of the world where Hepatitis A is more common. It is given in two separate doses, six to 12 months apart.

Partner Tip
Want to protect your baby? Go get your flu shot and Tdap booster too. It's always good to take one for the team.

Boosting your immune system. Many patients ask if there is something they can do to help their immune systems work more effectively. The best thing you can do to support your immune system is to give it the rest and nutrients it needs to function properly. In short, eat right and sleep well. Getting a professional or spouse massage regularly wouldn't hurt either.

Feel free to take extra Vitamin C, zinc, or Echinacea—we won't guarantee they will work, but they are safe during pregnancy. We do, however, discourage drinking green tea on a regular basis while you are pregnant. Yes, it is rich in antioxidants. And yes, the active ingredient, epigallocatechins (EGCG), may be beneficial in preventing some types of cancers. But EGCG also interferes with the way the body metabolizes folic acid (folate)—and folic acid is essential to prevent neural tube defects in babies.

International travel, exotic diseases, and you. If you are going somewhere outside the continental U.S. for a babymoon, be extra certain you do your homework. Some destinations carry infection risks that require vaccinations that may or may not be safe during pregnancy. We highly recommend that you go to cdc.gov/travel and check out the risks of your potential travel destination.

Now that you are sufficiently grossed out by all these germs, let's move on to a more "mature" subject: women who get pregnant at an, ahem, "advanced maternal age."

Advanced Maternal Age

Chapter 18

"Thirty-five is when you finally get your head together and your body starts falling apart."—Caryn Leschen

Congratulations! You are among a growing trend of moms-to-be who have a baby later in life. You're ecstatic . . . but concerned about all the risks you keep hearing about—from the media, from your friends and from your mother (who had three kids by the time she was 26!). We'll go over what you need to know as you dive into pregnancy as a more mature woman. Find information regarding additional tests you will be offered (Amniocentesis, CVS) is covered in detail in Chapter 5, Tests.

Advanced Maternal Age: What it means

Q. I don't feel old. Why am I labeled as "advanced maternal age" or AMA? Isn't 40 the new 30?

The definition of advanced maternal age (AMA) is any woman who will be 35 years of age or older at the time she gives birth to her baby.

Many women today choose to delay childbearing until later in life for a variety of reasons. More women are completing advanced degrees or are busy building careers in their late 20's and early 30's. Some women are getting married later in life. And women in their second and third marriages want to have additional children. Whatever the reason, it's trendy to have a baby after age 35.

ADVANCED AGE

? ?

Even if 40 is the new 30 for many of life's adventures, Mother Nature has not modified her definition when it comes to having babies. You still get the "AMA" rubber stamp on your medical record if you are 35 or over.

Factoid: In 1970, one in 100 babies were born to moms over age 35. Today, that number is one in seven.

Q. Are there any advantages to being an AMA mom?

Yes!

Your life experiences may make you more prepared for the rigors of parenthood. Mature parents-to-be are usually more educated and that translates into a more informed mom-to-be.

And, as an added bonus, you are more likely to be financially secure and have better health insurance.

DR B'S OPINION

"The one downside of becoming a parent after climbing the corporate ladder is that you are in for a real shock when your baby becomes the CEO of your house. This baby is going to rock your world. Relax . . . and enjoy it."

IS IT HARDER FOR ME TO BECOME PREGNANT?

Short answer: yes.

As a woman ages, she has more menstrual cycles where she does not release an egg (**OVULATE**). If there is no egg around to fertilize, there's no chance of becoming pregnant! There is a 20% chance of a 20 year-old couple getting pregnant in any one menstrual cycle. That drops to a three to five percent chance of this happening by the time a woman is 40.

Both egg quality and quantity begin to decline as a woman enters her 30's and 40's. And the older a woman gets, the more likely she is to have other issues that may make conception more difficult: **ENDOMETRIOSIS, UTERINE FIBROIDS, PELVIC INFLAMMATORY DISEASE**, previous pelvic surgery which could potentially scar the fallopian tubes, and chronic health conditions like diabetes or thyroid disease.

Bottom line: you'll probably still get pregnant, it just may take more time. It usually takes a woman over age 35 about 12 to 24 months to conceive.

Although the technical definition of "infertility" is no conception after one year of regular sexual intercourse, the real-life definition of infertility is shorter. The clock is ticking—and there is less time to sit around and see if a 35-year-old woman can become pregnant. The take-home message: schedule a consultation with your practitioner if you are over the age of 35 and have been trying regularly to conceive for six months without success.

Concerns during pregnancy

Q. Are there any more risks during pregnancy because I am a little older?

Yes, but the good news is that most women in their late 30's and early 40's end up having perfectly healthy babies. Don't let the list below freak you out.

Here are the risks to keep an eye on:

◆ *Miscarriage.* The risk is greater because AMA moms are more likely to have a fetus with a major genetic (chromosome) problem.

◆ *Gestational diabetes.* You are twice as likely to have gestational diabetes as your younger preggo friends.

◆ *High blood pressure.* There is a greater chance of both **GESTATIONAL HYPERTENSION** and **PREECLAMPSIA**.

◆ *Other medical problems.* You may have some pre-existing health problems that can complicate pregnancy (high blood pressure, lupus, diabetes, kidney problems).

◆ *Placenta problems.* **PLACENTA PREVIA** and placental insufficiency are more common.

◆ *Preterm delivery.* Women over age 35 are 50% more likely to deliver before 37 weeks.

◆ *Low birth weight.* Preterm delivery and having a low birth weight baby go together.

◆ *Stillbirth.* The risk is only *slightly* greater as you age. Women in their 20's have a four in 1000 chance of a stillbirth. Women 35 to 39 have a five in 1000 chance. Women 40 to 44 have a seven in 1000 chance. *(Anderson FW, Cleary-Goldman J, Joseph KS.)*

Reality Check

At 35 years of age, the risk of having a fetus with any chromosomal abnormality is one in 204. At age 40, that number is one in 63. At age 45, it is one in 19. *(ACOG)*

Q. Does my risk of miscarriage go up as I get older?

Yes. Miscarriage rates increase with a woman's age.

Studies show that a woman in her 20's has a one in ten chance of losing a recognized pregnancy to miscarriage. A woman who is 35 to 39 has a one in five chance. By the time a woman is 40 to 44 years old, she has a 50% chance of miscarrying.

The risk goes up primarily because the older you are, the more likely you will conceive a fetus with a major chromosomal defect.

About 85% of all miscarriages occur in the first trimester (no matter how old you are). *(Heffner L.)*

Q. I'm 36. Is there anything I can do to try to decrease my risk of complications once I get pregnant?

Most of these risks are out of your control. But having a pre-conception visit with your practitioner is helpful if you are not pregnant yet. That gives you a chance to discuss any pre-existing health conditions or medications you take regularly with your practitioner. You can start a prenatal vitamin, aim for an ideal body weight, exercise, cut out any bad habits (smoking, alcohol, illicit drugs), get any necessary vaccinations, and take good care of yourself.

But if you are like most of us who do not plan our pregnancies, start those healthy habits now and go to all your prenatal appointments with your practitioner.

Q. Are there any risks to the developing fetus due to my age?

Yes. Genetic defects aside, babies born to AMA moms have a slightly greater risk of having some birth defects. Note: we used the word SLIGHTLY, folks. Most babies are healthy and born with ten fingers and ten toes. *(Hollier LM, Reefhuis J.)*

Q. Should I do additional testing during pregnancy because of my age?

Yes. And the beauty of modern medicine is that every woman who is 35 or older does not automatically need to have an amniocentesis. Take a look at Chapter 5, Tests for information on chromosome testing options.

Reality Check

The American Congress of Obstetricians and Gynecologists (ACOG) recommends that women who will be 35 or older at the time of delivery be offered prenatal testing to diagnose (or, far more likely, rule out) Down syndrome and other chromosomal problems. Prenatal tests include amniocentesis and chorionic villus sampling (CVS). Most women who have these tests learn that their baby does *not* have a chromosomal problem.

Q. Are older moms and dads a double whammy?

Possibly.

Let's face it—if you are over age 35, it's likely your partner is too. If both mom and dad are of "advanced" age, there is a greater (although very small) risk of having a baby with a genetic defect. The chances of having a baby with Down syndrome go up significantly if a mother is 40 or older *and* the father is 35 or older. *(Fisch H.)*

It's worth your time to have genetic counseling if you are AMA and APA.

Reality check

If you put off childbearing until later in life, you are more likely to need fertility treatments. Over one-third of fertility treatments are performed on women over age 40.

Both advanced maternal age and fertility treatments increase your chances of having multiples. AMA and multiples are a recipe for a high-risk pregnancy.

Partner tip

Remember your partner may find being stamped as "advanced maternal age" a bit depressing. Treat any discussion of these issues with kid gloves. And do whatever it takes to remind your partner how young she really is!

Delivery Issues

Q. Are there any more risks during labor and delivery because of my age?

Yes. Because as much as you don't want to hear this—your body is older. But overall, you have a very low risk of encountering a problem!

Q. Is there any greater risk of having a C-section since I am older than 35?

Yes. Your odds of needing a C-section go up as your age does.

First-time moms over age 40 are twice as likely to have a Cesarean delivery compared to first-time moms under age 30. Here are the percentages of first-time moms who have a C-section, based on their age: *(Menacker F)*

- ◆ 47% of first-time moms over age 40
- ◆ 33% of first-time moms between 30–39
- ◆ 21% of first-time moms under age 30

HEY O-DADDY (OLDER DADDY)!

Okay guys, while you mostly hear about moms being older during pregnancy and the potential risks, you are not off the hook. For you, it's called Advanced Paternal Age (APA). Dads who are over the age of 40 at conception, have kids with a greater risk of *autism spectrum disorders* (almost six times the risk) and *Marfan syndrome* (as well as other autosomal dominant chromosome mutations).

There may also be a slightly increased risk of certain types of childhood leukemias and brain/spinal cord cancer in kids whose dads are older. There's a reason that the American Society of Reproductive Medicine recommends sperm donors be under age 40 (besides the fact that it's easier for younger guys to produce a specimen!).

Bottom line: your sperm are not getting any younger. If you compare a 30 year old to a 50 year old, older guys have fewer sperm, the sperm move around less and almost one in five sperm are abnormal. Older men lack antioxidant enzymes and that makes sperm more susceptible to mutations. *(Bianco A, Sartorelli EM.)*

If you are a father-to-be who is 50 or older, there is a greater risk of miscarriage or later fetal loss during pregnancy. The good news is that most babies born to more mature daddies are very healthy. Just ask Larry King or Woody Allen. *(Nybo AM)*

advanced maternal age

ADVANCED AGE

? ?

BOTTOM LINE. Ok, we realize some of this sounds quite depressing. But remember the vast majority of moms over 35 give birth to babies who are just fine. And thanks to modern medical science, many of the risks and concerns can be minimized or eliminated. So, do your best to have a positive outlook. The odds are in your favor!

Next up: all you need to know if you go into preterm labor.

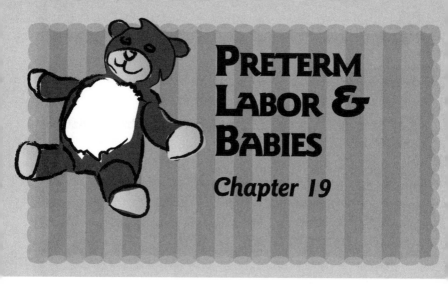

PRETERM LABOR & BABIES

Chapter 19

WHAT'S IN THIS CHAPTER

- ◆ HOW WILL I KNOW IF I AM IN PRETERM LABOR?
- ◆ WELCOME TO THE NICU
- ◆ BABIES BORN LESS THAN 34 WEEKS
- ◆ LATE PRETERM INFANTS

"Some babies are born in nine months, by the clock. Some babies are born, and they sit up and talk. Some babies are born, and no doctor is there. But some babies come in on a wing and a prayer."
—*Garrison Keillor*

No one is really prepared to have a baby *before* nine months of pregnancy, but it happens in about one in ten pregnancies. So this is reality. Think of this chapter as another one of those "this wasn't in the game plan" discussions.

Thanks to medical advances, practitioners can stall many preterm labors long enough to make delivery safer for the baby. Modern medicine has also come a long way in improving both the short- and long-term outcomes of babies who make a crash landing arrival.

This chapter will get you through the shock and awe of discovering you are delivering before you've had time to paint the nursery. It will answer the obvious questions swirling around in your head. Am I actually going to deliver this baby now? How long will my baby stay in the hospital? How sick will my baby be? What lies ahead for our family? This chapter, above all others, demonstrates why it's nice to have both an OB and a pediatrician here to help you with your pregnancy!

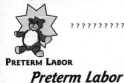

? ?

PRETERM LABOR

Preterm Labor

Q. How will I know if I am in preterm labor? What are the signs?

The signs of preterm labor often mimic the signs of full-term labor, only they happen before you have reached 37 weeks of pregnancy.

These symptoms include: *(ACOG)*

◆ Dull ache in your lower back.

◆ Episodes of hardening or tightening in the lower part of your belly that last 30 to 60 seconds.

◆ Menstrual-like cramping that either comes and goes or is constant.

◆ Increase in vaginal discharge (which may be blood-tinged).

◆ Feeling of pressure in your pelvis.

◆ Feeling like you need to pee or poop but nothing is coming out.

You may have any or all of these symptoms. If something seems awry, get it checked out.

Insider Secret
Be specific. Tell your practitioner exactly what you are feeling so she has a better idea of what is going on with your body. This is serious—it may save your baby.

Q. What causes preterm labor?

There are many possible causes of preterm labor.

These include bleeding within the uterus (**SUBCHORIONIC HEMORRHAGE** or **PLACENTAL ABRUPTION**), an over-distended uterus (**POLYHYDRAMNIOS** or multiple babies), bacterial infections and hormonal changes (possibly caused by fetal or maternal stress).

But often, docs can't find a reason for why a woman goes into preterm labor.

Reality Check
Premature births in the U.S. are on the rise. In 2007, 12.7% of all births were babies born before 37 weeks gestation. That's more than 500,000 live births a year. The price tag for their health care is $26 billion per year. *(Behrman RE.)*

Q. My first baby was born prematurely. What are the odds it will happen with this pregnancy?

Your risk is six to eight times greater than a woman who has never had a premature delivery. Your practitioner should keep a close eye on you!

Q. Is there any way to predict if I am at risk for going into preterm labor?

There are a few things that may put you at risk:

◆ Younger than 17 years of age.

- Older than 40 years of age.
- If you weighed less than 110 lbs. before becoming pregnant.
- Previous preterm birth.
- Pregnant with multiples.
- If you have a shortened cervix (your doctor can tell you that).
- Vaginal bleeding at any point during pregnancy.
- High blood pressure and protein in urine (**PREECLAMPSIA**).
- African-American.

As you can see by this list, most factors are out of your control.

Q. If I am at risk, is there anything to do to prevent preterm labor?

Short answer: some things (beyond praying) *may* help prevent labor.

Your practitioner may recommend **BED REST** (reclining and relaxing all day), **PELVIC REST** (no sex, tampons or douching), and having weekly visits with your doc.

Those extra visits will include frequent ultrasound measurements of your cervix until about 32 weeks. The shorter your cervix is before 32 weeks, the higher your risk of delivering early. After 32 weeks, your practitioner will measure it by doing regular vaginal exams. You may also have the **fFN TEST** (see Chapter 5, Tests) and will likely get screened for specific vaginal infections. In some situations, your practitioner may treat you with progesterone supplementation (see box below).

Q. What does bed rest really mean?

Yes, it means what is says!

If your doctor meant for you to be doing the laundry or shopping for groceries, it would not be called bed rest. Now, your doc may give you

---

USING PROGESTERONE TO PREVENT PRETERM BIRTH

It's a hot topic in OB circles: using progesterone to help prevent preterm birth.

A ground breaking 2003 study by the National Institutes of Health on this issue found progesterone significantly protected high-risk women against preterm birth. Since then, a number of other studies have confirmed this finding.

As a result, the American Congress of Obstetricians and Gynecologists now recommends it. Here is their official statement: "Progesterone supplementation for the prevention of recurrent preterm birth should be offered to women with a singleton pregnancy (only one baby in the uterus) and a prior spontaneous preterm birth due to spontaneous preterm labor or premature rupture of membranes. Current evidence does not support the routine use of progesterone in women with multiple gestations."

Translation: talk to your practitioner about progesterone supplements if you have delivered a preterm baby or had premature rupture of membranes in a previous pregnancy and delivered early. *(ACOG)*

some "get out of bed" passes here and there. But in general, you need to hang out in bed or on the couch.

This gives your cervix a break from the weight of your uterus, lowers your blood pressure, and forces you to rest. All these things can help your pregnancy progress a bit further and give your baby more time to mature.

Q. Is there a way to stop preterm labor once it starts?

Yes, but it depends on the individual situation.

The good news is that 80% of women who have signs and symptoms of preterm labor will *not* have a preterm delivery. Part of this depends on whether or not your practitioner identifies a treatable cause of preterm labor. It also depends on if you have any other complications with your pregnancy.

For example, if a woman comes into the hospital at 28 weeks with contractions occurring every five minutes and a cervix that is dilated to two centimeters, there is a good chance her labor may be stopped.

But suppose that same women comes into the hospital at 28 weeks, with contractions every five minutes, her cervix is five cm. dilated *and* she has moderate vaginal bleeding due to a placental abruption. In the latter case, it is likely that her labor will not stop. It is also likely that her OB will not try to stop her labor because it is safer for the fetus to deliver a little early than to remain in the uterus.

The point is—there are many variables that determine whose preterm labor gets treated and whose doesn't.

If your doctor decides to try to stop your preterm labor, she has a few medication choices. There is no clear "first-line drug" when it comes to treating preterm labor and your doctor will take many variables into account before selecting one to use. Below is a list of medications that are used to help treat preterm labor and some of their side effects:

Medications that can treat preterm labor *(Haerne AE.)*

MEDICATION TYPE	BRAND NAME	POSSIBLE MATERNAL SIDE EFFECTS
Beta-mimetic	Terbutaline	Fast heart rate, irregular heart rhythm, low blood pressure, fluid in lungs, an overall "jittery" feeling
Magnesium Sulfate		Flushing, lethargy, headache, double vision, dry mouth, fluid in lungs, heart failure (cardiac arrest)
Calcium channel blocker	Nifedipine	Flushing, headache, dizziness, nausea, low blood pressure
Prostaglandin Synthetase Inhibitors	Indomethacin Ketorolac Sulindac	Nausea, heartburn possible upset stomach/gastritis upset stomach

Factoid: A recent study showed that using intravenous (IV) magnesium sulfate to help stop preterm labor also reduces the chance that a preterm baby will have moderate or severe cerebral palsy. It is now standard treatment at many hospitals. *(Rouse DJ)*

Q. Do these medications work?

Yes, medication works for a *short* time. But this time is important time.

Most studies show that medication used to stop contractions (**TOCOLYT-ICS**) prolongs pregnancy for up to seven days. Is seven days really worth it? YES! Although that sounds like no time at all (particularly if you go into preterm labor at 27 weeks), seven days may buy enough time to prepare for a preterm delivery.

The biggest advantage is that you'll be able to take medication to help mature the fetus' lungs, brain and intestines. The medication is a steroid, usually given in two or four doses over a 24 to 48 hour period. It will also allow time for you to get a quick course in the consequences of having a premature baby with your OB, a perinatologist, and likely a neonatologist.

Besides medication, you will go on bed rest, have your contractions monitored, get tons of fluid either by mouth or IV, and stay in the hospital for close surveillance.

Q. Will I be able to go home or will I need to stay at the hospital?

If you are in preterm labor (regular uterine contractions with cervical dilation), you will most likely be admitted to the hospital. Your obstetrician and perinatologist will work together and develop a plan for the length of your stay, since that depends on many factors.

Premature Rupture of Membranes (PROM)

A few definitions first:
- *ROM* = Rupture of Membranes means your water bag breaks.
- *PROM* = Premature Rupture of Membranes means rupture of membranes occurs before labor begins.
- *PPROM* = Preterm Premature Rupture of Membranes means rupture of membranes occurs at less than 37 weeks gestation.

Reality Check

If you rupture your membranes prematurely (PPROM), you have a 60% to 70% chance of going into labor on your own and delivering within a week. It is rare for the fluid to stop leaking and for the pregnancy to continue. That's because up to 60% of women with PPROM develop an infection of the amniotic sac (**CHORIOAMNIONITIS**).

When the bag breaks, there is no longer a sterile protective barrier that keeps vaginal bacteria out of the uterus. This makes it easy for bacteria to enter the amniotic sac and uterus.

In fact, practitioners recommend immediate delivery if there is an obvious infection in the uterus (maternal fever, elevated maternal white blood cell count, foul-smelling amniotic fluid, rapid maternal heart rate, rapid fetal heart rate, non-reassuring fetal heart rate).

Q. I'm 30 weeks. My water broke but I'm NOT having contractions. What happens now?

In general, here is the step-by-step plan:

1. Your practitioner confirms you have broken your water bag (PPROM).
2. You get admitted to the hospital.
3. You are monitored to check your contraction pattern (or hopefully lack of one) as well as your baby's heart rate pattern.
4. You will get IV fluids for hydration.
5. You will get antibiotics to help prevent infection.
6. You will most likely get medication to stop contractions (if present).
7. You will get steroids (if indicated).
8. Then, we watch and wait.

If it looks like your baby is in trouble, your practitioner will recommend that you proceed to delivery. It's more likely you will have a C-section because fetuses born prematurely are often not in the head down position yet and there is also a higher risk of fetal distress, which will make your OB want your baby out sooner rather than later.

Q. Why does my doctor want to give me steroids? Will they help my baby?

Yes—if you are delivering between 24 and 34 weeks.

Steroids, formally known as *corticosteroids*, are a family of drugs that have a variety of therapeutic uses. (These steroids are very different than what some professional athletes use, by the way.)

If a preterm delivery is imminent, steroids are *the* single most beneficial thing your doctor can do for your baby.

Steroids cross the placenta and enter into the baby's system. They trigger the cells in the fetus' lungs, brain and intestines to mature. And when a baby is born prematurely, we worry most about these organs. Here are the concerns:

◆ Immature lungs cannot expand properly to hold air (**RESPIRATORY DISTRESS SYNDROME**).

◆ Immature brain has fragile blood vessels that bleed easily (**INTRAVENTRICULAR HEMORRHAGE**).

◆ Immature intestines have poor blood supply that can lead to injury and death of the tissues (**NECROTIZING ENTEROCOLITIS**).

Giving mom a dose of steroids (preferably within seven days of delivery) may help these organs mature and prevent these major complications of preterm babies. In short, steroids lower the risk of your preterm baby dying. The goal here is to get either two or four doses (depending on the type of steroid) before delivery.

Reality Check

More is not better. Depending on which steroid is used, women in preterm labor need just two or four doses before delivery. Giving multiple doses does not improve a baby's health outcome and can even lead to an increased risk of a newborn infection.

However, a "booster" dose of steroids may be given four to six weeks after the first course if you're still pregnant, still under 34 weeks, and still at increased risk of early delivery. The two-dose regimen has not been shown to increase any risk of fetal or newborn infection.

? ?

PRETERM LABOR

Q. My friend broke her bag at 32 weeks and her doctor gave her steroids. I am 35 weeks and just broke my bag. Why won't my doctor give them to me?

Steroids are most useful between 24 to 34 weeks.

If you are over 34 weeks, research shows there is no significant benefit. *(ACOG)* In most cases of PPROM, there is a "stressful event" like placental bleeding or infection that triggers the water bag to break. When there is stress, your fetus releases her own stress hormones (adrenaline), which accelerate lung, brain, and intestine maturation . . . just like the steroids.

And FYI, there is a gray zone (medicine is rarely black or white) between 32-34 weeks. Some experts recommend giving steroids to women with PPROM who fall in this category and others do not.

Q. I'm 30 weeks. My water broke and I am having contractions. What happens now?

It really depends on your particular situation.

Your doctor will look at your medical history, current vital signs and lab work, physical exam, and the health of the fetus (by fetal monitoring).

If you are in active labor and your cervix is five to six cm. dilated, medications will probably not help and you will be delivering a baby today. You will get IV antibiotics to protect the baby from infection.

But if you are in early labor and you have no other complications other than a broken water bag, your doctor may give you medication to stop labor.

Q. What caused my water bag to break so early?

There are many possible causes.

They include premature contractions, infection, second and third trimester bleeding, nutritional deficiency, smoking, an overdistended uterus (**POLYHY-DRAMNIOS**, multiple fetuses), having prior cervical surgery (LEEPs, cervical conization, cerclage), severe lung disease, or a history of amniocentesis.

In many cases, however, docs never identify a clear risk factor.

Factoid: If your water bag broke before 37 weeks with your first pregnancy, the risk of having it happen in any subsequent pregnancy is between 16% and 32%.

Q. What is the youngest age that a fetus can survive outside the womb?

Wow. This is a tough question. Experts look at both the baby's gestational age and their birth weight to determine this answer.

Babies under 26 weeks and those weighing less than 1.5 lbs. (750 grams) may survive outside the womb, but are likely to have some degree of lifelong health and/or neurological issues.

So it's not just about survival—it's about quality of life as well. And babies born before 24 weeks gestation have a very slim chance of survival.

Here are some stats to consider:

- ◆ Babies born at 23 weeks gestation have a 30% chance of survival.
- ◆ Babies born at 25 weeks gestation have a 75% chance of survival.

preterm labor

Survival rates by birthweight

Courtesy of Elsevier

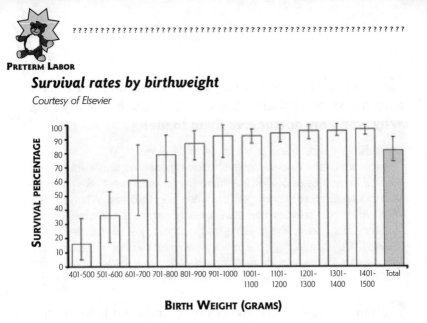

BIRTH WEIGHT (GRAMS)

- ◆ Babies born weighing one pound (400 to 500 grams) have an 11% survival rate.
- ◆ Babies born weighing 1.5 to 1.75 lbs. (700 to 800 grams) have a 75% survival rate. *(AAP, ACOG)*

We'll talk about life in the neonatal intensive care unit (NICU) later in this chapter and at Expecting411.com/extra. But the reality is that very premature newborns have the most serious health complications to overcome even if they survive delivery.

Any time a woman will potentially deliver a very premature baby (21 to 25 weeks gestation), parents-to-be should have an in-depth discussion with all health care team members (OB, perinatologist, neonatologist, pediatrician). The team can go over the baby's potential health outcome based on the age, estimated weight, and gender of the fetus.

When it comes to extremely preterm and low-birth weight babies, there will be a discussion on whether or not to perform rescue procedures on the baby (neonatal resuscitation). Example: a 0.8 lb. (400 gram) fetus at 22 weeks gestation has an extremely poor chance of survival. Many parents choose to avoid intervention. Other parents want providers to take all measures to aid survival.

If you are faced with this scenario, gather all the facts and ask questions to feel satisfied that you are making an informed decision. *(ACOG)*

Reality Check

Premature baby girls are stronger than baby boys. They have lower mortality rates as well as a lower risk of cerebral palsy.

Q. My doctor cannot stop my labor. Once the baby is born, will my baby be able to room in with me?

It depends on the maturity of the baby.

Usually babies beyond 35 to 36 weeks can stay with mom if they know how to breathe, eat, maintain their body temperature and do not have any risk of infection.

Some babies born between 34 to 36 weeks are observed in the NICU for 24 to 48 hours and then return to their mother's hospital room for the remainder of the stay.

Babies born even earlier than 34 weeks will stay in the NICU long after you have been discharged.

Q. What happens during/after delivery?

When delivery is imminent, the neonatal care team (neonatologist/neonatal nurse practitioner and neonatal nurse) arrives in your delivery suite or operating room. Your OB will hand your baby immediately over to them for care.

The first priorities for the team are to make sure your baby is breathing and his heart is beating. The team will perform CPR (cardiopulmonary resuscitation) and give medications, if necessary.

If your baby is very preterm, the team will place a tube into his throat to breathe for him, give him oxygen, and administer a medication (**SURFACTANT**) that helps keep the tiny air sacs in the lungs open.

The team will also dry your baby off and warm him up under a radiant warming exam table.

Once your baby is stabilized, you will be able to take a quick peek at him. But if your baby is ill, he will need to head to the NICU fairly quickly. You will get to visit with him (assuming the NICU is at your hospital) a few hours after delivery.

If you've had a C-section, though, you'll need to wait until at least the next day to visit in person. Make sure someone has a digital camera (or a good phone camera) to take some initial shots of your baby so that you don't actually have to wait an entire day to see him.

Neonatal Intensive Care Unit 411

Having your baby whisked away to the Neonatal Intensive Care Unit (NICU) is a scary, surreal experience that often follows a whirlwind, unexpected delivery. But once you get used to the place and your baby's amazing healthcare team, it becomes more familiar and less terrifying. At Expecting411.com/extra, we will go over the details of who cares for your baby, where you will stay, when you can visit the NICU and nurse your baby, what the typical health/growth/development issues are for premature babies, and, of course—when you will be able to take your baby home! We know you have a lot questions and concerns.

Late Preterm Infants (Babies born 34 to under 37 weeks)

Q. What is a late preterm infant?

Babies born between 34 weeks and under 37 weeks are considered premature, and get the designation "late preterm infant." Late preterm infants account for 70% of all preemies. They are the reason for the surge in prematurity rates in the past ten years.

The good news is that late preterm infants usually do not encounter the

preterm labor

major health complications that younger preemies do. But they still deserve special treatment. They are different than their full-term friends.

Q. Will my baby need to stay in the NICU?

Your baby will likely be cared for in the NICU if you deliver at 34 to 35 weeks. If you deliver in the 36th week, your baby may be able to room in with you and be cared for by your pediatrician and the nursery staff. But the medical staff will watch your baby to be sure he remembers to breathe, knows how to eat well enough to maintain a normal blood sugar, and can maintain his body temperature.

Check out Expecting411.com/extra for the health and growth issues that late preterm infants typically experience.

Q. My baby is a late preterm infant. Is there anything special I need to look out for?

Yes. Here is a list of his unique issues:

◆ *Neurologic:* About one-third of a baby's brain volume grows in the last eight weeks of gestation, so it's no surprise that your newborn is not as prepared as a full term baby to face the world. He'll probably be very sleepy and you'll need to awaken him for feedings. He may suck ineffectively, which can make feedings (especially breastfeeding) a real challenge. He may be kind of cranky, startle and have difficulty being soothed (don't get too discouraged). All of these things resolve, they just take a little time until your baby's brain and body matures.

◆ *Temperature regulation:* He may have trouble regulating his body temperature (besides having very little body fat to retain heat). Swaddle your baby with two or three receiving blankets and have him wear a hat for those first days after birth.

PREEMIE LINGO

Your baby's category based on his gestational age:

Late preterm:	34 to under 36 6/7 weeks gestation
Very preterm:	Under 32 weeks gestation
Extremely preterm:	At or below 25 weeks gestation

Your baby's category based on his birth weight:

Low birth weight (LBW):	Birth weight less than 2500 g (less than 5.5 lbs.)
Very low birth weight (VLBW):	Birth weight less than 1500 g (less than 3.3 lbs.)
Extremely low birth weight (ELBW):	Birth weight less than 1000 g (less than 2.2 lbs.)
"Micropreemies"	Birth weight less than 800 g (less than 1.8 lbs.)

◆ **Respiratory:** Your baby is being born around the time his lungs are maturing. If your baby is younger (34 to 35 weeks), he may have trouble breathing and need temporary breathing support. Due to neurologic immaturity, your baby is also at risk for **APNEA OF PREMATURITY** (forgetting to breathe)—see the section NICU ABC's online at Expecting411.com/extra.

◆ **Infectious Diseases:** Any preterm baby has a risk of a bloodstream infection (**SEPSIS**). Your baby may have lab work and other tests to rule it out.

◆ **Gastrointestinal:** Your baby will be a pokey eater in the beginning and so he won't poop very much. This, and an immature liver, make your baby more at risk of developing **JAUNDICE** than his full-term peers. And while term newborns may be jaundiced for the first four to five days of life, late preterm infants may have jaundice issues for the first five to seven days.

◆ **Growth/Nutrition:** Late preterm infants are difficult feeders. They are sleepy. They don't wake up on their own for feedings. They tire easily and fall asleep feeding. And their sucking ability, to put it bluntly, sucks.

So your baby is at risk for excessive weight loss/poor weight gain, which then leads to dehydration. To complicate matters even further, your baby is also at risk for low blood sugar in the first 24 hours of life—which would prevent just about anyone from having the energy to eat. Many late preterm infants need formula or expressed breast milk while they mature and learn to breastfeed. Supplements help reduce weight loss and give babies energy to learn to nurse.

Check out our companion book, *Baby 411*, for many tips on feeding a late preterm infant. See the back of this book for more info.

Reality Check
Take extra care when holding your newborn upright, as he has very poor head control and can collapse his airway.

Q. Will I be able to take my late preterm baby home when I am discharged from the hospital?

Maybe. It really depends on your baby's age and maturity.

And even if your pediatrician says he can leave with you, do not head out until your baby is at least 48 hours old. Here is what the American Academy of Pediatrics (AAP) says your baby needs to do to get his walking papers:

◆ Stable vital signs (body temperature, blood pressure, heart rate, and respiratory rate) for at least twelve hours before discharge.
◆ Proof he has the skill to eat by mouth (24 hours of successful feedings with coordinated sucking/swallowing/breathing).
◆ Formal breastfeeding assessment with a trained caregiver.
◆ At least one spontaneous poop.
◆ No significant dehydration.
◆ No significant jaundice.
◆ Follow-up planned with pediatrician in 24 to 48 hours.

The AAP developed these guidelines to decrease hospital readmissions in the first two weeks of life for dehydration, severe jaundice, lack of breathing (apnea), and infections. *(AAP, Hubbard E.)*

BOTTOM LINE: Even with late preterm infants, watch for developmental delays and subtle learning problems later in life.

Feedback from the Real World: Find a support network

Here are some specific tips to get through your NICU experience (and beyond) from seasoned parents of preemies:

◆ Become your child's advocate.
◆ Take breaks from the unit when you can.
◆ Rest when you can.
◆ Read to your child in a soft voice.
◆ Make relationships with other parents with children in the NICU.
◆ Learn the medications and orders written for your child.
◆ Trust the advice of your doctors, but don't be afraid to ask questions.
◆ Listen to advice from nurses. Nurses have lots of interaction with your baby and can be a huge asset during extensive stays in the hospital.
◆ Ask for help when you get home.
◆ Avoid public places during RSV season (October to April), especially the child's first season. (RSV is a respiratory virus that can cause serious breathing problems in former preterm babies.)
◆ Make sure to ask lots of questions and get well educated on your own.
◆ Be prepared to feel helpless and wonder if the staff is giving your baby the best care possible.
◆ Be with your baby as much as possible (both parents).
◆ Partners need to support each other. This is a critical time in your lives.
◆ Keep in mind how resilient babies are.
◆ Be clean, clean, clean–infections and the NICU don't mix.
◆ Be involved as much as possible – help the nurses with daily tasks.
◆ If your baby is born under two pounds, you can sign him up for Supplemental Security Income (SSI). This is a federal income support program. Go to ssa.gov/ssi/ for details.
◆ Keep your own medical records. You may need them for future reference.
◆ Keep an open dialogue with case managers and doctors and take notes to help you remember. The intensity of the situation makes it difficult to remember details of conversations.
◆ Don't ever give up.

Special thanks for these tips to Kelli Kelley, mom of two preemies and founder of the organization, A Hand to Hold.

Because preemies and multiple births often go together, we'll chat about twins, triplets, and more (oh my!) next.

MULTIPLES

Chapter 20

"When I have a kid, I want to put him in one of those strollers for twins, then run around the mall looking frantic."
—Steven Wright

Most pregnant couples reading this book are nervous about the prospect of caring for one newborn. Those parents have no idea how easy they have it.

You, however, have hit the daily double (or triple, or more). Your pregnancy will be different than your friends who are only carrying one fetus. There's more to it than getting bigger sooner or eating more than most teenage boys do.

Factoid: In the past 30 years, the number of twins born in the U.S. has risen by 65%. The number of triplets (or higher) have skyrocketed, up by 500%.

Fun Twin Facts

◆ *More twins are left-handed.* 18% to 22% of twins are left-handed compared with under 10% for non-twins.

◆ *Move over OctoMom:* The modern world record for giving birth to multiples is held by Leontina Albina from Chile, whose 55 children included three sets of triplets.

◆ *Cryptophasia:* Term for when twins develop their own "language" that only they understand.

Multiples, facts & figures

	TWINS	TRIPLETS	QUADRUPLETS
Average birth weight	2347 grams	1687	1309
Average gestational age at delivery	35.3 weeks	32.2	29.9
Percent with growth restriction	14-25%	50-60	50-60
Percent requiring admission to neonatal intensive care unit	25%	75	100
Average length of stay in neonatal intensive care unit	18 days	30	58
Percentage with major handicap	*	20	50
Risk of cerebral palsy (compared to singletons)	4 times	17	*
Risk of death by age 1 year (compared to singletons)	7 times	20	*

*Insufficient data. Source: ACOG.

Q. What's the difference between fraternal and identical twins? Does it matter?

The short answer: most twins are fraternal, which means they do not share all of their identical material. They are siblings with the same birthdays. Identical twins have exactly the same genetic material. The long answer: bear with us, this gets confusing.

Fraternal Twins (Dizygotic or DZ):

◆ Mom has two separate eggs (instead of just one) in her cycle and each egg gets fertilized by an individual sperm. In short: two eggs, two sperm.
◆ Two-thirds of all twins are fraternal.
◆ The babies do not share all of their genetic material. They are siblings with the same birthdays.
◆ The babies can be the same or different sex.
◆ They are "dizygotic" which means they are from two ("di") fertilized eggs ("zygotes"). With two fertilized eggs, there are always two placentas, two inner fetal membranes (amnion), and two outer fetal membranes (chorion). Technically, that's called **DIAMNIOTIC/DICHORIONIC** placentas.
◆ Women who used fertility medications that stimulate ovulation, in vitro fertilization, or embryo transfer are more prone to having fraternal twins.
◆ Women over 35 also have more fraternal twins.

Identical Twins (Monozygotic or MZ):

◆ Mom has one egg that gets fertilized by one sperm. But the fertilized egg spontaneously divides into two separate embryos. In short: one egg, one sperm, plus one extra split.
◆ Only one-third of all twins are identical.
◆ The babies have exactly the same genetic material.
◆ The babies must be the same sex.
◆ The placenta and fetal membranes of identical twins vary, depending on when that extra split occurs after fertilization. So identical twins can be:

MULTIPLES

1. DIAMNIOTIC, DICHORIONIC = 2 placentas, 2 amnions, 2 chorions.
2. DIAMNIOTIC, MONOCHORIONIC = 1 placenta, 1 chorion, 2 amnions (2 sacs).
3. MONOAMNIOTIC, MONOCHORIONIC = 1 placenta, 1 chorion, 1 amnion
(both babies are in the same sac—the rarest and most dangerous).

◆ Why do docs care about identical twins' fetal membranes? Identical
twins with just one chorion and amnion have more health risks and need
to be followed more closely.
◆ Identical twins have more birth defects (neural tube defects, abdominal
wall defects, urinary tract abnormalities).
◆ Identical monoamniotic-monochorionic twins may be mirror images.
One may be right handed and the other left handed. Or hair whorls
may go in exact opposite directions. They also have nearly identical
brain wave patterns on EEG.

Reality Check
Male and female twins are ALWAYS fraternal. They cannot be
identical because, clearly, they have different genetic material
when it comes to their plumbing!

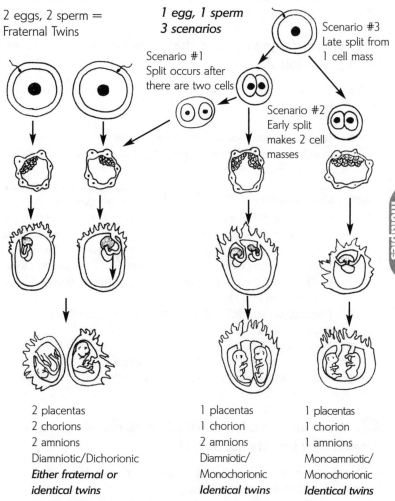

Dizygotic (DZ)	Monozygotic (MZ)	

Dizygotic (DZ)

2 eggs, 2 sperm =
Fraternal Twins

Monozygotic (MZ)

*1 egg, 1 sperm
3 scenarios*

Scenario #3
Late split from
1 cell mass

Scenario #1
Split occurs after
there are two cells

Scenario #2
Early split
makes 2 cell
masses

2 placentas	1 placentas	1 placentas
2 chorions	1 chorion	1 chorion
2 amnions	2 amnions	1 amnions
Diamniotic/Dichorionic	Diamniotic/	Monoamniotic/
	Monochorionic	Monochorionic
Either fraternal or	*Identical twins*	*Identical twins*
identical twins		

multiples

Reality Check

Your practitioner can usually figure out what type of twins you are having by ultrasound or at delivery. But if your same-sex twins have two placentas, two amnions, and two chorions (**DIAMNIOTIC/DICHORIONIC**), they can be either fraternal or identical. You can have the babies' DNA tested after birth to figure it out.

How'd this happen to me?

Q. Twins run in my family. What are the odds that I will have twins?

Identical twins happen randomly and do not run in families. *Fraternal* twins can be hereditary—but only if they run in the mother-to-be's family.

In the general population, the chance of having twins is between one in 80 to one in 250. Triplets occur by chance in one out of every 8000 pregnancies. But if you yourself are a fraternal twin, your chance of having twins goes up to one in 60. If fraternal twins run in your family, your chances increase as well. But the hereditary factor only pertains to a *woman's* family history. It doesn't matter if your husband has two sets of aunts who are twins and four sets of twin cousins once removed!

Q. Is there anything else that increases my chance of having multiples?

Other than assisted reproductive technology, here are the other factors that come into play:

◆ *Advanced maternal age.* Yes, older woman do have one advantage here—more hormones (specifically, follicle stimulating hormone or FSH)! FSH makes our eggs ripen and motivates the ovaries to work. As we age and our ovarian function declines, FSH levels rise to stimulate the ovaries. Extra FSH may cause more than one egg to be released per menstrual cycle, resulting in twins if both eggs are fertilized. Although women over the age of 35 are less likely to get pregnant in a menstrual cycle, they are more likely to have twins.

◆ *Race.* Your chances are greater if you are of African descent (one in 70). Your chances are lower if you are Japanese (one in 150) or Chinese (one in 300).

◆ *Previous pregnancies.* Your chances are greater if this is not your first pregnancy.

◆ *Previous pregnancy with twins.* Chances increase if you have already been pregnant with fraternal twins.

◆ *Taller women.* Women who are taller with a larger body frame have more twins.

Q. What are the odds of having multiples if I have been treated by a fertility specialist?

It really depends on what kind of treatment you have. Here is a general break down for having *fraternal* twins:

? ?

MULTIPLES

◆ Clomiphene citrate (Clomid) alone: 3% to 8% chance of multiples.
◆ Injectable ovulation induction medications (gonadotropins): 20%.
◆ In vitro fertilization (IVF): 20% to 40%—depending on how many embryos are transferred into your uterus.

But guess what? You also have better odds of *identical* (monochorionic) twins, too. The rate is about 3% to 5%, compared to a rate of 0.4% in the general population.

How does this happen? Example: you have two embryos placed into the uterus via IVF—but one decides to split— now you have three fetuses (one fraternal sibling, and two identical twins!). This little phenomenon is how some fertility patients end up with multiples beyond twins (higher order multiples). It also increases the complications.

Q. How early in my pregnancy will I know if I am carrying twins?

Docs can diagnose twins between six to ten weeks by ultrasound. If your practitioner doesn't do an ultrasound, she may still pick it up in the first trimester when the size of your uterus is larger than your dates. Then, she will refer you to have an ultrasound to confirm her suspicions.

What do I need to know?

Q. Why is carrying multiple babies considered a high-risk pregnancy?

Short answer: more babies = more pregnancy complications = more preterm deliveries.

Just about every pregnancy complication you hear about happens more often in women who are carrying multiples. That includes: **PREECLAMPSIA**, anemia, gestational diabetes, acute fatty liver, gallstones, blood clots, kidney infections, skin problems, premature rupture of membranes, preterm labor, and excessive bleeding after delivery. Whew! Yes, that is a long list. See Chapter 16, Complications, for details.

And babies who are born prematurely also have their unique set of issues (detailed in Chapter 19, Preterm Labor).

Fun, eh? Believe it or not, most women carrying multiples have healthy pregnancies and healthy babies. But we point these facts out to you to make you realize you have a special pregnancy that requires closer observation on your part and your doctor's.

Q. Are there any special tests or additional prenatal visits because I am carrying twins?

Yes. You visit your doctor more often, you get more tests, and you meet more doctors. Enter the perinatologist or maternal/fetal medicine specialist—a doctor who is a high-risk obstetric specialist.

Your doctor will watch for pregnancy complications and signs of preterm labor. It's also wise to have a perinatologist who will work with your obstetrician to ensure that any medical issues are identified early.

For the first 24 weeks, you will likely have the same number of office visits as your friends who are only carrying one baby. But from 22 to 28 weeks, you get to visit your OB or perinatologist every other week (as opposed to once a month).

Starting at 32 weeks, you will see your OB or perinatologist every week. If any complications arise, you may have even more appointments!

And yes, you get to do more tests. Here is what lies ahead:

1 MORE ULTRASOUND EXAMS. (Sorry, but many are with a vaginal probe). This allows docs to measure the length of your cervix to help identify your risk of preterm labor. You may also have regular ultrasounds every three to four weeks starting around 24 weeks to assess the growth of your babies and to look for other potential problems.

2 FETAL FIBRONECTIN TEST. Women at risk for preterm labor have higher than normal levels of fetal fibronectin. If it looks like you are at risk, your practitioner will likely do this test.

3 NON-STRESS TESTS. You will probably have these on a weekly basis starting at some point in your third trimester. Identical twins with one placenta and one sac are tested the earliest and the most often.

For a full discussion of these tests, see Chapter 5, Tests.

Q. Do pregnant moms of multiples have more morning sickness? I feel awful!

Yes! The more babies you carry, the more morning sickness you will have.

Morning sickness seems to be linked to elevated amounts of two hormones: beta-hCG and progesterone. When you are carrying multiple babies, your body makes more of these hormones. So, it's no surprise that you may have more "all-day" sickness. You are also at greater risk of having **HYPEREMESIS GRAVIDARUM.**

Q. Will I need to go on bed rest, stop working, exercising, or having sex any earlier in my pregnancy because I'm carrying multiples?

While most obstetricians and perinatologists will restrict certain activities for a multiples mom-to-be, there is very little scientific data to prove that these restrictions work.

Based on the precautionary principle alone, your doctor may recommend that you go on bed rest, restrict your activity, and go on pelvic rest. Yes, it may be horrible for your mental state. But think of it this way: it just might help your babies stay in your incubator for as long as possible.

Q. Am I going to gain more weight since I am carrying more than one baby?

Definitely. But take a cup-half-full view: you will also lose more after you deliver.

As a general rule, women carrying one baby should eat about 300

MULTIPLES

extra calories a day. A woman carrying twins should eat about 600 extra calories a day.

The Institute of Medicine's guidelines (based on pre-pregnancy weights) have special recommendations for moms-to-be of twins: *(Rasmussen KM.)*

DR B'S OPINION

"With multiples, the bigger your babies are at birth, the healthier they will be. Do what you need to do to give your babies the best shot!"

◆ A woman with a normal body mass index (BMI) before pregnancy should gain 37 to 54 lbs with a twins pregnancy.

◆ A woman who is overweight before pregnancy should gain 31 to 50 lbs.

◆ A woman who is obese before pregnancy should gain 25 to 42 lbs.

If you are carrying triplets, expect to gain 50 to 60 lbs. And you wild and crazy moms carrying quadruplets should gain up to 65 lbs.

Here is a key point: It's not only how much you gain, but when you gain it. You want to gain most of your weight in the first 28 weeks of your pregnancy. This is particularly important for women who were underweight before their pregnancy began. One of the leading research groups on pregnancy weight gain and newborn twins suggests the following "optimal" weight gain goals:

Weight gain goals in pounds per week *(Luke B.)*

(Based on your pre-pregnancy Body Mass Index or BMI)

PRE-PREGNANCY BMI	0-20 WEEKS	20-28 WEEKS	28 WEEKS TO DELIVERY
Underweight	1.25-1.75 lbs/wk	1.5-1.75 lbs/wk	1.25 lbs/wk
Normal	1-1.5	1.25-1.75	1
Overweight	1-1.25	1-1.5 1	1
Obese	0.75-1	0.75-1.25	0.75

We suggest you discuss your own personal weight gain goals with your obstetrician and perinatologist. One of the challenges: you may have already gained five to 12 lbs. from fertility medications if you conceived using one of many assisted reproductive technologies (IUI, IVF).

Your practitioner will keep an eye on everything and let you know if you are too far ahead or too far behind on the weight curve.

multiples

Q. I have twins and have been having a few contractions. My doctor wants to give me steroids. Why?

We go over this in detail in Chapter 19, Preterm Labor. But the bottom line is this: steroids help mature your babies' lungs, brains, and guts if they are born prematurely. They are the most beneficial if you get treated within seven days of delivery.

Q. Is it more likely that I will have premature babies?

Yes. 17% of all preterm births (occurring before 37 weeks) are from multiples. They account for 23% of all early preterm births (those that occur before 32 weeks). Here are the American statistics on deliveries: *(Hamilton BE.)*

◆ Twins deliver on average at 35 weeks.
◆ Triplets deliver on average at 32 weeks.

Insider Secret
Since you may deliver early, take your childbirth classes and hospital tour in your second trimester.

Q. Will my babies have any more health risks?

If you have identical twins with one placenta, they are at risk for something called **TWIN-TWIN TRANSFUSION SYNDROME** (see next question).

All types of identical twins are at slightly greater risk of birth defects including club foot, nervous system abnormalities and urinary tract abnormalities.

Even if the babies do not have major complications, many have a low birth weight or have been growth restricted (IUGR) in the womb.

Reality Check
Any set of multiples is at risk for having *discordant growth*. That means there is a greater than 20% difference in the size of the fetuses. Growth restriction happens in 14% to 25% of twins, while 50% to 60% of triplets and quads experience growth restriction.

Q. What exactly is twin-twin transfusion?

First of all, this only happens with identical twins that share a placenta (**MONOCHORIONIC**). The blood vessel connections within the placenta allow one twin to get more blood than the other one. The "recipient" twin gets more blood from the "donor" twin. It usually occurs and is diagnosed in the second trimester. And this is one of the things that your doc is looking for with all of those ultrasounds you are getting every few weeks!

The donor twin is significantly smaller. He may be anemic, with too little

DR B'S OPINION: PICK YOUR HOSPITAL CAREFULLY!

If you are having multiples, assume your babies will be coming earlier than planned. That means there is a decent chance your babies will need a special care nursery or NICU.

Think about that when you decide where to deliver. If you deliver in a community hospital and then your babies need to be transferred to a regional care center with a NICU across town or 50 miles away, you will not get to see your babies until you are discharged from the hospital. That may be a very long two to four days.

? ?

MULTIPLES

amniotic fluid and poor growth. At birth, this twin looks kind of pale and scrawny.

The recipient twin can be really big, have too much amniotic fluid, and too many red blood cells. At birth, this twin looks really pink and healthy. (In truth, the recipient twin is more likely to run into problems with jaundice, however.)

Twin-twin transfusion can lead to premature rupture of membranes and preterm labor. In rare, severe cases, one or both fetuses can die.

There are a few treatments that can be undertaken during pregnancy if either of the fetuses is at risk. None of them are risk free, but these are among the highest-risk pregnancies docs deal with. If this happens, your doctor and perinatologist will discuss this in detail with you.

Losing a fetus

Q. I had ART (assisted reproductive technology) and had three embryos transferred. All three took and now I am carrying triplets. What are the pros and cons of "selectively reducing" the number of babies I carry?

The official term is *multifetal pregnancy reduction*. This is obviously a touchy subject for anyone. It's a medical, ethical, and emotional dilemma for all parents-to-be and their practitioner.

Here is the health concern: when you start multiplying the number of fetuses in a pregnancy, you also multiply their health risks. Higher order multiples are smaller and are born earlier. They have a lower chance of survival and potentially face lifelong impairment. And the mom-to-be has greater risks as well when she is carrying more babies. Reducing the number of fetuses may improve the health of both the mother and her surviving babies.

Multifetal pregnancy reduction is really only a consideration with higher-order pregnancies (triplets or more). It's a bit riskier when fetal reduction is done with a twins or triplets pregnancy. In fact, there is a four to six percent chance of losing all the fetuses with a triplet to twin reduction. Pregnancy reduction may also be discussed when one of the fetuses is chromosomally or structurally abnormal.

If you choose reduction, the procedure is usually done at ten to 13 weeks. The fetus selected for termination may have a genetic or structural abnormality, or it may be in a safer location to reach in the womb. The doctor injects a medication into the fetus's heart to make it stop beating. The remnants of that fetal tissue do not interfere with the surviving fetuses. *(Evans MI.)*

Factoid: The United Kingdom only allows two embryos to be transferred in a woman under 40 years of age. It's called restricted embryo transfer. The U.S. currently has no laws on the books. But after the OctoMom, this may change in the near future!

Q. I've just learned that one of the fetuses has a very serious problem. Is there a way to terminate this pregnancy without risking the health of the other twin?

This is yet another difficult decision. This process is called **SELECTIVE FETAL TERMINATION**.

The procedure is similar to a multifetal pregnancy reduction. However, the risks of this procedure are greater because most selective fetal terminations are done later in pregnancy (between 16 to 22 weeks).

It's possible to lose the entire pregnancy if the abnormal fetus is situated in a difficult place (like lying over the cervix). But it is a decision based on risks. An abnormal twin with major malformations can put the healthy twin at risk. This is a very difficult decision to make. Ask for a referral to a support group or counselor who can be a resource for you.

FYI: Did you have ART (assisted reproductive technology)? Wondering about selection reduction or fetal termination? Head over to Expecting411.com/extra to read more.

Q. What if one of the twins dies in the womb. Will the other baby be okay?

It depends on when the loss occurs and if the babies share one placenta (**MONOCHORIONIC**).

The average rate of loss of a twin or triplet fetus is about six percent. The loss rate in higher-order multiples is probably much higher. If you lose a twin or triplet in the first trimester (**VANISHING TWIN**), the other fetus/fetuses usually do just fine.

It gets riskier for the surviving fetus/fetuses if the loss occurs *after* the first trimester. If the fetal death occurs after the first trimester and you are nowhere near delivery (at 20 weeks for example), your OB will probably watch you closely and let the pregnancy continue. This is particularly true if the fetal death has nothing to do with the uterus, placenta, or medical issues with mom.

If the fetal death occurs close to term, most experts recommend immediate delivery of the remaining fetus(es) because their survival is at risk.

The highest risk is for twins that share one placenta. That's because there are almost always connections between the blood vessels in the placenta. If one twin dies, the surviving twin experiences an immediate drop in blood pressure. And blood clots can form later on that may travel from the deceased twin to the live twin. This can cause major health problems for the surviving fetus.

Delivery issues

Reality Check

If you are having twins or higher order multiples, you need to deliver at a hospital with an obstetrician for the safety of you and your babies. So toss out any visions of a home birth and a midwife for this delivery.

Q. Will I be able to deliver twins vaginally?

Yes, it is possible if a few criteria are met. If you have had a vaginal

? ?

MULTIPLES

delivery before with a previous pregnancy, you have even better odds of avoiding a C-section.

Here's how the stars have to line up to make it work:

◆ The first twin to come out (also known as the *presenting twin* or "Twin A") must be facing head down (**VERTEX**).

◆ The second twin ("Twin B") is also facing head down (**VERTEX**).

◆ Or, if the second twin ("Twin B") is *not* facing head down, the first twin must be the same size or bigger than the second twin for a safe vaginal delivery.

It's possible to deliver the second twin, even if he is breech (head comes out last) as long as the first, larger, twin has paved the way. The last thing we want to do is to end up with a second twin whose head gets stuck in the birth canal.

Rarely, if you attempt a vaginal delivery with twins, you may deliver the first twin vaginally and need a C-section for the second. That's why docs deliver all twins in an operating room, not a regular delivery room.

If your twins are breech/vertex or breech/breech, your safest option is to have a C-section from the get-go.

Reality Check
42% of twins are both head down (vertex/vertex) at delivery.

If you are having triplets (or more!), check out Expecting411.com/extra for more info on childbirth.

Q. Is there any advantage to being the first born?

Other than bragging rights when they get older, there are a few medical reasons why the first twin often does better than the second.

The second twin (Twin B) is often in an abnormal position in the uterus (**BREECH** or **TRANSVERSE**), making delivery more difficult. Delivery of the second twin, particularly if the delivery is vaginal, can be risky because there are more cases of umbilical cord prolapse, placental abruption, and breech head entrapment with the second born.

Any of these situations can cause a temporary lack of oxygen to the baby's brain. And yes, that means there is a slightly greater risk of brain injury and cerebral palsy.

Q. How long is it between the first and second (and third...) deliveries?

If you are having a C-section, the deliveries of all babies occur within seconds or minutes of each other. Your doctor delivers one baby, cuts the cord, and hands the baby to the neonatal nurse. Then, she ruptures the second amniotic sac, delivers that baby and cuts its cord (and so on...).

But if you are delivering your twins vaginally, there can be a significant delay between the first and second baby. The average time between delivery of the first twin and second twin is 17 minutes. However, the time

MULTIPLES

? ?

between delivery of the first and second twin can range from just a minute or two . . . to many hours.

Factoid: Occasionally, twins have different birth dates. Sometimes one twin is born before midnight and the second twin is born after midnight!

Q. If I go into preterm labor, is it possible to deliver one twin and keep the other one from delivering until later?

Yes, but it is rare. If one twin delivers prematurely, the second twin usually delivers within hours.

Postpartum issues

Q. Am I going to have more trouble losing my pregnancy pounds?

That depends on how much weight you have gained. Most women carrying multiples gain more weight (ten pounds on average) than women carrying only one fetus. This means that there is more weight to lose.

Here's another good reason to breastfeed: you burn even more calories when you nurse or pump for two or more babies.

Start exercising as soon as you have your doctor's blessing. Walk or hike regularly with your kids. Put one in an infant carrier (like a Baby Bjorn) and one in a stroller, or both in a double stroller. It's a great way to burn calories and you'll get to spend time together. As they get a little older, you will also get to spend time picking leaves and goldfish crackers out of your hair afterwards. An added bonus.

Q. Will I be able to breastfeed multiples?

Yes. And every ounce counts.

Breast milk is the ideal nourishment for newborns, especially for those who may be born prematurely. Don't worry if you do not have enough breast milk to feed all your babies exclusively.

Insider Tip

Multiple needy newborns multiply the stress in the household. So, it shouldn't surprise you that moms of multiples are even more likely to suffer from postpartum depression. See Chapter 14, Postpartum, for signs of postpartum depression. Get professional help if you need it!

WHEN IT DOESN'T WORK

Chapter 21

"Perhaps, they are not stars in the sky, but rather openings where our loved ones shine down to let us know they are happy."
—Eskimo legend

This is the chapter no one really wants to read. If your pregnancy is progressing smoothly, you can just skip right past it.

But if your pregnancy ends abruptly, we will walk you down this road and help you to understand what happened, what happens next, and what you need to know to make key decisions.

Miscarriage

Q. What is a miscarriage?

A miscarriage (**SPONTANEOUS ABORTION**) is the loss of a pregnancy occurring before 20 weeks. More than 80% occur within the first 12 weeks, with most of those occurring before the eighth week.

Factoid: Your risk of having a miscarriage drops significantly if you make it past 15 weeks. Only six in every 1000 pregnancies miscarry after 15 weeks.

Q. How many pregnancies end up miscarrying?

This will shock you. *Up to 30% of all known pregnancies end as miscarriages.*

This rate may be even higher than what's reported because many women miscarry without even knowing they were pregnant. For example, you might be a few days late for your period and then have a heavier than normal period, with or without more cramping. This may have been a very early miscarriage.

Q. Why do miscarriages happen?

There are many reasons.

By far the most common reason is that the embryo or fetus is chromosomally abnormal. Remember we talked about mom and dad's chromosomes lining up (23 from the egg and 23 from the sperm) back in Chapter 1. Well, sometimes an embryo gets too many or too few chromosomes during this line up. Some embryos with chromosomal abnormalities can survive life outside the womb (such as Down syndrome). Others cannot. When survival is impossible, the body often spontaneously aborts that embryo.

The older the mother, the higher the risk of having a fetus with abnormal chromosomes. Thus, your risk of having a miscarriage also goes up as your age goes up. The general risk of having a fetus with any chromosomal abnormality at age 33 is one in 208, but at age 40, the risk increases to one in 40.

Other reasons for miscarriages include:
- A medical condition that interferes with successful pregnancy (lupus, diabetes, uncontrolled thyroid disease).
- Infection.
- Substance abuse (smoking, alcohol, marijuana, cocaine and others).
- Exposure to large doses of ionizing radiation.
- Trauma.

As you can see by the list, there are a few factors that you can control to ensure a successful pregnancy. There are also quite a few that are out of your control.

Q. Why do miscarriages happen more as women get older?

Older eggs mean more risk of damage to them.

Remember that we women are born with all of our eggs. They are buried deep within the ovaries until puberty and then each month when we ovulate, one of those eggs (and occasionally two) is released.

Women never make more eggs than what we were born with and all the eggs we do have are subject to all the exposures we have had during our lifetime (such as CT scans and x-rays).

As we get older, our eggs are more likely to have been "damaged" from some exposure that has occurred in the past. This can lead to embryos with abnormal chromosomes.

Q. What are some of the warning signs that a miscarriage may occur?

- Lower abdominal pain and vaginal bleeding.
- Painful cramping occurring every five to 15 minutes.
- Brown or bright red bleeding with or without abdominal pain.
- Increased mucousy discharge with pink or red streaks.
- Passing tissue from the vagina.
- Sudden decrease in the signs of "feeling pregnant."

If you are having any of these symptoms, discuss them with your doc.

DOESN'T WORK

Q. I am six weeks pregnant and have been having a small amount of vaginal bleeding. What is the chance I will have a miscarriage?

Twenty to 30% of pregnancies have some bleeding in the early part of pregnancy (first trimester). Of the early pregnancies (less than seven weeks) that have bleeding, 50% of those will go on to have a normal pregnancy and will ultimately deliver a baby. The other 50% will end in miscarriage. As you get farther along and approach the second trimester, you are less likely to miscarry, even if bleeding occurs.

Q. Is there anything I can do to prevent a miscarriage?

Unfortunately, in most cases, the answer is no. Your practitioner will likely recommend bed rest as well as pelvic rest. This means that he is recommending that you remain fairly sedentary (reclined on your bed, a couch or a big comfy chair) until your bleeding stops. It also means that you should refrain from intercourse, using tampons, douching or putting anything in the vagina until the bleeding stops.

Q. I am eight weeks along and I just passed a few large clots of blood. What do I do?

If you are having heavy vaginal bleeding at any point in your pregnancy, you should call your practitioner (day or night).

Although there is nothing docs can do to "save" a pregnancy before **VIABILITY** (23-24 weeks), there are a few things that your practitioner will do.

First, he will decide if you need to be seen right away or if the amount of bleeding you are having can wait to be evaluated. If this occurs during daylight hours, you will probably be asked to come into the office to have a pelvic exam and an ultrasound.

While waiting to see your practitioner, make sure you rest and drink a lot of water. Being active will only increase your bleeding. If you passed tissue (and you can stomach it) bring it in for your practitioner to examine. He may decide to send it out to a lab for further testing. This is especially important if you have a loss after the first trimester or if you have a history of recurrent miscarriages.

If this occurs in the middle of the night or on a weekend, you will likely be advised to go to the emergency room or an urgent care facility if your bleeding is severe.

Q. I'm six weeks pregnant and I've been having some bleeding. My doctor just confirmed that I miscarried (a complete abortion). How long will the bleeding last?

Your bleeding will probably continue for seven to ten days, although occasionally it can last for up to 14 days. It will be heaviest at the beginning and should become lighter and less red in color near the end.

If your bleeding lasts for more than 14 days, is associated with a fever or is heavier than a heavy period, you should contact your practitioner.

when it doesn't work

Q. I just miscarried. When will I get my period again?

Your next period should come four to six weeks after your miscarriage or D&C procedure (see box below). If you had irregular periods in the past, it may take longer. If you had normal periods in the past (every 28 to 30 days) and you haven't gotten your period within six weeks, call your practitioner.

Q. What is the name of the procedure to clear out any remaining tissues?

If you need a procedure to remove tissue after a miscarriage, you will either have a "D&C" (**DILATION AND CURETTAGE,** done before 12 weeks) or a "D&E" (**DILATION AND EVACUATION,** done after 12 weeks). Which one depends on how far along you were when you miscarried. Both are surgical procedures that remove the contents of the uterus.

Q. Where is the procedure done?

Many docs will do a D&C in their office if it is in the first trimester. Others prefer surgery centers. High-risk patients may have the procedure done at a hospital.

Q. Do I need to have any tests done first?

Before you have any procedure, your doctor needs to know a few things.

She will want to do an ultrasound (if you haven't already had one) to document that your pregnancy is in fact in the uterus and not in the fallopian tube or another abnormal location (**ECTOPIC PREGNANCY**). Also, there needs to be confirmation that the pregnancy has, in fact, ended (for example, no fetal heart rate).

Your practitioner also needs to know your blood type and Rh. If you are Rh negative (see Chapter 16, Complications, Complication #14), you will need an injection, called **RHOGAM**, at the time of your procedure.

Rhogam can be given up to 72 hours after the procedure but it is best to give it at the same time. This protects you from making antibodies that could potentially cross the placenta and harm a fetus in any future pregnancy.

Q. What does the procedure involve?

The D&C procedure itself is relatively simple. You are often given oral or IV pain medication. You will lie down on your back with your feet or knees placed in stirrups. Your doctor places a speculum in your vagina (just like when you get a Pap smear). Then, she cleans the cervix with a special type of soap to make things sterile.

If your practitioner is using local anesthesia to block the nerves in your cervix, she administers it now. It pinches and burns for a few seconds, very similar to getting a shot of novocaine at your dentist's office.

She then dilates your cervix using a series of small, thin instruments. Once the cervix has been dilated, in most cases, she will insert a suction device into the uterus and turn on the machine.

I warn my patients in advance that this part is pretty loud. If you have

I HAD A MISCARRIAGE. WHAT HAPPENS NEXT?

If you miscarry before six weeks, you will most likely need some rest at home and a few ibuprofen tablets.

But most other types of miscarriages require a surgical procedure to clear out any remaining products of conception. Here are those scenarios:

◆ **INCOMPLETE ABORTION**. After about six to seven weeks, this procedure reduces pain and amount of bleeding.

◆ **MISSED ABORTION.** This procedure removes all pregnancy tissue that has not been expelled from the uterus, despite the death of the embryo/fetus.

this done in your doctor's office, you may prefer to bring an iPod so you don't hear the noise. After most of the contents of the uterus have been removed, your doc inserts another instrument to check the walls of the uterus to make sure all products of conception have been removed.

That's it. The whole thing takes about ten minutes.

If you are having a D&E, you may be asked to come into your practitioner's office the day before the procedure to have something called laminaria placed into the cervical canal. Laminaria are thin dilators that are made out of seaweed. They absorb moisture from the cervix and vagina, and slowly expand over the next 12 hours so that the cervix begins to dilate. It makes further dilatation easier during the procedure the next day.

A D&E procedure usually takes longer than ten minutes and it is performed at an outpatient surgery center or hospital while you are under general anesthesia (asleep).

Q. Will I be uncomfortable?

Most practitioners performing D&Cs will give some kind of pain medication. If you have it done at your doctor's office, you will likely get oral pain medication (Ibuprofen, Vicodin, Percocet, Valium, Ativan—in different combinations, not all at once!). There is also an injection of a local anesthetic to numb the area, just like when the dentist numbs a tooth. You should be comfortable but you won't be "put to sleep." At most, you will feel a bit of cramping like a period.

If you have the procedure done at a surgery center or hospital with an anesthesiologist present, you will have IV pain medication and possibly anesthesia (again through an IV).

If you have a D&E procedure, you are given general anesthesia because this procedure is very painful.

Q. How long will I bleed afterwards?

This depends on how far along you are when you miscarry. Early miscarriages (under eight weeks) usually have a few days of bleeding after the procedure. The bleeding trails off and usually stops completely by seven to ten days. If you are farther along when you have your D&C or D&E, you may bleed for up to two weeks.

Q. I am seven weeks and just miscarried. My doctor said I had a "missed abortion." Should I have a D&C or just wait to miscarry naturally on my own?

It depends.

Most women who miscarry before seven to eight weeks have the option of miscarrying on their own. You wait for your body to begin the natural process of expelling the contents of the uterus. It involves some pretty intense cramping and heavy bleeding for a day or two, followed by lighter amounts of bleeding for up to seven to ten days afterwards. There is always a small risk that not all of the tissue will be passed and you will need a D&C.

If you miscarry later in pregnancy, often after eight to ten weeks, there is a lot of tissue that needs to be passed and the risk of having some of the tissue remain inside the uterus increases. The possibility of heavy bleeding, and even hemorrhage, rises as well. This is why most practitioners recommend a D&C for missed abortions that are more than eight weeks along.

The ultimate decision is yours. Some women do not want to undergo a surgical procedure and prefer to wait. If you decide to wait, you have two weeks for your body to take care of business. If nothing has happened after two weeks or so, your doctor may suggest a D&C to prevent infection or excessive bleeding leading to the inability to clot blood (a rare complication). Other women find it easier, both physically and emotionally, to get everything taken care of quickly.

Factoid: If your blood type is Rh negative, you will need Rhogam if you miscarry, regardless of whether you pass everything on your own or need a D&C. See earlier in the chapter for details.

Q. I'm worried that the D&C my doctor is recommending will make it harder for me to get pregnant again. Are there any risks to this procedure?

A D&C (dilatation and curettage) is the standard of care for incomplete abortions, missed abortions, miscarriages after about eight weeks, or when there is a need for specialized testing on the fetal tissue (see section on D&C's earlier in this chapter).

Your risk of having a complication is very low (about one percent) if a trained practitioner performs a D&C using sterile technique. The risks include infection (because no matter how sterile we are, bacteria are everywhere), bleeding (occasionally requiring medication and very rarely requiring a blood transfusion), and uterine perforation, which can occur when one of the surgical instruments makes a small hole through the wall of the uterus.

It is extremely rare to become infertile after having a D&C. You have an increased risk of infertility if you develop an infection of the uterine lining or you undergo vigorous scraping of the uterine walls (leading to scarring). Scarring is more likely if you have multiple D&C's, a postoperative infection, or a D&C after the first trimester.

Q. I went into my doctor's office for a routine visit at 18 weeks and she told me there wasn't a heartbeat. I'm

devastated and now have to have a D&E procedure. What can I expect physically afterwards?

Physically, it takes three to four weeks to recover from a D&E.

You will probably have moderate vaginal bleeding for up to seven days after your procedure. Following the heavier bleeding, expect some lighter bleeding or spotting for another few days to a week.

If you had normal monthly periods before the miscarriage, your period should resume four to six weeks after the procedure. If you haven't had a period by the sixth week, call your doctor.

Other symptoms include lower abdominal pain or cramping, similar to what you get with your period. These usually go away two to three days after the procedure. You may also have breast pain, engorgement or leaking. Try using ice packs and wrapping your breasts with a tight bandage or tight sports bra. This may last for about a week.

Your pregnancy hormones may continue to circulate for about a month after your miscarriage. It all depends on how advanced your pregnancy was when the miscarriage occurred.

Q. Is there anything I can do to decrease my risk of infection after the procedure?

Yes.

First, some practitioners give an antibiotic at the time of surgery. You can ask your practitioner if you will be receiving one.

After the procedure, you need "**PELVIC REST**" for two to four weeks (or until the bleeding stops). Pelvic rest means no tampons, douching or intercourse. It is also recommended that you avoid swimming pools, hot tubs and bathtubs.

Reality Check

You can shower after a D&C. It's the bathtub that's off limits.

Q. When will I be able to exercise again and return to all of my normal daily activities?

Your doc will tell you to take it easy and avoid exercise for a few days afterwards. Ease back into your activities. Remember you had surgery, even though you don't have a scar or stitches. Speak with your doctor for specific instructions on strenuous exercise and other activities.

Q. I am really sad about losing my pregnancy. Everyone keeps telling me that I will feel better, but I don't. Is this normal?

It is normal. MANY women go through it. You are grieving and there are several phases of emotions during this process.

You may feel shock, denial, guilt, depression, sadness, disbelief and anger. Sometimes, the extreme emotional pain causes physical symptoms, such as difficulty sleeping, loss of appetite, anxiety, fatigue and chest tightness. Don't ignore all of your emotions because they will only build up inside. Get through them and you will reach a phase of acceptance. It is okay to need help, counseling and in some cases, even medication.

During your healing process, situations will likely make you re-live the pain and sadness you felt at the beginning. You may find it hard to go to a friend's baby shower, see a mother nursing her child, or have a check up in your doctor's office in the same room where you were given the news that you miscarried. Allow yourself to go through these setbacks and allow time to heal.

Q. My husband doesn't seem to be sad about the fact that I just miscarried. Is that possible?

Men and women grieve differently.

While this isn't true in all cases, women typically are more expressive about their loss, feel the need to talk about it and are ten times more likely to ask for help or seek out counseling.

Men tend to use distraction as a technique to deal with grief and are more likely to investigate and problem solve than join a support group, go to therapy, or talk to their friends. A grieving man might bury himself in work or other projects and keep quiet, avoiding conversations with friends or family.

You also must realize that you were the one carrying the baby in your body. This allowed you, and not your partner, to form a unique bond. You saw and felt your body changing. Some women even report feeling a bond the second they get a positive pregnancy test. Partners may not experience real bonding until after the baby is born.

Recognize the differences in how you are each coping and grieving. Keep the lines of communication open. You need to let your partner know how you feel and vice versa. This way, you can both begin to heal in your own way.

Partner tip

Admit to your partner that you, too, are also grieving. You may not be in the mood to share your feelings, and that's okay. Just telling your partner that you are grieving privately will help.

Q. None of my friends have miscarried and I just don't know where to turn. Are there any resources for me?

It's so important to talk about what has happened and to voice your feelings and concerns. Sadness and anger are normal parts of healing and you have to let yourself go through these steps.

DR H'S OPINION

It may be stating the obvious, but having a miscarriage is tough on anyone. This is especially true for women who don't have any children yet. I can tell you from personal experience that the miscarriage I had prior to my first child being born was far more difficult emotionally than the one I had between my two children.

DOESN'T WORK

Talk with your practitioner to get all of your questions answered. Talk with your partner so you understand how the other is feeling. Here's a list of helpful books and websites for women who have miscarried.

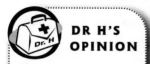

DR H'S OPINION

"Know that you are not alone. So many women have gone through one or more miscarriages. There is help and there is hope."

Books:
Miscarriage: Women sharing from the Heart by Shelly Marks, Marie Allen.
Miscarriage: A Shattered Dream by Sherokee Isle, Linda Hammer Burns
Surviving Pregnancy Loss: A complete sourcebook for women and their families by Rochelle Friedman and Bonnie Gradstein

Websites:
angelsinheaven.org
babyloss.com   miscarriagesupport.org.nz
mend.org   pain-heartache-hope.com

Q. I've had a miscarriage in the past and I just had another one at eight weeks. I am going in for a D&C tomorrow and my doctor wants to send the tissue to a lab to test the fetus' chromosomes. Is this a good idea?

Many things can cause a miscarriage, but abnormal chromosomes in the fetus are the most common explanation, by far.

Docs don't typically send the fetal tissue for testing for just one miscarriage because it is not likely to happen again and the testing can be expensive. If, however, a woman has had two or more miscarriages, many physicians recommend checking the fetus' chromosomes (karyotyping) to see if there is a chromosomal issue. If the chromosomes are normal, your practitioner knows to search for another cause.

Q. My doctor just did an ultrasound and told me I had a blighted ovum. What does that mean?

A blighted ovum means that there is an amniotic sac present, but no embryo. It is the cause of about 40% to 50% of all miscarriages occurring before 12 weeks. It is usually the result of a chromosomal abnormality. The pregnancy doesn't continue to grow, since there is some signal that "tells" the fertilized egg it would never develop into a healthy fetus.

Old Wives Tale
A miscarriage can be caused by exercise or carrying around a toddler. *False.* It is normal to feel some guilt after losing a pregnancy. Women rack their brains trying to pinpoint what past event led to the loss of their fetus. Was it bending over to pick up the plate that fell on the ground? Was it getting your hair colored? Was it the five-hour plane ride you took last week?

The truth is, none of these things cause a miscarriage. Miscarriages happen commonly and are often due to genetic reasons where the chromosomes are abnormal. It's very normal to feel guilty, but having a miscarriage is not your fault.

Q. Is there a way to prevent having a miscarriage?

Since most miscarriages result from chromosomal abnormalities, there is not much that can be done to prevent them.

Once you find out you are pregnant, do what you can to make your uterus the best possible home for your baby.

5 potentially treatable medical reasons for miscarriage

While many times there may not be an identifiable reason, it's worth doing a medical workup just in case. Here are five treatable medical disorders that increase the risk of miscarriage.

1. Celiac disease.
2. Lupus (Systemic Lupus Erythematosus).
3. Uncontrolled/undiagnosed thyroid disease.
4. Uncontrolled/undiagnosed diabetes.
5. Cigarette, alcohol or drug abuse.

If you have a chronic medical condition, try to plan your pregnancy when your disease is under control (as best as possible). A pre-pregnancy consult with your internist, obstetrician and a high-risk pregnancy specialist can be very important for planning a healthy pregnancy.

Q. Can stress can cause a miscarriage?

Some people think this is an old wives' tale, but there may be a wee bit of truth to it.

Recent studies show a relationship between stress and miscarriage as well as stress and preterm labor. *(Robinson JN.)* It's hard to prove stress causes miscarriage because we all have some level of stress in our daily lives. And most women give birth to healthy babies.

Here's what we know: stress increases the release of a hormone called cortisol. This hormone is being actively investigated as a link to miscarriage, preterm labor and other unfortunate pregnancy outcomes.

It's unlikely that the day-to-day stress you encounter will have any negative affect on your pregnancy. However, it is possible that major levels of stress that occur with the loss of a spouse or child, a divorce or major financial disaster could cause miscarriage or other pregnancy complications.

Q. I had a miscarriage. How long do I need to wait before trying to conceive again?

There is no amount of time that is perfect for everyone. But practitioners usually advise a woman to wait for two or three menstrual cycles before conceiving again. This is because it takes time for the lining of the uterus to fully regenerate and be healthy enough to carry another pregnancy.

DOESN'T WORK

WILL I MISCARRY AGAIN?

Here are the stats. But keep in mind that whatever your risk, there is a much greater chance that you will have a successful pregnancy rather than another miscarriage, no matter what your history is:

◆ One prior miscarriage: 20% chance of another miscarriage.
◆ Two prior miscarriages: 28% chance of another miscarriage.
◆ Three or more miscarriages: 43% chance of miscarriage.

The flip side is that a history of even one successful pregnancy improves your chances of being successful again.

◆ One live birth: 5% chance of miscarriage.
◆ More than one live birth: 4% chance of miscarriage.
◆ One live birth, and then one miscarriage: 6% chance of miscarriage.

Considering the frequency of miscarriage, about one in 36 women will have two miscarriages due to nothing more than chance. This is why many doctors will wait until a woman has had three or more consecutive miscarriages to begin a full investigation into the problem.

It's possible to improve your odds of success if you figure out why you have miscarried in the past. For example, if you had two miscarriages and then discovered that you had Hashimoto's thyroiditis (a form of thyroid disease), getting treated with thyroid replacement medication will lower your chance of having another miscarriage.

It is also important to take time to grieve your loss and be emotionally ready to go through another pregnancy.

But it really depends on your own situation. A very early pregnancy loss may differ from a loss in the second trimester. Check with your practitioner to see what she recommends.

Stillbirths

Q. What are the odds of carrying a baby to term, and then having the baby die in the womb before delivery?

This is called a stillbirth.

It's when the fetus dies after 20 weeks gestation. These occur in about one in 200 pregnancies. Term stillbirths (a stillbirth that occurs after 37 weeks) are much less common and occur in one out of every 1200 deliveries. The majority of stillbirths happen before labor begins. A very small percentage occur during labor and delivery.

Q. My doctor just told me that my baby is a stillborn. I'm in shock. What should I do?

when it doesn't work

DOESN'T WORK

? ?

This is one of the most difficult things for a woman/couple to ever go through. About 28,000 families in the United States suffer the loss of a viable baby prior to birth each year. There were no obvious problems in about half of those pregnancies.

Most couples are initially in shock. Everyone grieves differently, but it is very important to let yourself grieve.

Let yourself cry. Let yourself feel numb. Let yourself get angry. And then, let yourself heal.

And in the face of all this pain, you still have to deliver the baby. If you are not already in labor, you usually have to be induced to deliver vaginally or have a D&E (see info earlier in this chapter about this procedure). In some circumstances, it's also possible to wait until you go into labor on your own.

It's rare to have a Cesarean section for a stillbirth unless an unforeseen complication occurs during labor or delivery, or your previous deliveries were C-sections.

Doctors prefer to induce labor or perform the D&E as soon as possible after the diagnosis, although it is probably safe from a medical standpoint to wait up to two weeks. Waiting more than two weeks is dangerous because it increases your risk of developing a blood clotting problem or an infection in the uterus.

One important note: If you wait until you go into labor on your own or wait a week or two to be induced, it will affect how a baby looks at the time of delivery. This can be extremely distressing for parents so talk to your practitioner about this in advance.

Q. My best friend just had a stillbirth at 38 weeks. I am currently pregnant in my second trimester and am absolutely terrified that this will happen to me, too. Is there anything I can do to prevent a stillbirth?

Many stillbirths are not preventable. And having a stillbirth at term is rare.

But there are some things that can be done to decrease your risk. All women should do daily **FETAL KICK COUNTS** after about 26 weeks. Set aside some time each day to be aware of and/or record your baby's movements. You will begin to know when your baby is most active at about this time.

If you notice that your baby hasn't been as active or isn't moving at all after a 12 to 24 hour period, contact your practitioner.

Avoid smoking, alcohol and drug use during pregnancy. If you have been classified as "high risk," talk to your practitioner about whether you will need increased monitoring with ultrasounds and/or fetal heart rate monitoring (non-stress tests or NSTs).

If you have had a previous stillbirth, your practitioner will monitor you very closely with any subsequent pregnancy.

Having a stillborn baby is one of the most difficult things for a woman/couple to ever go through. We will walk you through this journey at Expecting411.com/extra.

DOESN'T WORK

Choosing Termination

Q. We just found out the fetus has a serious genetic defect. We are interested in terminating the pregnancy. What are the next steps?

The first step once you have learned that something may be wrong with your fetus is to speak with as many people as you can.

Schedule a consultation visit with your practitioner as well as a perinatologist (high-risk obstetric doctor) or genetic counselor if possible to make sure that you are fully educated before making a final decision. Do some research on the particular problem and bring questions. Getting a second opinion won't hurt either. Although questions will differ based on the individual condition, here are a few that may be helpful:

- What does this diagnosis/problem/condition mean?
- What organ systems are affected?
- Is there a chance that I will have a stillborn?
- Is there a chance the baby will die after birth?
- Will the baby need to have surgery? More than one?
- Is there any chance of intellectual disability?
- Is this condition something that we can accept/live with/embrace?
- Is this condition something that we are not prepared to accept/live with/embrace?

Once all of your questions have been answered, you will be able to make an informed decision. Mind you, it's never an *easy* decision. Even if you are quite sure that you would never want to deliver a baby with Trisomy 13, for example, your emotions may influence your decision.

Have a long talk with your partner. Sometimes, it is also helpful to talk with friends and family. For others, it is easier to talk with a therapist or religious advisor. If you have decided that termination is the right choice for you, the details of the procedure (D&C or D&E) itself are described earlier in this chapter.

Questions about pregnancy termination and molar pregnancies are covered at Expecting411.com/extra.

Don't forget to grieve

Even if you never got to know your baby, you formed a bond as a parent to your unborn child and you will have feelings of loss, guilt, and yes, even anger. Going through the grieving process is normal and a natural human emotion.

Everyone goes through it at their own pace and in their own way. And it doesn't matter if you lost your baby at eight weeks, 22 weeks or 34 weeks. It is a loss any way you look at it. Women who have miscarried often have many unanswered questions and it is extremely important to be in open communication with your practitioner, family and friends.

when it doesn't work

DOESN'T WORK

Here are two additional resources to connect with others who share the same experience.

nationalshareoffice.com
aplacetoremember.com

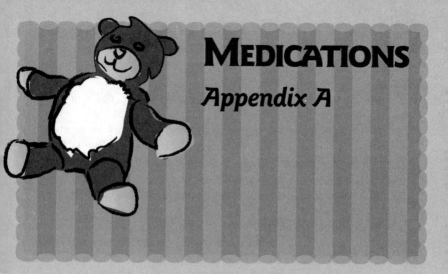

MEDICATIONS
Appendix A

There are several medications that are off limits or to be used with caution during pregnancy. Because the list is huge, look for detailed info on medication use during pregnancy and breastfeeding, as well as complementary/alternative therapies (herbs, homeopathic remedies, acupuncture) at Expecting411.com/extra. If you have questions, always ask your practitioner.

The most common over the counter medications you may be wondering about are listed here:

What can I take, doc?

Here's a summary of over the counter medications you can take for symptoms you might encounter:

SYMPTOM	OTC MEDICATION
Constipation	Docusate (Colace), Metamucil, Fibercon
Cough	Dextromethorphan (Robitussin DM)
Diarrhea	Loperamide (Imodium AD)
Flu symptoms	Acetaminophen and pseudoephedrine (Tylenol Cold)**, acetaminophen and diphenhydramine (Tylenol PM)
Headache, Fever	Regular strength acetaminophen (Tylenol)
Heartburn	Tums, Mylanta, Maalox, Rolaids, cimetidine (Tagamet), ranitidine (Zantac)
Hemorrhoids	Anusol HC, Tucks medicated pads (witch hazel pads)
Nasal congestion	Pseudoephedrine (Sudafed)**, diphenhydramine (Benadryl), cetirizine (Zyrtec), loratidine (Claritin— *not* Claritin D)*
Nausea	Vitamin B6 (100mg/day), Emetrol, Sea bands, ginger root capsules
Sore throat	Throat lozenges, Cepacol, salt water rinses

Notes:

- If your symptoms don't improve in three days, call your practitioner!
- *While Sudafed is safe to take during pregnancy for short periods of time (less than 48 hours), Claritin D is not. The "D" stands for decongestant, which is a higher dose than what is found in Sudafed.
- **Pseudoephedrine-containing products should be used for 48 hours or less.
- Regarding pain and fever-reducing medication: Avoid ibuprofen (Advil, Motrin) and naproxen (Aleve) throughout pregnancy. Ditto for baby aspirin after 28 weeks of pregnancy. And painkillers, like Vicodin and Tylenol #3 taken just prior to or just after conception, may be linked to certain birth defects. Take acetaminophen (Tylenol)—and even then—only when you really need it.

Helpful Hint

Some people use a combination of traditional care and complementary/alternative medicine or CAM (herbs, homeopathy, acupuncture, etc). Some CAM therapies are effective and safe. Others may be ineffective or downright dangerous. Our mantra is: show us the scientific evidence that a therapy is both safe and effective and we are happy to recommend it. Unfortunately, much of that data is lacking when it comes to CAM. Inform your practitioner of *any* therapies you are using that your practitioner has not prescribed.

Q. I took some medications before I knew I was pregnant. What effect will it have on the baby?

The answer depends on the specific medications you took. Most medications will not cause a serious problem for your fetus, especially if you stop using them once you know you are pregnant. Talk to your practitioner about any medications (over the counter, herbal, or prescription) you have been taking.

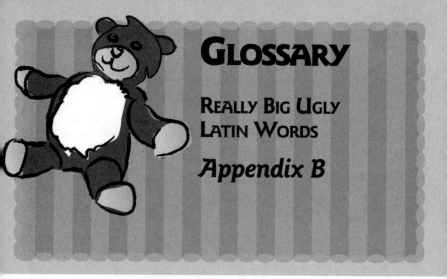

GLOSSARY

REALLY BIG UGLY LATIN WORDS

Appendix B

Abdominoplasty. A.k.a. "a tummy-tuck." A surgical procedure that helps tighten up loose fascia and muscles of the belly, while also removing excess skin and fat in the area.

ABO incompatibility. If mom has "O" blood type and her baby has type "A" or "B", the baby may be at risk of having a yellowing of the skin (jaundice) as a newborn. See **jaundice**.

Acid reflux. See GERD.

Acute fatty liver. A life-threatening condition where a pregnant woman's liver stops working.

Adnexae. Female organs—fallopian tubes and ovaries.

Adnexal torsion. The ovary and sometimes, the fallopian tube twists. Twisting cuts off the blood flow to these structures. This most often happens when an ovarian or tubal cyst is present. It's possible for everything to untwist on its own, but if it twists and gets stuck, surgery is required to untwist the ovary/fallopian tube, occasionally requiring removal.

Advanced maternal age. A woman who will be 35 years of age or older when she gives birth.

AFP. Stands for Alpha Fetoprotein. This is one of the hormones measured in both the Triple Screen and the Quad Screen tests.

Amniocentesis. A diagnostic test that can determine if a fetus has chromosomal defects. A thin needle goes through the skin into the uterus and a little bit of amniotic fluid is taken for analysis. The test is done between 15-20 weeks of pregnancy. This test is also done at times to determine whether a baby's lungs are mature enough to induce labor or perform a C-section at a time in pregnancy that is earlier than one week prior to the due date.

Amnioinfusion. Sterile water is injected into the uterus to help the umbilical cord float or to dilute thick meconium (if the fetus poops while still in the womb).

Amnion. Inner fetal membranes. The membranes that expand and enclose the embryo in a big, fluid filled space (the amniotic cavity). See below for amniotic fluid.

Amniotic fluid. Fluid that surrounds the fetus. It cushions the fetus, and allows

GLOSSARY

? ?

vital organs to grow and develop appropriately. The placenta makes some of it. And some of it is made from your unborn baby's urine.

Amniotic fluid embolism. A rare, serious condition where amniotic fluid (or other debris from the amniotic sac) ends up in the mother's blood. It can be fatal.

Analgesia. Medication that provides pain relief.

Anemia. Decreased ability of the red blood cells to carry an adequate amount of oxygen to body tissues. Various causes. Examples: iron-deficiency anemia, sickle cell anemia.

Anencephaly. A neural tube defect where there is partial or complete absence of the brain/skull.

Anesthesia. Medication that provides pain relief, immobilization, and/or sedation.

Anesthesiologist. Doctor who performs that epidural or spinal!

APGAR score. An assessment done at 1 and 5 minutes (and occasionally at 10 minutes) after delivery of your baby to see how he is transitioning to life outside the womb.

Apnea of prematurity. Babies who are born early may have temporary, prolonged pauses in their breathing. Preemies eventually outgrow this problem. Until they do, they are placed on a monitor with an alarm to warn parents if breathing stops.

ARDS (Adult Respiratory Distress Syndrome). A life-threatening emergency where there is fluid build-up in the lungs.

Areola or plural form, areolae. The colored tissue surrounding the nipples.

Atelectasis. A temporary situation where part of the lung tissue does not fully expand. Symptoms include shortness of breath or difficulty breathing.

Baby blues. From a few days after delivery to two weeks afterwards, you might be moody and irritable. But, you will have no trouble sleeping when you get the chance to.

Bacterial vaginosis. A bacterial overgrowth (overgrowth of Gardnerella vaginalis) that causes irritation (often itching and burning) of your external genital area and a fishy smelling discharge.

Bedrest. Exactly what it says. Resting and reclining 24/7.

Beta hCG. See Human chorionic gonadotropin.

Bicornuate uterus. Some women are born with a malformed uterus. This particular abnormality is a heart shaped womb with two "horns."

Bilirubin. A waste product of the body. It is broken down by the liver and intestines, and then excreted in our poop. When levels get too high, the body can't get rid of all of it via poop, and it collects in the skin—this is called jaundice.

Bishop score. A calculation that helps predict whether inducing labor will be successful.

Bladder infection. See urinary tract infection.

Blighted ovum. Fertilized egg attaches to the uterine wall, but an embryo never develops.

Bloody show. Blood-tinged vaginal discharge seen during labor.

Body Mass Index (BMI). This is a calculation to determine if your weight is appropriate for your height. See Expecting411.com (Bonus) to figure out what your BMI was before becoming pregnant. We don't measure BMI's during pregnancy.

Brachial plexus injury. Injury to the nerves supplying the shoulder, arm, and hand. Can occur in the fetus during a difficult delivery (ex: shoulder dystocia).

Braxton Hicks contractions. Your womb (uterus) is made out of muscle. You may feel your uterus flexing its muscles before you actually use them in labor. You will feel your uterus harden up and then relax. Those practice contractions are called Braxton-Hicks contractions. Some women, especially those who have had babies before, will feel these contractions in their second trimester. But, you are more likely to feel them in the third trimester.

Breech presentation. The baby's buttocks or foot/feet is the first body part preparing to exit the uterus. A procedure may be attempted to move the fetus (see external cephalic version). Or, a C-section is recommended.

C-section (Cesarean section): This is a surgical procedure used to deliver a baby. The obstetrician makes a small cut or incision in a woman's lower belly and uterus to remove the baby.

Carcinogen. A toxin that is known to cause cancer. Example: Arsenic, tobacco.

Cephalhematoma. Literally, a head bruise. This happens to newborns due to birth trauma. Some bruises are quite large and take one to two months to go away. Since the bruise is a collection of blood, it sometimes creates an additional bilirubin load (the breakdown product of red blood cells). This, in turn, can lead to newborn jaundice.

Cephalic. Refers to the head.

Cephalopelvic disproportion. Baby's head is too big to get through the mother's pelvic bones and thus, the birth canal.

Cerclage. Stitches temporarily placed in the cervix to keep it closed.

Cerebral palsy. Muscle and posture dysfunction that varies in severity, but does not get progressively worse.

Cervical insufficiency. Previously known as "cervical incompetence". Cervix begins to open (dilate) very early in pregnancy, often leading to loss of pregnancy. It happens between 13-24 weeks of pregnancy.

Cervix. The opening to your uterus (womb).

Chemical pregnancy. Your body makes enough pregnancy hormone to produce a positive pregnancy test, but not enough to produce a viable baby. You were pregnant, but a miscarriage occurred before anything could be detected by ultrasound.

Cholecystitis. Inflammation of the gallbladder.

glossary

Cholestasis of pregnancy. The normal flow of bile in the gallbladder and liver is decreased or stops altogether. The bile eventually enters the bloodstream and makes your skin turn yellow (see jaundice).

Chloasma. See melasma.

Chorioamnionitis. An infection of the amniotic sac.

Chorion. Fetal membranes that surround the embryo. Part of the choroin (the chorionic villi) invade the wall of the uterus and eventually form the placenta.

Chorionic Villus Sampling (CVS). A diagnostic test that determines whether or not a fetus has chromosomal defects. A thin catheter is placed into the uterus (either through the cervix or through the abdominal wall) and a small bit of tissue from the placenta is analyzed. The test is done between 10-13 weeks of pregnancy.

Chromosomes. Thin strands of DNA (genetic building blocks) that are found in most cells in our body. We get half of our chromosomes from our mom and half from our dad.

Clavicular fracture. Broken collarbone. It can happen to newborns during a difficult delivery. It happens more commonly if mom is small and baby is big or the baby's shoulder gets stuck during delivery. The bone heals nicely within six to eight weeks without a cast.

Cleft lip. A defect occurring during fetal development that causes a gap in the middle of the upper lip. It may or may not be associated with a cleft palate. See cleft palate.

Cleft palate. A defect occurring during fetal development involving the roof of the mouth, leaving an opening in the middle. It may be a partial defect, or a complete one that involves the lip as well. See cleft lip.

Clitoral hood. The tissue lying directly above the clitoris that is a popular place for body piercings. Ouch!

Clubfoot. A treatable condition where one or both feet turn in and downward.

Colposcopy. A simple procedure where a binocular microscope is used to look at the cells of the cervix.

Colostrum. Early breast milk. Some women begin producing and releasing it in their late second or third trimesters. This milk is rich with the antibodies you have made over your lifetime. It is lower in calories than the mature milk produced 3-5 days after delivery. It looks more clear and watery than mature milk.

Community hospital. A hospital designed to handle routine medical and surgical issues.

Conception. This is the moment when the egg and sperm meet. It is also called fertilization.

Congenital heart defect. This can be a defect in the formation of the muscle wall, valve, or a chamber of the heart. Many congenital heart defects are treatable with surgery.

Cord compression. The umbilical cord and its blood vessels get compressed because they cannot float around freely (sometimes from too little amniotic fluid). Less oxygen goes to the baby and the fetal heart rate may show a non-reassuring pattern (fetal distress).

Cord prolapse. The woman's cervix is open (dilated) and the baby's umbilical cord drops through it prior to delivery. This is serious stuff because it can reduce blood flow and oxygen to the baby. It most commonly seen in non-vertex presentations (when something other than baby's head is first—butt, knee, foot)

Corpus luteum. A cyst that forms on the ovary during pregnancy and secretes a hormone called progesterone.

CVS. See Chorionic Villus Sampling.

Deep Venous Thrombosis (DVT). A blood clot in the deep veins of the legs or pelvis.

Degenerating fibroid. Benign tumors that commonly grow in the uterus. They can enlarge during pregnancy and not get enough blood flow to sustain them. So, they begin to breakdown and become painful.

DHA. Stands for Docosahexaenoic acid. It is an Omega 3 fatty acid that is needed for brain, eye, and nervous system functioning.

Diabetes mellitus. A disease where the body either does not make enough insulin or does not utilize it to properly metabolize sugar.

Diamniotic/dichorionic. Twins who have two amniotic sacs, two chorions (fetal membranes), and two placentas. These twins can be identical or fraternal.

Diamniotic/monochorionic. Twins who have two amniotic sacs, one shared chorion (fetal membranes), and one placenta. These twins can only be identical.

Diaphragmatic hernia. An abnormal opening in the muscle (diaphragm) between the lungs and abdomen allows body organs to enter the lung cavity. This is a medical emergency at birth.

Diastasis Recti. See Rectus Diastasis.

Dilatation. The cervix begins to open to let the baby out. This ranges from closed (not dilated at all) to 10 centimeters (maximum dilation, occurring just before delivery occurs)

Dilation and Curettage. Procedure where the cervix is opened (dilated) and the contents within the uterus are removed (curettage).

Dilation and Evacuation. Procedure where the cervix is opened (dilated) and the contents within the uterus are removed (evacuation). This term applies to removal of a pregnancy within the uterus after the first trimester.

Disseminated Intravascular Coagulation (DIC). Serious blood clotting problem where tiny blood clots form throughout the body and block the blood flow to vital organs. The clots use up blood proteins needed to properly clot and excessive bleeding occurs.

Down Syndrome. Also known as Trisomy 21. Chromosomal defect where there are three chromosome 21's instead of two. It causes an intellectual disability as well as characteristic facial features and other deformities.

Ductus Arteriosus. This is a connection in the fetus between the major blood vessels connected to the heart (main pulmonary artery and the aorta). At birth, this connection usually closes off on its own.

Eclampsia. Seizures that occur in severe cases of preeclampsia.

Ectopic pregnancy. A fertilized egg should travel and eventually implant in a woman's uterus. If a fertilized egg implants in an incorrect location, outside of the uterus, it is called an ectopic pregnancy. It can implant in the fallopian tube, ovary, cervix or even in a woman's abdominal cavity. Since none of these places are fit for the embryo to grow, it usually dies within the first eight weeks. This is a medical emergency for a woman as it can cause severe bleeding (and yes, pain.)

Edema. Fluid accumulates in a body part, resulting in swelling of the area. Lay term: fluid retention.

EDC. Estimated date of confinement. In other words, how long you will be having company in your womb. Synonymous with EDD, estimated delivery date. EDD replaces EDC, which is an older, dated term, stemming from times when women really were confined for a period of time during and after giving birth.

EDD. See EDC.

Effacement. The cervix starts to thin out in preparation for birth. A normal cervical length is about 3 to 4 centimeters. When fully effaced (fully thinned out), the cervix can be as thin as a piece of paper.

Egg. A woman's contribution to the baby-making process. This is what is released from the ovary each month. Each egg contains half of the genetic material required to make a baby.

Elective C-section. A cesarean delivery that is planned before labor begins.

Embryo. This is what your unborn baby is called from the time of conception through the first eight weeks of development.

Emergency C-section. A cesarean delivery that is determined to be the best/safest mode of delivery. It can occur after labor is already in progress or may be the only mode of delivery in cases when labor has not yet begun (severe hemorrhage from a placenta previa at 34 weeks or non-reassuring fetal heart pattern found at an office visit).

Endometritis. Infection of the lining of the uterus. Symptoms include: fever, chills, lower abdominal pain, bleeding, uterine tenderness, and foul smelling discharge.

Endometriosis. Tissue from the lining of the uterus that inappropriately grows outside of the uterus. Patients can be symptom-free or suffer from severe pelvic pain.

Endometrium. Inner lining of your womb (uterus).

Engaged. When your baby's presenting body part moves down and settles into the pelvic cavity. Lay term: Lightening.

Engorgement. The milkman cometh. Period of excessive breast milk production around three to five days after childbirth. Women's breasts feel full and often uncomfortable until milk demand and milk supply even out.

Epidural anesthesia. Pain relief medication that numbs the nerves from the waist down. A thin catheter tube remains in place for the duration of labor and delivery, providing a continuous flow of medication.

Episiotomy. A surgical cut in the tissue of the vagina and perineum (the tissue between the vagina and rectum) to widen the opening. Performed just before delivery of the fetal head.

Epistaxis. Nosebleed.

Estimated Date of Delivery. See EDD.

Estimated Date of Confinement. See EDC.

Expanded AFP test. See Triple Screen.

External cephalic version. A procedure attempting to change a fetus' position before delivery by using ultrasound jelly and brute strength.

Failure to progress. The labor process does not advance as it should.

Fallopian tube. This is a muscular tube (one for each ovary) that is really an extension of the uterus. The fallopian tube sits right next to the ovary. A mature egg leaves the ovary and travels through the Fallopian tube to be either fertilized (a pregnancy occurs) or not (a menstrual period occurs).

Fatty liver. See acute fatty liver.

Fetal Alcohol Syndrome Disorders (FASD). A range of health issues that babies experience due to alcohol exposure in the womb.

Fetal growth restriction. See IUGR. A fetus that does not grow as much as expected. It can be due to a problem with the fetus, the mother, or the placenta.

Fetal fibronectin (fFN). This is a non-invasive test that screens for preterm labor. The fFN attaches your water bag to the inner lining of the uterus (endometrium). It starts to leak into the vagina when a woman is in preterm labor or is in danger of going into preterm labor.

Fetal hypoxia. Lack of oxygen to the fetus leading to brain cell death.

Fetal kick counts. Official definition—Relax for an hour and see if you can feel your baby kicking and moving around at least ten times. It is a sign that your baby is healthy and doing well. A more realistic goal—Be sure you feel movement within every 12 hour period. Do this every day around starting at about 26 weeks of pregnancy.

Fetus. This is what your unborn baby is called from nine weeks of development until he is born.

Fibroid, degenerating. See degenerating fibroid.

First trimester screening test. This is a non-invasive test that helps determine a woman's risk of having a baby with certain chromosomal defects.

Floppy baby syndrome. Abnormally low muscle tone due to a variety of medical or genetic conditions.

Full term. A baby who is born between 37–40 weeks gestation.

Fundal height. The measurement from your pubic bone to the top of your uterus. Your fundal height in centimeters should approximately equal your gestational week (ex: a baby who is 32 weeks should have a fundal height of approximately 30-34 cm).

Gastroenteritis. Stomach virus.

GERD (Gastroesophageal reflux disease). Lay terms: acid reflux or heartburn. Stomach acid comes up into the esophagus, causing burning discomfort/nauseated feeling/pain.

Gestation. The period of time that the embryo/fetus develops in the womb.

Gestational age. The number of weeks or days that the embryo/fetus has been in the womb. The countdown starts on the first day of your last menstrual period.

Gestational diabetes. Diabetes that occurs during pregnancy.

Gestational hypertension. High blood pressure that occurs during pregnancy.

Gingivitis. Bleeding, swollen gums.

Glucola test. This is a one hour test that screens all pregnant women for gestational diabetes. It is done at 24-28 weeks of pregnancy, in most cases. It involves consuming a sugary drink containing 50 grams of glucose and getting your blood drawn one hour later. If you fail this test, you get to take the three-hour glucose tolerance test. See Three-hour glucose tolerance test.

Group B Strep (GBS). A bacteria that most often lives in harmony with a woman in her gut/bowels and vagina. It occasionally causes a vaginal or urinary tract infection in mom. It can lead to serious infection for a newborn, though, if not properly treated.

Heartburn. See GERD.

HELLP Syndrome. A severe form of preeclampsia. H stands for hemolysis (red blood cells are broken down), EL stands for elevated liver enzymes, and LP stands for low platelets. Immediate delivery is necessary.

Hemoglobin electrophoresis. Special blood test that detects some of the inherited red blood cell abnormalities. See hemoglobinopathy.

Hemoglobinopathy. Inherited (genetic) red blood cell abnormality. Examples: sickle cell disease, thalassemia

Hemolytic anemia. There are several causes of red blood cell destruction that result in anemia. For newborns, it is due to mom's antibodies that attack and destroy his red blood cells.

Hemorrhoids. Swollen veins (varicose veins) around your anus. They are itchy and occasionally, they bleed. Aren't you glad you looked this one up?!

High-risk pregnancy. A pregnancy that is monitored more closely and more often, and one that is more likely to require specialized tests. Reasons for a high-risk pregnancy include: having multiples, a history of repeated miscarriages or an ectopic pregnancy, conceived with the help of a fertility specialist, having a chronic medical condition, being 35 years of age or older, or having a complication arise during pregnancy (gestational diabetes, gestational hypertension, etc).

Human chorionic gonadotropin (beta-hCG). Hormone produced by the placenta that turns a pregnancy test positive. It tells the body to build a nest for a growing baby and it tells the ovaries to stop producing mature eggs every month.

Hydronephrosis. Dilated or enlarged kidneys. It may be associated with a urinary tract obstruction or urinary reflux. It is often a transient/temporary finding on ultrasound in some fetuses that usually resolves after birth.

Hyperbilirubinemia. See jaundice.

Hyperemesis gravidarum. Constant nausea and vomiting that causes dehydration and weight loss. It's thought to be due to elevated hormone levels (particularly beta hCG) during pregnancy.

Hyperpigmentation. Area of the skin that has a darker color than normal. It occurs more commonly in darker skinned people.

Hypertension. High blood pressure.

Hyperthyroidism. Thyroid gland produces excess amount of thyroid hormone.

Hypoglycemia. Low blood sugar.

Hypopigmentation. Area of the skin that lacks color.

Hypothermia. Difficulty maintaining body temperature so body temperature gets too low. Premature babies usually have this problem.

Hypothyroidism. Thyroid gland does not produce adequate amounts of thyroid hormone.

Implantation. When your little peanut (embryo) attaches to the lining of the womb (uterus) and settles in.

Implantation bleeding. When the fertilized egg attaches to your womb (uterus), you may have some light spotting (mild vaginal bleeding). You may not even realize you are pregnant when this occurs because you have not missed your period yet.

Incompetent cervix. See cervical insufficiency.

Incomplete abortion. Some but not all, tissues of pregnancy pass. The tissue that remains can cause heavy bleeding. A D&C is often needed to remove the remaining tissue.

Incontinence. Lack of bladder control. Leaking urine. Fun.

Intertrigo. Skin chafing.

Intracranial hemorrhage. Bleeding within the skull or brain.

Intravenous fluid. A mixture of fluid and electrolytes (sodium, chloride, etc) that goes directly into a person's vein.

Intraventricular hemorrhage. A particular type of brain bleed (intracranial hemorrhage). Bleeding occurs within the brain's spinal fluid highway (ventricles). It occurs most commonly in babies born at or before 32 weeks ges-

glossary

tation, babies delivered vaginally, and those that have had asphyxia or occasionally severe birth trauma.

Isoimmunization. See Rh incompatibility.

IUGR (Intrauterine Growth Restriction). A small fetus who does not grow properly.

Jaundice. A yellowing of the skin and the whites of the eyes due to excess amounts of body waste (bilirubin) in the blood. It can be due to a liver problem or due to increased breakdown of red blood cells.

Kegel exercises. Exercises to help get your pelvic floor muscles back into shape.

Ketones. The breakdown products of fat.

Labor dystocia. A mother's cervix stops expanding (dilating) or the baby's head is too big for labor to continue without intervention.

Lanugo. Very fine, soft first hair found on the body of the fetus. It is often shed before delivery, but no worries if it is still present on your newborn.

Large for gestational age (LGA). Over 90th percentile birth weight compared to other babies born at the same age.

Last Menstrual Period (LMP). The first day you began bleeding in your monthly cycle before becoming pregnant.

Late Preterm Infant. A baby born at 34 weeks to 36 6/7 weeks of pregnancy.

Leukorrhea of pregnancy. Also known as vaginal discharge. Yellowish-white, thick and mucousy on the underwear. We know...yuck.

Lightening. As in "lightening your load." The lay term is "dropping". Your baby starts to head downward into your pelvis in preparation for being born. Some babies drop several weeks before delivery, others drop when labor begins. See engaged.

Linea alba. Translation: White line. Everyone has a line from the belly button to the top of the pubic hair. But, it's invisible when you aren't pregnant.

Linea nigra. Translation: Black line. A dark line from your belly button to your pubic hair that appears due to increased melanin production.

Lochia. Bloody discharge you will pass after delivery for about six weeks.

Macrosomic or macrosomia. Big baby, at least 8.5 pounds.

Mastitis. Breast infection usually caused by cracks in the nipples, blocked milk ducts, and germs that enter through the broken skin.

Meconium. Your baby's first poop. It's black and tarry and a real mess to clean up. Ideally, it is supposed to come out after your baby is born. Unborn babies who are under stress may pass their first meconium poop in the uterus prior to delivery. This can cause a temporary breathing problem at birth if the baby breathes it into his lungs.

Meconium aspiration syndrome. The baby's first poop ends up in his lungs. It can cause difficulty breathing and pneumonia. More commonly seen in babies that go past their due date.

Meconium-stained fluid. Amniotic fluid that is stained with baby poop (meconium). Seen after the amniotic sac is ruptured (you break your water bag) and the fluid begins to leak out.

Menstrual period. Also known as "your period". If an egg does not get fertilized by a sperm in a monthly cycle, the egg dies and the lining of the uterus that has been preparing to nurture a growing baby will slough off. The result is bleeding for 3-7 days.

Microcephaly. Small head size.

Miscarriage (spontaneous abortion). The loss of a pregnancy occurring before 20 weeks of pregnancy. There are specific types of miscarriage: complete abortion, incomplete abortion, inevitable abortion, missed abortion, recurrent abortion, threatened abortion.

Missed abortion. The fetus dies, but there is no pain or bleeding.

Molar pregnancy. A pregnancy that does not develop normally. Sometimes it is just pregnancy tissue (products of conception). Sometimes there is also an abnormal embryo growing, but it cannot survive. It can occasionally lead to a malignancy, but women are followed closely during and after molar pregnancies because of that potential.

Monochorionic. Twins who share one set of fetal membranes.

Monochorionic/monoamniotic. Twins share one set of fetal membranes, one placenta, and one amniotic sac. They can only be identical. This type of twin pregnancy is extremely high-risk.

Monounsaturated fats. Good fats—nuts, olives, avocados, olive and canola oil.

Mucous plug. The tissue that protects the cervix (opening to the uterus/womb) during pregnancy. It may fall out several weeks before you go into labor—so don't get too excited if you see it in your undies or in the toilet. It looks like a glob of snot. Double yuck! Some women never see it when it falls out. And, sometimes it comes out at delivery.

Multiparous. You have given birth before.

Neonatologist. A doctor who cares for ill and premature newborn babies.

Neural tube. The name for the beginnings of the brain, spinal cord, and nerves in an embryo or fetus.

Neural tube defect. Abnormality in the developing brain, spinal cord, and nervous system (the neural tube). Examples: spina bifida, anencephaly.

Nipple shells. Plastic devices placed over mom's nipple to help relieve soreness or help draw out flat or inverted nipples.

Nipple shield. A soft plastic artificial nipple that is placed over mom's nipple. It is used for two reasons 1) a baby has a larger target to latch onto and 2) a mother gains protection from baby's mouth to allow existing nursing-related injuries to heal.

Non-elective C-section. See emergency C-section.

Nonstress test (NST). A non-invasive test that looks for fetal well-being by examining the fetal heart rate.

Non-vertex presentation. A fetus who does not plan to come out head first. Stubborn little thing!

Nuchal cord. Umbilical cord is wrapped around the baby's neck. It's very common, and rarely a problem.

Nuchal lucency. Assessment to check the thickness of the back of a fetus' neck on ultrasound. It is done as part of the first trimester screening to assess for certain genetic syndromes.

Nulliparous. You have never delivered a baby before.

OA (Occiput Anterior). The typical position a baby is in at the time of delivery.

OP (Occiput Posterior). Baby is facing "sunny side up" at birth. This position can cause additional pain for the laboring mom (called back labor).

Oblique lie. Baby is lying diagonally when he is preparing to exit the womb.

Occiput transverse. The baby plans to come out head down, but her head is turned horizontally in relationship to her mother's pelvic bones. If she faces mom's left thigh, she is "right occiput transverse" or ROT. If she faces mom's right thigh, she is "left occiput transverse" or LOT.

Oligohydramnios. Too little amniotic fluid.

Ovarian cyst, ruptured. See ruptured ovarian cyst.

Ovary. Women are born with two of these tiny, oval shaped body organs. It's their job to store a woman's eggs. Each month, female hormones stimulate the ovary to mature one of the eggs (occasionally two) and ready it for fertilization.

Ovulation. When an egg leaves the ovary (home base) and makes the trek through the fallopian tube with the intention of meeting a nice sperm and uniting to become a baby.

Palpitations. When you sense your heart beating, like you had a double shot espresso.

Pancreatitis. Inflammation of the pancreas (an abdominal organ that releases enzymes that help in digesting food).

Pelvic Inflammatory Disease or PID. An infection of the uterus and fallopian tubes that can damage the female organs. Chlamydia and gonorrhea (sexually transmitted infections) are notorious for causing this problem. PID can lead to abscess formation, infertility, ectopic pregnancy, and chronic pain.

Pelvic rest. No sexual intercourse, no tampons, no douching.

Perinatologist. A physician who cares for women with high-risk pregnancies.

Period. See menstrual period.

Pfannenstiel incision. The name for the most common surgical cut made on the skin for a C-section. It is horizontal and made just low enough that you could still wear a bikini afterwards (if you so desire!).

Pitting edema. Fluid accumulation in the tissues that leads to swelling. If you press on a swollen area, the indentation remains. Press on the lower part of one of your legs just a few days before your due date and you'll see what we mean!

Placenta. Organ that interfaces between your body and your fetus while in your womb. It brings nourishment to and removes waste from the unborn baby (fetus). The umbilical cord, which contains blood vessels, is what serves as the conduit between the placenta and the fetus.

Placental abruption. Placenta pulls off the wall of the uterus prematurely. This compromises the fetus' blood flow and oxygen supply.

Placenta accreta. The placenta attaches too deeply to the inner layer of the uterus.

Placenta increta. The placenta invades too deeply and attaches to the muscle layer of the uterus.

Placenta percreta. The placenta attaches and invades through the muscle layer of the uterus, often growing into the bladder or other surrounding organs.

Placenta previa. If a fertilized egg implants in the uterus in an incorrect position (near the opening of the womb over the cervix), the placenta will then lie right over the cervix which can lead to significant bleeding in the later part of pregnancy.

Pneumonia. Lung infection.

Polyhydramnios. Too much amniotic fluid.

Polyunsaturated fats. Fats that include Omega 3 and Omega 6 fatty acids.

Postdates. A pregnancy that goes beyond 42 weeks, or more than 294 days after the first day of your last menstrual period.

Postdural puncture headache. Also known as a spinal headache. A complication of having epidural anesthesia that results in a pretty severe headache.

Postpartum: "Post" means after. Postpartum refers to the 6 week window after a woman gives birth.

Postpartum D & C. Procedure where the cervix is opened (dilated) and the contents of the uterus (may be left over placenta) are removed (curettage). Occurs after delivery to stop heavy bleeding. See retained products of conception or POC.

Postpartum depression. Severe fatigue, overwhelming feelings of sadness, trouble eating and sleeping after delivery.

Postpartum hemorrhage. Excessive bleeding after delivery. That means more than 500ml of blood loss in a vaginal delivery and more than 1 liter of blood loss after a C-section.

Postterm pregnancy. A pregnancy that goes beyond 42 weeks, or more than 294 days after the first day of your last menstrual period.

Precipitous labor. A rapid labor resulting in the birth of a baby in under three hours from start to finish.

Preconception: Before you are pregnant.

Preconception visit. This is a consultation appointment with your obstetrician/practitioner before you decide to become pregnant.

Preeclampsia. You develop high blood pressure after 20 weeks of pregnancy (you previously had normal blood pressure) and you have protein in your urine.

Premature Rupture of Membranes (PROM). You break your water bag before labor starts.

Prenatal: "Pre" means before and "natus" means birth. So, prenatal refers to the time after conception until birth. Some countries use the word antenatal and prenatal interchangeably. Confusing, we know.

Preterm Premature Rupture of Membranes (PPROM). You break your water bag before 37 weeks of pregnancy.

Public hospital. A hospital that provides services to all, regardless of ability to pay.

Pulmonary embolism (PE). A blood clot, usually from the legs (see deep venous thrombosis), obstructs the blood vessel to the lungs (the pulmonary artery). This can be life-threatening.

PUPPS (Pruritic Urticarial Papules and Plaques). Really itchy red patches on the belly, thighs, legs and arms.

Pyelonephritis. Kidney infection.

Quad screen. A blood test that looks at three specific hormones and one protein in a mother's blood made by the placenta and ovaries. It helps determine the likelihood of having a fetus with Down Syndrome, Trisomy 18, neural tube defects, and abdominal wall defects.

Quickening. Technical term for you feeling your baby kick or move around in the womb. It usually happens around 18-22 weeks gestation. Women who have been pregnant before may feel it as soon as 15-16 weeks.

Rectus Diastasis. A pregnant woman's expanding belly allows the area between the abdominal wall muscles to get bigger (creating a gap between the right and left sides). It is worse with multiples or repeated pregnancies. Consider doing Pilates after you deliver to help get those core muscles back in shape!

Respiratory Distress Syndrome (RDS). A premature baby whose lungs are not yet mature who has difficulty breathing on his own.

Retained products of conception or POC. Remnants of the placenta or amniotic membranes that are not expelled during delivery (or after a miscarriage). Their presence can interfere with the uterus contracting properly, and thus, lead to excessive bleeding (postpartum hemorrhage). A D&C is sometimes needed to remove the remaining tissue.

Retinal hemorrhage. Bleeding in the inner lining of the eye (retina).

Rh disease or isoimmunization or incompatibility. There is a blood type incompatibility between a mom who is Rh-negative and her fetus, who is Rh-positive. This can have serious affects on the fetus.

Rhogam. A medication given to a pregnant women who has an Rh-negative blood type to prevent her body from making antibodies to an Rh-positive fetus in a future pregnancy.

Ripe cervix. Your cervix is thinning or softening in preparation of labor.

Round ligament pain. Sharp pain in your abdomen or hip area, on one or both sides. Due to a rapidly growing uterus stretching some connections between the uterus and the abdominal wall.

Rupture of the amniotic sac. Lay term: "your water breaks". Clear, watery fluid. It does not smell like urine.

Rupture of membranes. See rupture of amniotic sac.

Ruptured ovarian cyst. The bursting of a fluid-filled sac on the surface of or in the ovary. It hurts.

Second trimester screening test. Also known as a multiple marker screening, a triple screen, or a quad screen (depending on how many substances are used in testing). "AFP" is one of the substances in the test. The screen aids in detecting Down Syndrome (Trisomy 21), Trisomy 18, defects in brain/spinal cord development (neural tube defects) and abdominal wall defects.

Selective fetal termination. The decision to end a pregnancy with an abnormal fetus in a multiple gestation pregnancy (twins, triplets, or more).

Sepsis. A serious bacterial infection in the bloodstream.

Shoulder dystocia. The baby's shoulder gets stuck behind mom's pubic bone during delivery. This is an emergency where multiple maneuvers are used to delivery the baby safely.

Sickle cell disease. Blood disorder where the red blood cells have an abnormal crescent shape. These cells get stuck in blood vessels and interfere with oxygen transport to the body tissues and organs.

Singleton. Carrying one baby during pregnancy.

Small for gestational age (SGA). A baby's birth weight is less than the 10th percentile compared to other babies born at the same number of weeks of pregnancy.

Smith-Lemli-Opitz syndrome. A genetic defect that results in abnormal cholesterol metabolism. Affected people have poor growth and intellectual disability.

Spina Bifida. A neural tube defect where part of the spinal cord tissue (rarely brain tissue) sits in an exposed sac. It is associated with hydrocephalus. See hydrocephalus.

Spinal anesthesia. Pain relief via a single injectionof medication into a specific area in the back, causing numbing from the waist down.

Spinal headache. See postdural puncture headache.

Spontaneous Abortion. See miscarriage.

Station. The measurement that compares where your baby's head is in relation to specific bones in your pelvis. It is a way that your practitioner can track your baby's descent into the birth canal.

Status asthmaticus. A severe asthma attack that can be life-threatening.

glossary

Stillbirth. A fetal death inside the uterus occurring after 22 weeks.

Stretch marks. Areas of the skin that begin as dark, purple/red streaks and eventually fade to pink/white/silver. The rapid growth of certain body parts (your breasts, your belly) causes a layer of skin to tear, resulting in these beautiful badges of courage.

Subchorionic hematoma. A collection of blood between the uterine wall and the fetal membranes. It can be a cause of vaginal bleeding.

Subgaleal hemorrhage. Bleeding between the skull bone and the layer of tissue overlying it. It happens to newborns at delivery, and can be quite serious. It's rare, but it happens more often in vacuum-assisted deliveries than in standard vaginal deliveries.

Sudden Infant Death Syndrome (SIDS). Infants who die in their sleep for no obvious reason. Risk factors include: moms who smoke, warm room temperature, fluffy bedding and pillow, and babies who sleep on their tummies.

Sulcal tears. Deep tears along the sides of the vagina after a vaginal childbirth.

Surfactant. A soapy substance produced by the lungs that keeps the tiniest airways (alveoli) open. Fetuses begin making surfactant around 26 weeks gestation. Because lung function is critical for survival, it is difficult for a fetus to survive before he begins making surfactant.

Symphysis pubic pain. Your pelvic bone hurts or it hurts to stand on one leg or walk.

Teaching hospital. A hospital that participates in the training of physicians and other health personnel.

Telangiectasias. Spider veins.

Teratogens. Any environmental exposure that causes a negative effect on the development of an embryo or fetus.

Three-hour glucose tolerance test. If you fail your one-hour glucola test, you get further testing to see if you really have gestational diabetes. In a nutshell, it involves getting four separate blood draws, drinking a really sugary drink (yes, again), and sitting in your practitioner's office or at a lab for three to four hours.

Thromboembolism. A blood clot forms in a blood vessel, then travels through the bloodstream and clogs up another blood vessel.

Thrombophilias. An inherited predisposition to making blood clots (thromboembolism).

Tocolytic medication or tocolytics. Medication used to stop preterm labor.

Transient Tachypnea of the Newborn (TTN). A newborn has some residual amniotic fluid in his lungs and thus breathes faster than normal to help clear it out. It is more common in C-sections. But, true to the name, it is temporary (transient).

Transvaginal ultrasound. Placing a probe into the vaginal canal to see an image of the womb, developing embryo/fetus and other female organs (ovaries/fallopian tubes). It is useful early in pregnancy.

Transverse lie. Fetus is lying sideways when he prepares to leave the womb. Not a good exit strategy. It is unsafe for both mother and baby, and a C-section is recommended.

Trimester. Your pregnancy lasts about 40 weeks. That time is divided into three stages or trimesters, and each is about 13 weeks. The first trimester is 0-13 weeks. The second trimester is 14-27 weeks. The third trimester is 28-40 weeks.

Triple Screen. This is a blood test that looks at three specific hormones in mom's blood made by the placenta and ovaries. It helps determine the likelihood of the fetus having Down Syndrome, Trisomy 18, neural tube defects, and abdominal wall defects. Test is most accurate between 16-18 weeks of pregnancy. Newer tests are now available—See Quad Screen.

Twin-twin transfusion syndrome. Twins who share one placenta (monchorionic) may have blood vessel connections that allow one twin to get a larger share of blood flow and nutrients ("recipient twin") and one twin to get less ("donor twin").

Type 1 Diabetes. See Diabetes Mellitus for details. Type 1 is caused by an insulin deficiency. There are not enough insulin-making cells in the pancreas because they have been destroyed. Type 1 Diabetes usually begins in childhood.

Type 2 Diabetes. See Diabetes Mellitus for details. Type 2 is primarily caused by the body's diminished response to insulin (resistance) as well as decreased insulin secretion. Type 2 Diabetes is more common in overweight and obese people.

Umbilical cord. The tissue that connects the placenta to the baby. It contains three blood vessels: one blood vessel brings nutrients, oxygen, and antibodies to the unborn baby and the other two send back the baby's waste products to its mom.

Umbilical cord prolapse. See cord prolapse.

Umbilicus. Belly button.

Unfavorable cervix. Your cervix is not ready to deliver yet.

Urethral sphincter. The muscle between the bladder and the urethra that prevents leakage of your urine.

Urinary incontinence. Inability to hold urine. Laughing and coughing make it worse in certain cases.

Urinary Tract Infection (UTI). Lay term: bladder infection. Bacterial infection in the urine.

Uterine atony. The uterine muscles are soft after delivery and do not contract. This can lead to excessive bleeding.

Uterine Didelphys. A double uterus. There is a double uterus and cervix. It is also possible to have additional duplications (example: vagina).

Uterine Fibroid. Benign smooth muscle tumor in the womb (uterus).

Uterine Fibroid, degenerating. See Degenerating fibroid.

Uterine rupture. The wall of the uterus opens, usually at the site of a previ-

glossary

ous uterine scar (ex: previous C-section).

Uterus. This is the female organ commonly known as the womb. It is where the developing baby grows until he/she is ready to be born.

Vagina. This is the muscular passageway between the opening of the womb (cervix) and the outside world. It is there for sexual intercourse and for menstrual bleeding. And, it is the birth canal that your baby will travel through if you deliver without needing a C-section.

Vaginal delivery: A baby is delivered after traveling through the birth canal (the vagina). The vagina is basically a muscular tube that goes from the uterus and cervix to the outside.

Vaginal discharge. See leukorrhea of pregnancy.

Vaginitis. Inflammation and irritation of the vagina. Itchy and red.

Vanishing twin. Death of one fetus early on in a twin pregnancy.

Varicella-zoster virus. The virus that causes both chickenpox and shingles.

Vasa previa. The blood vessels of the placenta are abnormally found coursing through the amniotic sac and lie directly over the cervix. This can occur when there are two lobes (pieces) of the placenta instead of one, or when there is an abnormal insertion of the umbilical cord into the placenta. Rupture of membranes may be life-threatening for the fetus.

Vasovagal event. Blood flow shifts away from the brain, causing someone to faint.

VBAC. Vaginal Birth After Cesarean.

Vernix. Cheesy substance that covers your unborn baby's skin to protect him from his watery environment. You'll see it on him once he is born.

Vertex. When your baby plans to be born with his head coming out first. This is the most common, and preferred position.

Viability. The age that a fetus is capable of surviving outside the womb. Ballpark is 23-24 weeks of pregnancy.

Vulva. The external female genitals. It includes both sets of "lips" or folds of tissue (called the labia majora and labia minora), the clitoris, and the outer part of the vagina.

Wound hematoma. A collection of blood at the site of an injury or surgical repair.

Yeast infection. Infection caused by. . .yeast (candida). Yeast likes warm, moist places where there is little competition from bacteria. It will often infect the vagina, nipples, and a baby's mouth. If inadequately treated, it can pass back and forth in a nursing mother/baby pair.

FOOTNOTES
Appendix C

Introduction: It's Blue

◆ American Congress of Obstetricians and Gynecologists. *Your Pregnancy and Birth,* 4th Ed. Washington, DC: ACOG;2005.

◆ Hacker NF, Moore JG. *Essentials of Obstetrics and Gynecology.* Philadelphia,PA: WB Saunders;1986.

◆ Sadler TW. *Langman's Medical Embryology,* 5th Ed. Baltimore, MD: Williams and Wilkins; 1985.

◆ visembryo.com.

Chapter 1: First Trimester

◆ Birnholz JC. The development of human fetal eye movement patterns. *Science.*1981 Aug 7;213(4508):679-81.

Chapter 5: Tests

◆ ACOG. Risk table for chromosomal abnormalities by maternal age at term. *ACOG Practice Bulletin.* Dec 2007;88.

◆ ACOG. Ultrasonography in pregnancy. *ACOG Practice Bulletin.* December 2004;58:858-867.

◆ Fretts RC. Evaluation of decreased fetal movements. In UpToDate. *UpToDate.* Basow DS (Ed). Waltham MA, 2009.

◆ Gabbe SG, Niebyl JR, Simpson JL. *Obstetrics: Normal and Problem Pregnancies,* 5th Ed. Philadelphia, PA: Churchill Livingstone Elsevier; 2007.

◆ Wilkins-Haug L, etal. Prenatal screening and diagnosis for fragile X syndrome. In UpToDate. Basow DS (Ed). UpToDate. Waltham, MA 2011.

Chapter 6: Nutrition

◆ American Medical Assn. Ama-assn.org/ama/no-index/about-ama/18641.shtml. Accessed February 15, 2010.

◆ August P. Prevention of preeclampsia. In UpToDate. Basow DS (Ed). *UpToDate.* Waltham MA, 2009.

◆ Bodnar LM, etal. Maternal Vitamin D deficiency increases the risk of preeclampsia. *J Clin Endo Metab.* 2007 Sep;92(9):3517-22. Epub 2007 May 29.

◆ Ebbeling CB, etal. Effects of decreasing sugar-sweetened beverage consumption on body weight in adolescents: a randomized, controlled pilot study. *Pediatrics.* Mar 2006;117:673-680.

FOOTNOTES

◆ Gabbe SG, Niebyl JR, Simpson JL. *Obstetrics: Normal and Problem Pregnancies,* 5th Ed. Philadelphia, PA: Churchill Livingstone Elsevier; 2007.

◆ Helland IB, etal. Maternal supplementation with very-long-chain n-3 fatty acids during pregnancy and lactation augments children's IQ at 4 years of age. *Pediatrics.* 2003; 111:e39-e44.

◆ Karmon A, Sheiner E. Pregnancy after bariatric surgery: A comprehensive review. *Arch Gyn OB.* 2008 May;277(5):381-8 Epub 2008 Feb 26.

◆ Kramer MS, Kakuma R. Energy and protein intake during pregnancy. *Cochrane Database of Systemic Reviews* 2003, Issue 4. Art. No: CD000032. DOI: 10.1002/14651858.CD000032.

◆ Northwestern Univ., Dept of Nutrition, 2008. Accessed February 15, 2010.

◆ Osmond C, Barker DJ. Fetal, infant, and childhood growth are predictors of coronary heart disease, diabetes, and hypertension in adult men and women. *Environmental Health Persp.* 2000 Jun;108 Suppl 3:545-5.

◆ Rasmussen SA, etal. Maternal obesity and the risk of neural tube defects: a meta-analysis. *Am J OB Gyn.* 2008;198:611.

◆ Smedts HP, etal. High maternal vitamin E intake by diet or supplements is associated with congenital heart disease in the offspring. *BJOG.* 2009 Feb;116(3):416-23.

◆ Stanhope KL, Havel PJ. Endocrine and metabolic effects of consuming beverages sweetened with fructose, glucose, sucrose, or high-fructose corn syrup. *Am J Clin Nutr.* 2008 Dec;88(6):1733S-1737S.

◆ Stothard KJ, etal. Maternal overweight and obesity and risk of congenital anomalies. *JAMA.* 2009: 301(6) 636-50.

◆ U.S. Dept of Health and Human Services and U.S. Dept of Agriculture. Dietary Guidelines for Americans, 2005. Healthierus.gov/dietaryguidelines accessed February 15, 2010.

◆ Weintraub AY, Levy A, Levi I, Mazor M, Wiznitzer A, Sheiner E. Effect of bariatric surgery on pregnancy outcome. *Int J Gynecol Obstet.* 2008;103:246-51.

Chapter 7: Environment

◆ ACOG Committee of Obstetric Practice. Guidelines for diagnostic imaging during pregnancy. *Obstetrics & Gynecology.* Sept 2004;299. Reaffirmed 2006.

◆ ACOG. Estimated Fetal Exposure From Some Common Radiologic Procedures. *ACOG Compendium.* 2008.

◆ American Academy of Pediatrics Technical Report: Mercury in the environment: implications for pediatricians. *Pediatrics.* 2001;108(1):197-205.

◆ Bouchard MF, etal. Prenatal exposure to organophosphate pesticides and IQ in 7- year-old children. Env Health Persp 119 (8). Aug 2011.

◆ Canfield RL, etal. Intellectual impairment in children with blood lead concentrations less than 10 mcg/dl. *NEJM.* 2003 Apr 17;348(16):1517-26.

◆ Centers for Disease Control at cdc.gov/nceh/clusters/fallon/organophosfaq.htm. Accessed February 15, 2010.

◆ Chang G. Substance use in pregnancy. In UpToDate. *UpToDate.* Basow DS (Ed). Waltham MA, 2009.

◆ Child Welfare Information Gateway at Childwelfare.org accessed June 18, 2009.

◆ Deltour I, etal. Time trends in brain tumor incidence rates in Denmark,

Finland, Norway, and Sweden, 1974-2003. *JNCI*. Dec 2009;101:1721-24.

◆ Engel SM etal. Prenatal exposure to organophosphates, paraoxonase 1, and cognitive development in childhood. Env Health Persp 119(8). Aug 2011.

◆ Food and Drug Administration at fda.gov, Environmental Protection Agency at epa.gov accessed February 15, 2010.

◆ Frazier LM. Reproductive disorders associated with pesticide exposure. *J Agromedicine*. 2007;12(1):27-37.

◆ Gillen-Goldstein J. Nutrition in Pregnancy. In UpToDate. *UpToDate*. Basow DS (Ed.) Waltham MA, 2009.

◆ Goldman RH. Occupational and environmental risks to reproduction in females. In UpToDate. *UpToDate*. Basow DS (Ed). Waltham MA, 2009.

◆ National Institute of Environmental Health Sciences at niehs.nih.gov/ emfrapid/booklet/home.htm accessed February 15, 2010.

◆ Norman RJ, Nisenblat V. The effect of caffeine on fertility and on pregnancy outcomes. In UpToDate. *UpToDate*. Basow DS (Ed). Waltham MA, 2009.

◆ Ownby D, etal. Exposure to dogs and cats in the first year of life and the risk of allergic sensitization at six or seven years of age. *JAMA*. 2002;288(8):963-972.

◆ Transportation Security Administration. TSA.gov. Accessed December 12, 2011.

◆ Turner MC, etal. Residential pesticides and childhood leukemia: a systematic review and meta-analysis. *Environmental Health Perspectives*. 118:33-41.

◆ Weiss B, etal. Pesticides. *Pediatrics*. 2004;113(4):1030-36.

Chapter 8: Lifestyles

◆ ACOG Committee on Obstetric Practice. Exercise during pregnancy and the postpartum period. ACOG Committee Opinion 267. *Obstetrics & Gynecology*.2002;99:171–173.

◆ ACOG Committee on Obstetric Practice. Air travel during pregnancy. *Obstetrics & Gynecology*. December 2001;264:410-411.

◆ Aronson ME, etal. Fatal air embolism in pregnancy resulting from an unusual sexual act. Obstet Gynecol 1967 Jul;30(1):127-30.

◆ Ashai S, etal. Pneumoperitoneum secondary to cunnilingus. NEJM. 1976 Jul 8;295(2):117.

◆ Breton C. Pre-Pregnancy And First Trimester Exposure To Maternal Smoking Affects DNA Methylation In The AXL Promoter" Presentation at American Thoracic Society, May 18, 2011, Abstract 18099.

◆ Camporesi EM. Diving and pregnancy. *Semin Perinatol*. 1996;20:292-302.

◆ Sterfield B. Physical activity and pregnancy outcome: review and recommendations. *Sports Medicine*. 1997;23:33–47.

◆ U.S. Dept of Labor and U.S. Equal Employment Opportunity Commission, accessed June 28, 2009.

Chapter 9: Spa Treatment

◆ Basow DS (Ed). Botulinum Toxin type A. In UpToDate. *UpToDate*. Basow DS (Ed). Waltham MA, 2009.

◆ Botoxcosmetic.com accessed Sept 21, 2008.

FOOTNOTES

? ?

◆ El Ghissani, etal. A review of human carcinogens—Part D: radiation. *Lancet Onc.* 2009;10:751.

◆ Hayden CGJ, Cross SE, Anderson C, Saunders NA, Roberts MS: Sunscreen penetration of human skin and related keratinocyte toxicity after topical application. *Skin Pharmacol Physiol.* 2005;18:170-174.

Chapter 10: Parenthood prep

◆ AAP Section on Hematology/Oncology and Section on Allergy/ Immunology Policy Statement. Cord blood banking for potential future transplantation. *Pediatrics.*2007; 119(1):165-170.

◆ ACOG Committee on Obstetric Practice and Committee on Genetics. Umbilical cord blood banking. ACOG Committee Opinion #399. *Obstetr Gynecol.*2008;111: 475-7.

◆ ACOG. Circumcision. ACOG Committee Opinion #260. *Obstetr Gynecol.* 2001;98:707-708.

◆ Centers for Disease Control. CDC.gov/pinkbook accessed July 28, 2009.

◆ Collins S, etal. Effects of circumcision on male sexual function: debunking a myth? *J Urol.* 2002 May;167(5):2111-2.

◆ Huston AC, etal. Mother's time with infant and time in employment as predictors of mother-child relationships and children's early development. *Child Development.* 2005;76(2):467-482.

◆ Immunization Action Coalition. Immunize.org accessed February 15, 2010.

◆ Kim D, etal. The effect of male circumcision on sexuality. *BJU Int.* 2006 Nov 28:PMID 17155977.

◆ Masood S, etal. Penile sensitivity and sexual satisfaction after circumcision:are we informing men correctly? *Urol Int.* 2005;75(1):62-6.

◆ MMWR. Sept 2, 2011. 60(34);1157-1163.

◆ Parentsguidecordblood.com accessed July 24, 2009.

◆ Ramnarace C. The truth about vaccines and autism. IVillage.com, September 2009.

◆ Shaikh N, etal. Epidemiology and risk factors for urinary tract infections in children. In UpToDate. *UpToDate.* Basow DS (Ed.) Waltham MA, 2009.

◆ Weiss H. *Curr Opin Inf Dis.* 2007 Feb;20(1):33-8.

Chapter 11: Breastfeeding

◆ Gabbe SG, Niebyl JR, Simpson JL. *Obstetrics: Normal and Problem Pregnancies,* 5th Ed. Philadelphia, PA: Churchill Livingstone Elsevier; 2007.

◆ Jenson D, etal. LATCH: a breastfeeding charting system and documentation tool. *J Ob Gyn Neonatal Nurs.*1994 Jan;23(1):27-32.

◆ Lawrence RA. *Breastfeeding: A Guide for the Medical Professional.* 5th ed. St Louis: Mosby, 1999.

◆ O'Connor NR, etal. Pacifiers and breastfeeding: a systematic review. *Arch Ped Adol Med.* 2009;163(4):378-382.

◆ Stuebe AM, etal. Lactation and incidence of premenopausal breast cancer: a longitudinal study. *Arch Int Med.* 2009 Aug 10;169(15):1364-71.

Chapter 12: Home Stretch

◆ ACOG Practice Bulletin. Fetal Macrosomia. *ACOG.* Nov 2000;2:663-673.

◆ ACOG. ACOG Committee Opinion #394. Cesarean delivery on maternal request. *Obstetr Gynecol.* 2007 Dec;110(6):1501.

- ACOG Practice Bulletin. *ACOG*. July 2004;54:748-757.
- Bakr AF, Abbas MM. Severe respiratory distress in term infants born electively at high altitude. *BMC Pregnancy and Childbirth*. 2006;6(4).
- Bishop EH. Pelvic scoring for elective induction. *Obstetr Gynecol*. August 1964;24(2):266-268.
- Cnattingius R, Cnattinguis S, Notzon RC. Obstacles to reducing cesarean rates in a low-cesarean setting: The effect of maternal age, height, and weight. *Obstet Gynecol*. 1998;92:501-506.
- HealthGrades, Obstetrics and Gynecology in American Hospitals, 2011.
- Liu S, Liston RM, Joseph KS, Heaman M, Sauve R, Kramer MS. Maternal mortality and severe morbidity associated with low-risk planned cesarean delivery versus planned vaginal delivery at term. Maternal Health Study Group of the Canadian Perinatal Surveillance System. *CMAJ*. 2007;176:455–60.
- McGuinness BJ, Trivedi AN. Maternal height as a risk factor for cesarean section due to failure to progress in labour. *Aust NZ J Obstet Gynaecol*. 1999;39:152-154.
- National Institutes of Health State of the Science Conference on Cesarean Delivery on Maternal Request in 2006, as quoted in the ACOG Committee Opinion, Number 394, December 2007.

Chapter 13: Labor Day

- ACOG. Analgesia and Cesarian delivery rate. ACOG Opinion 3339. *Obstetr Gynecology*. 2006;107:1487.
- Alderice F, etal. Techniques and materials for skin closure in caesarean section. *Cochrane Database Syst Rev*. 2003;(2):CD003577.
- Andersson O. Effect of delayed versus early umbilical cord clamping on neonatal outcomes and iron status at four months: a randomized controlled trial. BMJ 2011;343:bmj.d7157.
- Chaparro CM, etal. Effect of timing of umbilical cord clamping on iron status in Mexican infants: a randomized controlled trial. *Lancet*. 2006 Jun 17;367(9527):1997-2004.
- Macarthur AJ, Macarthur C, Weeks SK. Is epidural anesthesia in labor associated with chronic low back pain? A prospective cohort study. *Anesth Analg*. 1997;85:1066-1070.
- Ohel G, etal. Early versus late initiation of epidural analgesia in labor: does it increase the rate of cesarean section? A randomized trial. *Am J OB Gyn*. 2006 Mar;194(3):600-5.
- Russell R, Dundas R, Reynolds F. Long tern backache after childbirth:prospective search for causative factors. *BMJ*.1996;312:1384-1388.
- Strauss RG, etal. A randomized clinical trial comparing immediate versus delayed clamping of the umbilical cord in preterm infants: short-term clinical and laboratory endpoints. *Transfusion*. 2008 Apr(4);658-65. Epub 2008 Jan 10.
- Wong CA, etal. The risk of cesarean delivery with neuraxial analgesia given early versus late in labor. *NEJM*. 2005 Feb 17;352(7):655-65.

Chapter 14: Postpartum

- Dodd RY. Current risk for transfusion transmitted infections. *Curr Opin Hematol*. 2007;14(6):671-6.

◆ Dodd RY, Notari EP 4th, Stramer SL. Current prevalence and incidence of infectious disease markers and estimated window period risk in the American Red Cross blood donor population.*Transfusion*. 2002;42(8):975-79.

◆ Puryear L. *Understanding Your Moods When You're Expecting: Emotions, Mental Health, and Happiness—Before, During, and After Pregnancy*. Boston: Houghton Mifflin; 2007.

Chapter 15: 911

◆ Brown HL. Trauma in Pregnancy. *Obstetr Gynecol*. July 2009;114(1):147-160.

Chapter 16: Complications

◆ ACOG. Diagnosis and Management of Preeclampsia and Eclampsia. *ACOG Practice Bulletin*. January 2002;33:717-725.

◆ ACOG. Chronic hypertension in pregnancy. *ACOG Practice Bulletin*. July 2001;29:686-694.

◆ ACOG. Asthma in pregnancy. *ACOG Practice Bulletin* #90. Feb 2008.

◆ ACOG. Thyroid disease in pregnancy. *ACOG Practice Bulletin*. August 2002;37:741-750.

◆ ACOG. Pregestational diabetes mellitus. *ACOG Practice Bulletin*. March 2005;60:868-877.

◆ ACOG. Cervical Insufficiency. *ACOG Practice Bulletin*. 2003;48:793-801.

◆ ACOG. Fetal Macrosomia. *ACOG Practice Bulletin*. 2000;22:663-673.

◆ ACOG. Intrauterine Growth Restriction. *ACOG Practice Bulletin*. 2000;12:613-624.

◆ ACOG. Management of Postterm Pregnancy. *ACOG Practice Bulletin*. 2004;55:835-841.

◆ Gabbe SG, Niebyl JR, Simpson JL. *Obstetrics: Normal and Problem Pregnancies*, 5th Ed. Philadelphia, PA: Churchill Livingstone Elsevier; 2007.

◆ Kajantie E. Fetal origins of stress-related adult disease. *Annals NY Acad Sci*. Nov 2006;1083:11-27.

◆ March of Dimes, marchofdimes.com accessed September 17, 2009.

◆ National Institutes of Health. Nlm.nih.gov/medlineplus/ency/article/000896.htm accessed February 17, 2010.

◆ Norwitz ER. Postterm pregnancy. In UpToDate. *UpToDate*. Basow DS (Ed). Waltham MA, 2009.

◆ Robinson JN, Norwitz ER. Risk factors for preterm labor and delivery. In UpToDate. *UpToDate*. Basow DS (Ed). Waltham MA, 2009.

◆ Tam H, etal. Glucose intolerance and cardiometabolic risk in children exposed to maternal gestational diabetes mellitus in utero. *Pediatrics*.2008;122:1229-1234.

◆ Wu CS, etal. Preeclampsia and risk for epilepsy in offspring. *Pediatrics*.2008;122:1022-1078.

Chapter 17: Infections

◆ ACOG Committee Opinion. Prenatal and perinatal Human Immunodeficiency Virus testing: expanded recommendations. *ACOG*. September 2008;418:229-232.

◆ ACOG. Viral hepatitis in pregnancy. *ACOG Practice Bulletin*. 2007;

FOOTNOTES

? ?

86:304-318.

◆ ACOG. Perinatal viral and parasitic infections. *ACOG Practice Bulletin.* 2000; 20:650-662.

◆ *ACOG Today.* July 2004;48(6).

◆ Centers for Disease Control. Prevention and Control of Influenza. 4www.cdc.gov/mmwr/preview/mmwrhtml/rr53e430a1.htm accessed February 16, 2010.

◆ Centers for Disease Control, MMWR Oct 21, 2011

◆ Children's Hospital, Boston. Childrenshospital.org accessed Oct. 30, 2009.

Chapter 18: Advanced Maternal Age

◆ ACOG. Prenatal diagnosis of fetal chromosomal abnormalities. *ACOG Practice Bulletin.* May 2001;27:597-607.

◆ Anderson FWJ, Johnson TRB. Maternal mortality at Y2K. *Postgraduate Obstetrics and Gynecology.* 2000;20:1.

◆ Bianco A. Effect on advanced paternal age on fertility and pregnancy. In UpToDate. *UpToDate.* Basow DS (Ed). Waltham MA, 2009.

◆ Cleary-Goldman J, et al. Impact of Maternal Age on Obstetric Outcome. *Obstetrics and Gynecology.* May 2005;105(5):983-990.

◆ Fisch H, etal. The influence of paternal age on Down syndrome. *J Uro.* 2003 Jun;169(6):2275-8.

◆ Heffner L. Advanced maternal age—how old is too old? *NEJM.* November 2004;351(19):1927-1929.

◆ Hollier LM, Leveno KJ, Kelly MA, MCIntire DD, Cunningham FG. Maternal age and malformations in singleton births. *Obstet Gynecol.* 2000 Nov;96(5 Pt 1):701-6.

◆ Joseph KS, et al. The Perinatal Effects of Delayed Childbearing. *American Journal of Obstetrics and Gynecology.* June 2005;105(6):1410-1418.

◆ Menacker F. Trends in Cesarean Rates for First Births and Repeat Cesarean Rates for Low-Risk Women: United States, 1990-2003. *National Vital Statistics Reports.* September 22, 2005; 54(4).

◆ Nybo AM, etal. Advanced paternal age and risk of fetal death: a cohort study. *American Journal of Epidemiology.* 2004;160(12):1214-1222.

◆ Reefhuis J, Honein MA. Maternal age and non-chromosomal birth defects, Atlanta—1968-2000: teenager or thirty-something, who is at risk? *Birth Defects Res A Clin Mol Teratol.* 2004 Sep;70(9):572-9.

◆ Sartorelli EM, etal. Effect on paternal age on human sperm chromosomes. *Fertil Steril.* 2001 Dec;76(6):1119-23.

Chapter 19: Preterm labor and babies

◆ ACOG. Assessment of risk factors for preterm birth. *ACOG Practice Bulletin.* October 2001;31:709-716.

◆ ACOG. Management of preterm labor. *ACOG Practice Bulletin.* May 2003;43:765-773.

◆ ACOG. Premature rupture of membranes. *ACOG Practice Bulletin.* April 2007;80:281-293.

◆ ACOG Committee Opinion. Use of progesterone to reduce preterm birth. *ACOG.* October 2008;419:233-235.

◆ ACOG Committee Opinion #402: Antenatal corticosteroid therapy for fetal maturation. *Obstet Gynecol.* 2008;111:805.

footnotes

◆ ACOG. Perinatal care at the threshold of viability. *ACOG Practice Bulletin*. Sept 2002;38:751-758.

◆ American Academy of Pediatrics and the American Congress of Obstetrics and Gynecology. *Guidelines for Perinatal Care*, 6th Ed. Elk Grove Village, IL and Washington, DC: AAP and ACOG; 2007.

◆ AAP Clinical report: Late preterm infants: a population at risk. *Pediatrics*. 2007; 120(6):1389-1400.

◆ Behrman RE, Butler AS (Eds). *Preterm birth: causes, consequences, and prevention*. Washington, DC: The National Academies Press;2006.

◆ Blackman JA. NICU micropreemies: how do they fare? *Contemp Peds*.Feb 2007;24(2).

◆ Hearne AE, Nagey DA. Therapeutic agents in preterm labor;tocolytic agents. *Clin Ob Gyn*. 2000;43:787-801.

◆ Hubbard E, etal. The late preterm infant: a little baby with big needs. *Contemp Peds*. Mov 2007;24(11):51-59.

◆ Hurst NM, etal. Skin-to-skin holding in the NICU influences maternal milk volumes. *J Perinatol*.1997 May-June;(17)3:213-7.

◆ Moore ER, etal. Early skin-to-skin contact for mothers and their healthy newborn infants. *Cochrane Database Syst Rev*. 2007 Jul 18;(3):CD003519.

◆ Rouse DJ etal. A randomized, controlled trial of magnesium sulfate for the prevention of cerebral palsy. *NEJM*. 2008; 359:895.

Chapter 20: Multiples

◆ ACOG. Multiple gestation: complicated twin, triplet and high-order multifetal pregnancy. *ACOG Practice Bulletin*. October 2004;56:843-857.

◆ Evans MI, et al. International collaborative experience of 1789 patients having multifetal pregnancy reduction: a plateauing of risks and outcomes. *J Soc Gynecol Investig*.1996;3:23-6.

◆ Hamilton BE, etal. Births:preliminary data for 2005. *Natl Vital Stat Rep*. 2006 Dec 28;55(11):1-18.

◆ Luke B, etal. Body mass index—specific weight gains associated with optimal birth weights in twin pregnancies. *J Reprod Med*. 2003 Apr;48(4):217-24.

◆ Rasmussen KM, Yaktine AL (Eds). Institute of Medicine and National Research Council. *Weight gain during pregnancy: reexamining the guidelines*. Washington, DC: The National Academies Press; 2009 nap.edu/catalog/12584.html accessed February 17, 2010.

Chapter 21: When it doesn't work

◆ ACOG. Diagnosis and treatment of gestational trophoblastic disease. *ACOG Practice Bulletin*. June 2004;53:1201-1213.

◆ Robinson JN, Norwitz ER. Risk factors for preterm labor and delivery. In UpToDate. *UpToDate*. Basow DS (Ed).Waltham MA, 2009.

INDEX

index

Anti-herpes antibodies, 478
Antihistamines, 83, 90
Anti-inflammatories, 92, 364, 423, 439
Anti-itch creams, 104, 417
Anti-nausea medications, 222, 416, 423, 442
Antioxidants, 149, 177, 495
Antiphospholipid antibodies, 357, 430, 431, 439
Antiphospholipid syndrome, 357, 414, 430-431, 439, 463
Antipsychotics, 445, 446
Anti-seizure medications, 441
Antithrombin III deficiency, 414, 430-431
Anti-vaccine groups, 259, 262
Antiviral medications (AZT), 219, 471, 478, 479, 480
Anti-wrinkle creams, 234
    pregnancy/breastfeeding and, 242
Anxiety, 24, 290, 361, 409, 413, 415, 430, 444-445, 527
APA. See Advanced paternal age
APGAR scores, 340, 347, 351, 462, 464
    described, 538
Apnea of prematurity, 507, 508
    described, 538
Appendicitis, 191, 192, 394, 396, 398, 414, 420-421
ARDS. See Adult Respiratory Distress Syndrome
Areola, 85, 272, 273, 274, 276
    described, 538
Areolae, hair on, 100
ART. See Assisted reproductive technologies
Ashkenazi Jewish Genetic Panel (AJGP), 114, 115
    described, 121-122
Ashkenazi Jews: CF and, 121, 122
    Tay-Sachs and, 122
Aspirin, 232, 393, 431, 439, 463
Assisted-reproductive technologies (ART), 24, 31, 37, 517
Asthma, 87, 267, 361, 411, 412, 414
    described, 434
    NST and, 141
    pregnancy and, 434
    risk of, 185
    smoking and, 183
Atelectasis, 361, 367
    described, 538
Attention deficit disorder, 186, 199
Autism Science Foundation, 263
Autism spectrum disorder, 123, 124, 132, 441
    epidurals and, 342
    vaccines and, 262-263
Autoimmune antibodies, 430, 431
Autoimmune disease, 435, 439

Baby blues, 79, 383, 384
    described, 538
Baby bump, 54, 56, 369
Back pain, 18, 52, 53, 58, 67, 78, 94, 226, 397, 420, 452, 485
    chronic, 304, 342
    epidurals and, 342
    lifting and, 110
    low, 77, 107, 109, 207, 216, 225, 302, 395, 398, 399, 469
Bacteria, 29, 71, 164, 173, 178, 179, 182, 204, 234, 318, 337, 439, 468, 469, 501, 526
    avoiding, 181
    exposure to, 210
    harmful, 163
    infection with, 481
    sinuses and, 482
    spread of, 141
Bacterial meningitis, 261, 262
Bacterial vaginosis (BV), 486
    described, 486, 538
Bad habits, 9, 10, 21, 494
    stopping, 22, 183-187
Bariatric surgery, 158, 170, 171
Barium enemas, radiation from, 190
Barker Hypothesis, 170
Bathing, 215, 235, 236, 352
Bed rest, 217, 221, 342, 451, 454, 499-500, 523
    described, 538
    exercise and, 209
    multiples and, 514
    work and, 227
Behavior problems, 175, 186, 385
Belly: injuries to, 406
    rubbing, 53
    stretched out, 376
Belly Band, 58
Belly buttons, 70, 94, 103, 376, 420, 421
Belly pain, 31, 53, 67, 78, 393, 397, 420
Benadryl, 82, 83, 90, 104, 360
Beta-blockers, 436, 442
beta-hCG. See Human chorionic gonadotropin
Bicornuate uterus, 298, 415
    described, 447, 538
Bilirubin, 439
    described, 538
Biophysical profiles (BPP), 115, 143, 440, 455, 456, 463
Bipolar disorder, 384, 415, 445
Birth canal, 140, 280, 298, 311, 317, 322, 324, 327, 328, 458, 519
    presenting, 330
Birth control, 90, 217, 268, 278, 374
Birth defects, 47, 168, 171, 176, 189, 193, 211, 213, 298, 441, 446, 448, 454, 458

index

index

index

protein hydrolysate with iron, 258
  ready-to-feed, 258
  soy protein with iron, 258
Foundation for the Accreditation of
  Cellular Therapy, 248
Fragile X carrier screen, 114, 123
Fraternal twins, 510-512
  chance of, 512-513
Fruits, 25, 54, 152, 156, 157, 182, 195,
  202
  consuming, 101, 151, 153, 381
FSH, 512
FTP. *See* Failure to progress
Full Integrated Screening Test, 59, 127,
  130
Full term, 14
  described, 544
Fumes, exposure to, 196-198
Fundal height, 52, 58, 71, 461, 463
  described, 59, 544
Fungus, toenail, 240

Gallbladders, 47
  complications with, 394, 414, 416-
  421, 427
  inflammation of, 396, 498
  problems with, 414, 417, 419
Gallstones, 394, 396, 398, 420, 427,
  513
Gardnerella vaginalis, 486, 538
Gas, 23, 67, 76, 78, 89, 90, 163, 241,
  258, 278
  passing, 92, 222, 356
Gastric bypass surgery, 170
Gastroenteritis. *See* Stomach virus
Gastroesophageal reflux disease
  (GERD), 76, 89, 93, 258, 270, 434
  described, 544
Gastrointestinal tract, 90, 91, 163, 454,
  507
Gaucher's, 121
GBS. *See* Group B Strep
GDM. *See* Gestational diabetes
Generalized anxiety disorder (GAD),
  444
Genetic counseling, 35, 121, 127, 427,
  441, 494, 533
Genetic defects, 9, 35, 121, 123, 246,
  415, 431, 463, 517
  AMA and, 494
  described, 464
  termination and, 533
Genital area, 94, 341, 354
Genital infections, described, 485-486
Genitals, 61, 63, 97, 236
GERD. *See* Gastroesophageal reflux
  disease
German measles, described, 469-470
Germs, 173, 210
Gestation, 24, 31, 62, 121, 140, 296,
  399, 400, 499
  described, 13, 544

survivability and, 503-504
Gestational age, 13, 17, 45, 62, 295,
  431, 461, 462, 506
  described, 544
  large for, 415
Gestational diabetes (GDM), 53, 58,
  134, 136, 137, 142, 167, 171, 208,
  225, 290, 377, 414, 440, 462, 513
  AMA and, 493
  described, 437-438, 544
  exercise and, 211, 213
  risk factors for, 135, 437
Gestational hypertension, 209, 414,
  432-433, 545
  AMA and, 493
  described, 544
Giardia, 210, 484
Gingivitis, described, 544
Girl parts, 46
  changes for, 77, 94-99
  complications with, 414, 421-423
  healing of, 381
Girl problems, 468
  described, 485-486
Glucose, 117, 119, 153, 156, 166
  control, 437
  drinking, 135
  levels, 136, 137
Gonadotropins, 513
Gonorrhea, 31, 114, 119, 120
  described, 468-469
Grains, 152-153
  consuming, 15, 151
Graves' disease, 435, 436
Grieving, 527-528, 532, 533
Groin pain, 52, 53, 67, 77, 78, 107,
  108
Group B Strep (GBS), 65, 71, 315, 318,
  323, 467
  antibiotics for, 140
  described, 472, 544
  testing for, 139-140, 141
  vaginal/rectal culture, 114, 115
GTT. *See* Three-hour Glucose
  Tolerance Test
Gums: bleeding, 53, 67, 76, 78, 84,
  419, 428
  swollen, 53, 83, 84, 232
Gut, complications with, 414, 416-421
Guthrie, Robert, 253

Haiku Mama (Roy), quote from, 207
Hair: changes for, 77, 100-107
  coloring, 229-230
  growth of, 74, 100, 101, 230
  loss of, 101, 378, 435, 439
  postpartum, 377-378
Hair chemicals, avoiding, 230
Hair removal, pregnancy/breastfeed-
  ing and, 231, 241, 242
Hair removal creams: avoiding, 100,
  231

index

index

index

index

index

index

EXPECTING411.COM AND HOW TO REACH THE AUTHORS

Come visit us at Expecting411.com!

What's online?

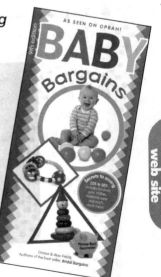

Subscribe to our blog. Read the latest news and studies on pregnancy!

Follow us on Twitter! Twitter.com/Expecting411

Become a fan on our Facebook page!

Join in the conversation with our popular message boards.

How to reach the authors:

◆ Email: authors@Expecting411.com

◆ Follow us on Twitter or post to our Facebook fan page!

More books by Windsor Peak Press

Baby Bargains: Secrets to saving 20% to 50% on baby gear! $17.95 (9th Edition). As seen on Oprah! Over 700,000 copies sold!

◆ Detailed reviews and ratings of baby gear, including strollers, car seats, cribs and more!

◆ In-depth money-saving tips!

◆ Dozens of safety tips to afford-ably baby-proof your home

See it at BabyBargains.com

web site

If yo ~~ked Expecting 411~~ .

Baby 411-

Clear Answers & Smart Advice For
Your Baby (5th edition). $14.95
As seen on Rachael Ray!
Inside you'll learn:

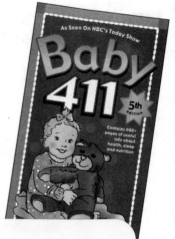

- ◆ **Sleep.** The best way to get your baby to sleep through the night.
- ◆ **First aid**—when to worry,

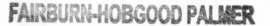